Closed-Loop Neurophysiology: Clinical Research

Closed-Loop Neurophysiology: Clinical Research

Edited by George Morris

STATES
ACADEMIC PRESS
www.statesacademicpress.com

States Academic Press,
109 South 5th Street,
Brooklyn, NY 11249, USA

Visit us on the World Wide Web at:
www.statesacademicpress.com

ISBN: 978-1-63989-114-6

Cataloging-in-Publication Data

Closed-loop neurophysiology : clinical research / edited by George Morris.
p. cm.
Includes bibliographical references and index.
ISBN 978-1-63989-114-6
1. Neurophysiology. 2. Nervous system--Diseases--Treatment. 3. Clinical neuropsychology. I. Morris, George.
RC349.8 .C56 2022
616.804 6--dc23

Table of Contents

Preface

This book aims to highlight the current researches and provides a platform to further the scope of innovations in this area. This book is a product of the combined efforts of many researchers and scientists, after going through thorough studies and analysis from different parts of the world. The objective of this book is to provide the readers with the latest information of the field.

Neurophysiology is the branch of physiology and neuroscience which is concerned with the study of nerve cells as they transmit and receive information. It focuses on the study of the brain and spinal cord, and their connection to the mental health. Some of the methods used for research in the field of neurophysiology are electrophysiological recordings such as voltage clamp, patch clamp, extracellular single-unit recording and recording of local field potentials. Closed-loop neuroscience is referred to as a field of study that considers the brain as a loop that interacts with itself and the environment in a relative manner. Closed loop neurophysiology is an upcoming field of science that has undergone rapid development over the past few decades. This book is a compilation of chapters that discuss the most vital concepts and emerging trends in this field. It is appropriate for students seeking detailed information in this area as well as for experts.

I would like to express my sincere thanks to the authors for their dedicated efforts in the completion of this book. I acknowledge the efforts of the publisher for providing constant support. Lastly, I would like to thank my family for their support in all academic endeavors.

Editor

1

Nanowire electrodes for high-density stimulation and measurement of neural circuits

Jacob T. Robinson[1]*, Marsela Jorgolli[2] and Hongkun Park[2,3]*

[1] Departments of Electrical and Computer Engineering and Bioengineering, Rice University, Houston, TX, USA
[2] Department of Physics, Harvard University, Cambridge, MA, USA
[3] Department of Chemistry and Chemical Biology, Harvard University, Cambridge, MA, USA

Edited by:
Ahmed El Hady, Max Planck Institute for Dynamics and Self Organization, Germany

Reviewed by:
Ahmed El Hady, Max Planck Institute for Dynamics and Self Organization, Germany
Bianxiao Cui, Stanford University, USA

***Correspondence:**
Jacob T. Robinson, Departments of Electrical and Computer Engineering and Bioengineering, Rice University, 6100 Main Street, MS 380, Houston, TX 77005, USA.
e-mail: jtrobinson@rice.edu;
Hongkun Park, Department of Chemistry and Chemical Biology and Physics, Harvard University, 12 Oxford St., Cambridge, MA 02138, USA.
e-mail: hongkun_park@harvard.edu

Brain-machine interfaces (BMIs) that can precisely monitor and control neural activity will likely require new hardware with improved resolution and specificity. New nanofabricated electrodes with feature sizes and densities comparable to neural circuits may lead to such improvements. In this perspective, we review the recent development of vertical nanowire (NW) electrodes that could provide highly parallel single-cell recording and stimulation for future BMIs. We compare the advantages of these devices and discuss some of the technical challenges that must be overcome for this technology to become a platform for next-generation closed-loop BMIs.

Keywords: brain machine interface (BMI), nanotechnology, nanowires, neuroengineering, electrophysiology

Today, brain-machines interfaces (BMIs) enable users to manipulate prosthetic limbs and computer interfaces by monitoring and processing their neural activity (Donoghue et al., 2007; Simeral et al., 2011). BMIs can also be used to treat neurological disorders such as Parkinson's disease (Volkmann, 2004), obsessive compulsive disorder (Bourne et al., 2012), and depression (Howland et al., 2011) by applying voltage or current pulses to specific regions deep within the brain—a treatment known as deep brain stimulation (DBS). As remarkable as today's BMI technology is, it is in many ways in its infancy. Future technology will seek to improve the precision with which external devices can be manipulated and the specificity of stimulation to the level of individual cells. These improvements will help expand the capabilities of neural prosthetics and extend the range of disorders that can be treated using DBS (Donoghue et al., 2007). To achieve these goals, the next generation of BMIs will need improved resolution for measurement and stimulation, as well as the ability to adjust their spatial and temporal stimulation patterns based on the current state of the neural activity (the devices with this latter capability are often termed "closed-loop" BMIs) (Stanslaski et al., 2012).

Currently, the large size and small number of electrodes in BMIs limits their stimulation and measurement resolution. State-of-the-art devices for DBS typically have 4–8 millimeter-sized electrodes (Stanslaski et al., 2012), whereas BMIs for neural recording typically use a few dozen electrodes that are 10–100 microns in diameter (Hochberg et al., 2006; Donoghue et al., 2007; Du et al., 2011) (**Figure 1A**). This density and feature size is a far cry from that of the human brain, which contains approximately one hundred billion neurons, each with diameter as fine as 10 microns (Williams and Herrup, 1988). In fact, a single square millimeter of brain tissue contains approximately one million neurons (Williams and Herrup, 1988). To match this number and density, future BMIs must feature smaller and denser electrode arrays in order to precisely monitor and control neural circuit activity. Furthermore, smaller electrodes (<1 micron in diameter) may also enable the recording of intracellular electrical signals of individual neurons (**Figure 1A**): compared to extracellular recording, these intracellular measurements will have improved signal to noise ratio and enable a clear cell-to-electrode registry (**Figures 1B–D**). Importantly, the improved signal to noise ratio also enables intracellular electrodes to record subthreshold neural activity (e.g., postsynaptic potentials) that can be used to determine the strength of synaptic connectivity.

Fortunately devices that match the feature size and density of neural circuits are routinely fabricated on silicon using contemporary nanofabrication techniques (Arden, 2002). This observation highlights the future role for semiconductor fabrication and nanotechnology as a platform for high-precision BMIs. Recently, these nanofabrication techniques have been used to create vertical nanowires (NWs) and nanotubes that can intracellularly stimulate and record the activity of neurons and other electrically active cells. Here we review this technology, highlight the

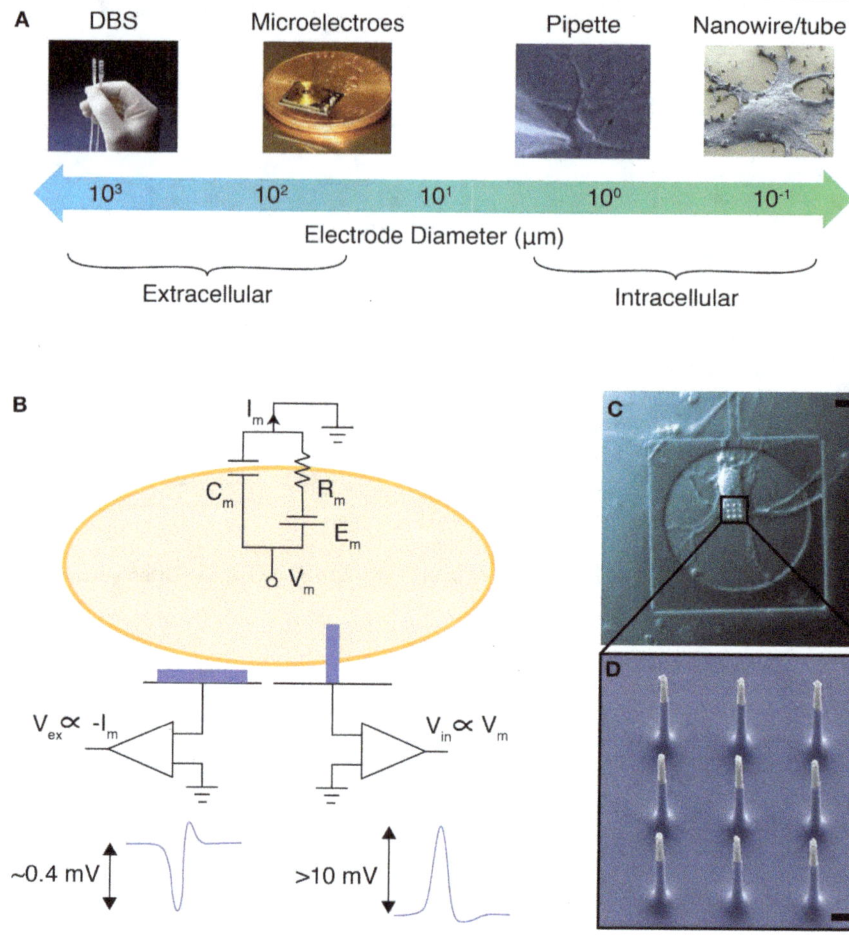

FIGURE 1 | NWs as intracellular electrodes. (A) The electrode diameters for various methods to record and stimulate neural activity. Electrodes with diameters less than 1 micron can be used as intracellular probes. Photo credits: DBS—EPDA.com, Microelectrodes—microsystems.utah.edu. **(B)** Equivalent circuit model for a cell on top of an extracellular (left) and intracellular (right) electrode. The membrane resistance, capacitance, and Nernst potential is shown as R_m, C_m, and E_m, respectively. The voltage recorded extracellularly (V_{ex}) is proportional to I_m, and typically has a magnitude of 0.4 mV for a neuronal action potential. The voltage recorded intracellularly (V_{in}), however, is proportional to V_m, and typically has a magnitude of greater than 10 mV for a neuronal action potential. **(C)** Optical microscope image of a rat cortical neuron grown on top of a vertical NW electrode, scale bar 10 microns. **(D)** Scanning electron micrograph of a set of vertical NWs, scale bar 1 micron. [**(C)** and **(D)** adapted from Robinson et al. (2012)].

characteristics that make NW electrodes an attractive platform for future BMIs, and comment on some of the challenges that face the development of these next-generation devices.

NWs AS INTRACELLULAR ELECTRODES

The electrical activity of neurons is most directly measured as the electrical potential across the cellular membrane. As a result, intracellular electrodes that can directly measure the membrane potential are widely considered the "gold standard" in neuronal recording. These high fidelity measurements, however, come at a cost. To monitor intracellular signals via traditional patch-clamp methods, glass micropipettes must be carefully aligned to the cellular membrane using manually controlled micromanipulators. Once the pipette is placed in contact with the cell, an intracellular electrical connection can be formed either by slowly driving the pipette through the cellular membrane or by applying negative pressure to seal the membrane against the pipette and then rupturing the circumscribed patch using a current pulse or a rapid impulse of negative pressure (**Figure 2A**). While this painstaking process is a commonly performed procedure, it is not scalable. As a result, today's BMIs are based on extracellular recording techniques that sacrifice the high fidelity of intracellular measurements for the sake of scalability. For instance, contemporary extracellular electrodes have array sizes approaching one hundred electrodes and can simultaneously measure the activity of dozens of individual neurons (Hochberg et al., 2006; Donoghue et al., 2007; Du et al., 2011).

While extracellular electrodes succeed in monitoring large numbers of neurons, there are potential challenges for using these devices as the basis for closed-loop BMIs. For instance, a single extracellular electrode records the spiking activity of many nearby cells. This makes it difficult to identify the activity that corresponds to each individual neuron. While a variety of computational techniques can be used to sort the recorded

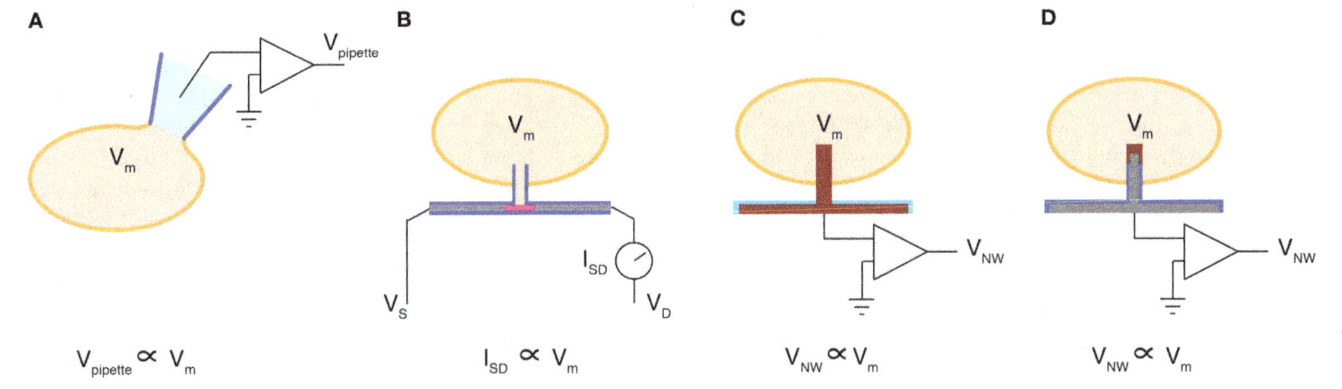

FIGURE 2 | Intracellular recording methods. (A) Whole cell patch pipette configuration measures a voltage ($V_{pipette}$) proportional to the membrane potential (V_m). **(B)** A vertical glass nanotube (blue) is grown on top of an FET (pink) that lies within an insulated NW (gray). When the nanotube penetrates the cellular membrane, the membrane potential can be measured as a change in the source-drain current (I_{SD}). **(C)** A platinum NW (red) is deposited on top of a platinum electrode (red) that is insulated by silicon nitride (blue). The voltage recorded at the NW (V_{NW}) is then proportional to the membrane potential. **(D)** A silicon NW (gray) insulated by glass (blue) is capped with a metallic film such as platinum (red). Similarly to **(C)**, V_{NW} is proportional to V_m, however in this configuration the NW sidewalls are insulated by glass, improving the amplitude of the measured signal and proving a surface for cell membrane fusion.

spikes based on their waveforms, this process typically requires a training period of several minutes, and must be repeated on a daily basis as the electrical coupling between the cells and extracellular electrode changes (Donoghue et al., 2007). Furthermore, typical signal to noise ratios are less than 10:1 (Hochberg et al., 2006; Donoghue et al., 2007; Du et al., 2011), and therefore slight degradation of the signal amplitude during chronic implantation leads to a gradual reduction in the number of individual neurons that can be recorded (Dickey et al., 2009). Stimulation using extracellular electrodes also lacks precise cell-to-electrode registry. During voltage or current pulses from an extracellular electrode, many cells in the vicinity of the electrode will be activated. This shortcoming ultimately limits the spatial accuracy of stimuli applied via extracellular probes.

To improve the cell-to-electrode registration, the size of the electrodes can be scaled down so that an individual electrode can interface to at most a single neuron (**Figure 1A**). This is the approach taken recently for vertical NW electrodes. Three recent papers have shown that these electrodes can be made small enough to penetrate the cellular membrane without compromising cell viability, and record or stimulate individual cells (Duan et al., 2012; Robinson et al., 2012; Xie et al., 2012). Thus silicon-based intracellular electrodes can provide both precise cell-to-electrode registration as well as large signal-to-noise ratios typically reserved for patch clamp recordings. Importantly, these NW devices can be fabricated using semiconductor nanofabrication techniques that can be scaled up to produce tens of thousands of recording sites in a single fabrication run, making this technology a potential platform for next generation BMIs requiring an increased number of electrodes.

Although the three recent demonstrations of vertical NW electrodes employed different fabrication strategies, each reported successful intracellular electrical measurements. Duan et al. used electron beam lithography to define nanoscale gold islands on the gate region of NW field-effect transistors (FETs). They used these islands as precursors for germanium (Ge) NW vapor-liquid-solid (VLS) growth (Duan et al., 2012). The Ge NWs were then coated with SiO_2 using atomic layer deposition and the Ge core was subsequently etched away using Hydrogen Peroxide. This process left a nanoscale glass tube leading the gate region of the NW FET (**Figure 2B**). The authors showed that when this glass nanotube penetrated the cellular membrane of a cardiomyocyte, the intracellular membrane potential could be recorded. In this configuration the cardiomyocyte membrane potential gates the NW FET such that the source-drain conductance maps to the intracellular membrane potential. One advantage of using the FET conductance to transduce the membrane potential is that the gain of the NW FET can be used to amplify the measured signal. An alternative strategy pursued by Robinson et al. used plasma etching to micromachine solid silicon (Si) NWs out of highly conductive silicon-on-insulator wafers (Robinson et al., 2012). The resulting Si NWs were then insulated by a thermally grown silicon oxide that was subsequently removed from the Si NW tips. The Si NW tips were coated with an evaporated platinum or gold film (**Figure 2D**). Unlike NW FETs, this approach requires amplifying electronics to boost the signal recorded by the Si NWs. At the same time, however, the Si NW electrodes can also be used to stimulate electrical activity by injecting current into the cell, thereby evoking neuronal action potentials on demand. Using the stimulation capabilities of the solid Si NWs, functional circuits can be reconstructed by systematically stimulating individual electrodes and recording the resulting response at another cell (Robinson et al., 2012). A third fabrication technique was employed by Xie et al. who used focused ion beams to deposit 100 nm diameter platinum NWs on top of planar platinum electrodes (Xie et al., 2012) (**Figure 2C**). The functionality of these devices were similar to those reported by Robinson et al. although Xie et al. used their device to monitor mitotic cardiac cells as opposed to primary neurons.

For each NW electrode device, care must be taken to secure a stable intracellular measurement. To improve the stability of the cell-electrode interface and promote NW penetration, Duan et al. coated their devices with a phospholipid (Duan et al., 2012). One drawback to this method is that the phospholipid coating prevents cells from being cultured directly on top of the electrodes. As a result, to test these devices cells were grown on a separate PDMS substrate, inverted, and aligned atop the devices for measurement. Alternatively, Robinson et al. and Xie et al. did not use a surface treatment to promote penetration and reported intracellular recordings in cells grown directly on top of the devices. Both groups reported that, at times, voltage pulses are required to permeabilize the membrane covering the electrode in order to achieve intracellular electrical coupling. Xie et al. showed that over time, the permeabilized membrane recovers; however, repeated application of voltage pulses can restore the intracellular electrical coupling. The observed time scale of this recovery is consistent with the kinetics of cell membrane electroporation for biomolecule delivery (Saulis et al., 1991).

FUTURE CHALLENGES FOR NW ELECTRODES *in vivo*

While electrically facilitated membrane permeabilization is adequate for *in vitro* studies, a long-term *in vivo* interface will likely require alternative approaches to stabilize the NW-cell interface. Potential surface treatments include the phospholipid coating used by Duan et al. and biomimetic surfaces developed by Almquist and Melosh (2010). While these methods have been successful in securing stable interfaces between cells and nanostructures, future studies should investigate their long term stability and biocompatibility *in vivo*.

In addition to stabilizing the cellular interface, future *in vivo* devices must also deal with the motion of the brain resulting from the expanding and contracting vasculature (Enzmann and Pelc, 1992). Improving the flexibility of the NW electrodes may help them function in living tissue like the brain. Recently Tian et al. have taken steps in this direction by embedding NW FETs in a flexible polymer matrix and releasing them from the rigid substrate (Tian et al., 2012). While these devices, which have only recently been reported, have yet to be used for intracellular measurements, this approach may allow intracellular electrodes to remain within the cell while the tissue moves. Supporting this idea are reports that vertical NWs can pin neurons in place and inhibit them from migrating away from NW electrodes (Xie et al., 2010). Such effects may help secure intracellular coupling *in vivo*. An alternative approach may be to imbed vertical silicon NWs in a PDMS or other polymeric matrix that can be peeled off the silicon substrate. Such methods have recently been used to create flexible photonic crystal cavities based on semiconductor NWs, and may be adapted to support vertical NW electrodes (Yu et al., 2013).

Another challenge to using NW electrodes *in vivo* is recording beyond the layer of dead cells and protective glia that surround implanted electrodes. Studies have reported the thickness of the dead cell layers to be approximately 40 microns (Chia and Levene, 2009). Therefore, to access healthy cells, the NWs electrodes must penetrate through this dead layer. One approach is to make long electrode shanks tipped with NW electrodes. Alternatively very high aspect ratio NWs can be fabricated using deep reactive ion etching and oxide thinning processes (Morton et al., 2008). Such high aspect ratio NWs will have increased flexibility (Li et al., 2009), which may help accommodate tissue movement.

Another concern for closed loop BMIs is the potential for crosstalk between stimulation and recording electrodes that could interfere with the feedback algorithms. Potential solutions to this problem fall primarily into two categories: (1) Recording hardware and/or software can be modified to reduce the crosstalk using techniques such as blanking, spectral filtering, or common mode rejection (Stanslaski et al., 2012) or (2) Stimulation can be performed optically using channel-rhodopsin (Erickson et al., 2008) or near-IR stimulation (Wells et al., 2005). The advantage of modifying the recording electronics is that there is no need to genetically modify neuronal populations or to employ optical sources and components. However, the added electronic elements needed to reduce crosstalk can increase the size and power consumption of the BMI. Optical stimulation, on the other hand, typically produces negligible electronic crosstalk, simplifying the design requirements and lowering the power consumption of the recording electronics.

Finally, to achieve the thousands to millions of recording sites that will be desired for future BMIs the number of electrodes must be increased. The NW electrodes described here have relied on a direct electrical connection to each electrode. This method, requiring a dedicated wire for each recording/stimulation site, is impractical for devices with large numbers of electrodes. Fortunately solutions to this "interconnect problem" have already been solved for semiconductor electronics. Image sensors, for instance, contain millions of pixels that can be read using only a few dozen connections. This reduced number of contacts is achieved by interleaving data from several pixels and transmitting it over a single wire. This multiplexing process can be implemented on-chip using complementary metal oxide semiconductor (CMOS) technology (Lei et al., 2011). Yet another advantage of silicon-based electrodes is that they can be readily coupled to back-side CMOS electronics using bonding or other post-processing methods such as those used for extracellular electrodes (Kim et al., 2009). The combination of NW electrodes and CMOS multiplexing will allow high-resolution BMIs to be created on a compact monolithic platform.

CONCLUSIONS

In the future, closed-loop BMIs will see improvements both to the hardware that interfaces to the neural circuits, and to the software that drives their activity. Ultimately this hardware may be able to stimulate and record the activity of thousands to millions of neurons with single-cell resolution. The high resolution combined with algorithms to identify the state of the neural circuit and predict its response to stimuli would provide a basis for new classes of BMIs that can accurately control neural circuits and translate this recorded activity into accurate manipulation of prosthetic devices. While there is currently no technology that can achieve such a high-resolution electrical interface, NW-based electrodes have made considerable progress toward this goal *in vitro*. To take the next step and employ nanotechnology for BMIs, efforts must be taken to improve the stability of the interface, flexibility of the electrodes, and compatibility with layers of dead cells and glia that accompany surgical implantation of electrodes. With these improvements, NW electrodes may become the preferred technology for high-resolution BMIs.

ACKNOWLEDGMENTS

This work was supported by an NIH Pioneer award (5DP1OD003893-03) and an NSF EFRI award (EFRI-0835947) to Hongkun Park.

REFERENCES

Almquist, B., and Melosh, N. (2010). Fusion of biomimetic stealth probes into lipid bilayer cores. *Proc. Natl. Acad. Sci. U.S.A.* 107, 5815–5820.

Arden, W. M. (2002). The international technology roadmap for semiconductors-perspectives and challenges for the next 15 years. *Curr. Opin. Solid State Mater. Sci.* 6, 371–377.

Bourne, S. K., Eckhardt, C. A., Sheth, S. A., and Eskandar, E. N. (2012). Mechanisms of deep brain stimulation for obsessive compulsive disorder: effects upon cells and circuits. *Front. Integr. Neurosci.* 6:29. doi: 10.3389/fnint.2012.00029

Chia, T., and Levene, M. (2009). Microprisms for *in vivo* multilayer cortical imaging. *J. Neurophysiol.* 102, 1310–1314.

Dickey, A. S., Suminski, A., Amit, Y., and Hatsopoulos, N. G. (2009). Single-unit stability using chronically implanted multielectrode arrays. *J. Neurophysiol.* 102, 1331–1339.

Donoghue, J. P., Nurmikko, A., Black, M., and Hochberg, L. R. (2007). Assistive technology and robotic control using motor cortex ensemble-based neural interface systems in humans with tetraplegia. *J. Physiol.* 579, 603–611.

Du, J., Blanche, T. J., Harrison, R. R., Lester, H. A., and Masmanidis, S. C. (2011). Multiplexed, high density electrophysiology with nanofabricated neural probes. *PLoS ONE* 6:e26204. doi: 10.1371/journal.pone.0026204

Duan, X., Gao, R., Xie, P., Cohen-Karni, T., Qing, Q., Choe, H. S., et al. (2012). Intracellular recordings of action potentials by an extracellular nanoscale field-effect transistor. *Nat. Nanotechnol.* 7, 174–179.

Enzmann, D. R., and Pelc, N. J. (1992). Brain motion: measurement with phase-contrast MR imaging. *Radiology* 185, 653–660.

Erickson, J., Tooker, A., Tai, Y.-C., and Pine, J. (2008). Caged neuron MEA: a system for long-term investigation of cultured neural network connectivity. *J. Neurosci. Methods* 175, 1–16.

Hochberg, L. R., Serruya, M. D., Friehs, G. M., Mukand, J. A., Saleh, M., Caplan, A. H., et al. (2006). Neuronal ensemble control of prosthetic devices by a human with tetraplegia. *Nature* 442, 164–171.

Howland, R. H., Shutt, L. S., Berman, S. R., Spotts, C. R., and Denko, T. (2011). The emerging use of technology for the treatment of depression and other neuropsychiatric disorders. *Ann. Clin. Psychiatry* 23, 48–62.

Kim, S., Bhandari, R., Klein, M., Negi, S., Rieth, L., Tathireddy, P., et al. (2009). Integrated wireless neural interface based on the Utah electrode array. *Biomed. Microdevices* 11, 453–466.

Lei, N., Ramakrishnan, S., Shi, P., Orcutt, J. S., Kam, L. C., and Shepard, K. L. (2011). High-resolution extracellular stimulation of dispersed hippocampal culture with high-density CMOS multielectrode array based on non-Faradaic electrodes. *J. Neural Eng.* 8:044003. doi: 10.1088/1741-2560/8/4/044003

Li, Z., Song, J., Mantini, G., Lu, M.-Y., Fang, H., Falconi, C., et al. (2009). Quantifying the traction force of a single cell by aligned silicon nanowire array. *Nano Lett.* 9, 3575–3580.

Morton, K. J., Nieberg, G., Bai, S., and Chou, S. Y. (2008). Wafer-scale patterning of sub-40 nm diameter and high aspect ratio (>50, 1) silicon pillar arrays by nanoimprint and etching. *Nanotechnology* 19, 345301.

Robinson, J. T., Jorgolli, M., Shalek, A. K., Yoon, M.-H., Gertner, R. S., and Park, H. (2012). Vertical nanowire electrode arrays as a scalable platform for intracellular interfacing to neuronal circuits. *Nat. Nanotechnol.* 7, 180–184.

Saulis, G., Venslauskas, M. S., and Naktinis, J. (1991). Kinetics of pore resealing in cell membranes after electroporation. *Bioelectrochem. Bioenerg.* 321, 1–13.

Simeral, J. D., Kim, S.-P., Black, M. J., Donoghue, J. P., and Hochberg, L. R. (2011). Neural control of cursor trajectory and click by a human with tetraplegia 1000 days after implant of an intracortical microelectrode array. *J. Neural Eng.* 8:025027. doi: 10.1088/1741-2560/8/2/025027

Stanslaski, S., Afshar, P., Cong, P., Giftakis, J., Stypulkowski, P., Carlson, D., et al. (2012). Design and validation of a fully implantable, chronic, closed-loop neuromodulation device with concurrent sensing and stimulation. *IEEE Trans. Neural Syst. Rehabil. Eng.* 20, 410–421.

Tian, B., Liu, J., Dvir, T., Jin, L., Tsui, J. H., Qing, Q., et al. (2012). Macroporous nanowire nanoelectronic scaffolds for synthetic tissues. *Nat. Mater.* 11, 1–9.

Volkmann, J. (2004). Deep brain stimulation for the treatment of Parkinson's disease. *J. Clin. Neurophysiol.* 21, 6–17.

Wells, J., Kao, C., Jansen, E. D., Konrad, P., and Mahadevan-Jansen, A. (2005). Application of infrared light for in vivo neural stimulation. *J. Biomed. Opt.* 10, 064003.

Williams, R. W., and Herrup, K. (1988). The control of neuron number. *Ann. Rev. Neurosci.* 11, 423–453.

Xie, C., Hanson, L., Xie, W., Lin, Z., Cui, B., and Cui, Y. (2010). Noninvasive neuron pinning with nanopillar arrays. *Nano Lett.* 10, 4020–4024.

Xie, C., Lin, Z., Hanson, L., Cui, Y., and Cui, B. (2012). Intracellular recording of action potentials by nanopillar electroporation. *Nat. Nanotechnol.* 7, 185–190.

Yu, C. L., Kim, H., De Leon, N., Frank, I. W., Robinson, J. T., McCutcheon, M., et al. (2013). Stretchable photonic crystal cavity with wide frequency tunability. *Nano Lett.* 13, 248–252.

2

The response clamp: functional characterization of neural systems using closed-loop control

Avner Wallach*

Department of Neurobiology, Weizmann Institute of Science, Rehovot, Israel

Edited by:
Ahmed El Hady, Max Planck Institute for Dynamics and Self Organization, Germany

Reviewed by:
Steve M. Potter, Georgia Institute of Technology, USA
Michele Giugliano, University of Antwerpen, Belgium

***Correspondence:**
Avner Wallach, Department of Neurobiology, Weizmann Institute of Science, 234 Herzl Street, Rehovot 76100, Israel.
e-mail: avnerw@tx.technion.ac.il

The voltage clamp method, pioneered by Hodgkin, Huxley, and Katz, laid the foundations to neurophysiological research. Its core rationale is the use of closed-loop control as a tool for system characterization. A recently introduced method, the *response clamp*, extends the voltage clamp rationale to the functional, phenomenological level. The method consists of on-line estimation of a response variable of interest (e.g., the probability of response or its latency) and a simple feedback control mechanism designed to tightly converge this variable toward a desired trajectory. In the present contribution I offer a perspective on this novel method and its applications in the broader context of system identification and characterization. First, I demonstrate how internal state variables are exposed using the method, and how the use of several controllers may allow for a detailed, multi-variable characterization of the system. Second, I discuss three different categories of applications of the method: (1) exploration of intrinsically generated dynamics, (2) exploration of extrinsically generated dynamics, and (3) generation of input–output trajectories. The relation of these categories to similar uses in the voltage clamp and other techniques is also discussed. Finally, I discuss the method's limitations, as well as its possible synthesis with existing complementary approaches.

Keywords: response clamp, control, closed-loop, physiology, psychophysics

MOTIVATION

A paramount goal of any neurophysiological study is to identify and characterize the function of neural systems. What kind of methodology can one employ in order to achieve this goal? A compelling option is to use the framework of control theory and signal processing, which engineers utilize to characterize artificial systems. The first step in this methodology is to define the system's input and output variables. Then, a set of signals is selected (e.g., step, pulse, or harmonic functions) and is applied to the system's input, while the output signal corresponding to each input is observed. Finally, the system is characterized in terms of its *input–output relations*, namely the conversion laws that dictate what kind of output arises in response to any given input (including novel, untested stimuli). Another realization of this approach is to use *noise* as input and to deduce the input–output relations using reverse correlations. This "open-loop" methodology is very efficient when simple systems are involved: a linear time-invariant (LTI) system (e.g., a classical resistor-capacitor circuit) may be fully characterized-based solely on its response to a single step function; simple non-linear elements, such as analog transistors in their "linear" regime, may also be studied using "small signal" (i.e., harmonic) analysis.

The application of such tools to biological systems, however, is severely limited. First, these systems are invariably composed of non-linear elements which exhibit sharp threshold phenomena, i.e., small changes in their input may cause abrupt and significant changes in their output. Second, biological systems are stochastic, with a response variance which is often comparable in magnitude to the response mean (Arieli et al., 1996). Finally, time and activity-dependent processes continuously change the properties of the system; such changes are referred to as inactivation, adaptation, habituation, learning, etc. Therefore, the history of activity impacts on the system's internal variables, which in turn affect future activity—and so forth. This internal feedback results in dynamic instabilities that are manifested in complex trajectories of the system's output.

This challenge was confronted by Hodgkin et al. (1952) in their analysis of the mechanisms underlying the generation of action-potentials. There, too, the dynamics of non-linear and history-dependent internal variables (in this case, membrane conductances) result in a complex voltage trajectory. The breakthrough in that study came with the development of a closed-loop technique called the *voltage clamp*, in which the system's output is stabilized by applying feedback control. Once the voltage is controlled, the dynamics of the membrane conductances were significantly simplified and could be measured by analyzing the control signal (i.e., the feedback current). This enabled comprehensive study and quantitative modeling of the system.

The essence of the clamp rationale, therefore, is to use control as a tool for system characterization; it inverts the experimental approach, determining the output of the system and observing the input signal required in order to obtain this desired output. One might expect this inverted system to simply reflect the behavior of the open-loop (i.e., current clamp) scenario, yet this is seldom the case in the non-linear, time-variant systems ubiquitous in physiology. The voltage clamp and other methods that emanated from it were extremely instrumental in elucidating the mechanisms of excitability. They did not, however, directly target the functionality of neural systems beyond the molecular level as the object of control.

The rationale of the voltage clamp technique was generalized to the study of neural systems at the functional, phenomenological level in a recently introduced method called the *response clamp* (Wallach et al., 2011). The current contribution aims at offering a comprehensive perspective of this method, its possible applications and extensions, as well as of its limitations. Note that, while termed a Review, this article does not attempt to provide an expansive outlook on the field of closed-loop methodology (for such a review of closed-loop physiology, for instance, see Arsiero et al., 2007).

THE RESPONSE CLAMP EXPOSES FUNCTIONAL STATE VARIABLES OF NEURAL SYSTEMS

The response clamp method utilizes a simple control procedure which allows robust manipulation of the system's response dynamics. First, a selected response feature is either directly measured or estimated from the system's activity. Then, a *Proportional-Integral-Derivative* (PID) controller (Levine et al., 1996) adjusts a stimulation parameter related to that feature in close-loop, so that the system's behavior converges to some desired pattern. The procedure eliminates the feedback from the system's response dynamics to its internal state dynamics. Moreover, these internal (and otherwise hidden) state dynamics are exposed to continuous measurement by analysis of the control signal. To demonstrate this let us use the example of clamping the response *probability*, which served in previously published studies (Marom and Wallach, 2011; Wallach and Marom, 2012).

Many excitable systems are characterized by an "all-or-none" response to external perturbation. While the responses themselves, once evoked, are stereotypical and uniform, the *probability* of evoking these responses is graded and depends on various stimulation parameters, as well as on the present state of the system. Some qualitative understanding of this dependence is required in order to establish control over the response probability; the easiest case is when the probability is monotonically related to some stimulus feature (e.g., intensity or contrast relative to the background). The most abundant form of such monotonic relationships in physiology and psychophysics is the *sigmoidal curve*, which exhibits threshold and saturation phenomena; several mathematical functions were used to model such sigmoidal relations, e.g., the *error function*, the *hyperbolic tangent* and the *logistic curve*. Let us consider the latter, which is characterized by a *threshold* parameter θ and a *dynamic range* parameter σ,

$$P(x;\, t) = \frac{1}{1 + e^{-\frac{(x(t)-\theta(t))}{\sigma(t)}}}, \tag{1}$$

where P is the response probability and x is the stimulation intensity (**Figure 1**). Note that small values of σ signify a steep sigmoid and therefore high sensitivity to changes in stimulation intensity [the maximal slope being $(4\sigma)^{-1}$].

Due to the monotonic nature of this relationship, the response probability may be controlled by continuously adjusting the stimulation intensity using a negative feedback loop; the PID algorithm of the response clamp is a simple and efficient way to realize this loop. If we choose 50% as our target response probability, it is readily apparent that the stimulation sequence produced by the controller must satisfy at all times $x(t) = \theta(t)$, i.e., the control signal in fact reflects the instantaneous threshold, a key functional state variable of the system. In practice this measurement contains some degree of inherent noise, since the system is stochastic and the response probability must be estimated using a finite number of samples.

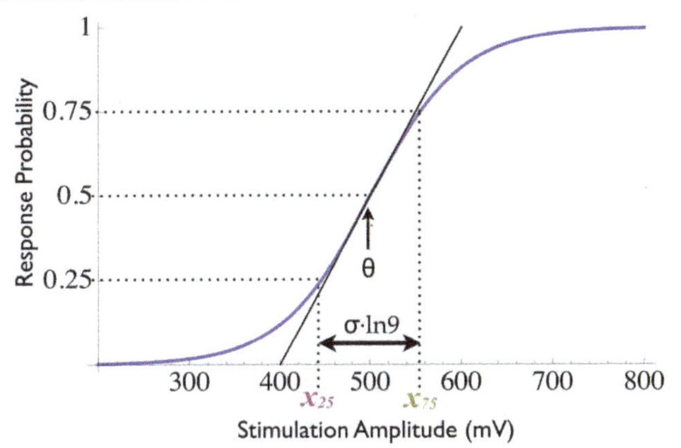

FIGURE 1 | Sigmoidal input–output relations. The response probability's dependence on stimulation intensity follows a sigmoidal function with two parameters (state variables): the threshold θ and the dynamic range σ (see Equation 1). When two response clamps are used, one controller may clamp to 0.75 and the other to 0.25, thus yielding measurements of two distinct loci on the response curve (denoted x_{75} and x_{25}, respectively). The mean of these measurements is the threshold, while their difference is proportional to the dynamic range.

Thus, using one response clamp controller, one locus on the input–output curve is tracked, providing a single-parameter characterization of these relations. A more detailed characterization is possible using multiple controllers, each clamping to a different value. The controllers take turns in stimulating the system (i.e., they are "time-multiplexed,") each using only the responses to its own stimuli in the control algorithm. This configuration provides non-simultaneous, mutually independent measurements of the system [see Wallach and Marom (2012) for details]. Thus, a multiple clamp set-up consisting of n controllers tracks n points in the input–output curve. Producing the state variables of interest from this set of measurements might require some "coordinate transform,"

$$\vec{S} = f\left(\vec{X}\right), \tag{2}$$

where $\vec{X}$ is the vector of measurements (i.e., the set of n control signals), f is some function and $\vec{S}$ is a vector of m state variables of interest ($m \leq n$). If, for example, the transform is linear, then

$$\vec{S} = \mathbf{T} \cdot \vec{X}, \tag{3}$$

where T is some $m \times n$ matrix.

In the example of the sigmoid relations presented in Equation (1), for instance, using two controllers enables tracking both the threshold and the dynamic range variables: the two controllers are used alternatingly, one clamps to 25% while the other to 75% response probability. Thus, the overall response is clamped to a constant 50% of the total stimulation and two distinct loci on the response curve, denoted x_{25} and x_{75}, are measured (see **Figure 1**). The two state variables $\theta(t)$ and $\sigma(t)$ are produced using the linear mapping[1]

$$\theta(t) = \frac{x_{75}(t) + x_{25}(t)}{2} \qquad \sigma(t) = \frac{x_{75}(t) - x_{25}(t)}{\ln 9}. \quad (4)$$

Figure 2A demonstrates typical recordings obtained using the double clamp procedure on isolated neurons *in vitro*. The state variables $\theta(t)$ and $\sigma(t)$ (in this case they are both expressed in mV), obtained using Equation (4), are presented in **Figures 2B,C.**

The use of multiple clamps, therefore, allows for a detailed, multiple-variable characterization of the system. This comes at the price of decreasing the temporal resolution of the measurements, since the total stimulation rate must be distributed between a number of controllers. Finally, multiple clamps may also be used to study structured or modular systems, e.g., the dynamics of coupling between interrelated systems or the integration of different inputs within the same system.

[1]This is a two-dimensional case of Equation (3), where $\vec{X} = \begin{pmatrix} x_{75} \\ x_{25} \end{pmatrix}$, $\vec{S} = \begin{pmatrix} \theta \\ \sigma \end{pmatrix}$ and $\mathbf{T} = \begin{pmatrix} 0.5 & 0.5 \\ (\ln 9)^{-1} & -(\ln 9)^{-1} \end{pmatrix}$

APPLICATIONS OF THE RESPONSE CLAMP

The possible applications of the method may be classified into three categories: (1) exploration of intrinsically generated dynamics (2) exploration of extrinsically generated dynamics, and (3) generation of input–output trajectories.

EXPLORING INTRINSICALLY GENERATED DYNAMICS

Let us return once more to our main source of inspiration, the voltage clamp technique. The studies pioneering this method, and many that followed, applied it on isolated systems (e.g., the giant squid axon) to observe the internal dynamics of ionic conductances at different voltage levels. Later, current fluctuations in microscopic, voltage-clamped membrane patches were analyzed to study the same issue at the molecular level, a technique termed "patch clamp" (Neher et al., 1978). In both cases, therefore, the voltage clamp was used to study the dynamics of the state variables with relations to changes in the clamped variable itself. Let us call such dynamics "intrinsic," as they are not related to some event occurring outside of the clamped system.

Similarly, the response clamp may be used to study the intrinsic dynamics of a system's state variables at the functional level. Such was the application of the response clamp in behavioral psychophysics (Marom and Wallach, 2011), where the subjects'

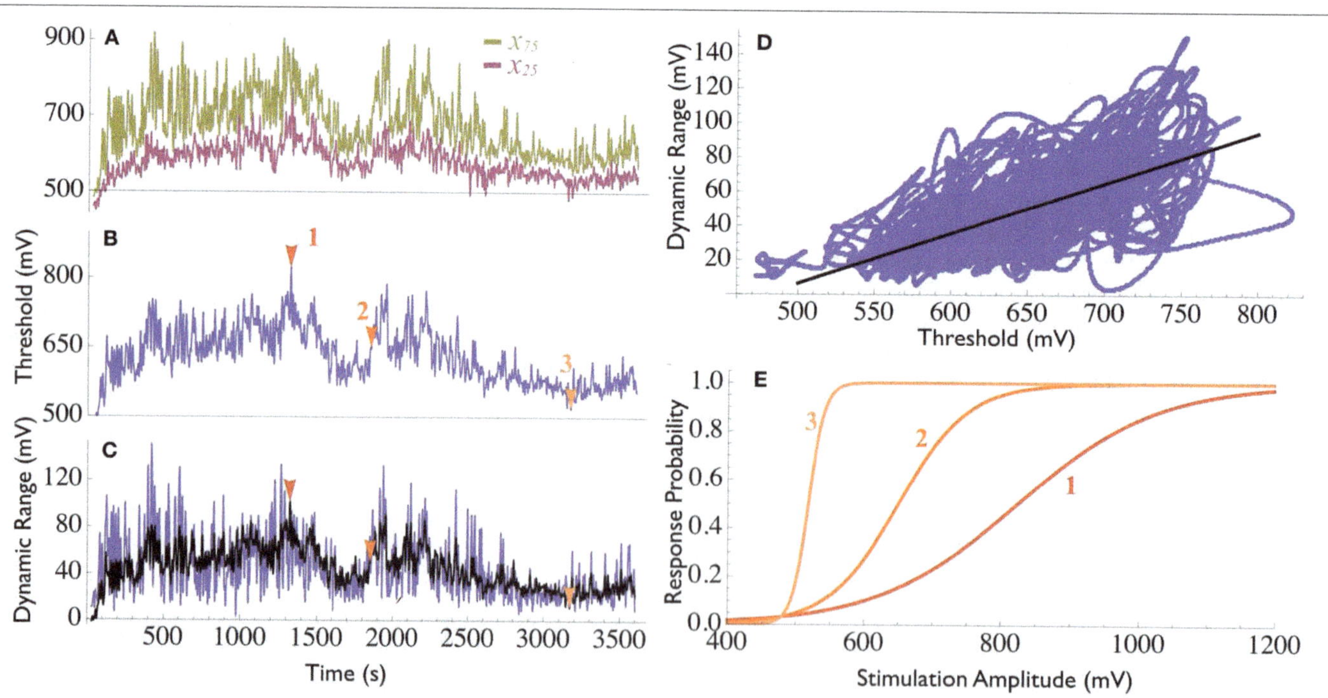

FIGURE 2 | Neuronal threshold and range dynamics. (A) Measurement of x_{75} (yellow) and x_{25} (purple) during 1 h of double clamping an isolated neuron *in vitro* (see Methods in Wallach et al., 2011). The two measurements are highly correlated. The neuronal threshold θ **(B)** and the dynamic range σ **(C)**, were computed using Equation (4) (blue line in both). **(D)** When the measurements are displayed in the threshold/range state plane, the significant correlations between them is evident. Fitting with a linear relation [Equation 5, black line in panel **(D)**, $R^2 = 0.52$] enables the estimation of the dynamic range based on the instantaneous threshold [black line in panel **(C)**]. **(E)** Examples to the instantaneous I/O relations (Equation 6) at three different points in time [marked with colored arrowheads in panels **(B)** and **(C)**]. The curve becomes stretched as the threshold increases. Note that as the threshold approaches the minimal value θ_0, the curve approaches a step-function, i.e., the neuron becomes a deterministic element.

response fluctuations in the clamped and unclamped scenarios were compared. The results suggest that these fluctuations are markedly restrained in closed-loop conditions, namely when the subject's actions have some (unconscious) effect on future stimuli. This led the authors to postulate that the well-documented trial-to-trial variability does not reflect, as previously suggested, an intrinsic "noise" process; rather, it stems from the unnatural open-loop experimental paradigm. The response clamp may be used in a similar manner to investigate the relations between psychophysical dynamics and brain activity (Monto et al., 2008), or to study the factors driving threshold fluctuations at the cellular, synaptic or network levels.

To further demonstrate how closed-loop analyses provide new insights into functional properties of a system, let us apply the double response probability clamp experiment discussed above to study intrinsic response dynamics of isolated neurons (Gal et al., 2010). By plotting the two derived state variables, θ and σ, against each other (**Figure 2D**), it becomes evident that the long term fluctuations of the dynamic range are highly correlated with those of the threshold. The relations between these two variables may thus be approximated using a linear expression, namely,

$$\sigma(t) = \alpha\,(\theta(t) - \theta_0)\,. \tag{5}$$

Equation (5) may be used to produce a smoothed estimate of σ based on the values of θ (black line in **Figure 2C**). The instantaneous input–output relations are therefore simplified in this case to a single state variable expression,

$$P(\bar{x}, \bar{\theta}(t)) = \frac{1}{1 + e^{-(\bar{x} - \bar{\theta}(t))/\alpha\bar{\theta}(t)}}, \tag{6}$$

where $\bar{x} = x - \theta_0$ and $\bar{\theta} = \theta - \theta_0$ are the *relative* stimulation amplitude and threshold, respectively. **Figure 2E** visualizes such instantaneous I/O relations in three different instants during the recording (marked with arrowheads in **Figures 2B,C**). This result is, in fact, quite expected, as scaling of sensitivity to changes with stimulation magnitude is a ubiquitous phenomenon in both physiology (Abbott et al., 1997) and psychophysics (e.g., the Weber–Fechner law, see Carterette and Friedman, 1974). Note that the offset parameter θ_0 has a biophysical significance: it is the threshold value at which the dynamic range becomes zero, i.e., the neuron becomes *deterministic* (the I/O relations become a step function). θ_0, therefore, is the minimal stimulation amplitude required to generate a spike at the maximal excitable state of the neuron, constituting an example to how analyses of intrinsic fluctuations of the system's state variables (reflected in the response clamps' control signals) yield novel findings as to the functional properties of the system.

EXPLORING EXTRINSICALLY GENERATED DYNAMICS

While much can be learned by studying isolated systems, neural systems are invariably embedded in networks and environments, where they interact with many external factors; any neuron, for instance, is affected by the activity of its peers via synaptic inputs converging onto it. The voltage clamp proved very beneficial in investigating the mechanisms of this communication by providing measurements of the *post synaptic currents* (Hagiwara and Tasaki, 1958): the membrane potential is held constant at some desired value, and changes in the feedback current *due to an external event* (e.g., an action potential generated in a neighboring cell) are measured. Using this application of the clamp, one may isolate individual input components (i.e., by clamping to a specific reversal potential) and separate them from the dynamics of the system itself (by preventing the generation of action potentials).

Similarly, the response clamp may be used to study changes in the functional behavior of systems due to interactions with their external environment. In a recently published paper (Wallach and Marom, 2012), the long-term effects of network events (brief episodes of synchronous, network-wide activity, also called "bursts" or "population spikes") on neuronal threshold were analyzed. Since the measurements are inherently noisy the effect of a single event was usually too small to observe and event-triggered averaging was applied. Using this procedure it was shown that network synchronous events induce a long lasting, bi-phasic deflection of the neuronal threshold. The results demonstrate interrelations between the dynamics at the two levels: the magnitude of the network event is reflected in the amplitude of the neuronal threshold deflection, while the relaxation of the threshold back to baseline is correlated with the recovery dynamics of network excitability.

These results demonstrate how the response clamp could be applied to the study of such extrinsically generated dynamics. Any measurable external influence on the clamped system (either subject to experimental control or autonomous) may be analyzed in a similar manner; the effects of various chemical compounds (such as neuromodulators or toxins) on overall cellular excitability, for instance, may be thus quantified. Similarly, the method may be implemented to study the interactions between different inputs to the same system: the response to one source may be clamped, and changes in the control signal due to activation of the second source may be recorded.

GENERATING INPUT–OUTPUT TRAJECTORIES

Like many other closed-loop stimulation techniques (e.g., Wagenaar et al., 2005; Arsiero et al., 2007; Rolston et al., 2010), the response clamp offers the capability to control the activity patterns of neural systems. This capability may, in and by itself, be useful in different experimental scenarios. In such cases, the control signal is not used for analysis; rather, the effect of the produced dynamics on other (non-clamped) variables is explored. The most notable derivative of the voltage clamp technique in this context is the *dynamic clamp* (Sharp et al., 1993), in which the current injected in a closed-loop effectively adds or removes conductance components to the cell; the contribution of these conductances to the overall system behavior, and not the injected current, is the subject of analysis in this method.

In the response clamp, it is this "overall system behavior" that is manipulated. For instance, let us assume that an isolated system is repetitively stimulated at rate f_{in}, and the response probability to this stimulation is clamped to some value p. The activity rate of this system, f_{out}, is therefore also clamped, since

$$f_{out} = f_{in} \cdot p. \tag{7}$$

Thus, by maintaining f_{in} constant and varying p, one may precisely produce desired activity patterns (see Figure 5 in Wallach et al., 2011). This may be useful if the clamped system serves as an input stage for downstream systems. Interestingly, Toettcher et al. (2011) recently suggested a similar approach (also using a PID-based algorithm) to control the dynamics of intracellular signaling pathways, thus generating a well-controlled, repeatable input to downstream components in the pathway.

Yet one may use this tool to do more than just control the output dynamics: by controlling both the clamped response and the input, regions of the *input–output space* may be efficiently covered. For instance, by jointly altering f_{in} and p (in opposite directions), one may observe the system's behavior at different input levels, while maintaining the output level (f_{out}) constant. Exploring various input–output combinations may elucidate the contributions of input-dependent effects (i.e., direct effects of stimulation) and activity-dependent effects to the overall behavior.

LIMITATIONS OF THE RESPONSE CLAMP AND COMPARISON WITH OTHER APPROACHES

COVERAGE OF THE TIME-SCALE SPECTRUM

The voltage clamp served as a source of inspiration and as a reference methodology for the development of the response clamp and its applications. However, a different range of time-scales is accessible in each of these two techniques. In voltage clamp, the controller (the feedback amplifier) is both extremely fast (i.e., its time-constant is much shorter than that of the clamped membrane) and powerful (i.e., the feedback gain is high) so that the clamp process is, for all practical purposes, instantaneous. Thus, the voltage clamp enables the investigation of even the fastest processes in the membrane (e.g., fast activation of sodium channels). Application of the voltage clamp to the study of extremely slow processes, however, is limited in several respects. First, voltage clamp is presently performed using physically invasive intracellular electrodes, a procedure which sets a practical upper bound to the duration of recordings. This technical limitation may be theoretically circumvented if a non-invasive realization of the method is invented (e.g., by harnessing optical techniques for both voltage measurements and current injection). However, voltage clamp is "invasive" in a different, more fundamental sense: as long as the cell is clamped, its natural behavior (i.e., emitting action-potentials) is completely shut-down. Thus, even if a non-invasive voltage clamp did exist, the results obtained using this technique would have little to do with natural long term dynamics of excitability.

The response clamp provides access to a range of time-scales which is complementary to those covered by the voltage clamp. On one hand, access to the very fast time-scales may be limited due to stimulation constraints (e.g., maximal possible stimulation intensity or rate) and to the time-scale of the control algorithm (determined by the various control parameters). On the other hand, the straightforward realization of the method using non-invasive means of stimulation and recording (e.g., extracellular electrodes), and the fact that the cell's natural spiking behavior remains intact, extends the experimental access into extremely long-term processes. By determining the time-scale of the clamped dynamics, the response clamp provides an experimental tool to separate processes of different time-scales governing the behavior.

APPLICABILITY TO CONTROLLABLE SYSTEMS

A prerequisite to any application of the response clamp is to establish reliable control of the response feature of interest by manipulation of some input parameter. In the systems studied so far, establishing this control was particularly straightforward since the input–output relations were monotonically non-decreasing (e.g., the sigmoidal curve in Equation 1). In systems where these relations are of a more complex nature (e.g., bell shaped or multi-modal), a more elaborate control algorithm is required (Astrom and Wittenmark, 1994). Moreover, in some systems the relevant input feature (the so called "receptive field") may be unknown. In such cases, some algorithm that finds this relevant input feature within the space of all possible inputs must be instated, in order for the clamp to be applicable. Such a combined solution is discussed in the next section.

REVERSE CORRELATION AND WHITE-NOISE ANALYSES

The response clamp demonstrates how closed-loop control may be used as a tool for system characterization. An important open-loop alternative which was already mentioned above is the *reverse correlation* approach. In this method the input–output relations of a system are exposed by computing various weighted statistics of the input variable, with the assigned weights derived from the output variable. The most common of these techniques is the *Spike-Triggered Average* (STA) and its extensions, which were used extensively in order to estimate the receptive fields of various neurons [see Simoncelli et al. (2004), and references therein]. When the input is under experimental control, approximated white-noise is usually applied, so that equal energy is applied across a broad range of time-scales (alternatively, whitening procedures may be used). This was shown to guarantee (under some additional restrictive conditions, see Paninski, 2003) that the estimation is unbiased.

There are several limitations to the use of reverse correlation methods. First, if the stimuli space is multi-dimensional, unbiased coverage of this space is very difficult experimentally, as the number of stimuli needed increase exponentially with each additional dimension [Benda et al. (2007) already purposed closed-loop stimulation as a method to efficiently sample this space when systematic, open-loop coverage is impractical]. More importantly, the underlying (and often unstated) assumption in these methods is that the system is feed-forward and static; the receptive field derived using STA is tightly related to the linear stage of *Linear-Nonlinear-Poisson* neuronal models, which do not account for refractoriness, output-dependent processes or threshold dynamics. Moreover, since the space of all possible output dynamics is not necessarily covered (e.g., high firing rates are rarely reached), such output-dependent effects may not be fully expressed in white-noise perturbation.

White-noise analysis, however, holds the considerable advantage of enabling identification of the input features to which the system is sensitive using very limited *a-priori* knowledge (e.g., the relevant modality). As it happens, this advantage precisely addresses the above mentioned impediment to the implementation of the response clamp, namely the need to identify a relevant and effective control variable. Thus, STA and the response clamp may be used in tandem, each method complementing the other: first, STA is implemented to expose the "static" or "baseline" receptive field; then, the response clamp uses this receptive field to produce the control variable, in order to expose the dynamic and output-dependent processes of the system.

COMPARISON WITH OTHER CLOSED-LOOP TECHNIQUES

Closed-loop control is, in itself, a widely accepted tool in many fields of research. Physiologists have employed closed-loop techniques and protocols to control aspects of neuronal activity at all levels of biological organization [see Arsiero et al. (2007) and references therein]. Already in the late 1960's, Eberhard E. Fetz showed that the activity of a single cortical neuron may be reinforced by applying closed-loop control of food pellets delivery (Fetz, 1969).

In psychophysics, a variety of procedures were developed over the past few decades in order to measure the psychometric threshold in closed-loop (Treutwein, 1995). The underlying assumption in all these procedures is that, in a given experiment, the threshold is *static*, and hence the procedure is stopped once it "converges" to a reliable estimate of this threshold. The key novelty in applying the response clamp to psychophysical investigations (Marom and Wallach, 2011), therefore, is in the analysis of post-convergence fluctuations of the threshold.

The fundamental difference between both the voltage- and response-clamp methods and other closed-loop techniques is that the control signal in all these techniques (be it food-pellet delivery rate, stimulation amplitude, etc.) is seldom used in order to gain access to the dynamics of hidden state variables. An interesting exception worth mentioning is a clinical method called *glucose clamp* (DeFronzo et al., 1979), developed in order to diagnose insulin secretion and resistance by analysis of the control signals (rates of glucose/insulin perfusion or infusion). This method, though rarely used in clinical practice, is considered the "gold standard" in the diagnosis of diabetes.

It should be stressed that the use of the PID control algorithm is, in and by itself, of no fundamental importance to the realization of the response clamp. This algorithm was chosen owing to its simplicity and generality; the PID is a pure-feedback, *model free* algorithm, and therefore little *a-priori* knowledge of the controlled system is required in order to implement it. Any other algorithm which efficiently clamps the system's response may be used. One might expect, for instance, that using other adaptive psychophysical protocols would yield similar results to those of Marom and Wallach (2011); rigorous examination of this prediction, however, is yet to be performed.

CONCLUDING REMARKS

The voltage clamp revolutionized the way physiologists study the mechanisms of excitability and synaptic communication. The response clamp method extends the clamp rationale toward functional characterization of neural systems. It offers a general framework for closed-loop exploration that may be implemented at any level of organization, using any available technique of measurement or perturbation. It may also be combined with complementary, open-loop approaches such as white-noise analysis. Finally, one may envision a paradigm in which voltage- or dynamic-clamp "command" is controlled in closed-loop by the response clamp algorithm. Such a multi-layered clamp set-up may aid in bridging the gap between mechanistic and functional characterization of neural systems.

ACKNOWLEDGMENTS

I am grateful to Dani Dagan and Shimon Marom for their valuable advice and assistance. The research leading to this review has received funding from the European Union Seventh Framework Program FP7 under grant agreement 269459 and was also supported by a grant of the Ministry of Science and Technology of the State of Israel and MATERA grant agreement 3-7878.

REFERENCES

Abbott, L., Varela, J., Sen, K., and Nelson, S. (1997). Synaptic depression and cortical gain control. *Science* 275, 221–224.

Arieli, A., Sterkin, A., Grinvald, A., and Aertsen, A. (1996). Dynamics of ongoing activity: explanation of the large variability in evoked cortical responses. *Science* 273, 1868.

Arsiero, M., Lüscher, H., and Giugliano, M. (2007). Real-time closed-loop electrophysiology: towards new frontiers in *in vitro* investigations in the neurosciences. *Arch. Ital. Biol.* 145, 193–209.

Astrom, K., and Wittenmark, B. (1994). *Adaptive Control.* Boston, MA: Addison-Wesley Longman Publishing Co., Inc.

Benda, J., Gollisch, T., Machens, C., and Herz, A. (2007). From response to stimulus: adaptive sampling in sensory physiology. *Curr. Opin. Neurobiol.* 17, 430–436.

Carterette, E., and Friedman, M. (1974). *Handbook of Perception.* Vol. 2. New York, NY: Academic Press.

DeFronzo, R., Tobin, J., and Andres, R. (1979). Glucose clamp technique: a method for quantifying insulin secretion and resistance. *Am. J. Physiol.* 237, E214.

Fetz, E. (1969). Operant conditioning of cortical unit activity. *Science* 163, 955–958.

Gal, A., Eytan, D., Wallach, A., Sandler, M., Schiller, J., and Marom, S. (2010). Dynamics of excitability over extended timescales in cultured cortical neurons. *J. Neurosci.* 30, 16332.

Hagiwara, S., and Tasaki, I. (1958). A study on the mechanism of impulse transmission across the giant synapse of the squid. *J. Physiol.* 143, 114–137.

Hodgkin, A., Huxley, A., and Katz, B. (1952). Measurement of current-voltage relations in the membrane of the giant axon of Loligo. *J. Physiol.* 116, 424.

Levine, W. S. (ed.). (1996). *The Control Handbook.* Boca Raton, FL: CRC press.

Marom, S., and Wallach, A. (2011). Relational dynamics in perception: impacts on trial-to-trial variation. *Front. Comput. Neurosci.* 5:16. doi: 10.3389/fncom.2011.00016

Monto, S., Palva, S., Voipio, J., and Palva, J. (2008). Very slow EEG fluctuations predict the dynamics of stimulus detection and oscillation amplitudes in humans. *J. Neurosci.* 28, 8268.

Neher, E., Sakmann, B., and Steinbach, J. (1978). The extracellular patch clamp: a method for resolving currents through individual open channels in biological membranes. *Pflugers Arch.* 375, 219–228.

Paninski, L. (2003). Convergence properties of three spike-triggered analysis techniques. *Network* 14, 437–464.

Rolston, J., Gross, R., and Potter, S. (2010). Closed-loop, open-source electrophysiology. *Front. Neurosci.* 4:31. doi: 10.3389/fnins.2010.00031

Sharp, A., O'Neil, M., Abbott, L., and Marder, E. (1993). Dynamic clamp: computer-generated conductances in real neurons. *J. Neurophysiol.* 69, 992.

Simoncelli, E., Paninski, L., Pillow, J., and Schwartz, O. (2004). Characterization of neural responses with stochastic stimuli. *Cogn. Neurosci.* 3, 327–338.

Toettcher, J., Gong, D., Lim, W., and Weiner, O. (2011). Light-based feedback for controlling intracellular signaling dynamics. *Nat. Methods* 8, 837–839.

Treutwein, B. (1995). Adaptive psychophysical procedures. *Vis. Res.* 35, 2503–2522.

Wagenaar, D., Madhavan, R., Pine, J., and Potter, S. (2005). Controlling bursting in cortical cultures with closed-loop multi-electrode stimulation. *J. Neurosci.* 25, 680.

Wallach, A., Eytan, D., Gal, A., Zrenner, C., and Marom, S. (2011). Neuronal response clamp. *Front. Neuroeng* 4:3 doi: 10.3389/fneng.2011.00003.

Wallach, A., and Marom, S. (2012). Interactions between network synchrony and the dynamics of neuronal threshold. *J. Neurophysiol.* 107, 2926–2936.

3

Adaptive enhancement of learning protocol in hippocampal cultured networks grown on multielectrode arrays

Alexey Pimashkin[1]*, Arseniy Gladkov[1,2], Irina Mukhina[1,2] and Victor Kazantsev[1,3]

[1] *Department of Neurodynamics and Neurobiology, Lobachevsky State University of Nizhny Novgorod, Nizhny Novgorod, Russia*
[2] *Normal Physiology Department, Nizhny Novgorod State Medical Academy, Nizhny Novgorod, Russia*
[3] *Laboratory of Nonlinear Processes in Living Systems, Institute of Applied Physics of the Russian Academy of Science, Nizhny Novgorod, Russia*

Edited by:
Ahmed El Hady, Max Planck Institute for Dynamics and Self Organization, Germany

Reviewed by:
Sergio Martinoia, University of Genova, Italy
Caleb Kemere, Rice University, USA
Robert E. Hampson, Wake Forest University Health Sciences, USA

***Correspondence:**
Alexey Pimashkin, Department of Neurodynamics and Neurobiology, Lobachevsky State University of Nizhny Novgorod, 23 Prospekt Gagarina, Nizhny Novgorod 603950, Russia.
e-mail: pimashkin@neuro.nnov.ru

Learning in neuronal networks can be investigated using dissociated cultures on multielectrode arrays supplied with appropriate closed-loop stimulation. It was shown in previous studies that weakly respondent neurons on the electrodes can be trained to increase their evoked spiking rate within a predefined time window after the stimulus. Such neurons can be associated with weak synaptic connections in nearby culture network. The stimulation leads to the increase in the connectivity and in the response. However, it was not possible to perform the learning protocol for the neurons on electrodes with relatively strong synaptic inputs and responding at higher rates. We proposed an adaptive closed-loop stimulation protocol capable to achieve learning even for the highly respondent electrodes. It means that the culture network can reorganize appropriately its synaptic connectivity to generate a desired response. We introduced an adaptive reinforcement condition accounting for the response variability in control stimulation. It significantly enhanced the learning protocol to a large number of responding electrodes independently on its base response level. We also found that learning effect preserved after 4–6 h after training.

Keywords: multielectrode arrays, hippocampal cultures, closed-loop, learning *in vitro*, learning in neural networks

INTRODUCTION

Neuronal networks formed in dissociated cultures grown on multielectrode arrays have been widely used as a biological model to monitor mechanisms of information encoding, synaptic plasticity, memory formation, and learning at the network level *in vitro* (le Feber et al., 2010; Frega et al., 2012; Maccione et al., 2012). Planar microelectrode systems permit simultaneous recording and electrical stimulation in different parts of the cultured neuronal network (Thomas et al., 1972).

After 2–3 weeks of spontaneous development the cultured neural networks display spontaneous burst discharges. The discharges consist of 0.1–1 Hz sequences of population bursts of 50–300 ms duration. Recent investigations showed that spatio-temporal patterns of spiking activity within the bursts are organized in a statistically repeatable and reproducible way (Raichman and Ben-Jacob, 2008; Pimashkin et al., 2011). Such repeatability indicated the presence of quite stable synaptic connectivity formed in the cultured network. External electrical stimulation modified the spiking pattern and, hence, induced long-term changes in the synaptic architecture of the underlying network. If the stimulation is applied with closed-loop conditions such changes may be directed to achieve a predefined profile of the evoked response. The latter can further be associated with navigating robots capable to implement simple behavioral tasks (Chao et al., 2008; Shahaf et al., 2008).

Low-frequency electrical stimulation in the form of pulse train (0.03–0.1 Hz) induced population burst responses over most of the neurons in the network during 50–300 ms after the stimulus artifact (Maeda et al., 1995; Wagenaar et al., 2004). Such stimulation did not change functional characteristics of the evoked response at both short and long-term periods (Chiappalone et al., 2008). However, spontaneous bursts can change their pattern after the low-frequency stimulation indicating changes in the network connectivity (Brewer et al., 2009; Bologna et al., 2010; Ide et al., 2010; le Feber et al., 2010). Increasing the stimulation frequency up to 1 Hz or higher led to suppression of the evoked responses (Jimbo et al., 1993; Shahaf and Marom, 2001; Eytan et al., 2003; Wagenaar et al., 2005; le Feber et al., 2010). Note, that tetanic stimulation with 10 Hz induced spike timing-dependent plasticity (STDP) in the culture network (Wagenaar et al., 2006a,b). Note also, that if signal propagation through synaptic pathways was blocked by applying 6-cyano-7-nitroquinoxaline-2,3-dione (CNQX) and (2R)-amino-5-phosphonovaleric acid (APV), the antagonists of *N*-methyl D-aspartate (NMDA) and α-amino-3-hydroxy-5-methyl-4-isoxazolepropionic acid (AMPA)-receptors, then the evoked spikes can be observed only at latencies shorter than 10 ms (Wagenaar et al., 2004). They represent a direct response on the excitation of an axon passing both the stimulation and the recording electrode, or on the excitation of a cell whose axon passes the recording electrode. Blocking Na^+ channels by tetrodotoxin (TTX) abolished all spontaneous and evoked activity in culture network. These results suggested that in normal conditions the stimulus evoked spikes with the latencies greater than 10 ms represented "network" spikes generated by signal propagation through the synaptic pathways of the culture network.

A closed-loop protocol of learning in cultured network of cortical neurons stimulated by low-frequency signal (0.3–1 Hz) was proposed by Shahaf and Marom (2001). Each stimulus response was defined as a number of evoked spikes appeared in 50 ± 10 ms post-stimulus interval. For continuous stimulation they introduced the response-to-stimulus ratio (R/S) for the single electrode. This quantity was defined as a moving average over 10 preceding responses. It characterized slow changes in the response caused by plasticity of synaptic pathways between neurons located near stimulating and recording electrodes. If the R/S value exceeded a certain threshold (R/S = 0.2 in Shahaf and Marom, 2001) the stimulation was stopped for 5 min providing the reinforcement. Then the cycle was repeated several times. Time interval needed to reach the threshold in each cycle was treated as adaptation time. The decrease of the adaptation time during the stimulation cycles was then interpreted as learning. Contrariwise, low-frequency stimulation in conditions without the reinforcement (e.g., open-loop conditions) did not induce the learning effect. Changes in the response was observed only on the trained electrode, whereas such effect was not found on the other electrodes. le Feber et al. (2010) found that closed-loop stimulation in cortical cultures induced significant changes in synaptic connectivity in contrast to the open-loop conditions. It was also noted that after training the spontaneous bursts were changed enhancing their correlation and synchrony (Li et al., 2007). This learning protocol was used in several other studies (Marom and Shahaf, 2002; Stegenga et al., 2009). It is important to note that only low-active electrodes recording one spike per 10 stimuli (e.g., with R/S = 0.1) were used for learning. Long-term changes were monitored for more than 30 cycles of stimulation. Electrodes with higher R/S (R/S = 0.5) were also examined for learning, but the learning effect was observed only during first six cycles of stimulation (Staveren et al., 2005).

In this paper we presented our results of learning experiments in hippocampal cultured networks on multielectrode arrays with closed-loop stimulation. Using adaptive and activity dependent reinforcement condition we found that the electrodes with relatively high response activity (R/S > 0.1) can be used for learning. Thus, the closed-loop stimulation could modify culture network synaptic pathways with relatively strong connections typically formed in spontaneous development. We also showed that the adaptive reinforcement significantly enhances the number of highly respondent electrodes (typically more than 50%) relative to the ones with lower response (R/S < 0.1) used in the previous studies.

MATERIALS AND METHODS

CELL CULTURING

Cell cultures were prepared from the hippocampus of C57Bl6 mice embryos at 18th prenatal day (E18) following standard procedures (Potter and DeMarse, 2001; Pimashkin et al., 2011). After trypsin treatment cells were dissociated by trituration and plated on 64-electrode arrays (Alpha MED Science, Japan), pre-coated with adhesion promoting molecules of polyethyleneimine (PEI). The final density of cell culture was about 15,000–20,000 cells/mm2. Note that in previous studies researchers used cultures with cell density of about 10,000–50,000 cells/mm2 (Shahaf and Marom, 2001) and 5000 cells/mm2 (le Feber et al., 2010). In both studies the cultures were plated from cortical cells. In similar learning experiments with hippocampal cultures the density was 2000 cells/mm2 (Li et al., 2007).

Cells were stored in culture neurobasal medium (Invitrogen 21103-049) with B27 (Invitrogen 17504-044), Glutamine (Invitrogen 25030-024) and fetal calf serum (PanEco κ055), under constant conditions of 37°C, 100% humidity, and 5% CO2 in air in an incubator (MCO-18AIC, SANYO). No antibiotics or antimycotics were used. Glial growth was not suppressed because glial cells were essential to long-term culture health. One half of the medium was changed every 2 days. Experiments were performed when neuronal networks were 3–6 weeks *in vitro* that permitted their functional and structural maturation (Eytan et al., 2003).

ELECTROPHYSIOLOGY

Extracellular potentials were collected through 64 planar platinum black electrodes simultaneously with the integrated MED64 system (Alpha MED Science, Japan). The 8 × 8 (64) microelectrode arrays with 50 μm × 50 μm size and the 150 μm spacing were used for recording at sampling rate of 20 kHz/channel (**Figure 1A**). Stimuli were generated using a four channels voltage/current stimulator (STG4004, MultiChannel Systems, Germany). Closed-loop conditions were performed by custom made software (Labview®) using real-time signal analysis and conditional stimulation.

SPIKE DETECTION

Detection of recorded spikes was based on threshold calculation of median of the signal according to the following formula:

$$T = N_S\sigma, \sigma = \text{median}\left(\frac{|x|}{0.6745}\right) \quad (1)$$

where x is the bandpass-filtered (0.3–8 KHz) data signal, σ is an estimate of the median normalized on the standard deviation of signal with zero number of spikes (Quiroga et al., 2004), and N_S is a spike detection coefficient determining detection threshold (Pimashkin et al., 2011). Standard deviation of signal containing Gaussian noise was equal to median of absolute values of the signal divided by 0.6745 which was a normalization of the median on the standard deviation.

Spike detection coefficient N_S permitted to take into account the contribution of different spike amplitudes. $N_S = 4$ was used for all data accounting spikes with amplitudes more than 20 μV. Minimal interspike interval was set to 1 ms. Detected spikes were then plotted in a raster diagram.

STIMULATION PROTOCOL

We used trains of biphasic rectangular voltage pulses (600 mV and 300 μs per phase, with positive phase first) at low-frequency in the range of 0.05–0.06 Hz. The value of stimulation frequency was chosen to induce bursting activity in the 20–500 ms post-stimulus interval (**Figure 1B**). Note that in previous studies the stimulation frequencies were significantly higher (0.1 Hz, 0.3 Hz, Shahaf and Marom, 2001; 0.2–0.33 Hz, le Feber et al., 2010) without any relation to spontaneous bursting frequency. In our experiments most of the stimuli with frequencies higher than 0.1 Hz did not evoked stable bursting activity. However, we found that stimulation at

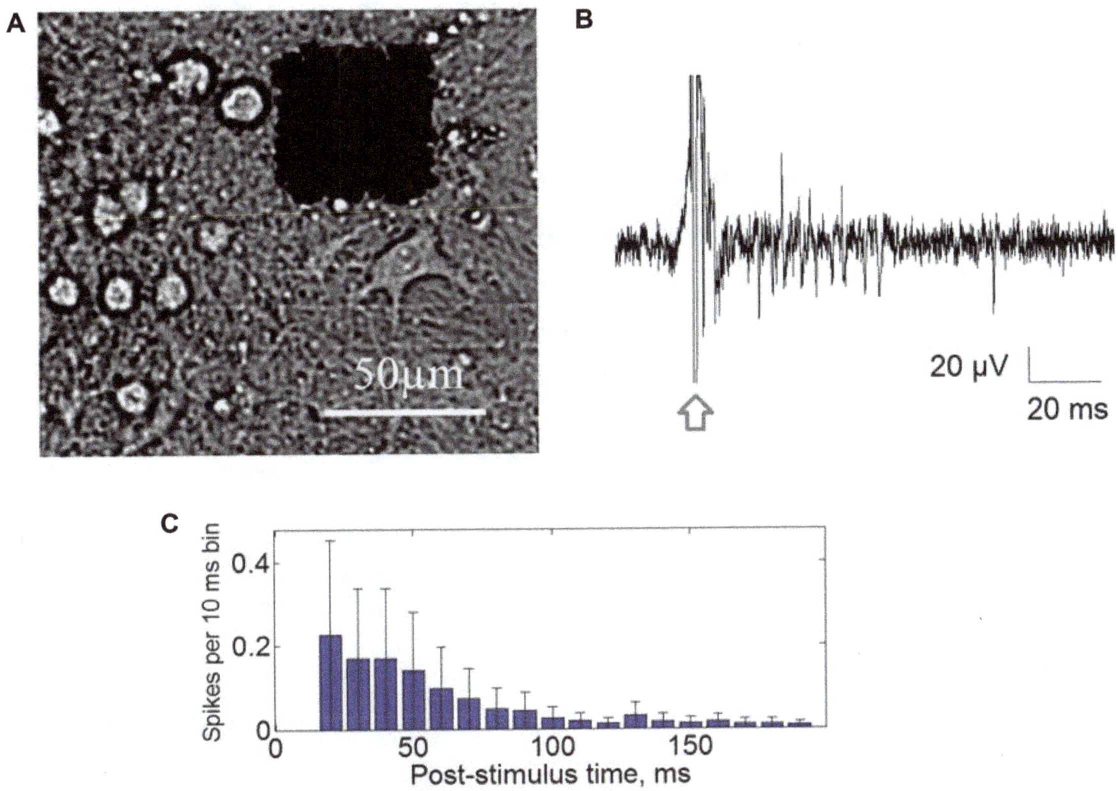

FIGURE 1 | (A) Cultured hippocampal cells grown on multielectrode array with 64 square electrodes with 50 µm size and 150 µm inter-electrode distance. **(B)** Post-stimulus response recorded from single electrode. Stimulation artifact marked by arrow. **(C)** Post-stimulus time histogram of the recorded spikes. Each bar represents average spike rate in 10 ms post-stimulus time interval ± standard deviation.

0.05 Hz and/or 0.06 Hz which is close to characteristic bursting frequency led to the evoked bursts. Note also, that technically the lower frequencies were also more preferable for the long-term stimulation because of the less influence on electrode disruption due to electrolysis.

Similarly, to previous studies we characterized the response by the response-to-stimulus ratio (R/S) calculated for each response and for each electrode. For our purpose, we counted the number of spikes detected in 40–80 ms post-stimulus interval on each electrode independently and then we defined R/S as the moving average across 10 preceding responses (Shahaf and Marom, 2001). This quantity indicated slow changes of the neuronal response over past 170–200 s.

Control stimulation (open-loop)

The control stimulation was performed during 75 min (five cycles of 10 min – stimulation, 5 min – rest) with 0.05 Hz stimulation frequency (150 stimuli) and with 0.06 Hz (180 stimuli). In more than 50% of the experiments (14 out of 24) the control stimulation was performed for 31 cycle (465 min ~7.5 h) to test the learning effect without reinforcement. After control stimulation the R/S values were calculated for each electrode.

The stimulation electrode first was chosen at random. If it evoked bursts recorded by the most of electrodes during stimulation for 5 min then the electrode was considered as stimulation electrode. If no bursting response was found, we tried another one. We considered only stably responding cultures, which during control stimulation did not significantly increase or decrease the total number of spikes in 20–300 ms post-stimulus interval for all recording electrodes. Slow changes of the responses were tested by estimating significant difference between the responses in the first and the last half of the recordings by Mann–Whitney rank-sum test ($p < 0.05$). If the sets of responses were not significantly different then the stimulation electrode was retained for further training, otherwise, we tested another electrode also chosen randomly or took another culture for the experiments. We also note, that most the cultures, in which the responses increased or decreased during control stimulation, demonstrated stable responses after several days. The responses were compared by relative changes of the mean value and of the standard deviation of the first and the last 30 stimuli responses in 20–300 ms interval normalized to the number of the spikes in the first 30 responses. Recording from each electrode was characterized by two statistical indicators: mean R/S value, M(R/S), and the R/S standard deviation, σ(R/S). The electrode for training was randomly chosen among the electrodes having M(R/S) value in the range of 0–8 with standard deviation in the range 0.1M(R/S) < σ (R/S) < 2 M(R/S) in control stimulation.

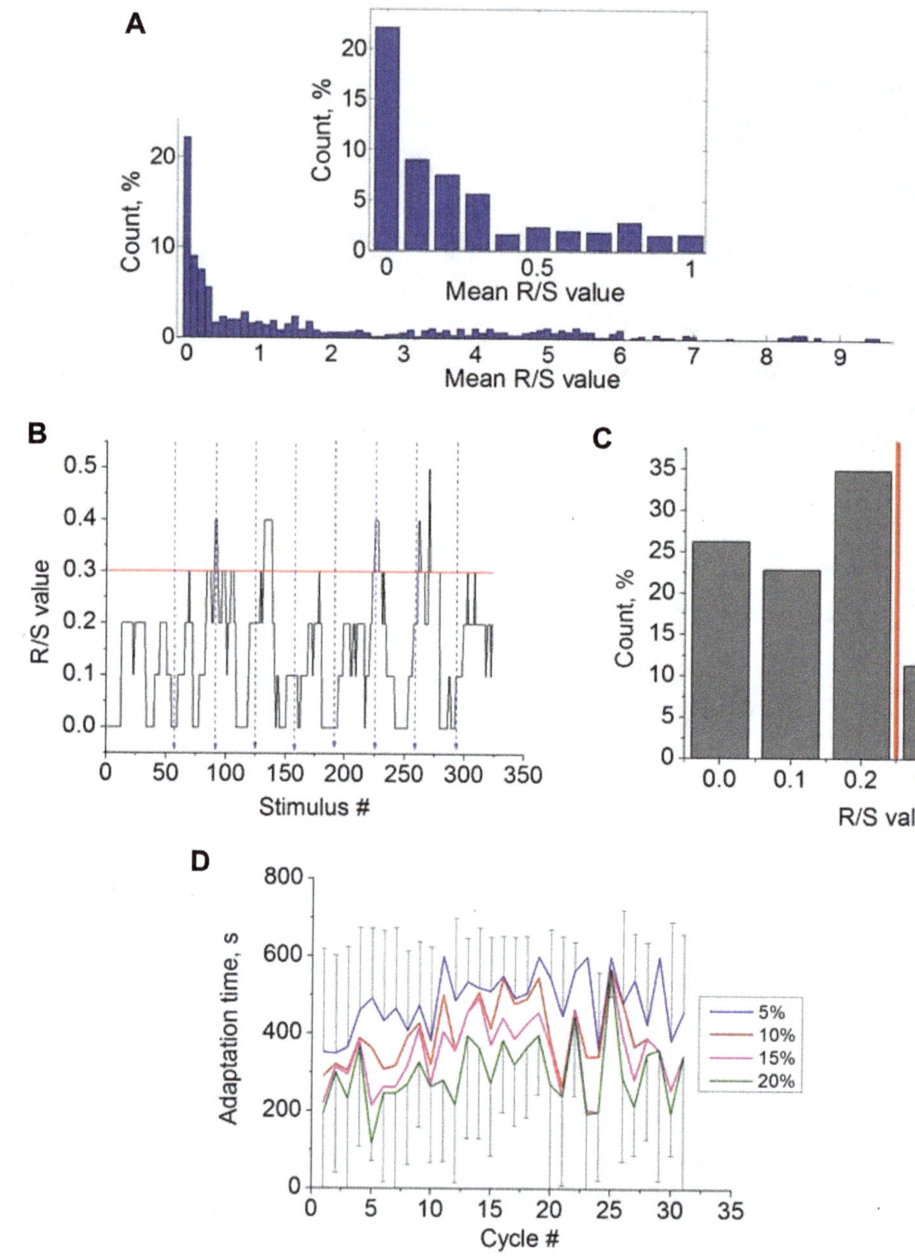

FIGURE 2 | (A) Average R/S values (M(R/S)) distribution for all recording electrodes during low-frequency stimulation (14 trials, $n = 10$ cultures). The inset shows the magnification of the histogram in the interval [0,1] of R/S values. **(B)** R/S values during several cycles of the control stimulation at selected electrode. Blue dashed lines illustrate the ends of the stimulation cycle. Red line shows the estimated R/S threshold value (see Materials and Methods). **(C)** Distribution of the R/S values from the selected electrode during control stimulation. Red line illustrates estimated R/S threshold value ($R/S_{Thr\%} = 15\%$). **(D)** Learning curves calculated for control experiments using different threshold estimation parameter $R/S_{Thr\%}$ - 5, 10, 15, and 20% ($n = 14$; see methods). Due to high variability of the characteristics the error bars (standard deviations) illustrated only for curves with $R/S_{Thr\%} = 5\%$ and $R/S_{Thr\%} = 20\%$.

Training stimulation (closed-loop)

Training stimulation was applied in closed-loop conditions. It started in one hour after the control stimulation. The training consisted of cyclic stimulation with continuous evaluation of the response. If the R/S value of the response to current stimulus exceeded a definite threshold then the stimulation stopped automatically. It provided the reinforcement for the culture targeting to achieve a required state. We introduced novel algorithm defining the R/S threshold for the reinforcement condition taking into account the responses in control stimulation. Such definition set different threshold values for different parts of the culture (e.g., different electrodes) involved in the training experiment. We took the highest 15% of the R/S values distribution for selected electrode, which was observed in control stimulation (example in **Figure 2C**). The lower boundary of that fraction of the distribution was assigned as the R/S threshold value. The threshold may also be referred as the 85th percentile. The percentage of the R/S values used for threshold estimation was defined as *threshold estimation parameter* $R/S_{Thr\%}$.

The training phase of the experiment consisted of sequence of the stimulation cycles with the same frequency and real-time evaluation of the R/S value on the selected electrode. If the R/S value of the activity from the selected electrode in response to stimulus reached the R/S threshold or if the stimulation time exceeds 10 min, then the stimulation was automatically stopped for 5 min completing the training cycle. Then the training cycle was repeated for 30–35 times. Thus the response of the neurons on the selected electrode altered the stimulation duration in each cycle. Time interval, from the beginning of the cycle to the moment where R/S value was found to be greater or equal to the R/S threshold was defined as *adaptation time*, $T_{R/S}$. The $T_{R/S}$ was monitored for each cycle and the sequence of $T_{R/S}$ values defined *learning curve.* Relative change of the $T_{R/S}$ during the experiment was defined as *adaptation time ratio*, $K(T_{R/S})$ and was estimated as mean $T_{R/S}$ in the last 10 cycles divided to the mean of the $T_{R/S}$ in the first 10 cycles. The decrease of the $T_{R/S}$ during the stimulation cycles $[K(T_{R/S}) < 0.5]$ was then treated as successful learning for the neurons on the selected electrode to generate the desired response on the stimulation. To compare the efficiency of the closed-loop stimulation parameters $K(T_{R/S})$ and $T_{R/S}$ were also calculated for control stimulation (e.g., the open-loop).

We also checked if the learning effect is stable in 4–6 h after the experiments by performing four cycle training stimulation.

At the longer time intervals (days or weeks) the cultures were changed significantly due to spontaneous development. In our experiments we reused some of them in not less than 2 days after the last training stimulation. When multiple experiments were performed on a single culture, we selected electrodes from different regions of the array for each new experiment to avoid possible influence of the previous stimulation experiments.

Spontaneous activity analysis

To analyze the effect of the stimulations on the state of the culture network we recorded spontaneous bursting activity during 10 min. We compared the average inter burst intervals, average number of spikes per burst and burst durations for the recordings before and after the stimulation experiments. Individual bursts detection was based on threshold estimation of basal spike rate activity as a total number of spikes observed in each 50 ms time bin (see Pimashkin et al., 2011 for more details). Statistical analysis of the bursting activity characteristics was performed by Mann–Whitney rank-sum test ($p < 0.05$).

RESULTS

OPEN-LOOP STIMULATION

First we analyzed responses of the culture on long-lasting (five cycles – 75 min and 31 cycles – 465 min) low-frequency stimulation (0.05, 0.06 Hz) of the stimulation electrodes that evoked population bursting response (see Materials and Methods). The stimuli were initially delivered through one randomly chosen electrode (**Figure 1B**). The dynamics of the evoked network response recorded from all electrodes was characterized by post-stimulus time histogram (PSTH). For each 10 ms time interval after the stimulus artifact a total number of the spikes recorded from all electrodes was calculated (**Figure 1C**). Maximum of the spike rate of the response was observed at 50–100 ms after stimulus.

Then, we analyzed the characteristics of the responses in the control stimulation (**Figure 2**). In our experiments we found that 31.13% of the electrodes (total 64) had $0 < M(R/S) \leq 0.1$ during the control stimulation (14 trials of long recordings, $n = 10$ cultures). The percentage of electrodes having $0 < M(R/S) \leq 10$ was 58.16% (**Figure 2A**). Particular electrodes for training stimulation were chosen among the electrodes with $0 < M(R/S) \leq 8$ (see Materials and Methods). Note that in previous studies only the activity from the electrodes with average R/S values during the control stimulation M(R/S) equal to 0.1 were chosen for training, and $R/S = 0.2$ was set as the R/S threshold (Shahaf and Marom, 2001; Li et al., 2007; Stegenga et al., 2009; le Feber et al., 2010).

Time dynamics of the R/S values for each stimulus response during the control stimulation is shown in **Figure 2B**. Ending moments of the 10 min stimulation cycles are marked by blue lines. Note that the responses were quite variable. The learning threshold was defined as the lower value from the highest 15% of R/S values referred as the 85th percentile of the R/S values (see Materials and Methods). The example of the R/S values distribution from the selected electrode and the R/S threshold is shown in **Figure 2C**. In other words, the threshold was set to detect quite rare and high rate responses. Note that for different electrodes the R/S thresholds were in range from 0.2 to 12 in different experiments.

After the threshold was defined the adaptation time $T_{R/S}$ can be estimated for each cycle. To confirm that the learning effect can be induced only in closed-loop conditions, we estimated a learning curve ($T_{R/S}$ for each cycle) for control stimulation (**Figure 2D**). The results show that adaptation time remains relatively stable. Next we analyzed the influence of the R/S threshold estimation parameter on the adaptation dynamics by setting different $R/S_{Thr\%}$ – 5, 10, 15, and 20% (95th, 90th, 85th, and 80th percentile, respectively). Note that the lower threshold is set the easier to reach the threshold by spontaneous fluctuations of the response. Hence, the adaptation curves for the lower thresholds were located lower (**Figure 2D**). However, changing the threshold did change qualitatively the adaptation dynamics.

CLOSED-LOOP STIMULATION

Next we made the experiments on training stimulation with the reinforcement (see Materials and Methods). In these conditions the stimulation were turned off when the learning threshold was reached at each cycle.

The adaptation dynamics for one experiment is shown in **Figure 3A**. The adaptation time for the case of successful learning (black curve) went down after several cycles of the training stimulation. We also found that some of the cultures could not be trained as illustrated by the red curve in **Figure 3A**. For those cultures the adaptation time was fluctuating with its maximal value for the whole duration of the stimulation. The training stimulation was applied for 17 different cultures in 24 experiments. **Figure 3B** shows average learning curve for the set of successful experiments.

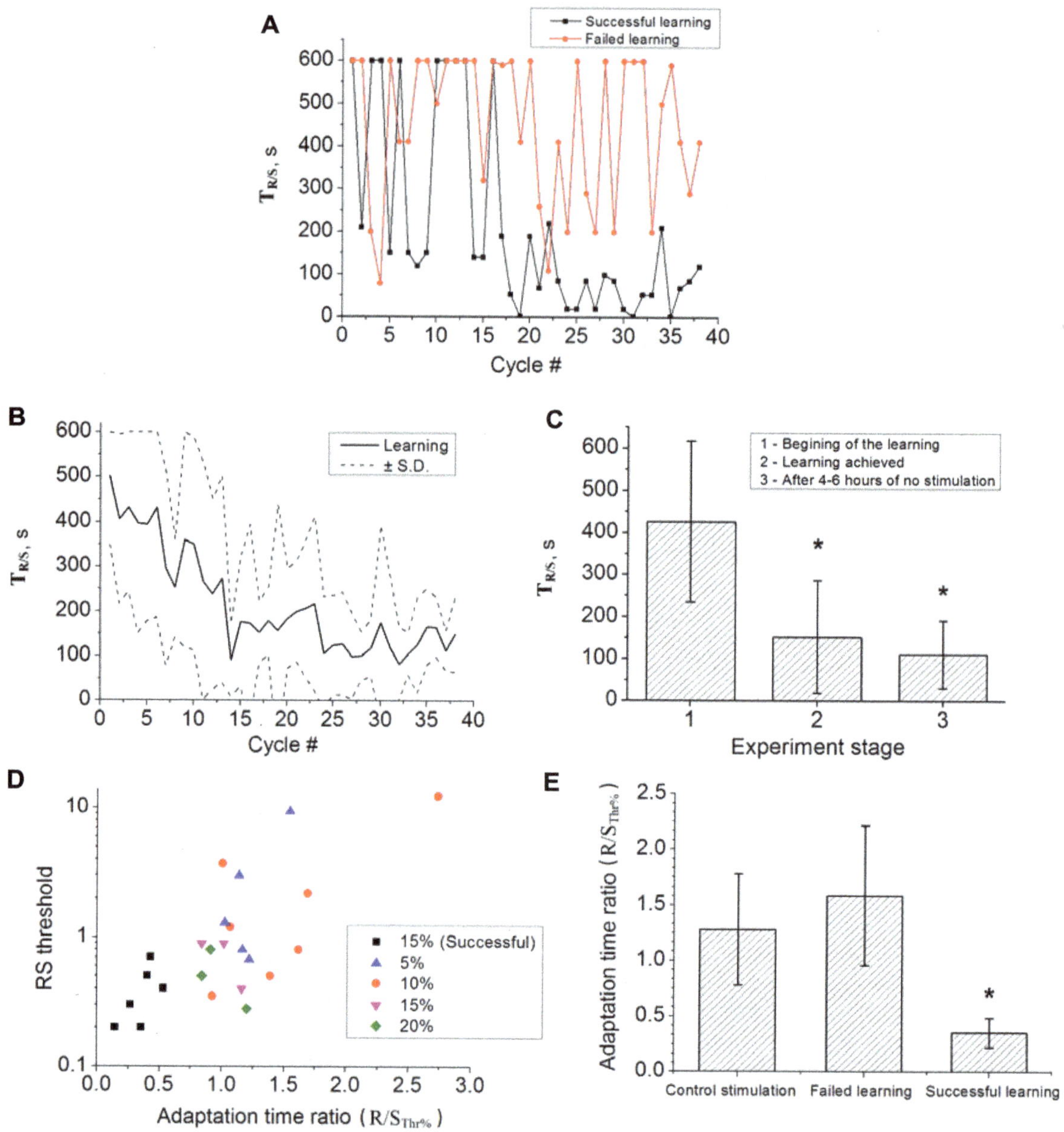

FIGURE 3 | (A) Learning curve in one successful experiment (black curve) and failure of learning in the other experiment (red curve). In the successful case the adaptation time significantly decreased. **(B)** Average learning curve (six experiments, six cultures). Dashed curves illustrates the standard deviation **(C)** Average adaptation time during five cycles at the beginning of the training experiment (1, $n = 6$), when learning is achieved (2, $n = 6$) and in 4–6 h after the end of main experiment (3, $n = 3$). Error bar corresponds to the standard deviation, statistical significance was tested by *t*-test ($p < 0.05$). **(D)** The R/S threshold values for successful (black markers) and failed (colored markers) learning experiments. The colored markers correspond to the use of different values of the threshold estimation parameter, $R/S_{Thr\%} = 5$, 10, 15, and 20% of R/S (see methods). In six experiments the learning was achieved using R/S threshold parameter 15% (out of 9 and out of 24 experiments in total). **(E)** Average adaptation time ratio for control stimulation, failed learning and successful learning. Error bar corresponds to standard deviation. The ratios of the successful learning were significantly different to the control stimulation (*t*-test, $p < 0.05$).

In contrast to the open-loop case (control stimulation) the adaptation time decreased indicating the learning effect. To quantify it we used the adaptation time ratio $K(T_{R/S}$; see Materials and Methods). If $K(T_{R/S})$ was lower than 0.6 then the training was considered as successful. We also analyzed the influence of the threshold estimation parameter (**Figure 3D**). Interestingly, that only the use of $R/S_{Thr\%} = 15\%$, induced the learning effect (black squares in **Figure 3D**). It was found in six of nine experiments for $n = 9$ cultures with absolute value of the R/S threshold less than 1. Similar statistics of about 50% successful experiments were reported in the previous studies (Shahaf and Marom, 2001; le Feber et al., 2010).

In the adaptation dynamics the decrease of time $T_{R/S}$ was typically observed after 10–14 stimulation cycles (see **Figures 3A,B**).

In two experiments it was decreased almost immediately after the second stimulation cycle. In average at the end of the training experiment the adaptation time became 110.62 ± 81.17. Note, that the average R/S values for the first and for the last 30 stimuli were not statistically different. In several experiments after 2–4 h of stimulation we obtained rather high $T_{R/S}$ values leading to higher deviations in the averaged values (**Figure 3B**).

To confirm that learning effect of the closed-loop stimulation may induced long-term changes (at the time scale of hours) we performed several experiments after main course of learning. The training stimulation of four cycles (60 min) was applied in 4–6 h after end of the main experiments. We found that in three of six cases the learning effect was preserved as illustrated in **Figure 3C**.

Next we addressed the question if the pattern of the response is changed due to the stimulation. We analyzed changes in the number of spikes recorded in the evoked response. **Figure 4A** illustrates these changes in one of the successful experiments. One can note that after learning the spike intensity of the response increased, e.g., more responses composed of doublets, triplets and more spikes were observed. The average increase over all successful experiments is illustrated in **Figure 4B**. We also analyzed the response from other responding electrodes as illustrated in **Figure 4C**. We found that after successful learning the activity of the whole culture network increased significantly.

Changes in spontaneous activity were monitored by 10 min recordings (see Materials and Methods). We calculated the average inter burst interval, average spikes per burst and burst duration as shown in **Figure 4D**. For each characteristic we did not find any significant difference comparing between the four different phases of the experiment (before the control stimulation, before and after training stimulation and after 4–6 h after main learning experiments).

DISCUSSION

We applied low-frequency stimulation to hippocampal culture network with on-line monitoring of the response-to-stimulus ratio (R/S) in open-loop and closed-loop conditions. The key response indicator was defined as average number of post-stimulus

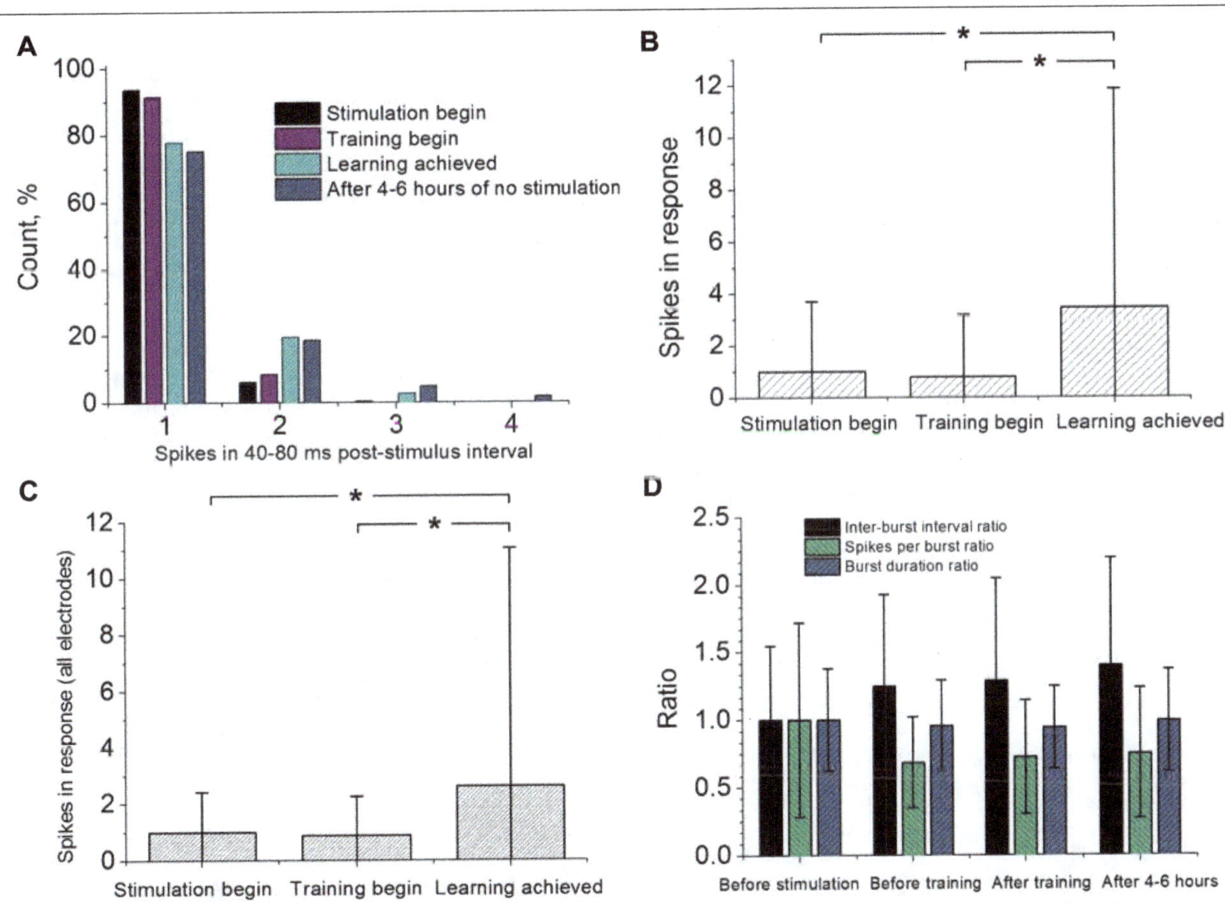

FIGURE 4 | (A) Response statistics of the neurons from training electrode represented by the number of spikes recorded in 40–80 ms post-stimulus interval. The responses were taken from 100 stimuli in the beginning of the control stimulation, beginning and ending of the training stimulation. Number of evoked spikes in 40–80 ms post-stimulus interval recorded from selected electrode **(B)** and from all recording electrodes **(C)**. The responses were taken from 100 stimuli in the beginning of the control stimulation, beginning and ending of the training stimulation. The quantities of the spikes were normalized to ones measured in control stimulation. **(D)** Spontaneous activity changes measured before the control stimulation, before and after training stimulation and after 4–6 h after main learning experiments. The quantities of the inter-burst intervals, spikes per burst and burst durations were normalized to ones measured in control conditions (before stimulation). The values were compared with the Rank-sum test ($p < 0.05$).

spikes per 10 stimuli in 40–80 ms time interval. Note that this interval corresponded to a peak in the post-stimulus histogram.

We found that learning in culture network can be achieved using an adaptive activity dependent reinforcement condition defined by the response-to-stimulus ratio (R/S) threshold value calculated from the statistics of control (e.g., the open-loop) stimulation. The threshold was estimated from the appearance of rare and high-rate responses in control stimulation (e.g., the highest 15% of the R/S values). Such responses may be associated with signal propagation along spontaneously activated and relatively strong synaptic pathways in the culture network. In other words, learning in our experiments means that particular synaptic pathways relative to particular stimulation electrode became "strengthen" to satisfy the reinforcement condition. In contrast to the previous studies in our approach we can use the electrodes with quite high basal activity in control simulation, $0 < M(R/S) < 0.5$. Note, that total number of such electrodes was quite high, $67 \pm 11\%$, which indicates that the learning protocol can be applied to rather large number of electrodes. Statistics of successful trials was about 50% which is comparable to earlier studies (Shahaf and Marom, 2001; le Feber et al., 2010).

Note, the R/S threshold, in fact, defines the reinforcement condition which is crucial for successful learning. In particular, we found that for lower values of the R/S threshold the learning effect was not achieved at all (**Figure 3D**). It is explained by the fact that the high variability of basal responses in culture network led to the increase of the fraction of random over-threshold responses that fails the learning effect which is concerned with regular changes in synaptic pathways in the network.

It is believed that learning effect is associated with structural and functional plasticity of underlying neuronal networks. In simple words synaptic connections are modified due to closed-loop stimulation to achieve an adaptive state defined by the reinforcement condition. In earlier studies low-activity electrodes were typically used (Shahaf and Marom, 2001; le Feber et al., 2010). Their activation implied that synaptic connections accompanying the electrodes were strengthened after the stimulation. Our results eventually demonstrated that not only weak connections between stimulating and recording electrodes can be increased but also well-functioning synaptic pathways can be modified for active electrodes.

Previous studies (Shahaf and Marom, 2001; Li et al., 2007) demonstrated that such training was quite selective. Only neurons on the trained electrodes increased the number of spikes in the response and hence the R/S value. In our experiments we found some increase of the responses from all electrodes (**Figure 4C**) and increase from the trained (selected) electrode (**Figure 4B**). However, the difference of this increase was not significant indicating the absence of the selectivity. We assume that it happened because of the overall activity (mean R/S) and R/S threshold were higher than in the previous studies. Setting higher reinforcement conditions for reaching the threshold in our learning protocol may require stronger modification of the overall synaptic connectivity (hence lower selectivity) to achieve learning.

Another important question was for how long time the synaptic changes can be preserved in the network after learning. We checked the response of our six trained cultures after 4–6 h and found that learning effect preserved in three of six samples (**Figures 3C,E**). Thus, the training stimulation in closed-loop conditions may induce long-term changes in structure and functions of culture network synaptic connectivity. We also found that spontaneous activity of the trained cultures was relatively stable and did not change significantly after learning experiments, e.g., we did not find statistical difference in the characteristics of the spontaneously generated bursts (inter-burst intervals, spikes per burst and burst durations).

ACKNOWLEDGMENTS

This research was supported by The Ministry of education and science of Russia, projects No. 8055, 14.B37.21.0927, 14.B37.21.1073, 14.B37.21.1203, 14.132.21.1663, 11.519.11.1003, Grant for Leading Scientists (No. 11.G34.31.0012), by the Russian President Grant No. MK-4602.2013.4 and MCB Program of Russian Academy of Science.

REFERENCES

Bologna, L. L., Nieus, T., Tedesco, M., Chiappalone, M., Benfenati, F., and Martinoia, S. (2010). Low-frequency stimulation enhances burst activity in cortical cultures during development. *Neuroscience* 165, 692–704.

Brewer, G. J., Boehler, M. D., and Ide, A. N. (2009). Wheeler Chronic electrical stimulation of cultured hippocampal networks increases spontaneous spike rates. *J. Neurosci. Methods* 184, 104–109.

Chao, Z. C., Bakkum, D. J., and Potter, S. M. (2008). Shaping embodied neural networks for adaptive goal-directed behavior. *PLoS Comput. Biol.* 4:e1000042. doi: 10.1371/journal.pcbi.1000042

Chiappalone, M., Massobrio, P., and Martinoia, S. (2008). Network plasticity in cortical assemblies. *Eur. J. Neurosci.* 28, 221–237.

Eytan, D., Brenner, N., and Marom, S. (2003). Selective adaptation in networks of cortical neurons. *J. Neurosci.* 23, 9349–9356.

Frega, M., Pasquale, V., Tedesco, M., Marcoli, M., Contestabile, A., Nanni, M., et al. (2012). Cortical cultures coupled to micro-electrode arrays: a novel approach to perform in vitro excitotoxicity testing. *Neurotoxicol. Teratol.* 34, 116–27

Ide, A. N., Andruska, A., Boehler, M., Wheeler, B. C., and Brewer, G. J. (2010). Chronic network stimulation enhances evoked action potentials. *J. Neural Eng.* 7, 16008.

Jimbo, Y., Robinson, H., and Kawana, A. (1993). Simultaneous measurement of intracellular calcium and electrical activity from patterned neural networks in culture. *IEEE Trans. Biomed. Eng.* 40, 804–810.

le Feber, J., Stegenga, J., and Rutten, W. L. C. (2010). The effect of slow electrical stimuli to achieve learning in cultured networks of rat cortical neurons. *PLoS ONE* 5:e8871. doi: 10.1371/journal.pone.0008871

Li, Y., Zhou, W., Li, X., Zeng, S., and Luo, Q. (2007). Dynamics of learning in cultured neuronal networks with antagonists of glutamate receptors. *Biophys. J.* 93, 4151–4158.

Maccione, A., Garofalo, M., Nieus, T., Tedesco, M., Berdondini, L., and Martinoia, S. (2012). Multiscale functional connectivity estimation on low-density neuronal cultures recorded by high-density CMOS Micro Electrode Arrays. *J. Neurosci. Methods* 207, 161–171.

Maeda, E., Robinson, H. P. C., and Kawana, A. (1995). The mechanism of generation and propagation of synchronized bursting in developing networks of cortical neurons. *J. Neurosci.* 15, 6834–6845.

Marom, S., and Shahaf, G. (2002). Development, learning and memory in large random networks of cortical neurons: lessons beyond anatomy. *Q. Rev. Biophys.* 35, 63–87.

Pimashkin, A., Kastalskiy, I., Simonov, A., Koryagina, E., Mukhina, I., and Kazantsev, V. (2011). Spiking signatures of spontaneous activity bursts in hippocampal cultures. *Front. Comput. Neurosci.* 5:46. doi: 10.3389/fncom.2011.00046

Potter, S. M., and DeMarse, T. B. (2001). A new approach to neural cell culture for long-term studies. *J. Neurosci. Methods* 110, 17–24.

Quiroga, R., Nadasdy, Q., and Ben-Shaul, Y. (2004). Unsupervised spike detection and sorting with wavelets and superparamagnetic clustering. *Neural Comput.* 16, 1661–1688.

Raichman, N., and Ben-Jacob, E. (2008). Identifying repeating motifs in the activation of synchronized bursts in cultured neuronal networks. *J. Neurosci. Methods* 170, 96–110.

Shahaf, G., Eytan, D., Gal, A., Kermany, E., Lyakhov, V., Zrenner, C., et al. (2008). Order-based representation in random networks of cortical neurons. *PLoS Comput. Biol.* 4:e1000228. doi:10.1371/journal.pcbi.1000228

Shahaf, G., and Marom, S. (2001). Learning in networks of cortical neurons. *J. Neurosci.* 21, 8782–8788.

Staveren, G. W., Buitenweg, J. R., Marani, E., and Rutten, W. L. C. (2005). The effect of training of cultured neuronal networks, can they learn? *Proc. Neural Eng.* 328–331.

Stegenga, J., Le Feber, J., Marani, E., and Rutten, W. L. C. (2009). The effect of learning on bursting. *Biomed. Eng.* 56, 1220–1227.

Thomas, C. A. Jr., Springer, P. A., Loeb, G. E., Berwald-Netter, Y., and Okun, L. M. (1972). A miniature microelectrode array to monitor the bioelectric activity of cultured cells. *Exp. Cell Res.* 74, 61–66.

Wagenaar, D. A., Madhavan, R., Pine, J., and Potter, S. M. (2005). Controlling bursting in cortical cultures with closed-loop multielectrode stimulation. *J. Neurosci.* 25, 680–688.

Wagenaar, D. A., Pine, J., and Potter, S. M. (2004). Effective parameters for stimulation of dissociated cultures using multi-electrode arrays. *J. Neurosci. Methods* 138, 27–37.

Wagenaar, D. A., Pine, J., and Potter, S. M. (2006a). An extremely rich repertoire of bursting patterns during the development of cortical cultures. *BMC Neurosci.* 7:11. doi: 10.1186/1471-2202-7-11

Wagenaar, D. A., Pine, J., and Potter, S. M. (2006b). Searching for plasticity in dissociated cortical cultures on multi-electrode arrays. *J. Negat. Results Biomed.* 5:16.

4

A Hebbian learning rule gives rise to mirror neurons and links them to control theoretic inverse models

A. Hanuschkin[1,2], S. Ganguli[3] and R. H. R. Hahnloser[1,2]*

[1] Institute of Neuroinformatics, University of Zurich and ETH Zurich, Zurich, Switzerland
[2] Neuroscience Center Zurich (ZNZ), Zurich, Switzerland
[3] Department of Applied Physics, Stanford University, Stanford, USA

Edited by:
Ahmed El Hady, Max Planck Institute for Dynamics and Self Organization, Germany

Reviewed by:
Yang Dan, University of California, USA
Klaus R. Pawelzik, University Bremen, Germany

***Correspondence:**
R. H. R. Hahnloser, Institute of Neuroinformatics, University of Zurich and ETH Zurich, Winterthurerstrasse 190, CH-8057 Zurich, Switzerland
e-mail: rich@ini.phys.ethz.ch

Mirror neurons are neurons whose responses to the observation of a motor act resemble responses measured during production of that act. Computationally, mirror neurons have been viewed as evidence for the existence of internal inverse models. Such models, rooted within control theory, map-desired sensory targets onto the motor commands required to generate those targets. To jointly explore both the formation of mirrored responses and their functional contribution to inverse models, we develop a correlation-based theory of interactions between a sensory and a motor area. We show that a simple eligibility-weighted Hebbian learning rule, operating within a sensorimotor loop during motor explorations and stabilized by heterosynaptic competition, naturally gives rise to mirror neurons as well as control theoretic inverse models encoded in the synaptic weights from sensory to motor neurons. Crucially, we find that the correlational structure or stereotypy of the neural code underlying motor explorations determines the nature of the learned inverse model: random motor codes lead to causal inverses that map sensory activity patterns to their motor causes; such inverses are maximally useful, by allowing the imitation of arbitrary sensory target sequences. By contrast, stereotyped motor codes lead to less useful predictive inverses that map sensory activity to future motor actions. Our theory generalizes previous work on inverse models by showing that such models can be learned in a simple Hebbian framework without the need for error signals or backpropagation, and it makes new conceptual connections between the causal nature of inverse models, the statistical structure of motor variability, and the time-lag between sensory and motor responses of mirror neurons. Applied to bird song learning, our theory can account for puzzling aspects of the song system, including necessity of sensorimotor gating and selectivity of auditory responses to bird's own song (BOS) stimuli.

Keywords: mirror neurons, inverse problem, linear models, songbird, sensory motor learning

INTRODUCTION

Complex vertebrate motor behaviors are generated by dedicated cortical circuits. The organization of these circuits and the plasticity rules that lead to their development and that guarantee their maintenance are functionally related to neural activity in single units and across larger populations (Gallese et al., 1996; Rizzolatti et al., 1996; Rizzolatti and Craighero, 2004; Harvey et al., 2012). For example, neural activity often strongly co-varies with motor behavior, allowing for estimation of detailed limb movement parameters from mere single-neuron recordings (Georgopoulos et al., 1986; Schwartz et al., 1988) and facilitating neural prosthesis (Santhanam et al., 2006; Ethier et al., 2012). However, in other cases, the amount of firing variability in single neurons can be dramatically dissociated from behavioral variability. For example, in songbirds, two distinct premotor areas are responsible for the generation of different aspects of the same vocal behavior. On the one hand, the cortical area HVC is involved in generating stereotyped adult song; lesions of HVC lead to degradation of typical adult song toward more unstructured subsong typical of very young birds (Nottebohm et al., 1976; Aronov et al., 2008). On the other hand, its counterpart, the lateral magnocellular nucleus of the anterior nidopallium (LMAN) in very young birds is involved in subsong production and in adults it is involved in the production of very subtle song variability that is barely noticeable to the human ear (Aronov et al., 2008). Lesions of LMAN in juveniles abolish song learning (Bottjer et al., 1984), and lesions in adults reduce the already small variability of adult undirected songs (the songs not direct toward another bird), manifest for example by reduced fluctuations of sound pitch (Kao et al., 2005; Stepanek and Doupe, 2010).

These lesion studies ascribing differential roles of HVC and LMAN to song production, are paralleled by findings from electrophysiology. In HVC of singing birds, single principal neurons fire highly stereotyped spiking patterns associated with a given song syllable, with precision of individual action potentials in the sub millisecond range (Hahnloser et al., 2002; Kozhevnikov and Fee, 2007). By contrast, in LMAN of birds singing undirected songs, neurons fire very variable spike patterns, patterns that fluctuate on a trial-to-trial basis between loosely timed high-frequency bursts of action potentials and no spiking at all (Olveczky et al., 2005; Kao et al., 2008). Thus, stereotyped adult song is subserved by precise firing in HVC whereas subtle variability of adult song is subserved by large firing variability in LMAN, **Figure 1**. The diverse neural codes in LMAN and HVC are integrated in a dedicated nucleus that mediates both differential influences from these stereotypy and variability generators. Both HVC and LMAN project to the robust nucleus of the arcopallium (RA), which is the cortical output nucleus that directly innervates syringeal and respiratory motor neurons.

Whether stereotyped or variable, internal motor patterns responsible for generating behavior cannot be fully understood without considering the sensory input reaching the motor system.

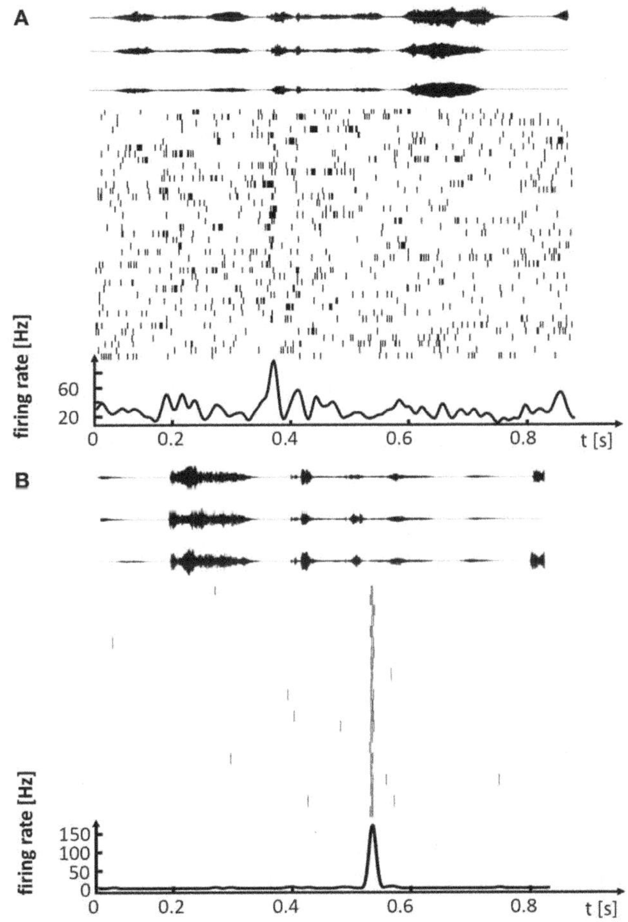

FIGURE 1 | Spiking activity in single neurons of singing zebra finches, illustrating (A) a variable premotor code in LMAN and (B) a stereotyped code in HVC. (A) Spike raster plot of LMAN projection neuron aligned to 41 renditions of the stereotyped song motif. Three exemplary sound oscillograms of the motif are shown on top. The neuron produces single spikes and spike bursts at different times in each rendition of the motif. The motif-averaged firing rate is shown at the bottom. **(B)** Spike raster plot of HVC projection neuron aligned to 22 renditions of the stereotyped song motif (in a different bird), three exemplary motif oscillograms are shown on top. In each rendition of the motif the neuron produces a brief burst of spikes at precisely the same time.

Indeed, the very development of motor systems as well as the formation of motor plans are profoundly shaped by sensory inputs. For example, the development of the mirror neuron system depends on sensorimotor experience (Catmur, 2012) and, the successful development of birdsong depends on intact HVC and LMAN activity during sensory exposure (Basham et al., 1996; Roberts et al., 2012).

We have learned much about the integration of sensory inputs into motor systems from single neuron studies examining responses during motor production and during matched sensory states. Among the key findings are mirror neurons that fire similarly when an animal executes a motor act and when it sees or hears another animal perform that same act. For example, mirror neurons in F5 of monkey premotor cortex fire both when the monkey touches an object and sees another subject touch that object (Rizzolatti et al., 1996; Rizzolatti and Craighero, 2004). Mirror neurons also exist in HVC of songbirds; these neurons fire at a precise time in the song, both when the bird sings the song and when it hears a similar song produced by another bird (Prather et al., 2008).

Mirror neurons establish a link between the observation of an act in another and self-generation of that same act. Such a remarkable correspondence between sensory and motor roles in single neurons has led to numerous suggestions about the function of mirror neurons in communication, imitation learning, cultural learning, and language development (Rizzolatti and Craighero, 2004; Oztop et al., 2012). Most importantly, mirrored responses have been proposed to be causally related to streams of motor and sensory activity (Oztop et al., 2006, 2012). A recent proposal is to tie properties of the mirror neuron system to correlative learning rules (Cooper et al., 2012). Accordingly, sensory responses in mirror neurons could develop from the contingency of motor-related firing and its sensory consequences feeding back to motor areas. Here we develop this idea and propose a simple mathematical theory of mirror neuron formation from correlational learning rules. To examine the critical role of motor variability, we study, based on earlier work (Hahnloser and Ganguli, 2013), mirror neuron formation for both motor codes with strongly correlated firing patterns among neurons, as in HVC, as well as for motor codes with uncorrelated firing patterns among neurons, as in LMAN.

We are particularly interested in relating mirror neuron properties to their computational role in control theoretic inverse models. Mirror neurons have previously been recognized as direct evidence of inverse models, which are models that transform desired sensory states into motor commands that can achieve those states and may be used for action generation (Oztop et al., 2012). From the control-theoretic perspective, internal inverse models give rise to mirrored responses because of the precise correspondence between a desired sensory target, the motor commands for producing that target, and the resulting sensory feedback. We pursue this idea and elucidate the conditions under which inverse models can arise from correlational learning during sensory feedback-dependent motor explorations.

We assume inverse models form in a context without prior knowledge of structure of either the motor apparatus or the delayed sensory feedback. We design an eligibility-weighted correlational learning rule that allows for the formation of both inverse models and mirror neurons. In the rule we propose, synaptic strengthening depends on contiguous co-activation of pre-and postsynaptic neurons, whereas synaptic weakening depends on heterosynaptic competition between sensory afferents innervating the same motor neuron. We argue that from a synaptic perspective, this rule is considerably simpler and more plausible than previously proposed rules and computational approaches toward systems-level inverse models based on error backpropagation (Jordan and Rumelhart, 1992). Our rule is most closely related to direct inverse model approaches (Miller, 1987; Slotine, 1987), in which, however, the possibility of unknown feedback delays has not been adequately addressed. Most importantly, we find that whether the formed mirror neuron system and inverse model is suitable for action imitation depends on the correlational structure of the neural code associated with motor production. Whereas a variable (explorative) motor code leads to causal inverse models and is suitable for mirror-neuron dependent action imitation, a stereotyped (repetitive) motor code leads to predictive inverse models and is not suitable for action imitation. Thus, our work provides an interesting link between the correlational structure of motor behavior, its underlying neural code, and fine-grained temporal properties of mirror neuron responses and their suitability for flexible action imitation.

Furthermore, these conceptual connections suggest a set of natural experiments designed to probe for the existence, and characterize the causal nature of, inverse models by measuring the fine grained temporal properties of the sensory and motor responses of mirror neurons. As we discuss below, when applied to the bird song system, these experiments make a specific, testable prediction about the existence and temporal properties of mirror neurons in the variable motor circuit LMAN, as well as explain the origin of previously observed temporal properties of mirror neurons in the stereotyped motor circuit HVC.

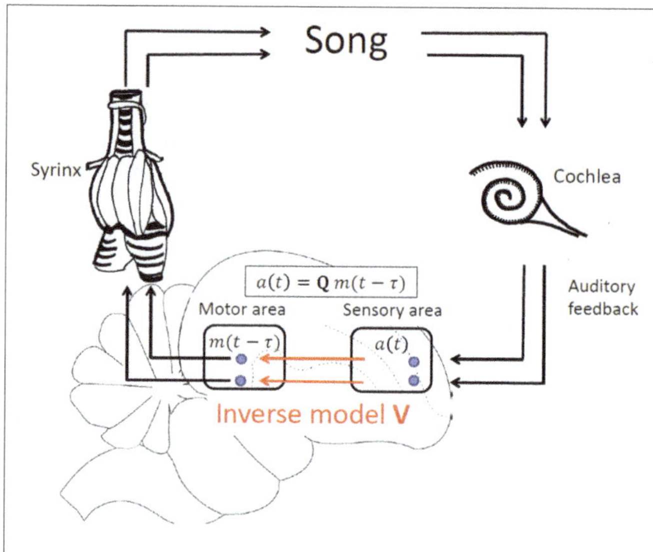

FIGURE 2 | Delayed feedback and inverse model, illustrated by vocal production in birds. In our model of delayed sensory feedback the auditory response $a(t)$ in a sensory area at time t depends linearly on motor activity $m(t-\tau)$ in a motor brain area at an earlier time $t-\tau$ according to $a(t) = \mathbf{Q}m(t-\tau)$, where $\mathbf{Q}$ is the unknown motor-sensory mapping and τ the unknown delay of auditory feedback. An inverse $\mathbf{V}$ is a mapping from sensory neurons back onto motor neurons that inverts the action of $\mathbf{Q}$: $\mathbf{V} = \mathbf{Q}^{-1}$.

RESULTS

A LINEAR FRAMEWORK

We develop our theory in a simple linear framework in which the sensory response $a(t)$ in a sensory brain area at time t is a vector of firing rates that is linearly related to the motor cause $m(t-\tau)$ at an earlier time $t-\tau$, where $m(t-\tau)$ is a vector of firing rates in a motor area such as HVC or LMAN. The *time delay of sensory feedback* $\tau = \tau_m + \tau_a$ is the sum of the time τ_m needed to translate motor activity into behavioral (vocal) output and the time τ_a it takes for a vocalization to elicit a sensory response. We assume a linear *motor-sensory mapping* modeled by the matrix $\mathbf{Q}$, allowing us to specify the form of delayed sensory feedback as $a(t) = \mathbf{Q}m(t-\tau)$, **Figure 2**.

Note that for simplicity we assume linearity of the motor-sensory mapping $\mathbf{Q}$. However, the simple linearity assumption inherent in $\mathbf{Q}$ need not be inconsistent with the existence of non-linearities between motor neuron activity and behavioral output (for example, song) and also with non-linearities between behavioral output and sensory responses. While it is the case that each of these transformations is highly non-linear, the dimensionality of motor behavior patterns realizable by muscle activity, or recorded by early sensory responses, is much smaller than the dimensionality of sensory or motor activity patterns deep within the cortex, by virtue of the fact that cortical motor and sensory neurons largely outnumber the few muscles and sensory receptors involved in the composite motor to sensory feedback loop. So for example, within the bird song system, it is thus probable that the low dimensional, composite non-linear transformation from cortical motor patterns, to muscle activity in the syrinx, to song, to cochlear response, back to cortical sensory feedback, could be well-approximated by a direct high dimensional linear map from the cortical motor area back to the cortical sensory area. This is in exact analogy to the theory of support vector regression approaches from machine learning, in which low dimensional non-linear maps can be well-approximated by high dimensional linear maps (Smola and Schölkopf, 2004). Thus, for our purposes, all we assume is that there exists at least one high dimensional linear map from cortical motor patterns to cortical sensory feedback patterns that approximates the composite feedback pathway implemented through the non-linear processes of motor generation and perception.

Now, an inverse model in this context is a mapping $\mathbf{V} = \mathbf{Q}^{-1}$ expressed in the synaptic weights $\mathbf{V}$ from sensory onto motor neurons. Such a mapping allows sensory neurons to postdict the possible motor cause m^a of a sensory target (vector) a (either driven externally, recalled from memory, or resulting from a planning strategy) according to $m^a = \mathbf{V}a$. Such a postdiction ability of inverse models can be used in feedforward motor control in which the appropriate stream of motor commands $m^a(t)$ can be computed for a given desired sensory target sequence $a(t)$ according to $m^a(t) = \mathbf{V}a(t)$.

The goals of our theory are to outline a biologically plausible, local mechanism for learning of the synaptic mapping **V** and to characterize the associated emergence of mirror neurons in this process.

ELIGIBILITY-WEIGHTED HEBBIAN LEARNING

We designed a simple learning rule in which potentiation of sensory-to-motor synaptic connections **V** arises from correlated firing in pairs of sensory and motor neurons. Because sensory feedback is delayed, synapses must be able to detect correlated firing within some non-zero time window, which we achieve by introducing an eligibility trace $e(s)$ that establishes a link between activity at time t in a motor neuron and activity in a sensory neuron at a later time $t + s$ (see also **Figures 3A,C**). The eligibility trace modulates the change in synaptic strength associated with correlated pre- and postsynaptic firing—it is a biophysical process that resides on the postsynaptic side of **V** synapses and is triggered by activity (i.e., spikes) in the postsynaptic (motor) neuron. Intuitively, we imagine that the spiking of a motor neuron, elicited for example from an internal source of motor variation that generates exploratory motor behavior, triggers the eligibility trace that in turn makes all synapses from sensory neurons onto that motor neuron eligible for future modification. Thus, if the delayed sensory feedback arrives to the sensory area within the window of eligibility, sensory to motor synapses can potentially learn to postdict the motor cause by correlating the current sensory feedback with past motor activity that might have generated it. We further assume that the eligibility is monotonically decaying in time, implying that sensory inputs preferentially connect onto motor neurons that were recently and reliably activated rather than motor neurons that were activated a long time ago. Necessarily, the decay of the eligibility trace must be slow enough to be able to attribute significant eligibility to sensory inputs with motor-to-sensory delays τ, which we subsume in the condition $e(\tau) \gg 0$.

The full correlational learning rule describing changes in synaptic strength V_{ij} from auditory neuron j onto motor neuron i reads:

$$\delta V_{ij} = \int_0^\infty ds\left[e(s)m_i(t-s)a_j(t)\right] - \hat{m}_i(t)a_j(t), \qquad (1)$$

where $\hat{m}_i(t) = \sum_k V_{ik}a_k(t)$ is the (silently) postdicted motor activity, corresponding to the summed auditory input to neuron

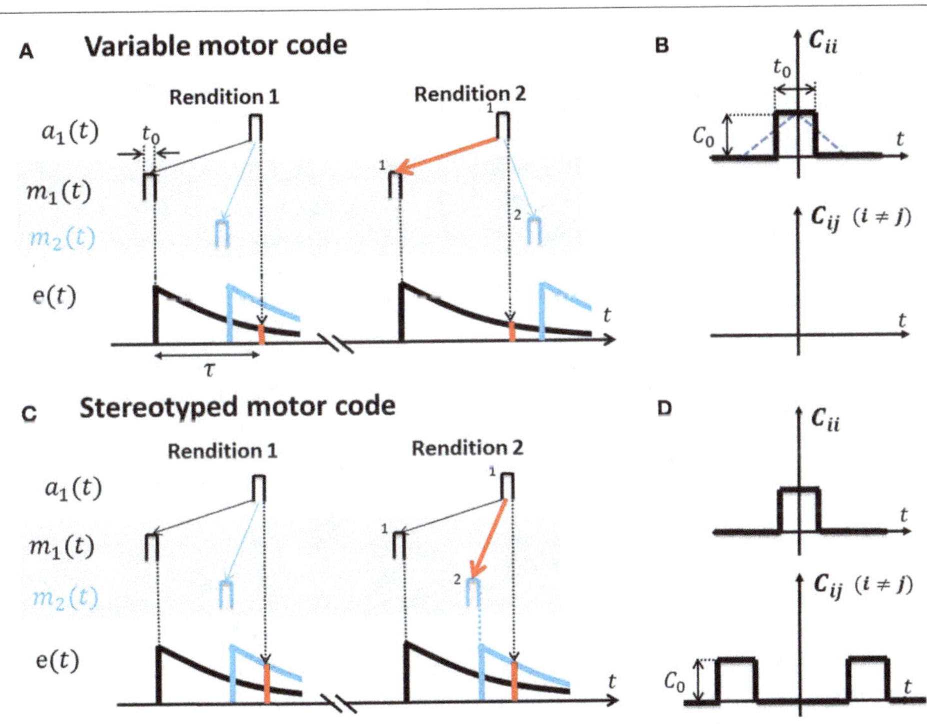

FIGURE 3 | Cross-correlation functions for variable and stereotyped motor codes. (A) In a variable motor code $m(t)$ (shaded area). Activity bursts m_1 (black) and m_2 (blue) of width t_0 in two example motor neurons occur at diverse time lags relative to each other across renditions of the song motif. Auditory tuning in the shown sensory neuron is such that it responds a_1 to bursts m_1 after a time lag τ. Repeated co-activation $m_1 \rightarrow a_1$ and non-zero eligibility $e(\tau)$ (red bar) at time lag τ leads to increased synaptic weight V_{11} (red arrow) and to a causal inverse. Lack of correlation between m_2 and a_1, as well as heterosynaptic competition, prevents V_{21} from similarly increasing (blue thin arrow). **(B)** The cross-correlation function $C_{ij}(t)$ for variable codes is flat except the auto-correlation peak at zero time lag (motor activity is uncorrelated among neuron pairs). Note: based on square activity pulses in motor neurons in **(A)** the true cross-correlation shape is triangular (blue dotted line) which we approximate by a square pulse of width $t_0 \simeq 10\,ms$. The auto-correlation peak height is C_0. **(C)** In a stereotyped motor code $m(t)$ (shaded area), bursts m_1 (black) and m_2 (blue) occur at a fixed time lag relative to each other across renditions of the song motif (traveling pulse of activity). Repeated co-activation $m_2 \rightarrow a_1$ at higher eligibility (red bar) than the eligibility of $m_1 \rightarrow a_1$ leads to strengthening of synapse V_{21} (red arrow) and to a predictive inverse. **(D)** The cross-correlation function $C_{ij}(t)$ for stereotyped codes peaks also at non-zero time lags.

i at time t. The subtractive term $\hat{m}_i a_j$ provides an equal time heterosynaptic depression (Lynch et al., 1977; Chistiakova and Volgushev, 2009) among all sensory afferent synapses onto a motor neuron. The strength of this depression depends on the amount of presynaptic activity but does not depend directly on postsynaptic activation. The utility of such depression is not only to stabilize activity but also to force synaptic connections towards inverse mappings as we will see. Note that we assume **V** synapses are "silently" correlating pre- and postsynaptic activity in Equation 1, i.e., **V** synapses do not contribute either to postsynaptic depolarization or to postsynaptic hyperpolarization. In other words, while the inverse model is being learned, the motor activity $m_i(t)$ is entirely driven by some other source than the afferent auditory input. Thus, from the perspective of extracellular physiology, it would appear that sensory feedback arriving to the motor area through the inverse model, is gated out of the motor area while that motor area is engaged in internally generated motor explorations.

In the following we examine the outcome of this learning rule in response to various forms of motor codes, with the goal of computing the synaptic weight matrix **V** at a steady-state of the learning rule, $\frac{d}{dt}\langle \mathbf{V} \rangle = 0$, where $\langle \rangle$ denotes averaging over time (e.g., over different renditions of the song). To simplify the calculations, we assume motor codes with narrow spike-train cross-correlation functions, i.e., the width t_0 of spike-train cross-correlation functions is much smaller than the characteristic decay time of the eligibility trace. Although such functions have not been extensively studied due to the difficulty of simultaneously recording from several neurons during singing, narrow cross-correlation is plausible for RA and HVC neurons because pseudo simultaneous recordings can be constructed from serial recordings thanks to high firing stereotypy in these cells, yielding cross-correlation widths on the order of 10 ms (Leonardo and Fee, 2005). Note that in LMAN, because of high firing variability, similar estimation of cross-correlation width is virtually impossible.

We model motor codes with diverse inherent levels of randomness. We model stereotyped motor codes by assuming that spike-train cross correlations extend over large time lags, in agreement with a traveling pulse of activity (Hahnloser et al., 2002; Harvey et al., 2012). We model variable motor codes by assuming that cross-correlations vanish except in a peak at zero time lag (white noise assumption), **Figure 3B**.

A VARIABLE NEURAL CODE YIELDS CAUSAL INVERSES

If motor activity is uncorrelated among different neuron pairs, the resulting sensory to motor map $\mathbf{V} = e(\tau)t_0\mathbf{Q}^{-1}$ equals the inverse of **Q** weighted by the eligibility at time lag τ (Equation A5, for the derivation see Appendix A3). Hence, **V** is a causal inverse that maps sensory representations onto their motor causes (in **Figure 3A**, auditory neurons map onto those motor neurons whose firing correlates most strongly with their own).

For example, during singing the motor cause $m_1(t-\tau)$ (say a neuron that generates a 4 kHz tone) will frequently be followed by auditory response $a_1(t)$ (a 4 kHz detector neuron), leading to strengthening of synapse V_{11}. By contrast, due to high variability of the motor code, associations between $m_2(t-\tau)$ (say a neuron that generates a 3 kHz tone) and $a_1(t)$ are much less frequent (because the bird randomizes the production of 3 and 4 kHz tones). Hence, synapse V_{21} from the 4 kHz detector onto the 3 kHz generator will lose to synapse V_{11} due to heterosynaptic competition (**Figure 3A**).

A STEREOTYPED NEURAL CODE YIELDS PREDICTIVE INVERSES

If the motor code is stereotyped and different motor neuron pairs are correlated at even very large time lags (extending over the full range of the eligibility trace and possibly beyond), then $\mathbf{V} \simeq e(0)t_0\mathbf{H}^{\tau}\mathbf{Q}^{-1}$ is approximately a concatenation of the inverse of **Q** and a shifter matrix $\mathbf{H}^{\tau}$ that maps motor activity at one time onto motor activity at a time lag τ later, i.e., **V** is a predictive inverse of **Q** (Equation A10). Under a predictive inverse **V**, a sensory neuron maps onto those motor neurons that were most recently active (and reliably follow in activation other motor neurons that give rise to the sensory neuron's response).

For example, during singing, the motor cause $m_1(t-\tau)$ of a 4 kHz tone will frequently occur before the cause $m_2(t)$ of a 3 kHz tone (because the bird produces stereotyped downsweep syllables). Hence, the 4 kHz auditory detector response $a_1(t)$ will find much higher eligibility in motor neuron 2, leading to strengthening of V_{21} at the expense of V_{11}, i.e., the 4 kHz detector neuron connects onto the 3 kHz generator neuron (**Figure 3C**).

LACK OF RESPONSE TO PERTURBED AUDITORY FEEDBACK AND SELECTIVITY FOR THE BOS

During Hebbian learning of **V** in Equation 1 we required that synapses **V** are not able to drive spike responses in motor neurons during singing (**V** synapses learn silently). The main intuitive reason for the necessity of silent learning is that the learning goal of the inverse model synapses are to silently correlate the motor and sensory streams, without perturbing the motor stream that would result if sensory feedback were to pass through and drive spikes in the motor area. If the inverse model synapses allowed sensory feedback to significantly drive motor spikes, then the incoming sensory signals would serve to drive motor activity resulting in cyclic motor output with cycle time approximately equal to τ, i.e., birds would unavoidably produce repetitive motor output (stuttering).

Interestingly, there is much evidence for the gating out of sensory information in song motor nuclei. Principal motor neurons in LMAN and HVC do not respond to playback of white noise stimuli during singing (Leonardo, 2004; Kozhevnikov and Fee, 2007) and during states of high arousal (Cardin and Schmidt, 2003), though there are reports of distorted feedback responses in HVC interneurons in Bengalese finches (Sakata and Brainard, 2008). Lack of feedback sensitivity in principal motor neurons is usually ascribed to a form of gating caused by specific thalamic or neuromodulatory mechanisms (Dave et al., 1998; Schmidt and Konishi, 1998; Shea and Margoliash, 2003; Cardin and Schmidt, 2004; Coleman et al., 2007; Hahnloser et al., 2008), see also the Discussion.

By contrast, LMAN (Doupe and Konishi, 1991; Doupe, 1997; Solis and Doupe, 1999; Roy and Mooney, 2007) and HVC neurons (Katz and Gurney, 1981; Margoliash, 1983, 1986; Williams and Nottebohm, 1985) respond to auditory stimulation while birds are anesthetized or asleep, which we model as gating on of **V** synapses, i.e., we assume that auditory responses in motor neurons are driven via the learned inverse models.

The puzzling observation of the gating out of sensory inputs to motor areas during motor exploration, is naturally accounted for in our theory by necessity of correlating the current presynaptic sensory stream with past postsynaptic motor streams, to learn an unbiased inverse model (of unperturbed motor stream).

Also, interestingly, in both HVC and LMAN sensory responses are strongest for bird's own song (BOS) stimuli compared to other stimuli including the tutor song or the BOS played back in reverse time (McCasland and Konishi, 1981; Margoliash, 1986; Lewicki, 1996; Solis and Doupe, 1999). Such selectivity follows naturally from our model assumptions: for both stereotyped and variable motor codes, the mappings, whether causal or predictive, can only invert sensory responses that lie in the image of **Q** and cannot invert the full space of responses orthogonal to the image of **Q**. Such a restriction arises because only sensations that could arise through combinations of previously experienced sensory feedback during singing can actually be inverted into appropriate motor commands. In other words, the inverse model synapses map prior sensory feedback generated by the bird's own previous song into appropriate motor commands, but necessarily fails to map sensory activity patterns that are very different from the BOS into coherent motor patterns. Thus, assuming HVC and LMAN can be thought of as downstream of the output of an inverse model, our Hebbian learning rule generating inverse models can naturally account for the preference of sensory responses in HVC and LMAN for BOS; sounds very different from BOS are not appropriately inverted, and therefore presumably do not lead to coherent activation of motor patterns via sensory inputs propagating through the inverse model synapses.

INVERSE MODELS AND SENSORIMOTOR MIRRORING

The Hebbian learning rule in Section Eligibility-Weighted Hebbian Learning determines the wiring of sensory afferents into motor areas based on sensorimotor experience. How could one experimentally test for the existence of such wiring without painstaking, detailed inspection of anatomical connections and characterization of the sensorimotor mapping **Q**? Here we outline the design of experiments to probe for the existence of either causal or predictive inverse models. We propose to record from single neurons both in sensory and motor states and to compare motor activity and sensory-evoked responses using cross-correlation functions: as we will show, the time lag of peak cross correlation provides evidence for either predictive or causal inverses.

In such mirroring experiments that we propose, a single neuron is first recorded during singing and then during playback of the just recorded songs while the bird is asleep in the dark (during which the auditory gate is open and motor neurons become responsive to auditory stimuli, presumably through an inverse model from an upstream sensory area). In our model, sensory responses $m_i^a(t) = \hat{m}_i(t) = \sum_k V_{ij} a_j(t)$ during playback are driven via synaptic weights **V** (assumed to be at a steady-state of Equation 1, $\frac{d}{dt}\langle \mathbf{V} \rangle = 0$). Computing the cross-correlation functions Corr(s) of the sensory response $m_i^a(t)$ with motor activity $m_i(t)$ (as a function of time lag s) yields that (see **Figure 4**):

1. For variable neural codes we have that $m_i^a(t) = e(\tau)t_0 m_i(t-\tau)$ and the cross-correlation function Corr(s) is 0 except at time lags $s \in \left[\tau - \frac{t_0}{2}, \tau + \frac{t_0}{2}\right]$ thus the peak correlation is near the sensorimotor time lag τ. In other words, for causal inverses the cross-correlation function between motor activity and sensory-evoked response peaks near time lag τ. That is, causal inverses are associated with large mirroring offsets equal to the loop delay τ. The reason is that the auditory response $m_1^a(t) \propto m_1(t-\tau)$ to song playback lags the song generating motor activity by a time lag τ. Intuitively, in a causal inverse model, if a motor neuron's activity is time locked to a particular song feature, it must fire before that feature in the motor production state, but after that feature in the sensory response state. This yields a temporal lag, or mirroring offset between the two (song-aligned) spike trains of a neuron recorded during motor production and during sensory exposure.
2. For stereotyped neural codes we have that $m_i^a(t) \simeq e(0)t_0 m_i(t)$ and the cross-correlation function Corr(s) as a function of the time lag s is proportional to the eligibility trace $e(s)$. Thus, assuming a monotonic decay of eligibility, Corr(s) peaks at time lag $s = 0$. In other words, for predictive inverses the cross-correlation function peaks near zero time lag and predictive inverses are associated with close to zero mirroring offsets. The reason is that the auditory response $m_1^a(t) \propto m_1(t)$ to song playback shows no lag with respect to the song generating motor activity. Intuitively, in a predictive inverse model, sensory feedback from a past motor action maps to concurrent motor activity in a stereotyped motor stream, which necessarily occurs after the motor activity that caused the sensory feedback. Thus, the past song elicits the firing of a motor neuron that generates future song. This implies that for any neuron there is no lag between its sensory and motor responses; the motor and sensory-evoked spikes of a motor neuron downstream of a predictive inverse model occur at the same time relative to song.

For derivations and model assumptions see Appendices A2–A4. In particular, here we assumed no synaptic delay between auditory and motor neuron, though this assumption can be relaxed. In summary, for both stereotyped and variable motor codes, sensory responses mirror motor activity. The amount of randomness in the motor code dictates the time lag of peak cross-correlation between motor activity and sensory-evoked responses, which we refer to as the *mirroring offset*. The mirroring offset thus serves as an important experimental observable that provides a window into fundamental differences in the types of inverse models that are computed by Hebbian learning, **Figure 4**.

Note that variable motor codes are associated with weaker mirroring than stereotyped codes, i.e., the cross-correlation functions for variable codes exhibit lower peak amplitudes than cross-correlation functions associated with stereotyped codes: In our model, the ratio of peak cross correlation is given by the eligibility at time lag τ divided by the eligibility at time lag zero (Equation A12 derived in the Appendices A3, A4). Thus, the steeper the

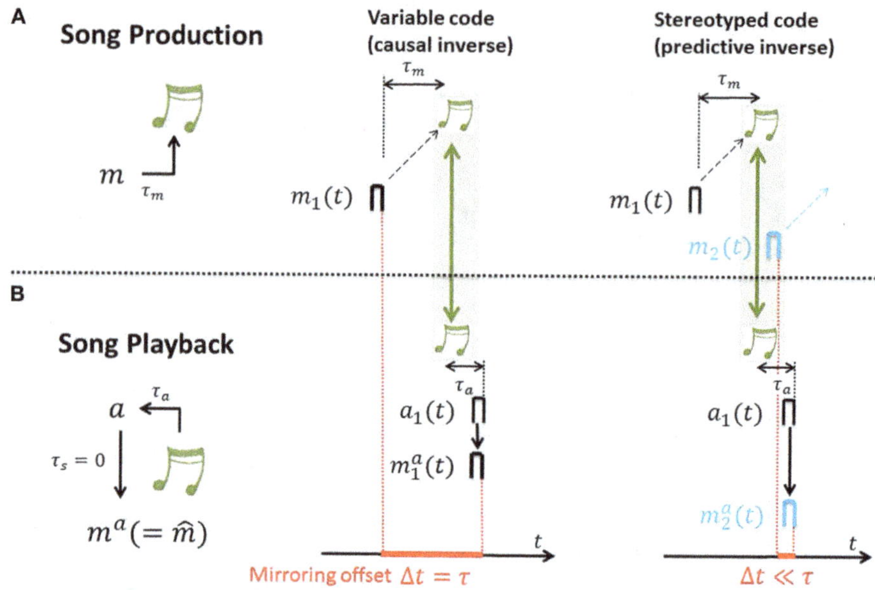

FIGURE 4 | The mirroring offset is determined in recordings of neural activity across (A) singing and (B) auditory stimulation by song playback; the offset (red) is large for causal inverses (middle column) and close to zero for predictive inverses (right column). (A) During singing, a motor-neuron burst m_1 drives a song feature (green notes) after a time delay τ_m. **(B)** Playback of that song feature leads to auditory response a_1 after a time delay τ_a. And, auditory response a_1 leads to motor neuron response m_1^a in case of a causal inverse (middle column) and to motor neuron response m_2^a in case of a predictive inverse (right column) after an additional time lag τ_s (spike propagation time from auditory to motor area) that is assumed to be 0 for simplicity. Thus, after alignment of motor activity and sensory response with song (green arrows), in the case of a causal inverse, the mirroring offset Δt defined as the time lag between motor activity and playback response (red bar with extension set by red dashed lines) is equal to the sensory feedback delay $\tau = \tau_m + \tau_a$, whereas in the case of a predictive inverse the mirroring offset Δt is close to 0. The reason for the 0 offset associated with a predictive inverse is that the auditory burst a_1 driving the playback response m_2^a is selective to the sound feature that during singing was generated by the much earlier burst m_1 in a different neuron (black burst in **(A)**, right panel), but not the feature generated by m_2 (blue burst in **(A)**, right panel).

eligibility trace, the weaker the mirrored response in case of variable motor codes. By contrast, the shape of the eligibility trace is expected to have almost no influence in case of stereotyped codes.

Note that the auditory response $m_i^a(t) = \sum_k V_{ik}\, a_k(t)$ in a motor neuron to song playback is mathematically identical to the (silently) postdicted motor activity $\hat{m}_i(t) = \sum_k V_{ik}\, a_k(t)$ defined after Equation 1, and used in learning the inverse model. Nevertheless, we use different symbols for these quantities to disentangle their meaning, i.e., the former being a superthreshold sensory response elicited in a quiet non-singing state of the bird, the latter being a subthreshold subtractive term that stabilizes synaptic learning during singing. The biophysical underpinnings of these two terms might largely be identical, with the silent nature of the posticted activity arising from some form of response gating (see also the Discussion).

GRADIENT DESCENT

We note that the learning rule in Equation 1 corresponds to gradient descent on the following error function:

$$\mathrm{E}(t) = \frac{1}{2} \sum_i \int_0^\infty \left[m_i(t-s) - \sum_k \mathrm{V}_{ik} a_k(t) \right]^2 e(s) \mathrm{d}s \qquad (2)$$

For a derivation, see Appendix A1. Thus, synaptic weights **V** converge such as to yield optimal postdiction $\hat{m}_i(t) = \sum_k V_{ik}\, a_k(t)$ of motor activity from sensory feedback. The origin of our eligibility-weighted Hebbian learning rule with heterosynaptic competition, from gradient descent of an energy function, confers a degree of robustness to the learning, as well as suggests generalizations to situations in which the synaptic transformation from sensory to motor areas is non-linear.

PROBABILISTIC MODELS

More realistic neuron models are non-linear and contain spikes that are potentially probabilistic and certainly binary events. Also, more realistically, we may want to explicitly model intrinsic noise in motor and sensory-related responses rather than deal with motor variability only through their effects on cross correlations. As a first step to dealing with such realism, we have derived two probabilistic neuron models in which inverse models and mirroring can be studied in similar manners as in the linear model, outlined in the following.

In one of these models we calculate the influence of probabilistic (binary) responses on the strength of mirroring. We consider a random motor area that at any time can only be in one of two possible states $M = 1$ and $M = 0$ with prior probability $p(M = 1) = \frac{1}{2}$. Assume analogously that the sensory area is such that a particular sensory feature is either detected ($S = 1$) or not detected ($S = 0$). We then model the relationship between motor activity and sensory consequence in terms of conditional dependencies between these two random variables. We assess the strength of mirroring in this model in terms of the cross-correlation coefficient between the two random variables (as derived in Appendix A5) and find the following result:

(A) For perfect auditory tuning (sensory neurons exhibit no noise to repeated sensory stimulation) the cross-correlation coefficient is given by the difference between the probabilities that the detected sensory feature is driven by the motor area vs. not driven by it. In other words, mirrored responses are proportional to the strength with which a single motor neuron contributes toward generation of the detected feature.

(B) In case of equal intrinsic noise in motor and sensory systems we find that the correlation coefficient is positive and proportional to the squared difference between the probabilities that the detected sensory feature is driven by the motor area vs. not driven by it.

Thus, the simple probabilistic model shows that the strength of mirroring may also be strongly reduced by the amount of intrinsic noise present in sensory and motor systems.

DISCUSSION

We have presented a simple model for the development of mirror neuron systems that is mathematically tractable, allowing us to relate mirror neuron properties such as the correlative strengths and the time lag of peak mirrored responses to the stereotypy (the correlation structure) of motor-related firing. Mirroring properties depend on the variability of the neural motor code which may be dissociated from apparent variability of the motor behavior as is the case in LMAN neurons that fire highly variable spike patterns despite high song stereotypy in adults. Our conclusions are valid for arbitrary sensory systems, provided they are able to signal sensory feedback from motor actions with sufficient sensitivity matched to the behavioral richness generated by the motor system (and of course provided that sensory afferents are subject to correlative Hebbian learning). In our derivation we have assumed that cross-correlation functions among motor neuron pairs are narrow, which was a simplifying assumption that allowed us to derive simple analytical forms of the sensory-to-motor mapping **V** and of mirroring properties. Approximate inverses should also result for motor codes with more complex time dependence, because by construction, the learning rule we considered corresponds to a gradient-descent rule that achieves minimal inversion error.

Although inverse models are attractive as models for vocal learning (Guenther et al., 2006; Hahnloser and Ganguli, 2013), they have previously been judged to be inappropriate for vocal learning in songbirds because of mainly two reasons: (1) young birds require many song repetitions with auditory feedback (Doya and Sejnowski, 2000), and (2) the learning schemes proposed either used a biologically implausible algorithm (Jordan and Rumelhart, 1992) or assumed the preexistence of an approximate inverse model (Kawato, 1990). Here we suggested a resolution to both of these issues and shown that in contrary to previous beliefs, inverse models constitute a potentially plausible framework for vocal learning in birds, too: the many song explorations used by young birds could be required to actually learn the high dimensional inverse model; and, the correlational learning we proposed is quite plausible and simple (but non-trivial nevertheless). This suggests potentially opening up the hypothesis space for learning rules operating within cortico-basal ganglia circuits, in both mammalian and bird song systems, to include models spanning the range from pure reinforcement learning (RL) to pure inverse model learning. Of particular interest would be intermediate learning rules that synergistically incorporate both dopamine-dependent plasticity thought to underlie RL as well, as Hebbian based plasticity shown here to mediate inverse model learning, in order to implement sophisticated model-based RL strategies. For example, a simple proposal would be that dopamine delivered to striatal synapses from the ventral tegmental area (VTA) might not be released purely nonspecifically, but instead might be delivered by an inverse model that can partially map errors in sensory coordinates to errors in motor coordinates, thereby guiding learning in ways more sophisticated than pure RL (O'Reilly and Frank, 2006).

The key to learning causal inverse models is motor variability. In motor areas such as HVC that fire stereotyped patterns, auditory afferents cannot disentangle cause-and-effect, leading to preferential formation of predictive inverses rather than causal ones. Predictive inverses have limited usefulness for action imitation from action observation, because under a predictive inverse, observation of a particular motor gesture will lead to imitation of the subsequent gesture in the imitator's motor repertoire, which may not be part of the actions to be imitated. For example, if a bird repeatedly sings *ABCD* during formation of the inverse and wants to later imitate repetitions of *ABDB*, then its predictive inverse will constrain it to produce repetitions of *BCDA* because perception of *A* maps to production of *B*, perception of *B* maps to production of *C*, etc.

Small temporal delays between motor activity and activity evoked by playback of BOS or BOS-resembling sounds have been reported previously. Prather et al. (2008) showed there is a small mirroring offsets of just a few milliseconds in HVC_X neurons of awake swamp sparrows and report similar (not quantified) results in Bengalese finches. Furthermore, Dave and Margoliash (2000) observed a small time lag of auditory-evoked activity also in RA neurons of sleeping zebra finches. Both these experimental findings reflect a predictive inverse. While predictive inverses have limited usefulness for action imitation they might provide stability in sequential vocalization. Indeed Sakata and Brainard report that perturbation of auditory feedback can change song syntax in Bengalese finches (Sakata and Brainard, 2006, 2008; Hanuschkin et al., 2011). By contrast, a causal inverse revealing itself by a large mirroring offset is maximally useful for song imitation. Indeed, preliminary results indicated a large non-zero mirroring offsets in LMAN (Giret et al., 2012).

An important element of our theory is the eligibility trace. To endow Hebbian learning with such a trace is necessary in realistic situations in which effects (sensory feedback) follow their cause (motor command) with some non-zero time lag arising from signal propagation delays, from twitch times of muscles, and from sensory and synaptic receptor latencies. In humans such a lag could span up to several hundreds of milliseconds, whereas in birds it may be as short as several tens of milliseconds. Eligibility traces also appear in RL theories (Seung, 2003; Fiete et al., 2007) and seem to be a general prerequisite for learning in the context of delayed feedback or delayed reward. We can imagine that neurons and synapses may hold decaying eligibility traces in terms of dedicated molecules such as calcium. Action potential generation is associated with rapid calcium entry that decays over the time course from several hundreds of milliseconds to a few seconds (McGeown et al., 1996; Wallace et al., 2008). The monotonic decay of intracellular calcium is well-suited to modeling a monotonically decaying eligibility trace. However, a monotonic decay of eligibility harbors both advantages and disadvantages. The disadvantage, as discussed, is the problem associated with stereotyped motor generators that can only hold predictive inverse models; to make inverse models causal, motor variability is required. Another way to guarantee causal inverse models—even under stereotyped motor explorations—would be to consider eligibility traces that do not monotonically decay but that peak at precisely the time delay inherent in closed sensorimotor feedback loops. The main caveat of such eligibility traces is that it may be questionable whether different muscles recruited for the same behavior must necessarily be associated with the same sensorimotor delay—and it is presently unclear how such variable delays could be matched to variable eligibility traces across synapses in a way that would ensure the learning of a causal inverse model. Moreover, phenomena such as speech co-articulation make it unlikely that there exists a constant sensorimotor delay across a large range of premotor neurons. The advantage, on the other hand, of a decaying eligibility trace is that sensorimotor contingencies and inverses can be learned regardless of sensorimotor latencies, providing robustness of sensorimotor learning.

Convergence of the sensory to motor synaptic weights toward inverses depends on details of the heterosynaptic competitive term. Heterosynaptic competitive terms have a certain appeal because of the useful normalization they provide (Fiete et al., 2010). In the context of this work, such terms imply locally available information at a single synapse about sensory inputs to other synapses. Though this information need not be provided instantaneously, we can only speculate about possible mechanisms for sharing such information among different synapses onto the same postsynaptic neuron. One possibility is that some form of intracellular signaling conveys this information. Another possibility to be explored is whether there exists an entire class of such competitive terms with a similar effect. For example, provided that motor and sensory codes are sufficiently sparse, it is conceivable that very simple subtractive terms might suffice for inverse formation. Whether other (even simpler) competitive terms result in approximate inverses needs to be further explored. We would like to point out preliminary evidence that inverses can be learned with Hebbian rules that include no heterosynaptic competitive terms (Senn and Pawelzik, pers. communication).

Our Hebbian learning theory has been analyzed so far in linear circuits, but we have indicated ways to overcome linearity by pinpointing extensions of our work to include nonlinear mappings and probabilistic neuron models. Further work will be required to test whether our correlative learning approach is suitable also for inverse model learning employing detailed biophysical models of the avian syrinx.

ACKNOWLEDGMENTS

We acknowledge support by the European Research Council (ERC-Advanced Grant 268911) and the Swiss National Science Foundation (Grant 31003A_127024), and support from the Swartz, Sloan, and Burroughs-Wellcome foundations, and Defense Advanced Research Projects Agency (DARPA). R. H. R. Hahnloser thanks Walter Senn for helpful discussions on inverse models and S. Ganguli thanks Michael Brainard and Kris Bouchard for useful discussions on birdsong learning, and the transition from causal to predictive inverse models.

REFERENCES

Aronov, D., Andalman, A. S., and Fee, M. S. (2008). A specialized forebrain circuit for vocal babbling in the juvenile songbird. *Science* 320, 630–634. doi: 10.1126/science.1155140

Basham, M. E., Nordeen, E. J., and Nordeen, K. W. (1996). Blockade of NMDA receptors in the anterior forebrain impairs sensory acquisition in the zebra finch (*Poephila guttata*). *Neurobiol. Learn. Mem.* 66, 295–304. doi: 10.1006/nlme.1996.0071

Bottjer, S., Miesner, E., and Arnold, A. (1984). Forebrain lesions disrupt development but not maintenance of song in passerine birds. *Science* 224, 901–903. doi: 10.1126/science.6719123

Cardin, J. A., and Schmidt, M. F. (2003). Song system auditory responses are stable and highly tuned during sedation, rapidly modulated and unselective during wakefulness, and suppressed by arousal. *J. Neurophysiol.* 90, 2884–2899. doi: 10.1152/jn.00391.2003

Cardin, J. A., and Schmidt, M. F. (2004). Auditory responses in multiple sensorimotor song system nuclei are co-modulated by behavioral state. *J. Neurophysiol.* 91, 2148–2163. doi: 10.1152/jn.00918.2003

Catmur, C. (2012). Sensorimotor learning and the ontogeny of the mirror neuron system. *Neurosci. Lett.* 540, 21–27. doi: 10.1016/j.neulet.2012.10.001

Chistiakova, M., and Volgushev, M. (2009). Heterosynaptic plasticity in the neocortex. *Exp. Brain Res.* 199, 377–390. doi: 10.1007/s00221-009-1859-5

Coleman, M. J., Roy, A., Wild, J. M., and Mooney, R. (2007). Thalamic gating of auditory responses in telencephalic song control nuclei. *J. Neurosci.* 27, 10024–10036. doi: 10.1523/jneurosci.2215-07.2007

Cooper, R. P., Cook, R., Dickinson, A., and Heyes, C. M. (2012). Associative (not Hebbian) learning and the mirror neuron system. *Neurosci. Lett.* 540, 28–36. doi: 10.1016/j.neulet.2012.10.002

Dave, A. S., and Margoliash, D. (2000). Song replay during sleep and computational rules for sensorimotor vocal learning. *Science* 290, 812–816. doi: 10.1126/science.290.5492.812

Dave, A. S., Yu, A. C., and Margoliash, D. (1998). Behavioral state modulation of auditory activity in a vocal motor system. *Science* 282, 2250–2254.

Doupe, A. J. (1997). Song- and order-selective neurons in the songbird anterior forebrain and their emergence during vocal development. *J. Neurosci.* 17, 1147–1167.

Doupe, A. J., and Konishi, M. (1991). Song-selective auditory circuits in the vocal control system of the zebra finch. *Proc. Natl. Acad. Sci. U.S.A.* 88, 11339–11343.

Doya, K., and Sejnowski, T. (2000). "A computational model of avian song learning," in *The New Cognitive Neurosciences*, 2nd Edn, ed M.

S. Gazzaniga (Cambridge, London: MIT Press), 469–484.

Ethier, C., Oby, E. R., Bauman, M. J., and Miller, L. E. (2012). Restoration of grasp following paralysis through brain-controlled stimulation of muscles. *Nature* 485, 368–371. doi: 10.1038/nature10987

Fiete, I. R., Fee, M. S., and Seung, H. S. (2007). Model of birdsong learning based on gradient estimation by dynamic perturbation of neural conductances. *J. Neurophysiol.* 98, 2038–2057. doi: 10.1152/jn.01311.2006

Fiete, I. R., Senn, W., Wang, C. Z. H., and Hahnloser, R. H. R. (2010). Spike-time-dependent plasticity and heterosynaptic competition organize networks to produce long scale-free sequences of neural activity. *Neuron* 65, 563–576. doi: 10.1016/j.neuron.2010.02.003

Gallese, V., Fadiga, L., Fogassi, L., and Rizzolatti, G. (1996). Action recognition in the premotor cortex. *Brain* 119, 593–609. doi: 10.1093/brain/119.2.593

Georgopoulos, A., Schwartz, A., and Kettner, R. (1986). Neuronal population coding of movement direction. *Science* 233, 1416–1419. doi: 10.1126/science.3749885

Giret, N., Kornfeld, J., Ganguli, S., and Hahnloser, R. (2012). "Delayed mirrored activity in the Zebra finch song system," in *Proceeding of 609.15/FFF53 Society for Neuroscience Meeting*, (New Orleans).

Guenther, F. H., Ghosh, S. S., and Tourville, J. A. (2006). Neural modeling and imaging of the cortical interactions underlying syllable production. *Brain Lang.* 96, 280–301. doi: 10.1016/j.bandl.2005.06.001

Hahnloser, R., and Ganguli, S. (2013). "Vocal learning with inverse models," in *Principles of Neural Coding*, eds S. Panzeri and P. Quiroga (Boca Raton, FL: CRC Taylor and Francis), 547–564.

Hahnloser, R. H. R., Kozhevnikov, A. A., and Fee, M. S. (2002). An ultra-sparse code underlies the generation of neural sequences in a songbird. *Nature* 419, 65–70. doi: 10.1038/nature00974

Hahnloser, R. H. R., Wang, C. Z.-H., Nager, A., and Naie, K. (2008). Spikes and bursts in two types of thalamic projection neurons differentially shape sleep patterns and auditory responses in a songbird. *J. Neurosci.* 28, 5040–5052. doi: 10.1523/jneurosci.5059-07.2008.

Hanuschkin, A., Diesmann, M., and Morrison, A. (2011). A reafferent and feed-forward model of song syntax generation in the Bengalese finch. *J. Comput. Neurosci.* 31, 509–532. doi: 10.1007/s10827-011-0318-z

Harvey, C. D., Coen, P., and Tank, D. W. (2012). Choice-specific sequences in parietal cortex during a virtual-navigation decision task. *Nature* 484, 62–68. doi: 10.1038/nature10918

Jordan, M. I., and Rumelhart, D. E. (1992). Forward models: supervised learning with a distal teacher. *Cogn. Sci.* 16, 307–354. doi: 10.1207/s15516709cog1603_1

Kao, M. H., Doupe, A. J., and Brainard, M. S. (2005). Contributions of an avian basal ganglia-forebrain circuit to real-time modulation of song. *Nature* 433, 638–643. doi: 10.1038/nature03127

Kao, M. H., Wright, B. D., and Doupe, A. J. (2008). Neurons in a forebrain nucleus required for vocal plasticity rapidly switch between precise firing and variable bursting depending on social context. *J. Neurosci.* 28, 13232–13247. doi: 10.1523/jneurosci.2250-08.2008

Katz, L. C., and Gurney, M. E. (1981). Auditory responses in the zebra finch's motor system for song. *Brain Res.* 221, 192–197. doi: 10.1016/0006-899391073-8

Kawato, M. (1990). "Feedback-error learning neural network for supervised motor learning," in *Advanced Neural Computer*, ed R. Eckmiller (North-Holland: Elsevier), 365–372.

Kozhevnikov, A. A., and Fee, M. S. (2007). Singing-related activity of identified HVC neurons in the zebra finch. *J. Neurophysiol.* 97, 4271–4283. doi: 10.1152/jn.00952.2006

Leonardo, A. (2004). Experimental test of the birdsong error-correction model. *Proc. Natl. Acad. Sci. U.S.A.* 101, 16935–16940. doi: 10.1073/pnas.0407870101

Leonardo, A., and Fee, M. S. (2005). Ensemble coding of vocal control in birdsong. *J. Neurosci.* 25, 652–661. doi:10.1523/jneurosci.3036-04.2005

Lewicki, M. S. (1996). Intracellular characterization of song-specific neurons in the zebra finch auditory forebrain. *J. Neurosci.* 16, 5855–5863.

Lynch, G. S., Dunwiddie, T., and Gribkoff, V. (1977). Heterosynaptic depression: a postsynaptic correlate of long-term potentiation. *Nature* 266, 737–739. doi: 10.1038/266737a0

Margoliash, D. (1983). Acoustic parameters underlying the responses of song-specific neurons in the white-crowned sparrow. *J. Neurosci.* 3, 1039–1057.

Margoliash, D. (1986). Preference for autogenous song by auditory neurons in a song system nucleus of the white-crowned sparrow. *J. Neurosci.* 6, 1643–1661.

McCasland, J. S., and Konishi, M. (1981). Interaction between auditory and motor activities in an avian song control nucleus. *Proc. Natl. Acad. Sci. U.S.A.* 78, 7815–7819. doi: 10.1073/pnas.78.12.7815

McGeown, J. G., Drummond, R. M., McCarron, J. G., and Fay, F. S. (1996). The temporal profile of calcium transients in voltage clamped gastric myocytes from Bufo marinus. *J. Physiol.* 497(Pt 2), 321–336.

Miller, W. I. (1987). Sensor-based control of robotic manipulators using a general learning algorithm. *IEEE J. Rob. Autom.* 3, 157–165. doi: 10.1109/jra.1987.1087081

Nottebohm, F., Stokes, T. M., and Leonard, C. M. (1976). Central control of song in the canary, *Serinus canarius*. *J. Comp. Neurol.* 165, 457–486. doi: 10.1002/cne.901650405

Olveczky, B. P., Andalman, A. S., and Fee, M. S. (2005). Vocal experimentation in the juvenile songbird requires a basal ganglia circuit. *PLoS Biol.* 3:e153. doi: 10.1371/journal.pbio.0030153

O'Reilly, R. C., and Frank, M. J. (2006). Making working memory work: a computational model of learning in the prefrontal cortex and basal ganglia. *Neural Comput.* 18, 283–328. doi: 10.1162/089976606775093909

Oztop, E., Kawato, M., and Arbib, M. (2006). Mirror neurons and imitation: a computationally guided review. *Neural Netw.* 19, 254–271. doi: 10.1016/j.neunet.2006.02.002

Oztop, E., Kawato, M., and Arbib, M. A. (2012). Mirror neurons: functions, mechanisms and models. *Neurosci. Lett.* 540, 43–55. doi: 10.1016/j.neulet.2012.10.005

Prather, J. F., Peters, S., Nowicki, S., and Mooney, R. (2008). Precise auditory-vocal mirroring in neurons for learned vocal communication. *Nature* 451, 305–310. doi: 10.1038/nature06492

Rizzolatti, G., and Craighero, L. (2004). The mirror-neuron system. *Annu. Rev. Neurosci.* 27, 169–192. doi: 10.1146/annurev.neuro.27.070203.144230

Rizzolatti, G., Fadiga, L., Gallese, V., and Fogassi, L. (1996). Premotor cortex and the recognition of motor actions. *Cogn. Brain Res.* 3, 131–141.

Roberts, T. F., Gobes, S. M. H., Murugan, M., Ölveczky, B. P., and Mooney, R. (2012). Motor circuits are required to encode a sensory model for imitative learning. *Nat. Neurosci.* 15, 1454–1459. doi: 10.1038/nn.3206

Roy, A., and Mooney, R. (2007). Auditory plasticity in a basal ganglia-forebrain pathway during decrystallization of adult birdsong. *J. Neurosci.* 27, 6374–6387. doi: 10.1523/jneurosci.0894-07.2007

Sakata, J. T., and Brainard, M. S. (2006). Real-time contributions of auditory feedback to avian vocal motor control. *J. Neurosci.* 26, 9619–9628. doi: 10.1523/jneurosci.2027-06.2006

Sakata, J. T., and Brainard, M. S. (2008). Online contributions of auditory feedback to neural activity in avian song control circuitry. *J. Neurosci.* 28, 11378–11390. doi: 10.1523/jneurosci.3254-08.2008

Santhanam, G., Ryu, S. I., Yu, B. M., Afshar, A., and Shenoy, K. V. (2006). A high-performance brain-computer interface. *Nature* 442, 195–198. doi: 10.1038/nature04968

Schmidt, M. F., and Konishi, M. (1998). Gating of auditory responses in the vocal control system of awake songbirds. *Nat. Neurosci.* 1, 513–518. doi: 10.1038/2232

Schwartz, A. B., Kettner, R. E., and Georgopoulos, A. P. (1988). Primate motor cortex and free arm movements to visual targets in three-dimensional space. I. Relations between single cell discharge and direction of movement. *J. Neurosci.* 8, 2913–2927.

Seung, H. S. (2003). Learning in spiking neural networks by reinforcement of stochastic synaptic transmission. *Neuron* 40, 1063–1073.

Shea, S. D., and Margoliash, D. (2003). Basal forebrain cholinergic modulation of auditory activity in the zebra finch song system. *Neuron* 40, 1213–1226.

Slotine, J.-J. E. (1987). On the adaptive control of robot manipulators. *Int. J. Rob. Res.* 6, 49–59. doi: 10.1177/027836498700600303

Smola, A., and Schölkopf, B. (2004). A tutorial on support vector regression. *Stat. Comput.* 14, 199–222. doi: 10.1023/B:STCO.0000035301.49549.88

Solis, M. M., and Doupe, A. J. (1999). Contributions of tutor and bird's own song experience to neural selectivity in the songbird anterior forebrain. *J. Neurosci.* 19, 4559–4584.

Stepanek, L., and Doupe, A. J. (2010). Activity in a cortical-basal ganglia circuit for song is required for social context-dependent vocal variability.

J. Neurophysiol. 104, 2474–2486. doi: 10.1152/jn.00977.2009

Wallace, D. J., Meyer, S., Astori, S., Yang, Y., Bausen, M., Palmer, A. E., et al. (2008). Single-spike detection *in vitro* and *in vivo* with a genetic Ca^{2+} sensor. *Nat. Methods* 5, 797–804. doi: 10.1038/nmeth.1242

Williams, H., and Nottebohm, F. (1985). Auditory responses in avian vocal motor neurons: a motor theory for song perception in birds. *Science* 229, 279–282.

APPENDICES

A1. GRADIENT DESCENT DERIVATION OF ELIGIBILITY-WEIGHTED HEBBIAN LEARNING

We can derive the learning rule in Equation 1 by gradient (steepest) descent on an error function E. The differential change $\delta\mathbf{V}$ in synaptic weight is proportional to the gradient and we can write:

$$\delta\mathbf{V} = -\frac{dE}{d\mathbf{V}}. \tag{A1}$$

The error function $E_i(t)$ for neuron i we define as the square difference between motor activity $m_i(t-s)$ and postdicted motor activity $\hat{m}_i(t) = \sum_k V_{ik}\, a_k(t)$, weighted by the eligibility associated with the time lag s.

$$E_i(t) = \frac{1}{2}\int_0^{\infty} ds\left[m_i(t-s) - \sum_k V_{ik}\, a_k(t)\right]^2 e(s)$$

The total error is simply the sum of errors over all neurons $E = \sum_i E_i$.

By taking the gradient with respect to the i, j th weight only we find

$$\frac{dE_i}{dV_{ij}} = -\int_0^{\infty} ds\left[m_i(t-s) - \sum_k V_{ik}\, a_k(t)\right] e(s)a_j(t)$$

$$= -\int_0^{\infty} ds\left[e(s)m_i(t-s)\, a_j(t) + \sum_k V_{ik}a_k(t)\, a_j(t)e(s)\right].$$

Assume a normalized eligibility trace $\left(\int_0^{\infty} e(s)ds = 1\right)$:

$$\frac{dE_i}{dV_{ij}} = -\int_0^{\infty} ds\, e(s)m_i(t-s)\, a_j(t) + \sum_k V_{ik}\, a_k(t)\, a_j(t).$$

$$\Rightarrow \delta V_{ij} = \int_0^{\infty} ds\, e(s)m_i(t-s)\, a_j(t) - \sum_k V_{ik}\, a_k(t)\, a_j(t) \tag{A2}$$

A1.1. Extension to non-linear network

Note that our linear approach can be extended by introducing a nonlinear function f in the auditory to motor mapping in Equation 2:

$$E = \frac{1}{2}\sum_i \int_0^{\infty} ds\left[m_i(t-s) - f\left(\sum_k V_{ik}\, a_k(t)\right)\right]^2 e(s)$$

$$\Rightarrow \delta V_{ij} = \int_0^{\infty} ds\left[m_i(t-s) - f_i\right] f_i'\, a_k(t)e(s),$$

$$= \int_0^{\infty} ds\, m_i(t-s)f_i'(t)\, a_k(t)e(s) - f_i(t)f_i'(t)\, a_k(t)$$

Where $f_i = f\left(\sum_k V_{ik}\, a_k(t)\right)$ and $f_i' = df\left(\sum_k V_{ik}\, a_k(t)\right)/dV_{ij}$.

A1.2. Probabilistic derivation of Hebbian learning rule

We derive a version of the Hebbian learning rule in Equation 1 that is based on the following probabilistic Boltzmann neuron model. For simplicity, we do not include the time dependence in the derivation ($\tau = 0$). The auditory feedback response a given a motor activation m is given by the conditional probability

$$P_{\mathbf{Q}}(a|m) = \frac{e^{a^T\mathbf{Q}m}}{Z_{\mathbf{Q}}(m)},$$

parameterized by the matrix $\mathbf{Q}$, which is the motor-sensory mapping (as before) and where

$$Z_{\mathbf{Q}}(m) = \sum_a e^{a^T\mathbf{Q}m}$$

is the partition function. The posterior probability of m is given by

$$P_{\mathbf{Q}}(m|a) = \frac{P_{\mathbf{Q}}(a|m)P(m)}{P(a)}.$$

In a sensory state, auditory responses in motor neurons are driven via synapses $\mathbf{V}$ according to the probabilistic model:

$$P_{\mathbf{V}}(m|a) = \frac{e^{m^T\mathbf{V}a}}{Z_{\mathbf{V}}(a)}$$

with partition function

$$Z_{\mathbf{V}}(a) = \sum_m e^{m^T\mathbf{V}a}.$$

The error function in Equation 2 is replaced by the Kullbach-Leibler (KL) divergence between $P_{\mathbf{Q}}(m|a)$ and $P_{\mathbf{V}}(m|a)$:

$$\begin{aligned}
D_{KL}\left(P_{\mathbf{Q}}(m|a), P_{\mathbf{V}}(m|a)\right) &= \sum_m P_{\mathbf{Q}}(m|a)\ln\left(\frac{P_{\mathbf{Q}}(m|a)}{P_{\mathbf{V}}(m|a)}\right)\\
&= \sum_m P_{\mathbf{Q}}(m|a)\left[\ln\left(P_{\mathbf{Q}}(m|a)\right)\right.\\
&\quad \left.- \ln\left(P_{\mathbf{V}}(m|a)\right)\right]\\
&= \sum_m P_{\mathbf{Q}}(m|a)\left[\ln\left(P_{\mathbf{Q}}(m|a)\right)\right.\\
&\quad \left.+ \ln\left(Z_{\mathbf{V}}(a)\right) - m^T\mathbf{V}a\right]
\end{aligned} \tag{A3}$$

Before taking the derivative of D_{KL} we compute the derivative of the partition function:

$$\begin{aligned}
\frac{\partial}{\partial V_{ij}} Z_{\mathbf{V}}(a) &= \sum_m e^{m^T\mathbf{V}a} \frac{\partial}{\partial V_{ij}} m^T\mathbf{V}a = \sum_m e^{m^T\mathbf{V}a} m_i\, a_j\\
&= Z_{\mathbf{V}}(a)a_j \sum_m P_{\mathbf{V}}(m|a)m_i\\
&= Z_{\mathbf{V}}(a)a_j\langle m_i|a\rangle_m,
\end{aligned}$$

based on which it follows that

$$\frac{\partial}{\partial V_{ij}}\ln(Z_{\mathbf{V}}(a)) = \frac{1}{Z_{\mathbf{V}}(a)}\frac{\partial}{\partial V_{ij}} Z_{\mathbf{V}}(a) = a_j\langle m_i|a\rangle_m.$$

Using this relationship and Equation A3 we can calculate the derivative of the KL-divergence with respect to V_{ij}:

$$\begin{aligned}
&\frac{\partial}{\partial V_{ij}} D_{KL}(P_Q(m|a), P_V(m|a)) \\
&= \frac{\partial}{\partial V_{ij}} \sum_m P_Q(m|a) \left[\ln (P_Q(m|a)) + \ln (Z_V(a)) - m^T V a \right] \\
&= \sum_m P_Q(m|a) \left(\frac{\partial}{\partial V_{ij}} (\ln (Z_V(a))) - m_i a_j \right) \\
&= \sum_m \frac{P_Q(a|m)P(m)}{P(a)} \left(\frac{\partial}{\partial V_{ij}} (\ln (Z_V(a))) - m_i a_j \right) \\
&\Rightarrow \left\langle - \frac{\partial}{\partial V_{ij}} D_{KL}(P_Q(m|a), P_V(m|a)) \right\rangle_a \\
&= \sum_{a,m} P_Q(a|m)P(m) \left(m_i a_j - \frac{\partial}{\partial V_{ij}} (\ln (Z_V(a))) \right)
\end{aligned}$$

Thus, the gradient decent leads to

$$\Rightarrow \delta V_{ij} = m_i a_j - \frac{\partial}{\partial V_{ij}} (\ln (Z_V(a))) = \left[m_i - \langle m_i | a \rangle_m \right] a_j$$

This is the probabilistic analog of Equation A2, in which the silent postdictive motor activity $\hat{m}_i$ is replaced by the conditional expectation $\langle m_i|a\rangle_m$ of activity in motor neuron i given the sensory response a.

A2. CORRELATION OF MOTOR ACTIVITY DETERMINES AVERAGE SYNAPTIC CHANGE

The average synaptic change under learning rule Equation A2 satisfies

$$\begin{aligned}
\langle \delta V_{ij} \rangle &= \int_0^\infty \langle m_i(t-s) a_j(t) \rangle e(s) ds - \left\langle \sum_k V_{ik} a_k(t) a_j(t) \right\rangle \\
&= \int_0^\infty \left\langle \sum_k m_i(t') Q_{jk} m_k(t' + s - \tau) e(s) \right\rangle ds \\
&\quad - \left\langle \sum_{kml} V_{ik} Q_{kl} Q_{jm} m_m(t-\tau) m_l(t-\tau) \right\rangle,
\end{aligned}$$

where we have substituted $t' = t - s$. We can write this equation as

$$\langle \delta \mathbf{V} \rangle = \left[\int_0^\infty e(s) \mathbf{C}(s-\tau) ds - \mathbf{VQC}(0) \right] \mathbf{Q}^T, \qquad \text{(A4)}$$

where $C_{ij}(s) = \langle m_i(t) m_j(t+s) \rangle$ is the cross-correlation matrix of motor activity at time lag s. In the following we assume without loss of generality that the delay τ_s of synaptic transmission between auditory and motor neurons is negligibly small.

A3. VARIABLE MOTOR CODE

A3.1. V is a causal inverse

We assume a motor code with a narrow correlation function that is non-zero only for small t_0.

$$\mathbf{C(s)} = \begin{cases} \mathbf{1} C_0 \text{ for } |s| < t_0/2 \\ 0 \text{ otherwise} \end{cases}$$

Where $\mathbf{1}$ is the unity matrix and C_0 is a positive constant. The steady state solution $\langle \delta \mathbf{V} \rangle = 0$ of Equation A4 leads to

$$\int_0^\infty e(s) \mathbf{C}(s-\tau) ds - \mathbf{VQC}(0) = 0.$$

Assuming that the eligibility trace is constant over short time intervals of duration t_0 (over which the correlation function is non-zero) yields

$$\Rightarrow e(\tau)\, t_0 \mathbf{1} C_0 - \mathbf{VQ1} C_0 = 0$$

$$\Longleftrightarrow \mathbf{VQ} = e(\tau) t_0 \mathbf{1}$$

This implies that the auditory to motor mapping $\mathbf{V}$ is proportional to the inverse of $\mathbf{Q}$ weighted by the eligibility at time lag τ:

$$\mathbf{V} = e(\tau) t_0 \mathbf{Q}^{-1} \qquad \text{(A5)}$$

Thus, $\mathbf{V}$ is a causal inverse, at least when restricted to the image of $\mathbf{Q}$.

A3.2. Variable motor codes are associated with large mirroring offsets

We simulate a mirroring experiment in which we cross correlate in a given neuron the motor activity $m_i(t)$ and the activity $m_i^a(t)$ that results from observation of the motor act (achieved in birds by song playback though a loudspeaker).

The auditory response in motor neuron i is given by

$$\begin{aligned}
m_i^a(t) &= \sum_j V_{ij} a_j(t) \\
&= \sum_j (\mathbf{VQ})_{ij} m_j(t-\tau) \\
&= e(\tau) t_0 \sum_j \delta_{i,j} m_j(t-\tau). \\
&= e(\tau) t_0\, m_i(t-\tau),
\end{aligned}$$

Where $\delta_{i,j}$ is the Kronecker-Delta, ($\delta_{i,j} = 1$ for $i = j$ and $\delta_{i,j} = 0$ otherwise). Note that relative to song (either produced by the bird or played through the loudspeaker) the playback-evoked activity $m_i^a(t)$ is shifted with respect to the motor activity $m_i(t-\tau)$ by a time shift τ (as illustrated in **Figure 4**). The cross correlation

Corr(s) between sensory-evoked and motor generated activity is defined as,

$$\text{Corr}(s) = \frac{1}{T'}\int_0^{T'} m_i(t)m_i^a(t+s)\text{d}t = \langle m_i(t)m_i^a(t+s)\rangle \quad \text{(A6)}$$

Where T' is the duration of the motor behavior (e.g., the song motif or song). Inserting the expression for the motor activity evoked by the auditory response into Equation A6 yields,

$$\begin{aligned}\text{Corr}(s) &= \langle m_i(t)e(\tau)t_0\, m_i(t-\tau+s)\rangle \\ &= \begin{cases} e(\tau)t_0C_0 & \text{for } |s-\tau| < t_0/2 \\ 0 & \text{otherwise}\end{cases} \end{aligned} \quad \text{(A7)}$$

Thus, the cross correlation is nonzero in a small time centered around τ. The peak cross-correlation value is given by the eligibility trace at time lag τ.

$$\text{CorrPeak} = t_0C_0e(\tau)$$

Note that our calculations are valid in principle for mean-subtracted $m_i(t)$. In case of non-mean subtracted m_i we should replace the cross correlation in Equation A6 by the cross covariance to obtain the same findings. However, in practice, mean subtraction is not necessary because the peak location (the mirroring offset) is independent of the mean.

A4. STEREOTYPED MOTOR CODES

A4.1. V is a predictive inverse

We describe the motor activity by a traveling pulse $m_i(t) = \eta\left(\frac{i}{\omega} - t\right)$ with speed ω, where

$$\eta(t) = \begin{cases} 1 & \text{for } |t| < t_0/2 \\ 0 & \text{otherwise}\end{cases}$$

and $t_0 = 1/\omega$. The cross-correlation matrix for such a traveling pulse is a triangular pulse of height t_0/T and width $2t_0$ which we approximate by a square pulse of width t_0, $C_{ij}(s) \simeq \frac{t_0}{T}\eta\left(\frac{i-j}{\omega} + s\right)$ in the following (illustrated in **Figure 3D**). To facilitate comparison of inverses associated with stereotyped and variable motor codes, we assume their peak correlations are identical, i.e.,

$$C_0 = \frac{t_0}{T}.$$

At a steady state $\langle\delta\mathbf{V}\rangle = 0$, Equation A4 yields

$$\int_0^\infty e(s)\mathbf{C}(s-\tau)\text{d}s - \mathbf{VQC}(0) = 0.$$

Assuming again that the eligibility trace is constant over short time intervals of width t_0, we find

$$\Rightarrow e\left(\tau - \frac{i-j}{\omega}\right)t_0 = \mathbf{VQ}.$$

Given sensory input $a_j(t)$ and the inverse map $\mathbf{V}$, the auditory-evoked activity $m_j^a(t)$ is proportional to the eligibility trace:

$$\begin{aligned} m_i^a(t) &= \sum_j \text{V}_{ij}\, a_j(t) \\ &= \sum_j (\mathbf{VQ})_{ij}\, m_j(t-\tau) \\ &= e\left(t - \frac{i}{\omega}\right)t_0, \end{aligned} \quad \text{(A8)}$$

defined for $t \geq \frac{i}{\omega}$.

By approximating the eligibility trace only by its maximum value $e\left(t-\frac{i}{\omega}\right) = e(0)\eta\left(t-\frac{i}{\omega}\right)$ we have that approximately

$$m_i^a(t) \simeq e(0)t_0\, m_i(t), \quad \text{(A9)}$$

and so the playback-evoked activity $m_i^a(t)$ is roughly identical to motor activity $m_i(t)$ (as illustrated in **Figure 4**).

To compute the matrix **V** we use the same approximation for the eligibility trace to obtain

$$\frac{1}{t_0}(\mathbf{VQ})_{ij} \simeq e(0)\eta(i-j-\tau) = e(0)\mathbf{H}_{ij}^\tau,$$

where we have set $\omega = 1$, and where **H** is a shifter matrix (also called cyclic permutation or circulant matrix), e.g., for $n = 4$:

$$\mathbf{H} = \begin{pmatrix} 0 & 1 & 0 & 0 \\ 0 & 0 & 1 & 0 \\ 0 & 0 & 0 & 1 \\ 1 & 0 & 0 & 0 \end{pmatrix}.$$

With this approximation we find that the synaptic mapping

$$\mathbf{V} \simeq e(0)t_0\mathbf{H}^\tau\mathbf{Q}^{-1} \quad \text{(A10)}$$

is the inverse of the motor map shifted in time by τ, i.e., **V** maps sensory activity evoked by motor activity at time t onto motor activity at time $t+\tau$. In other words, the sensory lag is compensated and sensory-evoked motor activity at time t predicts motor activity at time t. Hence, **V** is a predictive inverse.

A4.2. Stereotyped motor codes are associated with small mirroring offsets

Based on the sensory-evoked activity $m_i^a(t)$ derived in Equation A8 we find for the cross-correlation function Corr (s) between motor activity $m_i(t)$ and sensory-evoked activity $m_i^a(t)$:

$$\begin{aligned}\text{Corr}(s) &= \frac{1}{T}\int_0^T m_i(t)m_i^a(t+s)\text{d}t \\ &= \frac{t_0}{T}\int_0^T \eta\left(\frac{i}{\omega} - t\right)e\left(t - \frac{i}{\omega} + s\right)\text{d}t \\ &= \frac{t_0^2}{T}e(s) = t_0C_0e(s). \end{aligned} \quad \text{(A11)}$$

Thus, the cross-correlation function is proportional to the eligibility trace. If the eligibility trace is monotonically decaying we find that the peak of Corr(s) occurs at $s = 0$ and is given by

$$\mathrm{CorrPeak} = t_0 C_0 e(s).$$

In other words, stereotyped neural codes are associated with zero mirroring offsets.

The ratio of peak cross correlation for variable (A6) and stereotyped (A10) motor codes is given by

$$r = \frac{e(\tau)}{e(0)}, \quad \text{(A12)}$$

implying that the more stereotyped a neural code, the stronger is the observed mirroring effect.

A5. MIRRORED RESPONSE STRENGTH IN A PROBABILISTIC MODEL

In the following we define a probabilistic model of a motor neuron that allows us to compute the mirroring strength, i.e., the correlation between motor activity and sensory-evoked activity. We assume a minimal model in which a neuron has only two states $R = 1$ (active) and $R = 0$ (inactive). In addition, we assume two behavioral states $B = 1$ (behavioral feature present), and $B = 0$ (behavioral feature absent). During motor production, the degeneracy of the motor code quantified by the conditional probability of neural activity given that the feature of interest is present during the behavior (e.g., the finger is extended or the song pitch is high) is

$$P_M(R = 1|B = 1) = p_1$$

and the probability that the neuron is active while the behavioral feature is absent (intrinsic noise) is

$$P_M(R = 1|B = 0) = p_2.$$

Hence, the average motor response [for prior $P(B = 1) = 1/2$] is given by

$$\langle R \rangle_{\text{motor}} = \sum_i 1 \times P_M(R = 1|B = i)P(B = i) = \frac{1}{2}(p_1 + p_2) = p.$$

In the sensory state (during observation of the behavior), the reliability of a response quantified by the conditional probability of triggering a sensory response given presence of the behavioral feature in the stimulus is given by,

$$P_S(R = 1|B = 1) = q_1$$

and the probability of a sensory response without the behavioral feature (intrinsic noise) is:

$$P_S(R = 1|B = 0) = q_2.$$

The parameters p_1, p_2, q_1, and q_2 can be freely chosen in this minimal model, for example $q_2 = p_2$ if intrinsic noise in sensory and motor states are assumed to be equal.

The average response in the sensory state is given by

$$\langle R \rangle_{\text{sensory}} = \frac{1}{2}(q_1 + q_2) = q.$$

The correlation between sensory and motor responses in this cell is

$$\langle R_{\text{motor}} R_{\text{sensory}} \rangle = \sum_i 1 \times P_M(R = 1|B = i)P_S(R = 1|B = i) \times P(B = i) = \frac{1}{2}(p_1 q_1 + p_2 q_2).$$

And, the correlation coefficient between motor- and sensory-evoked response is

$$\mathrm{CorrCoeff} = \frac{\langle R_{\text{motor}} R_{\text{sensory}} \rangle - \langle R_{\text{motor}} \rangle \langle R_{\text{sensory}} \rangle}{\sqrt{\langle R_{\text{sensory}} R_{\text{sensory}} \rangle \langle R_{\text{motor}} R_{\text{motor}} \rangle}} = \frac{\frac{1}{2}(p_1 q_1 + p_2 q_2) - pq}{\sqrt{p(1-p)q(1-q)}}.$$

We can discuss the following special cases:

- perfect sensory tuning ($q_1 = 1,\ q_2 = 0$, no instrinsic noise in sensory state):

$$\mathrm{CorrCoeff} = \frac{p_1 - p_2}{2\sqrt{p(1-p)}}$$

- same tuning and same intrinsic noise in motor and in sensory states ($q_1 = p_1,\ q_2 = p_2$):

$$\mathrm{CorrCoeff} = \frac{(p_1 - p_2)^2}{4p(1-p)}$$

In summary, the strength of mirrored responses scales linearly or quadratically with the contrastive probability that neural responses are locked to the behavioral feature vs. spontaneously driven.

5

Statistics of neuronal identification with open- and closed-loop measures of intrinsic excitability

Ted Brookings[1]*, Rachel Grashow[2] and Eve Marder[1]

[1] *Volen Center and Biology Department, Brandeis University, Waltham, MA, USA*
[2] *Environmental Health Department, Harvard School of Public Health, Boston, MA, USA*

Edited by:
Ahmed El Hady, Max Planck Institute for Dynamics and Self Organization, Germany

Reviewed by:
Scott Hooper, Ohio University, USA
Farzan Nadim, New Jersey Institute of Technology, USA
Ronald L. Calabrese, Emory University, USA

****Correspondence:***
Ted Brookings, Volen Center and Biology Department, Brandeis University, Volen Center MS 013, 415 South Street, Waltham, MA 02454, USA.
e-mail: ted.brookings@googlemail.com

In complex nervous systems patterns of neuronal activity and measures of intrinsic neuronal excitability are often used as criteria for identifying and/or classifying neurons. We asked how well identification of neurons by conventional measures of intrinsic excitability compares with a measure of neuronal excitability derived from a neuron's behavior in a dynamic clamp constructed two-cell network. We used four cell types from the crab stomatogastric ganglion: the pyloric dilator, lateral pyloric, gastric mill, and dorsal gastric neurons. Each neuron was evaluated for six conventional measures of intrinsic excitability (intrinsic properties, IPs). Additionally, each neuron was coupled by reciprocal inhibitory synapses made with the dynamic clamp to a Morris–Lecar model neuron and the resulting network was assayed for four measures of network activity (network activity properties, NAPs). We searched for linear combinations of IPs that correlated with each NAP, and combinations of NAPs that correlated with each IP. In the process we developed a method to correct for multiple correlations while searching for correlating features. When properly controlled for multiple correlations, four of the IPs were correlated with NAPs, and all four NAPs were correlated with IPs. Neurons were classified into cell types by training a linear classifier on sets of properties, or using *k*-medoids clustering. The IPs were modestly successful in classifying the neurons, and the NAPs were more successful. Combining the two measures did better than either measure alone, but not well enough to classify neurons with perfect accuracy, thus reiterating that electrophysiological measures of single-cell properties alone are not sufficient for reliable cell identification.

Keywords: clustering algorithms, multiple correlations, feature selection, stomatogastric ganglion, identified neurons, dynamic clamp, half-center oscillator, Morris–Lecar model

INTRODUCTION

A major step in elucidating the connectivity of nervous system circuits is identifying the neurons in the circuit. In the case of small invertebrate circuits neuronal identification is often straightforward (Getting and Dekin, 1985; Getting, 1989; Marder and Calabrese, 1996; Marder and Bucher, 2001, 2007; Kristan et al., 2005), using a combination of neuronal projection patterns, position, firing patterns, size, and color. This has facilitated the establishment of the connectivity diagrams of the circuits underlying stereotyped behaviors in a variety of animals (Mulloney and Selverston, 1974a,b; Selverston et al., 1976; Getting et al., 1980; Selverston and Miller, 1980; Getting, 1981; Hume and Getting, 1982; Hume et al., 1982; Miller and Selverston, 1982a,b; Pearson et al., 1985; Katz, 1996; Marder and Calabrese, 1996; Perrins and Weiss, 1996; Schmidt et al., 2001; Sasaki et al., 2007; Calabrese et al., 2011).

In contrast, developing relatively unambiguous connectivity diagrams for circuits with larger numbers of neurons such as those found in most vertebrate nervous systems has been historically more difficult, partially because neuronal identification has been challenging. This is starting to change with the advent of new genetic and molecular techniques. Nonetheless, classification of neurons into types and subtypes is not yet routine in larger networks (Jonas et al., 2004; Sugino et al., 2006; Toledo-Rodriguez and Markram, 2007; Miller et al., 2008; Okaty et al., 2011a,b), and a variety of electrophysiological measures are often used to classify neurons in types and subtypes.

The use of electrophysiological measurements alone for identification can be potentially problematical, as many neurons can change their activity patterns as a function of neuromodulation and activation of modulatory pathways (Dickinson et al., 1990; Meyrand et al., 1991; Weimann et al., 1991; Weimann and Marder, 1994). Moreover, recent work has shown that the same identified neurons can show large ranges in the values of many conventional measures of intrinsic excitability (intrinsic properties; IPs) in different animals (Grashow et al., 2010). In this study we compare directly the utility of six IPs with less conventional measures obtained by introducing a biological neuron into an artificial network with an oscillatory model neuron, and analyzing the resulting activity (network activity properties, NAPs). IPs are obtained via open-loop stimulation, whereas the NAPs are obtained in closed loop: the dynamic clamp injects current into the biological neuron based on the state of the model neuron, which is in turn affected by the biological neuron. The NAPs nevertheless constitute a measure of the biological neuron's properties, because the model neuron is standardized, and thus differences in NAPs between experiments must originate in differences in the neurons themselves.

Our hypothesis was that a measure of intrinsic excitability that challenges a biological neuron with a time-varying closed-loop stimulation might better reveal its essential properties than more static measures. To this end, we searched for relationships between IPs and NAPs, and asked if either was effective in predicting the neuron's cell type.

Grashow et al. (2010) searched for relationships between IPs and NAPs, as pairwise correlations. We expected whole sets of properties to give more information about neuronal identity than individual properties, therefore we asked the related but distinct question: can the IPs be reconstructed from NAPs, and vice versa? Thus for each IP we chose a subset of NAPs and performed a linear regression to fit the IP with the chosen NAPs. We then searched for the subset of NAPs that gave the least regression error per degree of freedom. This search for the most relevant set of properties, known as "feature selection" (see Materials and Methods), found a small set of NAPs that correlated highly with each IP; and when applied conversely, a small set of IPs that correlated highly with each NAP. We were then confronted with the problem of assessing the significance of the correlation that we had discovered. Consequently, one of the goals of this paper was to develop a statistical procedure to correctly assess the significance of multiple correlations, especially those that arise from feature selection.

While Grashow et al. (2010) showed that IPs and NAPs differ across cell types, here we attempt to deduce neuronal type from properties. We trained linear classifiers to test if neuronal types fall into different (linearly separable) regions of property-space. We used k-medoids clustering to test if neuronal identity could be blindly discovered, looking only at the properties. One challenge of this approach is that the result of a clustering algorithm is the assignment of each cell to an essentially unlabeled cluster index, making assessment of clustering accuracy an issue. Particularly problematic is determining if differing clustering results from two different sets of properties are significant or merely statistical flukes. Therefore another goal was to develop a procedure to assess the significance of differences in clustering results.

MATERIALS AND METHODS

The majority of the raw data used for these analyses was published in Grashow et al. (2010), and then supplemented with additional experiments. All experiments were done on identified neurons of the stomatogastric ganglion (STG) of the crab *Cancer borealis*. For each neuron we measured six traditional IPs, and with dynamic clamp, four NAPs. Details of the experimental methods are identical to those previously published (Grashow et al., 2010). Here we reiterate the essential details.

ELECTROPHYSIOLOGY

Recordings and current injections were performed in discontinuous current-clamp mode with sample rates between 1.8 and 2.1 kHz. Input resistance was measured as the slope of the voltage–current (VI) curve in response to hyperpolarizing current injections, (voltage was measured after the neuron reached steady state). The frequency–current (FI) curve was measured as the response to depolarizing current injections (typically between 0 and 1 nA). In the STG cells that we assayed, the FI curve had a characteristic shape that was curved at lower injected currents, but became approximately linear at higher injected currents. We computed FI slope by fitting a line to the linear region of the FI curve. This linear region was determined by fitting a line to the FI curve, then progressively eliminating the point with the lowest current injected, until the residual error was small or only three points remained. The residual error was considered acceptable if the sum of squared error divided by the degrees of freedom (number of points minus two) was less than 2.0. Spike frequency at 1 nA was read from the FI curve. Minimum voltage with zero injected current was taken from a trace where the neuron was not perturbed (in silent cells, this would be the resting membrane potential).

CONSTRUCTING THE HYBRID CIRCUIT

Real-time Linux dynamic clamp (Dorval et al., 2001), version 2.6, was run on an 800-MHz Dell Precision desktop computer. STG neurons were incorporated into a hybrid network with a simulated Morris and Lecar (1981) model. The biological neuron and the Morris–Lecar model neuron were connected with mutually inhibitory synapses, and artificial hyperpolarization-activated inward current (I_h) was added to the biological neuron. The maximal conductance of the synapse from the model to the STG cell was $\bar{g}_{syn}$. The maximal conductance of the synapse from the biological cell to the Morris–Lecar cell was $2 \times \bar{g}_{syn}$. The maximal conductance of the I_h current was $\bar{g}_h$. $\bar{g}_{syn}$ and $\bar{g}_h$ were each independently varied from 10 to 100 nS in 15 nS steps, forming a seven-by-seven grid from every possible combination.

Identically to the procedures in Grashow et al. (2010), the Morris–Lecar model contained a non-inactivating Ca^{2+} conductance and a non-inactivating K^+ conductance, in addition to a leak conductance. The membrane voltage of the Morris–Lecar neuron was determined based on the following equations:

$$C\frac{dV}{dt} = -\bar{g}_{leak}\left(V - E_{leak}\right) - \bar{g}_{Ca}M\left(V - E_{Ca}\right) - \bar{g}_K N\left(V - E_K\right)$$

$$\frac{dN}{dt} = \tau_N\left(N_\infty - N\right)$$

$$\frac{dM}{dt} = \tau_M\left(M_\infty - M\right)$$

$$M_\infty = \frac{1}{1 + \exp\left(\frac{-(V - V_{1/2,Ca})}{V_{slope,Ca}}\right)}$$

$$N_\infty = \frac{1}{1 + \exp\left(\frac{-(V - V_{1/2,K})}{V_{slope,K}}\right)}$$

$$\tau_N = \tau_{0K}\,\mathrm{sech}\left(\frac{V - V_{1/2,K}}{2V_{slope,K}}\right)$$

The values of the fixed parameters are in **Table 1**. C was the membrane capacitance of the Morris–Lecar model neuron. $\bar{g}_{Ca}$, $\bar{g}_K$, and $\bar{g}_{leak}$ were the maximal conductances for the Ca^{2+}, K^+, and leak conductances, respectively. $V_{1/2,Ca}$ was the half-activation voltage of the Ca^{2+} conductance and $V_{slope,Ca}$ was the slope of the activation curve for gCa^{2+}. E_{Ca} was the reversal potential for the Ca^{2+} current, and τ_M was the time constant for M, the activation variable of the Ca^{2+} conductance. $V_{1/2,K}$ was the half-activation of the K^+ current, $V_{slope,K}$ was the slope of the activation curve

Table 1 | Values of parameters for the Morris–Lecar model cell, artificial hyperpolarization-activated currents, and artificial inhibitory synapses.

MORRIS–LECAR PARAMETERS	
C	10 nF
$\bar{g}_{Ca}$	200 nS
E_{Ca}	100 mV
$V_{1/2,Ca}$	−20 mV
$V_{slope,Ca}$	15 mV
τ_M	1 us
$\bar{g}_K$	200 nS
E_K	−80 mV
$V_{1/2,K}$	−20 mV
$V_{slope,K}$	15 mV
τ_{OK}	500 ms
$\bar{g}_{leak}$	50 nS
E_{leak}	−60 mV
***I_h* PARAMETERS**	
$\bar{g}_h$	10–100 nS
E_h	−10 mV
$V_{1/2}$	−50 mV
s_R	7 mV
c_R	0.33 Hz
V_{kR}	−110 mV
s_{kR}	−13 mV
SYNAPSE PARAMETERS	
$\bar{g}_{syn}$	10–100 nS
E_{syn} (bio postsynaptic)	−70 mV
E_{syn} (model postsynaptic)	−80 mV
τ_{syn}	100 ms
$V_{1/2}$	−45 mV
V_{slope}	5 mV

for the K^+ conductance and E_K was the reversal potential of K^+. τ_{OK} is the scale factor for the time constant for N, the activation variable of the K^+ current. E_{leak} is the reversal potential for the leak current.

The artificial I_h (Buchholtz et al., 1992; Sharp et al., 1996) was described by the equations:

$$I_h = \bar{g}_h R\left(E_h - V\right)$$

$$\frac{dR}{dt} = k_R\left(R_\infty - R\right)$$

where

$$R_\infty(V) = \frac{1}{1 + \exp\left[\left(V - V_{1/2}\right)/s_R\right]}$$

$$k_R(V) = c_R\left\{1 + \exp\left[\left(V - V_{kR}\right)/s_{kR}\right]\right\}$$

where $\bar{g}_h$ (varied from 10 to 100 nS) was the maximal conductance of I_h; R was the instantaneous activation; R_∞ was the steady-state activation; E_h was the I_h reversal potential; $V_{1/2}$ was the half-maximum activation; s_R was the step width; c_R was the rate constant; V_{kR} was the half-maximum potential for the rate; and s_{kR} was the step width for the rate.

The artificial inhibitory graded transmission synapse from the Morris–Lecar model to the biological cell was based on Sharp et al. (1996) and was described by the following equations:

$$I_{syn} = \bar{g}_{syn} \cdot S \cdot \left(E_{syn} - V_{post}\right)$$

$$\left(1 - S_\infty\right)\tau_{syn}\frac{dS}{dt} = \left(S_\infty - S\right)$$

where

$$S_\infty\left(V_{pre}\right) = \begin{Bmatrix} \tanh\left[\left(V_{pre} - V_{1/2}\right)/V_{slope}\right] & \text{if } V_{pre} > V_{1/2} \\ 0 & \text{otherwise} \end{Bmatrix}$$

where $\bar{g}_{syn}$(varied from 10 to 100 nS) was the maximal synaptic conductance; S was the instantaneous synaptic activation; S_∞ was the steady-state synaptic activation. The reversal potential of the synaptic current, E_{syn}, had different values in the two synapses: −80 mV when the biological neuron was postsynaptic, and −70 mV when the Morris–Lecar model was postsynaptic. V_{pre} and V_{post} are the presynaptic and postsynaptic potentials, respectively; τ_{syn} was the time constant for synaptic decay; $V_{1/2}$ was the synaptic half-activation voltage and V_{slope} was the synaptic slope voltage.

ASSAYING HALF-CENTER ACTIVITY

Network activity was classified into one of four categories. If the biological cell did not fire action potentials and had no oscillation, the network was "silent." If the biological cell had no spikes but did have a slow membrane potential oscillation, the network was "model dominated." If the biological cell fired action potentials, the network was either "half-center" or "bio-dominated." In half-center networks, the biological cell had slow membrane potential oscillations, and the predominant flow of synaptic current was from the bursting cell (the biological cell, then the model cell in alternation) to the non-bursting cell greater than 90% of the time.

FINDING CORRELATIONS BETWEEN NAPs AND IPs

For each IP, we searched for subsets of NAPs that were highly correlated with it. Conversely for each NAP we searched for subsets of IPs that were highly correlated with it. Both analyses were required because the problem is inherently asymmetric: it is possible for each individual NAP to be well-explained by a linear combination of IPs, but conversely have no individual IP that is well-explained by a linear combination of NAPs. We describe the algorithm to find subsets of NAPs that are highly correlated with an IP; the converse algorithm is identical, only with the data sets swapped.

We formed matrices M_{IP} and M_{NAP}, whose rows denote identity and whose columns denote different IPs and NAPs respectively. We z-scored each matrix column to eliminate the effects of scaling and offset. For each IP (column of M_{IP}) we searched for a subset of NAPs (columns of M_{NAP}) and linear coefficients that approximated the column of M_{IP}. For a given subset of NAPs we formed a reduced matrix R_{NAP} that contained only the columns corresponding to the properties we chose, then performed linear regression to find the best linear coefficients. We assessed the quality of this fit, or "prediction error" as mean square error per degree of freedom, where the number of degrees of freedom was the number of rows (STG neurons) minus the number of columns of R_{NAP} (properties in the subset). We associated this prediction error with the subset of NAPs, and found the best subset of NAPs by minimizing the prediction error with greedy feature selection.

GREEDY FEATURE SELECTION

The greedy algorithm is a heuristic approach to searching a large space of candidate features. It quickly selects a very good subset of features, although not necessarily the best. We initialized the greedy algorithm by creating an empty set of features, and declaring its prediction error to be infinite. We then proceeded iteratively as follows:

1. Form every subset of features that can be created by adding either one or two new properties to the current best subset.
2. Compute the prediction error of all the new subsets.
3. If any has a prediction error lower than the current best subset, select the subset with the lowest prediction error as the new best, and iterate again; otherwise stop.

At the end of iteration, the output of the greedy algorithm was the best subset of features and their prediction error.

ASSIGNING *p*-VALUES TO CORRELATIONS

Given enough properties, we expect to see large correlations between some of them, even if they are merely random numbers. This is exacerbated by the greedy algorithm, because it discovers the largest correlations and ignores small ones. To determine whether the correlations in the data were large enough to be likely real, we computed the probability that equally large correlations would be found randomly in uncorrelated data.

Correlations in data are related to ordering. Independently scrambling the order of rows of M_{IP} and rows of M_{NAP} eliminates any correlations between IPs and NAPs, while preserving their distributions as well as the relationships within the IPs and within the NAPs. Performing the greedy search for correlations on these scrambled data returns the prediction errors for correlations between unrelated data. Because there are many ways to scramble the rows, we did this repeatedly (10,000 scrambled trials) and obtained an empirical estimate of the null distribution for prediction errors. The *p*-value of a correlation arising randomly is the proportion of prediction errors in the null distribution that is lower than the prediction error from the unscrambled data.

CORRECTING FOR MULTIPLE CORRELATIONS

Because of the need to assign many *p*-values, we expected that several might yield apparently "significant" results by chance, thus *p*-values needed to be adjusted to compensate for this problem. We describe a method for evaluating and correcting *p*-values obtained from scrambled data, that is conceptually similar to the Holm–Bonferroni correction (Holm, 1979; Aickin and Gensler, 1996) for multiple comparisons. A fit to scrambled data is expected to occasionally produce outliers with very low errors, although it is not clear that these outliers would be concentrated on any particular IP or NAP. Thus to determine if our best fit is likely due to chance, we compare our best fit to the best fit for each scrambled trial, regardless of which property gave the best fit in the different scrambled trials.

Therefore we started by sorting the prediction errors from the correlation search into increasing order. Then we proceeded iteratively as with the Holm–Bonferroni technique, starting with the best fit (least prediction error). We sorted the prediction error from each scrambled trial into increasing order, generating an empirical estimate of the null distribution of the best fit. The adjusted *p*-value for the fit was the proportion of scrambled best fits that had lower error. If the adjusted *p*-value did not meet the significance criterion ($p < 0.05$) the fit and all higher error fits were not significant and the iteration stopped. Otherwise the fit was significant, and the corresponding property was removed from consideration in future *p*-values, both in the scrambled and unscrambled data. For example, if property P_3 was the best fit and was found to be significant, then P_3 would be removed from each scrambled trial regardless of whether it was the best fit for that scrambled trial. Then the iteration would continue with the next best fit. In this way (similar to Holm–Bonferroni), the best overall fit is compared to the best of N scrambled fits, the second-best is compared to $N-1$, etc., until one of the fits is not significant. Furthermore, the data being removed from consideration are data that have already been shown to have correlations significantly better than chance.

LINEAR CLASSIFICATION

Linear classifiers were constructed of four binary classifiers, one for each neuronal type. Each binary classifier computed the likelihood that a set of properties belonged to a cell corresponding to the classifier's type. The likelihood function for binary classifiers was a logistic function acting on a linear function of *z*-scored neuronal properties (Bishop, 1996; Taylor et al., 2006). If there are N properties, then the likelihood L was calculated as

$$L(\vec{w}) = P\left(w_0 + p_1 * w_1 + p_2 * w_2 + \ldots + p_N * w_N\right),$$

where p_n are the *z*-scored properties, w_n are the weights (w_0 is an offset), and P is the logistic function,

$$P(x) = \frac{1}{1+\exp(-x)}.$$

The weights for all binary classifiers were trained simultaneously using the whole dataset (or a subset if we were using cross-validation). To minimize the weights, we used a "soft max" function

$$S = \frac{L_{\text{correct}}}{L_{DG} + L_{PD} + L_{GM} + L_{LP}},$$

where L_{DG}, L_{PD}, L_{GM}, and L_{LP} were the likelihoods computed for each cell type, and L_{correct} is the likelihood for the correct cell type for a given cell. When training the classifier, we maximized the sum of the log-likelihood of S over the whole dataset (or a subset if we were using cross-validation),

$$\vec{w} = \arg\max \sum_{k \in \{\text{neurons}\}} \log\left(S_k(\vec{w})\right)$$

The optimization was performed using an iterative line-search method (Bishop, 1996), initialized with Fisher's linear discriminant (Bishop, 1996). When determining the results of the trained classifier, we determined the cell type as the one with the greatest likelihood.

To determine how well linear classification generalized, we used leave-two-out cross-validation. Thousand trials were conducted. In each trial the properties for two randomly chosen neurons were selected to be test data, and a linear classifier was trained on the remaining data. After the classifier was trained, the test data were classified. The cross-validation accuracy was the proportion of test data that were classified correctly.

FINDING CLUSTERS

We used k-medoids (Hastie et al., 2009) to categorize blindly STG neurons based on their z-scored properties. We set $k = 4$ and measured distance between points using L_1 (taxicab) norm. The k-medoids algorithm was initialized using the same procedure as k-means++ (Arthur and Vassilvitskii, 2007). Because the initialization is not deterministic, we used 200 trials, using the results of the trial that had the smallest average distance from each point to its medoid.

The results of the clustering allow construction of a contingency table called a "confusion matrix." The rows of the matrix correspond to STG cell type, the columns to cluster label, and the entries are the number of cells so categorized [e.g., the gastric mill (GM), 2 entry corresponds to the number of GM cells grouped into cluster 2]. Cluster labels were assigned the cell identity that maximized the proportion of cells correctly identified (proportion correct). Mutual information (MI) was computed as in Vinh et al. (2009). Adjusted mutual information (AMI) was computed as

$$AMI = \frac{MI - \overline{MI}}{MI_{max} - \overline{MI}},$$

where $\overline{MI}$ is the expected value of MI for a random clustering, and MI_{max} is the maximum possible MI. MI_{max} was computed as in Vinh et al. (2009). We computed $\overline{MI}$ as the mean of the distribution of MI for random clustering, generated using a bootstrap technique.

GENERATING THE DISTRIBUTION OF MUTUAL INFORMATION VIA BOOTSTRAP

We modeled the confusion matrix as being generated by binomial random numbers [e.g., if two out of 13 dorsal gastric (DG) neurons were in cluster 1, the DG,1 entry was modeled as binomial random with a maximum value of 13 and an expectation value of 2]. From a given confusion matrix, we randomly generated synthetic confusion matrices using the same binomial distributions for each entry, and computed MI from these synthetic confusion matrices. We used 10,000 synthetic confusion matrices to generate an empirical distribution of MI. Because the clustering algorithm will always place at least one cell in every cluster, any synthetic confusion matrices with a column of all zeros were discarded and regenerated. To generate the MI distribution for real data sets, we used the confusion matrix generated by the results of the k-medoids algorithm. To generate the MI distribution for clustering of random data sets, we used a confusion matrix with identical columns, and rows that summed to the number of cells in our actual data set (e.g., the sum of the DG row was equal to the number of DG cells in our data).

COMPUTING *P*-VALUES FOR DIFFERENCES IN CLUSTERING

We did not seek to compute a rigorous probability that one set of properties is inherently superior to another with regard to clustering performance. Instead we asked if the difference in MI between two clustering results (MI_{low} and MI_{high}) can be plausibly ascribed merely to fluctuations in the number of cells in each cluster. To compute p between two clusterings, we used the bootstrap method to obtain the distribution of MI_{low}. We then calculated p as the proportion of synthetic MI_{low} that is greater than the actual MI_{high}. We called differences with $p < 0.05$ "significant."

SOURCE CODE

Source code implementing the statistical methods that we developed is hosted permanently at http://www.bio.brandeis.edu/MarderLabCode/

RESULTS

The STG of the crab *C. borealis* has 26–27 neurons, that can be reliably identified according to their projection patterns (Marder and Bucher, 2007). Each STG has two pyloric dilator (PD) neurons, one lateral pyloric (LP) neuron, four GM neurons, and one DG neuron. The data in this paper come from 55 neurons (PD $n = 13$; LP $n = 15$; GM $n = 14$; DG $n = 13$). The PD and LP neurons are part of the circuit that generates the fast (period ~1 s) pyloric rhythm and the GM and DG neurons are part of the circuit that generates the slow (period 6–10 s) GM rhythm.

Conventional IPs were measured by injecting current steps and ramps into individual neurons to measure input resistance, spike threshold voltage, FI slope, spike frequency with 1 nA injected current, spike height, and minimum voltage with zero injected current. **Figure 1A** shows a recording of a DG neuron in response to a current ramp, showing the voltage at threshold and the spike height. **Figure 1B** shows the same cell in response to depolarizing current pulses of different amplitudes. **Figure 1C** shows the plot of spike frequency vs. injected current. Spike frequency with 1 nA injected current can be read directly from this plot, while the linear fit (blue line) allows determination of FI slope. **Figure 2** summarizes all of the IPs that went into the analysis, with the new data points in color, and those from the prior study (Grashow et al., 2010) in gray. Note that the variance of each measure is considerable, and there is a great deal of overlap across cell types.

Because of the overlap in these measures even across neurons with very different characteristic behaviors during ongoing network activity, we reasoned that a set of properties that better captured the potential dynamics of the neurons in a closed-loop dynamic network might be more useful in characterizing these neurons than the conventional, open-loop IPs shown in **Figure 1**.

Stomatogastric ganglion neurons are part of circuits that are rhythmically active, so we sought a measure that would place these neurons into a rhythmically active circuit under experimenter control. Therefore we used the dynamic clamp to create two-cell circuits: one cell being the neuron to be evaluated, the second a standard model neuron used in all experiments. **Figure 3** shows the result of a dynamic clamp experiment in which an isolated DG neuron was coupled with reciprocal inhibition to a Morris–Lecar model neuron (Morris and Lecar, 1981; Grashow et al., 2010), and the strength of the synaptic conductances ($\bar{g}_{syn}$) and an imposed

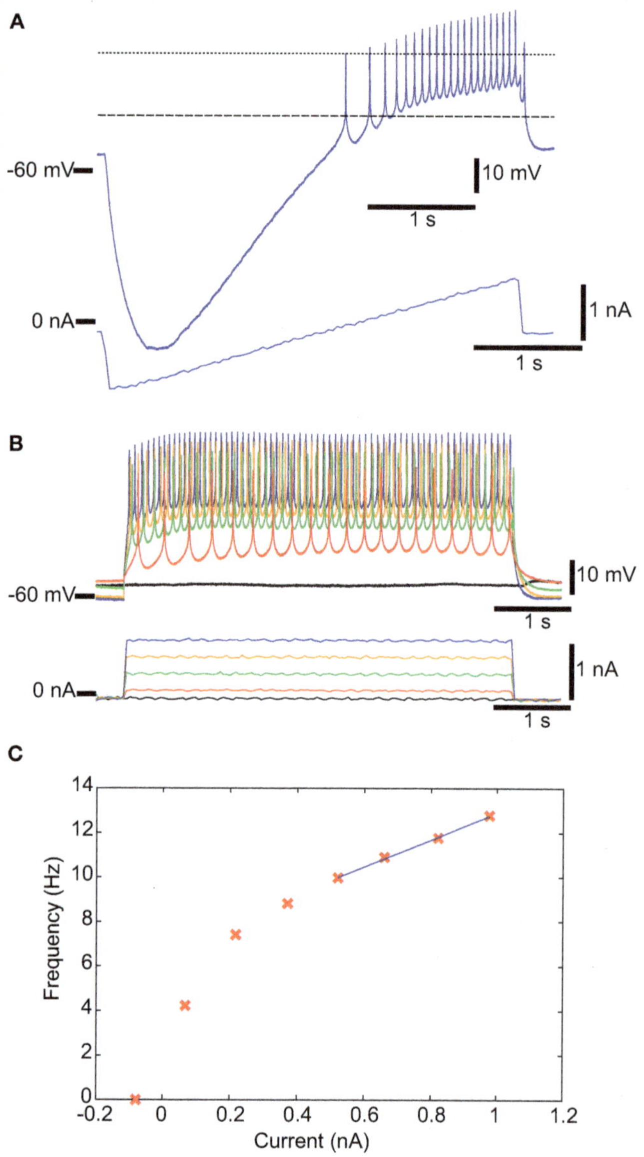

FIGURE 1 | Traditional IPs for one DG neuron. (A,B) Membrane potential is shown in the top trace, and injected current in the bottom trace. **(A)** Spike threshold voltage is the voltage at the point of maximum curvature (dashed line) before the first spike in response to a ramp of injected current. **(B)** The FI curve was obtained by measuring spike frequency in response to depolarizing current steps. **(C)** FI Slope is the slope of the best-fit line to the linear region of the FI curve. For this DG neuron, the four rightmost points were used (see Materials and Methods). The spike rate in response to 1 nA of injected current is (in this case) the last data point.

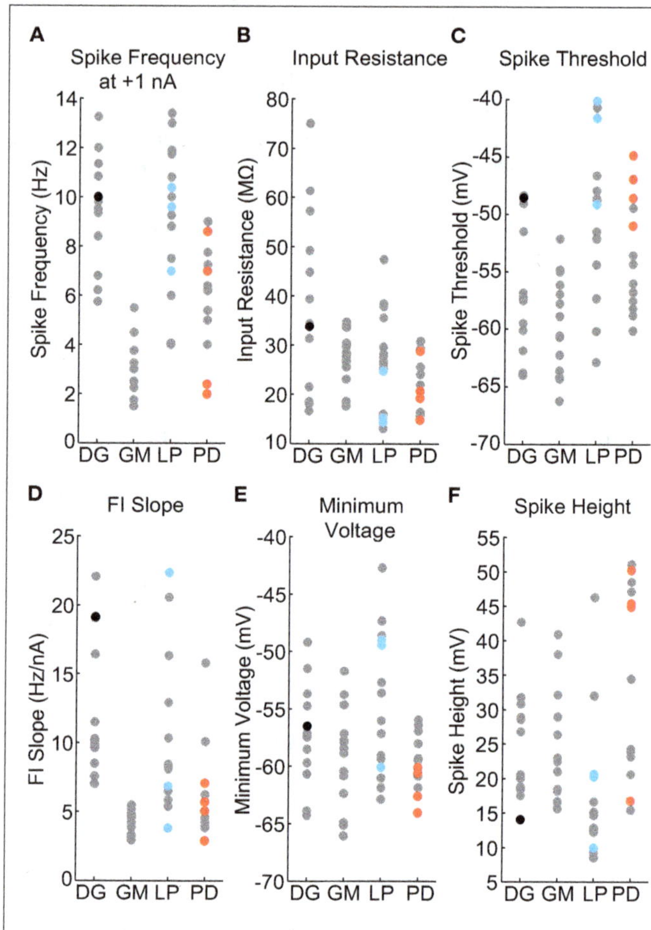

FIGURE 2 | Values of IPs, by neuron type. New data points are in color, and those from the prior study (Grashow et al., 2010) are in gray. **(A)** Spike frequency with 1 nA injected current. **(B)** Input resistance. **(C)** Spike threshold voltage. **(D)** Frequency–current slope. **(E)** Minimum voltage with zero injected current. **(F)** Spike height.

I_h conductance ($\bar{g}_h$) were varied. A schematic of this circuit is shown in **Figure 3A**. **Figure 3B** shows the behavior of the model neuron and the biological neuron in the uncoupled state, and **Figures 3C,D** show different patterns of resulting network activity. **Figure 3E** illustrates the case in which the model and biological neurons are firing in alternating bursts of activity, or half-center oscillations. We obtained NAPs exclusively by examining networks with half-center activity, because these were precisely the networks that exhibited rhythmic activity with the complex mix of spiking and slow membrane potential oscillations that characterizes the membrane potential trajectories that STG neurons display during ongoing pyloric and gastric mill rhythms.

Figure 3F shows a map of the network behavior as $\bar{g}_{syn}$ and $\bar{g}_h$ were varied. The map positions that produced half-center alternating bursts are shown in the red dots. For each of the 55 experiments, we used these maps to calculate the proportion of map positions that resulted in half-center activity. In the map shown in **Figure 3F**, this proportion was 11/49. For each set of parameters that gave half-center activity (map positions with alternating bursts) we calculated the half-center frequency and the number of spikes/burst in the biological neuron (**Figure 3G**). Because each biological neuron used had a different set of IPs, we expected that the map produced with each one would be different. The hypothesis was that features of these maps and of their half-center behavior (size, location, burst frequencies, number of spikes/burst of half-center activity) would constitute a data set that might more reliably capture the neurons' dynamics, and consequently their cellular identity, than the conventional measures of intrinsic excitability.

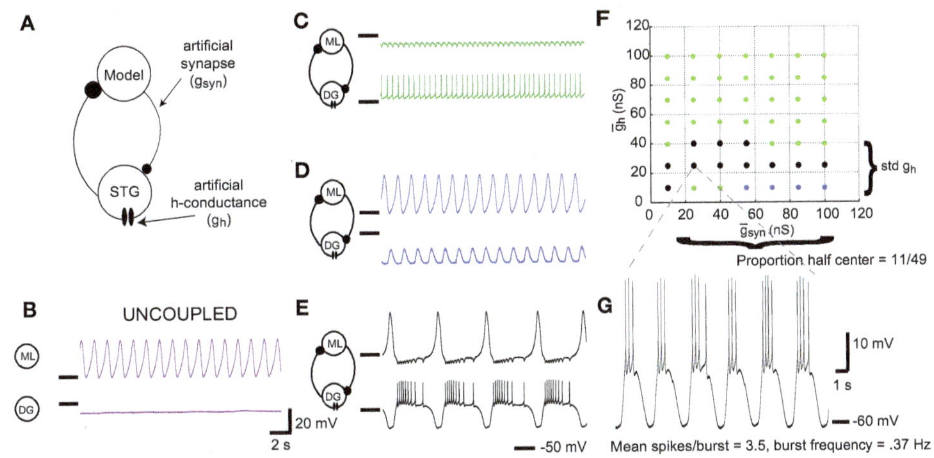

FIGURE 3 | Network activity of the artificial circuit depends on ($\bar{g}_{syn}, \bar{g}_h$) parameter values. (A) Schematic for two-cell synthetic circuit. A model Morris–Lecar neuron is connected to a biological STG neuron (either DG, GM, LP, or PD) via artificial mutual inhibitory synapses. Dynamic clamp simulated the synapses, as well as injecting artificial *h*-conductance into the STG neuron. **(B)** Voltage traces from uncoupled ($\bar{g}_{syn} = 0$, $\bar{g}_h = 0$)Morris–Lecar model (top) and DG neuron (bottom). **(C–E)** Voltage traces from connected circuit with different ($\bar{g}_{syn}$, $\bar{g}_h$) parameter values. Colors denote network activity classification: green traces denote networks dominated by the DG neuron, blue denotes networks dominated by the Morris–Lecar neuron, and red denotes networks exhibiting half-center oscillations. **(C)** $\bar{g}_{syn} = 70$, $\bar{g}_h = 55$. **(D)** $\bar{g}_{syn} = 85$, $\bar{g}_h = 10$. **(E)** $\bar{g}_{syn} = 40$, $\bar{g}_h = 40$. **(F,G)** NAPs are representative of a biological neuron's overall response to all of the ($\bar{g}_{syn}$, $\bar{g}_h$) parameter values in a map. **(F)** The proportion of half-center networks is trivially obtained from the map. Std $\bar{g}_h$ is the SD of $\bar{g}_h$ values among half-center networks. **(G)** Spikes per burst and half-center frequency are both obtained from individual networks, then averaged over all half-center networks.

Figure 4 presents the data from all of the half-centers found in the 55 experiments analyzed. In most of the maps half-center activity was found in a horizontal swath, indicating that half-center activity was more sensitive to $\bar{g}_h$ than to $\bar{g}_{syn}$. The SD of $\bar{g}_h$ provides a measure of the width of the horizontal swath. **Figure 4A** shows that although the variance of this measure for each cell type is considerable, the PDs had a larger SD than the other cell types. The proportion of half-centers in the 55 neurons is shown in **Figure 4B**. The mean half-center frequency was higher in the PD neuron set of networks (**Figure 4C**), and mean number of spikes/burst was lowest in the networks made with GM neurons (**Figure 4D**).

We refer to the four measures – "SD of $\bar{g}_h$," "proportion of half-center networks," "mean half-center frequency," and "mean spikes per burst" – as NAPs. There are many conceivable network properties; however we restricted the analysis to a handful that were simple to measure and that we reasoned would be related to both IPs and cell identity.

CORRELATIONS BETWEEN NAPs AND IPs

We first asked if there is any predictive relationship between these measures of network activity and conventional IPs. For each IP, we searched for the subset of NAPs that best predicted it (see Materials and Methods). Conversely, we looked for the subset of IPs that best predicted each NAP.

To assess the significance of any correlations we repeated the predictive analysis on 10,000 shuffled trials (see Materials and Methods). In a shuffled trial, we scrambled the cell identity while preserving the distribution of individual properties. The shuffled trials provided an empirical estimate of the null distribution for prediction error; and because the null distribution was estimated from trials with multiple correlations, we were able to correct for multiple correlations and calculate adjusted p-values (see Materials and Methods).

The results of this analysis are detailed in **Table 2. Figure 5** shows selected scatter-plots of several properties vs. the values predicted by their best-fit linear combination. Three of the six IPs were significantly predicted by NAPs, and all of the NAPs were significantly predicted by IPs. However, the R^2 values of the correlations were low, indicating weak predictive value.

LINEAR CLASSIFIER

We next asked whether we could reliably determine the identity of the four neuron types using the six measurements of IPs (**Figure 2**), using the four measurements of NAPs taken from the dynamic clamp networks (**Figure 4**) or by combining the two sets of data together. Given the large range of these measurements within a cell type and the overlap of the values across the cell types, it is clear that no single measure would reliably allow the identification of the neurons.

To identify neuron types by their properties, the different cell types must have properties that segregate into different clusters. To check if this is the case, we attempted to train a linear classifier to determine neuronal identity based on a given set of z-scored properties. The classifier was constructed of four binary linear classifiers, one for each neuronal class. Binary classifiers estimated the likelihood that a neuron's properties corresponded to the binary classifier's STG type. The likelihood was a number between zero and one; whichever binary classifier returned the highest likelihood "won," and the overall classifier then determined that the properties belonged to a neuron of the corresponding type.

Conceptually, for a set of N properties, a linear classifier describes four $N - 1$ dimensional oriented hyperplanes (one for each binary classifier), with all the neurons of the correct type on the "plus" side of a hyperplane, and the remaining neurons on the "minus" side. In practice, the situation may be less straightforward, with all four hyperplanes being in compromise positions,

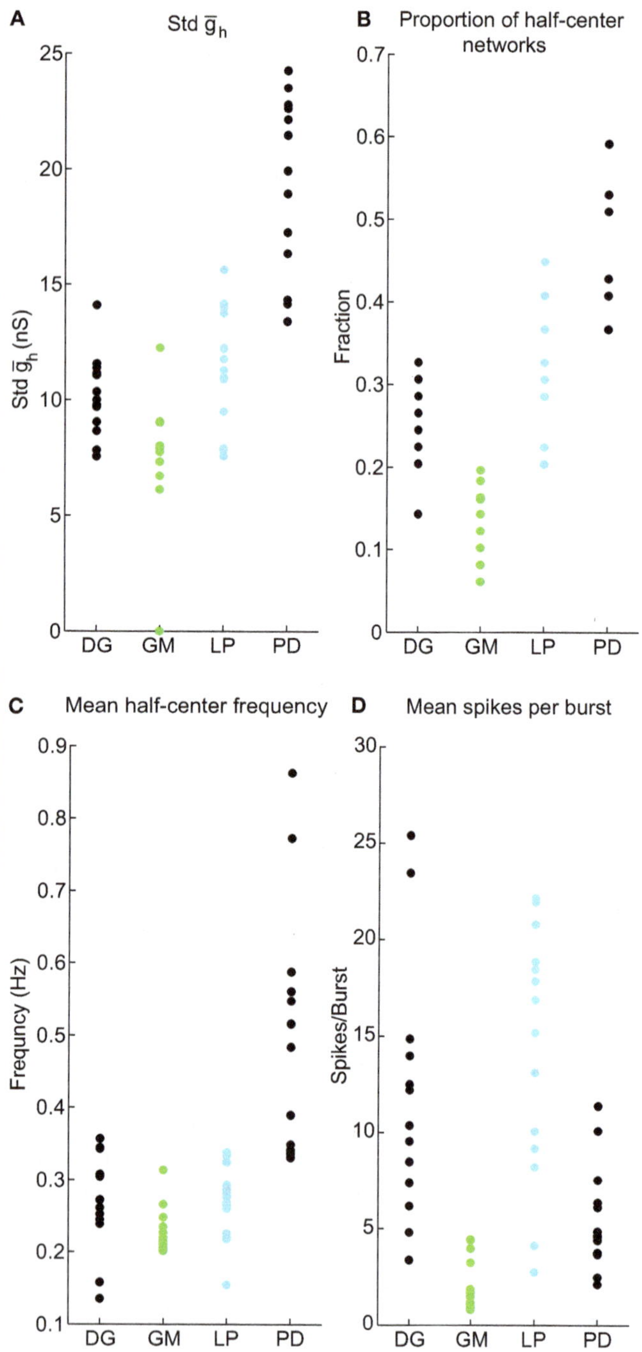

FIGURE 4 | Values of NAPs, by neuron type. (A) Std $\bar{g}_h$. **(B)** Proportion of half-center networks. **(C)** Mean half-center frequency. **(D)** Mean spikes per burst.

allowing their pooled information to determine identity. In such a situation, placement, and orientation of hyperplanes may depend on outlier points, especially when the number of cells is small but N is large.

We trained a linear classifier for each set of properties. The classifier based on IPs identified 85% of cells correctly, the classifier based on NAPs identified 84% correctly, and the combined properties classifier identified 100% of cells correctly (**Figure 6**). However, these high accuracies were partially due to overfitting outlier points. When we tested the generalizability of these classifiers with leave-two-out cross-validation (see Materials and Methods), the accuracy of each classifier dropped somewhat: IPs classified 64% correctly, NAPs 68%, and the combined data 78%. Thus only by combining the two data sets can the cell types be distinguished on the basis of properties, and even then the boundary between them is complex and dependent upon the position of outlier points.

FINDING CLUSTERS

Ideally, one would like to identify neuron types blindly, not merely verify that they fall into properties of clusters. This approach would be applicable to a system where cells cannot be unambiguously identified as they can in the STG. We used the k-medoids algorithm (Hastie et al., 2009) with $k = 4$ to find clusters of properties. However, clusters do not directly correspond to any particular cell type (i.e., after running k-medoids, a cell is labeled "cluster 2" not "GM"). To address this issue, we computed two measures of accuracy. We assigned cluster labels to cell identity to maximize the number of cells that are correctly categorized, and computed the "proportion correct." This number is necessarily in the interval between $1/k$ and 1. We also computed the MI between the cluster labels and the cell identities. By appropriately scaling the MI we computed the AMI which has a maximum value of one, and an expected value of zero for random numbers. In addition to our real data, we applied the clustering technique to a synthetic set of properties generated from Gaussian random numbers, to illustrate chance results. We used a bootstrap technique to estimate p-values for significant differences in MI between clusterings.

Both of the accuracy measures (MI/AMI and proportion correct) showed the same general trends. No set of properties was able to correctly identify all cells. When we performed k-medoids clustering on Gaussian random numbers, as expected we obtained no information (proportion correct = 0.29, MI = 0.089, AMI = −0.002). Real neuronal properties were able to obtain significant information: for IPs proportion correct = 0.60, MI = 0.36, and AMI = 0.21; for NAPs proportion correct = 0.69, MI = 0.72, and AMI = 0.49; and for both sets joined proportion correct = 0.84, MI = 0.90, and AMI = 0.62. The results of clustering on the combined properties are depicted in **Figure 7A**. All sets of STG properties achieved results significantly better than random numbers, with $p < 0.001$. The differences between sets of properties were also significant (NAPs vs. IPs $p = 0.01$, combined properties vs. IPs $p < 0.001$, combined properties vs. NAPs $p = 0.03$). The quantification of accuracy is summarized in **Figure 7B**. Together these results show that NAPs encode more information about cell identity than traditional IPs, but both sets contain distinct information (**Figure 7C**).

DISCUSSION

Establishing reasonable and reliable methods for classifying and characterizing neurons has been a far thornier practical problem than might have been predicted from first principles. While there

Table 2 | Correlations between IPs and NAPs.

IP	R^2	Adjusted *p*-value	Best fit with	NAP	R^2	Adjusted *p*-value	Best fit with
Spike rate + 1 nA	0.65	<0.001	Mean spikes per burst, proportion half-center, std $\bar{g}_h$	**Mean spikes per burst**	0.68	<0.001	Spike rate + 1 nA, min v, spike thresh V, FI slope
Spike threshold voltage	0.46	<0.001	Mean spikes per burst, mean half-center frequency, proportion half-center	**Mean half-center frequency**	0.54	<0.001	Spike thresh V, min v, FI slope, spike rate + 1 nA
Minimum voltage	0.34	0.0017	Mean spikes per burst, proportion half-center	**Std $\bar{g}_h$**	0.54	<0.001	Spike height, spike thresh V, min v, spike rate + 1 nA, FI slope, input resistance
Spike height	0.20	N.S.	Std $\bar{g}_h$, mean spikes per burst	**Proportion half-center**	0.48	<0.001	Spike thresh V, min v, spike rate + 1 nA, spike height, FI slope, input resistance
Input resistance	0.14	N.S.	Std $\bar{g}_h$ mean spikes per burst				
FI slope	0.10	N.S.	Mean spikes per burst				

Each property (in bold) was fit with one or more properties from the other data set. The optimal set of fitting parameters was determined via greedy feature selection. We list the resulting R^2, adjusted p-value, and optimal fitting properties for each property. p-Values are adjusted for multiple correlations and the feature-selection process.

are large and uniquely identifiable neurons in small invertebrate nervous systems and in the spinal cords of fish and frogs, in most regions of the vertebrate central nervous system and in many brain areas in invertebrates, cell identification cannot be achieved by size or location of the neurons alone. The electrophysiological firing patterns of many neurons change (Dickinson et al., 1990; Weimann et al., 1991), either as a consequence of neuromodulation, development, or disease. Transmitter phenotype (Borodinsky et al., 2004) and transcription factor expression (William et al., 2003; Wienecke et al., 2010) are often developmentally or activity regulated, complicating the use of a single chemical marker to identify neurons, although chemical markers may be sufficient at times (Zagoraiou et al., 2009). Neuronal projection patterns to distant targets such as muscles or other brain regions often provide unambiguous identification, but when multiple cell types are entangled in local circuits, even projection patterns may not be sufficient. These issues are further confounded by the large variance measured in a variety of properties of individual neurons (Getting, 1981; Hume and Getting, 1982; Swensen and Bean, 2005; Schulz et al., 2006, 2007; Goaillard et al., 2009; Tobin et al., 2009; Grashow et al., 2010). This raises the question of whether combining multiple measures can serve to better cluster or identify neurons, and if so, what kinds of assays are potentially more useful than conventional measures of intrinsic excitability.

In this study we used six conventional measures of neuronal IPs and four measures of how neurons behaved in an artificial network to determine whether any or all of these measures could correctly cluster and identify neurons whose identity was already known. This exercise highlighted a number of difficulties that, to a greater or lesser degree, will potentially plague investigators wishing to use electrophysiological measures to identify neurons. It is clear from the variance in each of the IPs across individual neurons of the same class and from the overlap of these values across cell types, that no single measure would reliably serve to identify the neurons (**Figure 2**; Grashow et al., 2010). Therefore, our goal was to determine whether the combined set of electrophysiological measures would reliably allow us to cluster the neurons into groups that mapped correctly with their identity.

One might naively think that increasing the number of electrophysiological measures performed for each neuron would increase the likelihood of proper identification. This might appear to be especially the case if each measure probes a different essential feature of the cell's performance. For that reason, we chose to embed each neuron in an artificial network that we reasoned would test its dynamic behavior differently than the conventional measures of excitability. Nonetheless, increasing the number of measures made for each neuron tested comes with a statistical cost, as each additional increases the likelihood of finding spurious correlations. Because it is necessary to correct for this before assigning statistical significance, adding measures that even partially sample the same biophysical attributes to a neuron may be more counterproductive than helpful. For some cell types a different set of measured IPs or NAPs might be more useful than those studied here. Nonetheless, our point is simply to say that "more is not necessarily better." To this end, in choosing the NAPs that we included, we used our biological intuition to select four that appeared to be relatively functionally independent of each other, and we discarded many other potential network measures that might have added relatively little to the analysis and added a substantial multiple comparison statistical burden. Obviously, these problems are more acute with relatively modest-sized data sets, such as that analyzed here, and become less acute with data sets with *n*'s in the several thousand (at which point it is also possible to use additional methods).

Because STG neurons can be recorded from intracellularly for many hours it was experimentally feasible for us to ask whether these NAPs would be useful in neuron characterization. We were surprised that the networks did not provide more information than they did, and we do not expect or recommend that

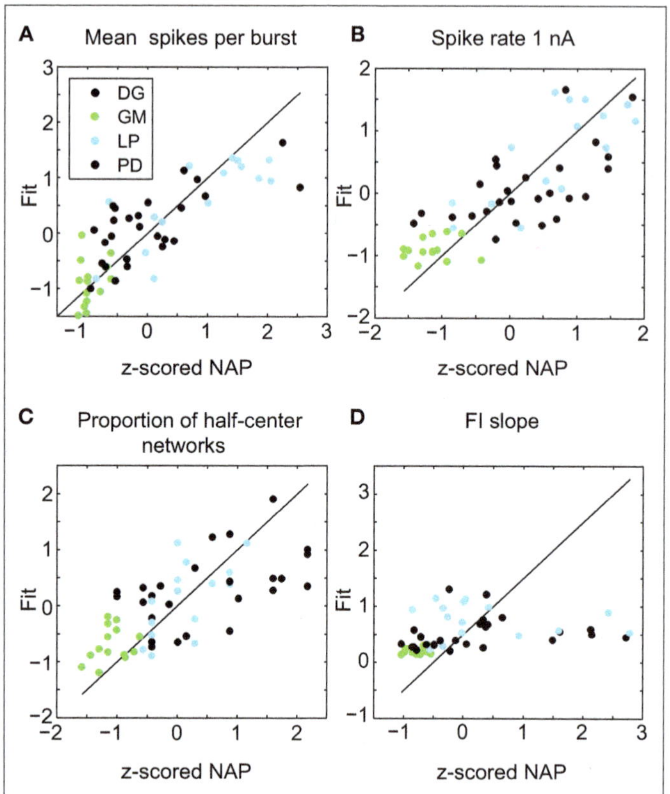

FIGURE 5 | Sample fits of *z*-scored neuronal properties. Value of the property being fit (x) vs. value predicted by the best regression (y). The line $y = x$ corresponds to a perfect fit. **(A)** Mean spikes per burst was best fit simultaneously to spike rate 1 nA, minimum voltage, spike threshold voltage, and FI slope ($R^2 = 0.68$, $p < 0.001$). **(B)** Spike rate 1 nA was best fit simultaneously to mean spikes per burst, proportion of half-center networks, and std $\bar{g}_h$ ($R^2 = 0.65$, $p < 0.001$). **(C)** Proportion of half-center networks was best fit simultaneously to spike threshold voltage, minimum voltage, spike rate 1 nA, spike height, FI slope, and input resistance ($R^2 = 0.48$, $p < 0.001$). **(D)** FI slope had no significant correlations, but was best fit with mean spikes per burst ($R^2 = 0.10$, $p > 0.05$).

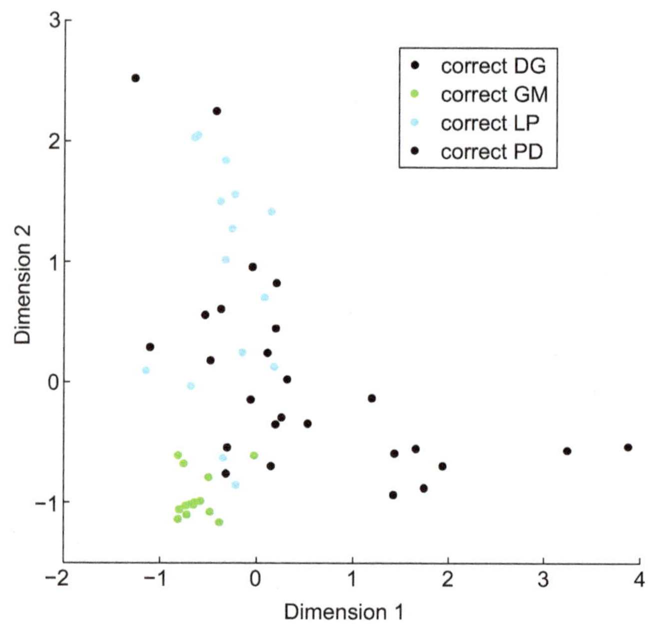

FIGURE 6 | A linear classifier can be trained to correctly identify cell type. Hundred percentage of neurons were correctly identified when a linear classifier was trained on combined IPs and NAPs. To visualize the grouping of neurons by property, we projected the 10-dimensional space of properties down to two dimensions. Analogously to the results of Principal Component Analysis, we determined components (combinations of properties) that pointed along directions of particular interest. These directions (Dimension 1 and Dimension 2) were chosen to provide maximal spacing between the different neuronal types.

an investigator working in systems where recordings cannot be maintained for many hours attempt the same process, although other closed-loop measures that are less time-consuming could be devised.

We assessed significance of correlations with a custom bootstrapping method that combines shuffled trials and the Holm–Bonferroni correction for multiple comparisons. It is commonly assumed that correlations do not need to be corrected because they are only indicative of interesting relationships, not a rigorous test in themselves. However, the process of finding correlations may be *too* effective – if it can find seemingly strong correlations in random data, then there may be confusion between correlations that are indicative of real relationships, and those that are most likely spurious.

Data-mining commonly produces large spurious correlations. When we simply applied a Pearson correlation test, every correlation was "significant" and there were several p-values less than 10^{-10}. Using shuffled trials properly accounts for the power of data-mining and dramatically increased the magnitude of the p-values (many were still highly significant). Building Holm–Bonferroni into the procedure allowed further correction for investigating many properties.

Although these two methods (comparing to shuffled trials, and adjusting p-values with the Holm–Bonferroni method) are commonly used separately, we are not aware of them being used together as done here. However, we believe it is necessary to combine them because we had no *a priori* hypothesis about which correlations were likely to be most significant. After searching a data set for correlations we find several with varying strengths, and want to know which correlations are weak enough that they could plausibly be drawn from the distribution of expected spurious correlations. To do this it was necessary to keep track of all the correlations for each shuffled trial, and therefore integrate the multiple comparisons correction into the shuffled trial structure.

The results of our correlation analysis appear to differ from Grashow et al. (2010) which analyzed much of the same data. However it should be borne in mind that the two analyses ask different questions. Grashow et al. (2010) asked, "What are the pairwise relationships between these different properties?", while here we asked "How well can we reconstruct one set of properties from the other?" Both are potentially interesting questions, and have their strengths and weaknesses.

Grashow et al. (2010) tested all possible pairwise correlations (48 total) between larger property sets. Because of this,

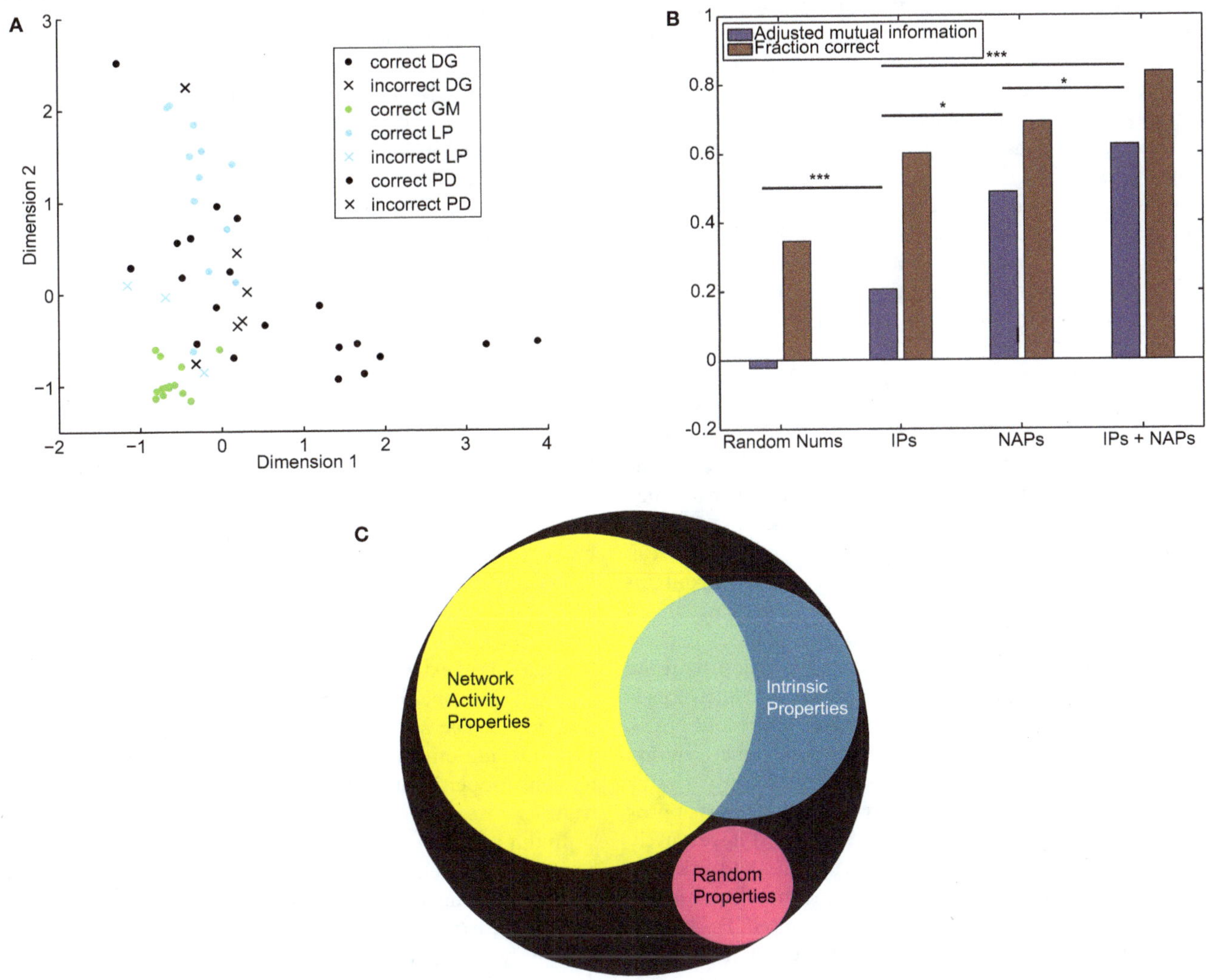

FIGURE 7 | IPs and NAPs partially encode neuronal identity. **(A)** *k*-Medoids clustering was applied to the combined IPs and NAPs of STG neurons. Filled circles denote correctly classified neurons, Xs denote errors. The 10-dimensional space is projected down to two dimensions that best separate the different neuronal types. **(B)** Adjusted mutual information (blue) and proportion correct (red) by property type. *p*-Values between clustering results are computed by the technique described in Section "Materials and Methods." $*p < 0.05$, $***p < 0.001$. **(C)** A Venn diagram depicting the information encoded by the two sets of properties, assuming improved encoding of the combined sets is due to non-overlapping mutual information. The area of the black circle depicts perfect encoding of cell identity, while the magenta circle describes the mutual information expected from a set of randomly generated properties.

their correction for multiple comparisons was quite large. We searched for the best linear reconstruction for each property (10 total), thus incurring a smaller penalty for multiple comparisons. However the approach here may not find all the correlations that are of potential interest. For instance, if an NAP is highly correlated with two IPs, and those two IPs are highly correlated with each other, then this approach is unlikely to discover that the NAP is correlated with both IPs. More likely it would only discover one of them. This is because adding the second IP will decrease the degrees of freedom without substantially improving the fit, leading the combination to be heavily discounted by the feature-selection algorithm. Thus some of the differences between the two studies result from asking different questions.

However, some differences between the studies were due to improvements in methodology. As is often done, Grashow et al. (2010) computed adjusted *p*-values by using the Pearson correlation coefficient test for normally distributed data, then applying the Holm–Bonferroni correction for multiple comparisons. These data exhibit deviations from normality (e.g., **Figure 2F**, where LP exhibits substantial skew, and PD appears to be bimodal) and thus the Pearson correlation test is not fully appropriate. Furthermore the Holm–Bonferroni correction may be overly conservative because it does not account for potential relationships between the different quantities whose correlation is being tested. Here, basing the significance test on scrambled trials, we avoided making assumptions about the distribution of the data. By incorporating the adjustment for multiple correlations into the scrambled trials, we directly computed the approximate null distribution for the nth-best correlation. This enabled us to compute a p-value that is conservative enough to account for multiple correlations without being unnecessarily over-conservative.

In general, the methods we used – searching for correlations and clustering – decrease in effectiveness as the dimensionality they must work in (the number of properties) increases. Increasing dimensionality increases the probability of finding correlations between random numbers, making corrections for multiple correlations more severe and therefore decreasing the ability to detect real correlations. Clustering algorithms suffer from a host of problems referred to collectively as "the curse of dimensionality" (Bishop, 1996; Beyer et al., 1999; Hinneburg et al., 2000; Houle et al., 2010), which cause them to find the "wrong" clusters. It is especially difficult if extraneous dimensions are added, because algorithms naturally tend to break up clusters at essentially meaningless gaps in the extraneous dimensions. We decreased the number of properties we considered to avoid this problem as much as possible.

In this analysis the information pertaining to cell identity can be thought of as a Venn diagram (**Figure 7C**), with IPs containing some information, NAPs containing more information, and some overlap between the two sets. It is possible that because we used six measures of IPs, thus a higher dimension than the NAPs, they are merely falling afoul of the curse of dimensionality and thus unfairly penalized when compared to the four NAPs. However, when the two sets are grouped together the resulting set of properties has still higher dimensionality and outperforms either one separately, suggesting that the Venn diagram is appropriately representing the data. Looking at the raw MI if we naively assume that non-overlapping information combines additively, we see that the NAPs contain roughly twice as much information as the IPs, and that roughly half the information in the IPs is in the overlapping region of the Venn diagram (**Figure 7C**). Thus the NAPs do capture the neuronal dynamics of each cell type better than the conventional measures of IPs, although we cannot perfectly identify neurons only by their properties. The success of NAPs suggests that closed-loop dynamic current perturbations yield greater information about cell identity than static perturbations. However, the properties extracted from this perturbation must be chosen carefully, because the size of the data sets will never be large enough to search through the essentially infinite space of all possible properties.

We used k-medoids, one of the simplest clustering algorithms (Andreopoulos et al., 2009), but not always the best. The k-medoids algorithm is nearly the same as the k-means algorithm, however clusters are represented by one of the members of the cluster (called the "medoid," and chosen to minimize distance to other members of the cluster) rather than the mean of members of the cluster. k-Medoids is more robust to outliers than k-means (Andreopoulos et al., 2009; Hastie et al., 2009) and is applicable in situations when computing mean objects is impossible or undesirable. k-Medoids is slower than k-means with very large data sets [selecting the medoid is $O(N^2)$ while computing the mean is $O(N)$]. However, as is common for electrophysiology, the data set studied here is small and we expect plentiful outliers due to the variability in neurons and noise inherent in measuring neuronal properties. In principle, more sophisticated density-based (Sander et al., 1998), nearest-neighbor-based (Ertöz et al., 2003; Bohm et al., 2004; Pei et al., 2009; Kriegel et al., 2011), or correlation-based (Kriegel et al., 2008) methods are capable of determining the number of clusters, recognizing extraneous dimensions, and finding clusters with complex shapes. When deciding on the methods we would use for this paper, we conducted pilot tests for a variety of clustering algorithms on synthetic data sets of a size comparable to our IPs and NAPs. In these pilot tests, we found that the more sophisticated clustering algorithms were less successful at identifying cluster membership (i.e., neuronal identity) correctly. With small data sets, there were inevitably extraneous large density fluctuations or extraneous correlations, therefore for this study, k-medoids was superior by virtue of being simpler, but this would certainly change with a larger data set. These results suggest that with a large number of neurons and a small number of highly relevant properties, identifying cells via clustering is likely to be fruitful.

In this analysis we implemented corrections for multiple comparisons and methods to determine the statistical significance of the resulting correlations. In many studies reporting correlations, corrections for multiple correlations were not made. Obviously, if the correlations are robust, they will persist after the appropriate corrections are made. Nonetheless, it is likely that some reported correlations in the literature would not have survived a more rigorous statistical analysis. Of course, it is essential to remember that a weak correlation may point to a fundamental biological insight, while a strong correlation may not always help illuminate an underlying biological process.

ACKNOWLEDGMENTS

We thank Dr. Adam Taylor for useful discussions. This work was supported by MH467842, T32 NS07292, and NS058110 from the National Institutes of Health.

REFERENCES

Aickin, M., and Gensler, H. (1996). Adjusting for multiple testing when reporting research results: the Bonferroni vs Holm methods. *Am. J. Public Health* 86, 726–728.

Andreopoulos, B., An, A., Wang, X., and Schroeder, M. (2009). A roadmap of clustering algorithms: finding a match for a biomedical application. *Brief. Bioinformatics* 10, 297–314.

Arthur, D., and Vassilvitskii, S. (2007). "k-Means++: the advantages of careful seeding," in *Proceedings of the Eighteenth Annual ACM-SIAM Symposium on Discrete Algorithms*. (New Orleans, LA: Society for Industrial and Applied Mathematics), 1027–1035.

Beyer, K., Goldstein, J., Ramakrishnan, R., and Shaft, U. (1999). When is "nearest neighbor" meaningful?" in *Database Theory – ICDT'99*, eds C. Beeri and P. Buneman (Berlin: Springer), 217–235.

Bishop, C. M. (1996). *Neural Networks for Pattern Recognition*. Oxford: Oxford University Press.

Bohm, C., Railing, K., Kriegel, H. P., and Kroger, P. (2004). "Density connected clustering with local subspace preferences," in *ICDM '04. Fourth IEEE International Conference on Data Mining, 2004*, Piscataway, 27–34.

Borodinsky, L. N., Root, C. M., Cronin, J. A., Sann, S. B., Gu, X., and Spitzer, N. C. (2004). Activity-dependent homeostatic specification of transmitter expression in embryonic neurons. *Nature* 429, 523–530.

Buchholtz, F., Golowasch, J., Epstein, I. R., and Marder, E. (1992). Mathematical model of an identified stomatogastric ganglion neuron. *J. Neurophysiol.* 67, 332–340.

Calabrese, R. L., Norris, B. J., Wenning, A., and Wright, T. M. (2011). Coping with variability in small neuronal networks. *Integr. Comp. Biol.* 51, 845–855.

Dickinson, P. S., Mecsas, C., and Marder, E. (1990). Neuropeptide fusion of two motor pattern generator circuits. *Nature* 344, 155–158.

Dorval, A. D., Christini, D. J., and White, J. A. (2001). Real-time linux dynamic clamp: a fast and flexible way to construct virtual ion channels in living cells. *Ann. Biomed. Eng.* 29, 897–907.

Ertöz, L., Steinbach, M., and Kumar, V. (2003). "Finding clusters of different sizes, shapes, and densities in noisy, high dimensional data," in *Proceedings of the Third SIAM International Conference on Data Mining,* eds D. Barbará and C. Kamath (San Francisco: Society for Industrial and Applied Mathematics), 12.

Getting, P. A. (1981). Mechanisms of pattern generation underlying swimming in Tritonia. I. Neuronal network formed by monosynaptic connections. *J. Neurophysiol.* 46, 65–79.

Getting, P. A. (1989). Emerging principles governing the operation of neural networks. *Annu. Rev. Neurosci.* 12, 185–204.

Getting, P. A., and Dekin, M. S. (1985). Mechanisms of pattern generation underlying swimming in TRITONIA. IV. Gating of central pattern generator. *J. Neurophysiol.* 53, 466–480.

Getting, P. A., Lennard, P. R., and Hume, R. I. (1980). Central pattern generator mediating swimming in tritonia. I. Identification and synaptic interactions. *J. Neurophysiol.* 44, 151–164.

Goaillard, J. M., Taylor, A. L., Schulz, D. J., and Marder, E. (2009). Functional consequences of animal-to-animal variation in circuit parameters. *Nat. Neurosci.* 12, 1424–1430.

Grashow, R., Brookings, T., and Marder, E. (2010). Compensation for variable intrinsic neuronal excitability by circuit-synaptic interactions. *J. Neurosci.* 30, 9145–9156.

Hastie, T., Tibshirani, R., and Friedman, J. (2009). *The Elements of Statistical Learning: Data Mining, Inference, and Prediction.* New York: Springer Verlag, 515–520.

Hinneburg, A., Aggarwal, C. C., and Keim, D. A. (2000). "What is the nearest neighbor in high dimensional spaces?" in *Proceedings of the 26th International Conference on Very Large Data Bases* (San Francisco: Morgan Kaufmann Publishers Inc.) 671675, 506–515.

Holm, S. (1979). A simple sequentially rejective multiple test procedure. *Scand. J. Stat.* 6, 65–70.

Houle, M., Kriegel, H.-P., Kröger, P., Schubert, E., and Zimek, A. (2010). "Can shared-neighbor distances defeat the curse of dimensionality?" in *Scientific and Statistical Database Management,* eds M. Gertz and B. Ludäscher (Berlin: Springer), 482–500.

Hume, R. I., and Getting, P. A. (1982). Motor organization of tritonia swimming. II. Synaptic drive to flexion neurons from premotor interneurons. *J. Neurophysiol.* 47, 75–90.

Hume, R. I., Getting, P. A., and Del Beccaro, M. A. (1982). Motor organization of tritonia swimming. I. Quantitative analysis of swim behavior and flexion neuron firing patterns. *J. Neurophysiol.* 47, 60–74.

Jonas, P., Bischofberger, J., Fricker, D., and Miles, R. (2004). Interneuron diversity series: fast in, fast out – temporal and spatial signal processing in hippocampal interneurons. *Trends Neurosci.* 27, 30–40.

Katz, P. S. (1996). Neurons, networks, and motor behavior. *Neuron* 16, 245–253.

Kriegel, H.-P., Kröger, P., Sander, J., and Zimek, A. (2011). Density-based clustering. *Wiley Interdiscip. Rev. Data Min. Knowl. Discov.* 1, 231–240.

Kriegel, H.-P., Kröger, P., Schubert, E., and Zimek, A. (2008). "A general framework for increasing the robustness of PCA-based correlation clustering algorithms," in *Scientific and Statistical Database Management,* eds B. Ludäscher and N. Mamoulis (Berlin: Springer), 418–435.

Kristan, W. B. Jr., Calabrese, R. L., and Friesen, W. O. (2005). Neuronal control of leech behavior. *Prog. Neurobiol.* 76, 279–327.

Marder, E., and Bucher, D. (2001). Central pattern generators and the control of rhythmic movements. *Curr. Biol.* 11, R986–R996.

Marder, E., and Bucher, D. (2007). Understanding circuit dynamics using the stomatogastric nervous system of lobsters and crabs. *Annu. Rev. Physiol.* 69, 291–316.

Marder, E., and Calabrese, R. L. (1996). Principles of rhythmic motor pattern generation. *Physiol. Rev.* 76, 687–717.

Meyrand, P., Simmers, J., and Moulins, M. (1991). Construction of a pattern-generating circuit with neurons of different networks. *Nature* 351, 60–63.

Miller, J. P., and Selverston, A. I. (1982a). Mechanisms underlying pattern generation in lobster stomatogastric ganglion as determined by selective inactivation of identified neurons. II. Oscillatory properties of pyloric neurons. *J. Neurophysiol.* 48, 1378–1391.

Miller, J. P., and Selverston, A. I. (1982b). Mechanisms underlying pattern generation in lobster stomatogastric ganglion as determined by selective inactivation of identified neurons. IV. Network properties of pyloric system. *J. Neurophysiol.* 48, 1416–1432.

Miller, M. N., Okaty, B. W., and Nelson, S. B. (2008). Region-specific spike-frequency acceleration in layer 5 pyramidal neurons mediated by Kv1 subunits. *J. Neurosci.* 28, 13716–13726.

Morris, C., and Lecar, H. (1981). Voltage oscillations in the barnacle giant muscle fiber. *Biophys. J.* 35, 193–213.

Mulloney, B., and Selverston, A. I. (1974a). Organization of the stomatogastric ganglion in the spiny lobster. I. Neurons driving the lateral teeth. *J. Comp. Physiol.* 91, 1–32.

Mulloney, B., and Selverston, A. I. (1974b). Organization of the stomatogastric ganglion in the spiny lobster. III. Coordination of the two subsets of the gastric system. *J. Comp. Physiol.* 91, 53–78.

Okaty, B. W., Sugino, K., and Nelson, S. B. (2011a). Cell type-specific transcriptomics in the brain. *J. Neurosci.* 31, 6939–6943.

Okaty, B. W., Sugino, K., and Nelson, S. B. (2011b). A quantitative comparison of cell-type-specific microarray gene expression profiling methods in the mouse brain. *PLoS ONE* 6, e16493. doi:10.1371/journal.pone.0016493

Pearson, K. G., Reye, D. N., Parsons, D. W., and Bicker, G. (1985). Flight-initiating interneurons in the locust. *J. Neurophysiol.* 53, 910–925.

Pei, T., Zhu, A. X., Zhou, C., Li, B., and Qin, C. (2009). Detecting feature from spatial point processes using collective nearest neighbor. *Comput. Environ. Urban Syst.* 33, 435–447.

Perrins, R., and Weiss, K. R. (1996). A cerebral central pattern generator in *Aplysia* and its connections with buccal feeding circuitry. *J. Neurosci.* 16, 7030–7045.

Sander, J., Ester, M., Kriegel, H.-P., and Xu, X. (1998). Density-based clustering in spatial databases: the algorithm GDBSCAN and its applications. *Data Min. Knowl. Discov.* 2, 169–194.

Sasaki, K., Due, M. R., Jing, J., and Weiss, K. R. (2007). Feeding CPG in *Aplysia* directly controls two distinct outputs of a compartmentalized interneuron that functions as a CPG element. *J. Neurophysiol.* 98, 3796–3801.

Schmidt, J., Fischer, H., and Buschges, A. (2001). Pattern generation for walking and searching movements of a stick insect leg. II. Control of motoneuronal activity. *J. Neurophysiol.* 85, 354–361.

Schulz, D. J., Goaillard, J. M., and Marder, E. (2006). Variable channel expression in identified single and electrically coupled neurons in different animals. *Nat. Neurosci.* 9, 356–362.

Schulz, D. J., Goaillard, J. M., and Marder, E. E. (2007). Quantitative expression profiling of identified neurons reveals cell-specific constraints on highly variable levels of gene expression. *Proc. Natl. Acad. Sci. U.S.A.* 104, 13187–13191.

Selverston, A. I., and Miller, J. P. (1980). Mechanisms underlying pattern generation in the lobster stomatogastric ganglion as determined by selective inactivation of identified neurons. I. Pyloric neurons. *J. Neurophysiol.* 44, 1102–1121.

Selverston, A. I., Russell, D. F., Miller, J. P., and King, D. G. (1976). The stomatogastric nervous system: structure and function of a small neural network. *Prog. Neurobiol.* 7, 215–290.

Sharp, A. A., Skinner, F. K., and Marder, E. (1996). Mechanisms of oscillation in dynamic clamp constructed two-cell half-center circuits. *J. Neurophysiol.* 76, 867–883.

Sugino, K., Hempel, C. M., Miller, M. N., Hattox, A. M., Shapiro, P., Wu, C., Huang, Z. J., and Nelson, S. B. (2006). Molecular taxonomy of major neuronal classes in the adult mouse forebrain. *Nat. Neurosci.* 9, 99–107.

Swensen, A. M., and Bean, B. P. (2005). Robustness of burst firing in dissociated Purkinje neurons with acute or long-term reductions in sodium conductance. *J. Neurosci.* 25, 3509–3520.

Taylor, A. L., Hickey, T. J., Prinz, A. A., and Marder, E. (2006). Structure and visualization of high-dimensional conductance spaces. *J. Neurophysiol.* 96, 891–905.

Tobin, A. E., Cruz-Bermudez, N. D., Marder, E., and Schulz, D. J. (2009). Correlations in ion channel mRNA in rhythmically active neurons. *PLoS ONE* 4, e6742. doi:10.1371/journal.pone.0006742

Toledo-Rodriguez, M., and Markram, H. (2007). Single-cell RT-PCR, a technique to decipher the electrical, anatomical, and genetic determinants of neuronal diversity. *Methods Mol. Biol.* 403, 123–139.

Vinh, N. X., Epps, J., and Bailey, J. (2009). "Information theoretic measures for clusterings comparison: is a correction for chance necessary?" in *Proceedings of the 26th Annual International Conference on Machine Learning* (Montreal, QC: ACM), 1073–1080.

Weimann, J. M., and Marder, E. (1994). Switching neurons are integral members of multiple oscillatory networks. *Curr. Biol.* 4, 896–902.

Weimann, J. M., Meyrand, P., and Marder, E. (1991). Neurons that form multiple pattern generators: identification and multiple activity patterns of gastric/pyloric neurons in the crab stomatogastric system. *J. Neurophysiol.* 65, 111–122.

Wienecke, J., Westerdahl, A. C., Hultborn, H., Kiehn, O., and Ryge, J. (2010). Global gene expression analysis of rodent motor neurons following spinal cord injury associates molecular mechanisms with development of postinjury spasticity. *J. Neurophysiol.* 103, 761–778.

William, C. M., Tanabe, Y., and Jessell, T. M. (2003). Regulation of motor neuron subtype identity by repressor activity of Mnx class homeodomain proteins. *Development* 130, 1523–1536.

Zagoraiou, L., Akay, T., Martin, J. F., Brownstone, R. M., Jessell, T. M., and Miles, G. B. (2009). A cluster of cholinergic premotor interneurons modulates mouse locomotor activity. *Neuron* 64, 645–662.

6

Real-time system for studies of the effects of acoustic feedback on animal vocalizations

Mike Skocik[1] and Alexay Kozhevnikov[1,2]*

[1] Department of Physics, Pennsylvania State University, University Park, PA, USA
[2] Department of Psychology, Pennsylvania State University, University Park, PA, USA

Edited by:
Ahmed El Hady, Max Planck Institute for Dynamics and Self Organization, Germany

Reviewed by:
Ahmed El Hady, Max Planck Institute for Dynamics and Self Organization, Germany
Noah Cowan, Johns Hopkins University, USA

***Correspondence:**
Alexay Kozhevnikov, Department of Physics, Pennsylvania State University, University Park, PA, USA. Department of Psychology, Pennsylvania State University, University Park, PA, USA.
e-mail: akozhevn@phys.psu.edu

Studies of behavioral and neural responses to distorted auditory feedback (DAF) can help shed light on the neural mechanisms of animal vocalizations. We describe an apparatus for generating real-time acoustic feedback. The system can very rapidly detect acoustic features in a song and output acoustic signals if the detected features match the desired acoustic template. The system uses spectrogram-based detection of acoustic elements. It is low-cost and can be programmed for a variety of behavioral experiments requiring acoustic feedback or neural stimulation. We use the system to study the effects of acoustic feedback on birds' vocalizations and demonstrate that such an acoustic feedback can cause both immediate and long-term changes to birds' songs.

Keywords: acoustic feedback, animal vocalizations, behavioral neuroscience, sensory feedback, real-time data processing

INTRODUCTION

Distorted auditory feedback (DAF) is used for assessing the effects of auditory input on vocal production. Presenting DAF and assessing its effects on the song and on the neural activity have been used in songbirds to study the mechanisms of song production and learning (Leonardo and Konishi, 1999; Sakata and Brainard, 2006; Andalman and Fee, 2009; Keller and Hahnloser, 2009; Tschida and Mooney, 2012). Human speech is sensitive to certain types of DAF (Lee, 1950; Houde and Jordan, 1998), and DAF is used to study speech mechanisms. It is often desirable to have real-time DAF, i.e., to rapidly (in a few milliseconds or faster) detect the occurrence of specific acoustic elements in vocalization and present an auditory stimulus once the target acoustic element is detected.

In this paper, we describe an automated system for real-time DAF and demonstrate its use to study both the immediate and the long-term effects of DAF on the song of Bengalese finches. The system uses open-source software and, therefore, is extremely flexible and customizable by the user. It has a significantly lower cost than commercial systems.

Songbirds use auditory feedback to learn to sing when they are young and to maintain their songs in adulthood (Konishi, 1965; Brainard and Doupe, 2000). Long-term exposure to DAF has been shown to cause song degradation in songbirds (Okanoya and Yamaguchi, 1997; Woolley and Rubel, 1997; Leonardo and Konishi, 1999). Some bird species' songs exhibit immediate sensitivity to acoustic input. For these birds, DAF can have an immediate effect on the timing and acoustic structure of the song (Sakata and Brainard, 2006). Analyzing the effects of DAF can yield new understanding of the neural organization of the song and the mechanisms of song learning (Brainard and Doupe, 2000). To study the questions about the effects of time-localized DAF on birdsong, it is important to be able to deliver DAF with high temporal precision in relation to vocalization. To do this, it is necessary to rapidly and reliably detect the specific acoustic elements of the bird's song and, after detection of the acoustic element, generate an acoustic output.

It is a challenging technical task for an acoustic feedback system to be real-time. Real-time performance is most easily achieved with analog systems (Cynx and Von Rad, 2001), but digital systems offer significant advantages in terms of convenience and flexibility. However, the advantages of a digital system are accompanied by the difficulties of making a digital system have small and constant processing delays. The system has to perform analog-to-digital conversion, fast analysis of the recently acquired data and digital-to-analog conversion, and these operations have to take place with reliable timing and concurrently with saving the acquired data. Custom-made DAF systems have been developed and used in behavioral studies (Leonardo and Konishi, 1999; Kao et al., 2005), but their real-time processing characteristics have not been reported. Oftentimes, custom-made systems have significant and not well-controlled delays, especially for systems based on PC's running Windows. Commercial systems for real-time acoustic processing are available but are expensive.

We developed a real-time DAF system based on a PC running Linux and the Real-Time eXperiment Interface (RTXI) software (Lin et al., 2010) and a National Instruments A/D card. The system is low-cost (the cost is only the cost of the hardware, the software is free). The system is capable of A/D bandwidth of over 30 kHz with real-time processing of acoustic signals.

METHODS

A PC with an Intel i7 six-core processor (2.66 GHz) and 4 GB or RAM running Ubuntu Linux 2.6.29.4-rtai with RTXI version 1.1.2 and a National Instruments PCIe-6251 A/D card is used. The A/D card receives audio input from a microphone (AudioTechnika PRO-44, used with Behringer Shark DSP110 microphone amplifier). The output is sent to a speaker amplifier (SLA-1, Applied Research and Technology); the output of the amplifier is connected to a speaker.

The Data Recorder software within RTXI is custom modified. The simplified diagram of signal processing is shown in **Figure 1**. The system has two modes of operation—a non-triggered (idle) mode and a triggered (active) mode. At the core of the modified software is the circular buffer that takes data points one-by-one from the data acquisition engine once they become available. In the non-triggered mode [**Figure 1 (top)**], the system continuously (every 1 ms) computes the rms of the last 10 ms of the input signal. If the signal rms exceeds the threshold, the system is switched into triggered mode.

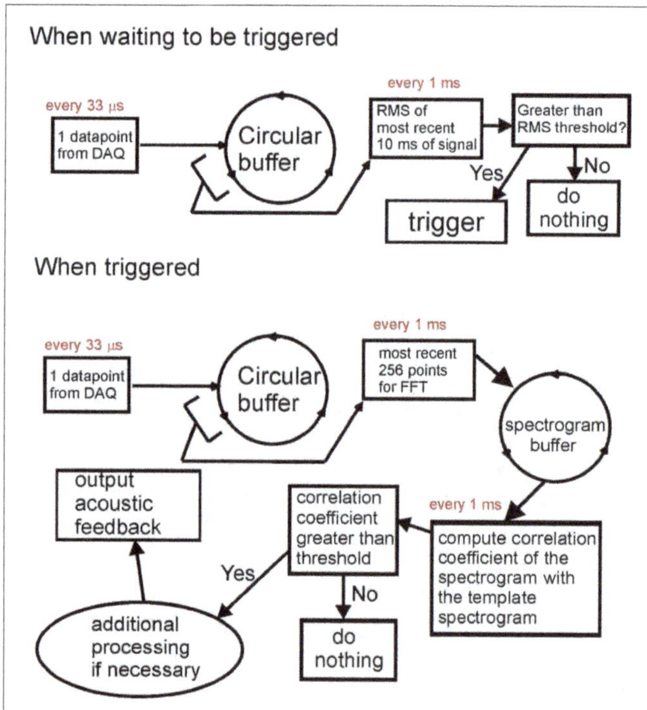

FIGURE 1 | Block diagram of the acoustic feedback system. When not triggered **(top)**, the system computes the rms of the input signal. When the rms exceeds the threshold, the system is triggered. When triggered **(bottom)**, the system computes the spectrogram of the most recent 20 ms of signal and computes the correlation coefficient of this spectrogram with the spectrogram of the template sound (e.g., song syllable). The template sound is detected when the correlation coefficient exceeds a threshold value; in this case, acoustic feedback can be generated. Both the input and the acoustic output are saved to the computer hard drive.

In triggered mode, the system does real-time processing of auditory data. In **Figure 1 (bottom)**, we show the processing done for recognizing the song syllable of a Bengalese finch. The FFT of the past 256 data points (~8.4 ms) is computed every 1 ms and stored in an FFT circular buffer. Every 1 ms, the spectrogram of the most recent 40 ms of the input signal is obtained from the FFT circular buffer. A correlation coefficient between the input signal spectrogram and the spectrogram of the template is computed. If the correlation coefficient exceeds the threshold, the system detects the occurrence of the target song syllable, and acoustic feedback can be generated, or further processing can be done. While generating acoustic feedback, the system keeps going through all of the above steps, but is disallowed from registering another detection to prevent it from triggering on its own output.

The presence of the data circular buffer allows very fast access to chunks of the most recent data for processing without affecting the timing of the data acquisition process. The FFT circular buffer also allows extremely fast computations of the spectrograms of the sound (computing the spectrogram is a computationally-intensive task). This enables the system to recognize complex vocal elements based on their spectrogram (e.g., frequency sweeps) without compromising the timing. While triggered, every 1 s, the system computes the rms of the previous 200 ms of the input signal to check if the acoustic input is still present. If the rms is below a threshold (no signal), the system goes into the idle mode. While triggered, the system continually saves all the data acquired in a separate array and saves the data to the hard drive once it is switched back to idle mode. A more detailed description of this system, along with the source code, is available at http://www.phys.psu.edu/~akozhevn/ac_feedback/.

RESULTS

We tested the performance of our DAF system in several tasks which are often needed in behavioral experiments using acoustic feedback. We also used the system to assess the effects of acoustic feedback on the song of Bengalese finch. All animal procedures were carried out in accordance with the locally approved IACUC protocol.

DELAY BETWEEN INPUT AND OUTPUT TEST

A simple task is generating acoustic feedback when the input level exceeds a certain threshold. Although this task may be too simple for most behavioral experiments, the delay in the system between detecting the crossing of the threshold and producing the output is a useful figure for indicating how fast the system can be when it is solely converting A/D and D/A and saving data without any complex data processing.

The system was programmed so that, once the input exceeded a fixed threshold, the acquired input signal was sent to the D/A output with no extra processing. A square wave with the amplitude exceeding the threshold was applied to the input; the delay between the input and the output was measured with the digital oscilloscope. The measured delay between the output and the input was $27 \pm 9\,\mu s$ (mean ± SD, min = $9\,\mu s$, max = $43\,\mu s$). The sample rate was 30.3 kHz, so the observed delays corresponded to a delay of 1 data point between the input and the output.

The observed variations of the delay are due to the difference in timing between the external input signal and the timing of the A/D events. In all cases, however, the delay between the input and the output does not exceed 1 datapoint. Therefore, the system has real-time capability.

DETECTION OF SPECIFIC VOCAL ELEMENTS IN THE BIRD'S SONG

A typical task in experiments using acoustic feedback is detection of a certain "template" sound. The template can be either a sound of a certain frequency or a more complex combination of frequencies, frequency sweeps, etc. Once the template is detected, the acoustic feedback can be played back to the animal. This task is computationally intensive because one needs to compute the characteristics of the recently acquired input signal, then compare these with the characteristics of the template and, if the input is sufficiently similar to the template, decide that the detection has occurred and generate acoustic output. The computation has to be done fast enough to enable real-time performance and not interfere with the data acquisition process.

Common techniques that have been used for detecting acoustic elements are spectrogram-based techniques (Leonardo and Fee, 2005) and feature-based techniques (Tchernichovski et al., 2000). In a spectrogram-based approach, the spectrogram of the recently acquired signal is computed and compared to the template spectrogram. A common way to accomplish this is to compute the correlation coefficient between the two spectrograms. Detection of the template sound occurs if the correlation coefficient exceeds a threshold value.

We tested the performance of the system for detection of specific syllables in the song of a Bengalese finch. The Bengalese finch song consists of a sequence of syllables separated by silences (inter-syllable gaps) (**Figure 2**). The acoustic structure of the song syllables is fairly stable; the main source of variability from one song to another is the sequence of syllables in each song (Honda and Okanoya, 1999).

To detect a specific song syllable, the system continuously computes the correlation coefficient of the spectrogram of the most recent 20 ms segment of the acquired signal with the spectrogram of a 20-ms syllable template (see Methods, **Figure 1**). The target syllable is detected by the system when the correlation coefficient exceeds the threshold value of 0.8. The value of the threshold was chosen by examining the target syllable detections by the DAF system in a set of about 20 songs and comparing the detected syllable occurrences with the actual occurrences of the target syllables determined by visual examination of the song spectrograms. If the threshold is set too high, the probability of missing the target syllable increases. Setting the threshold too low increases the probability of false positive detections. After the syllable detection, acoustic feedback (either white noise or the song syllable) can be played back to the bird.

Typical performance of the system on the real-time syllable recognition task is shown in **Figure 2**. The top spectrogram shows "detection only" mode—the system detects the target syllable in real time, but no playback is generated. The bottom spectrogram shows detection and playback generation—after detecting the target syllable, the system plays back another song syllable

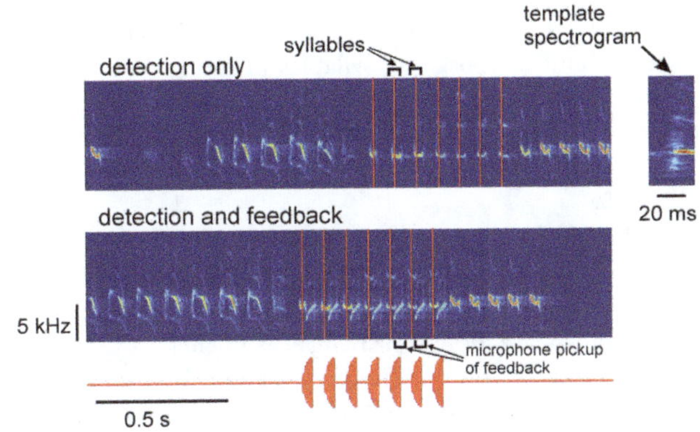

FIGURE 2 | Top: spectrogram of the song of a Bengalese finch and the times of occurrence of one of the song syllables. The system was programmed to only detect the occurrences of the target syllable in real time, no acoustic feedback was generated. The detection times are shown as vertical red lines. **Bottom:** the system is detecting the target syllables (vertical red lines) and is generating acoustic feedback after detection. The acoustic feedback waveform is shown below. The feedback signal is one of the birdsong syllables; the acoustic feedback pickup by the microphone is visible on the spectrogram. The zoomed-in spectrogram of the template is shown on the right.

to the bird. The vertical red lines indicate the detection times of the target syllable. The zoomed-in spectrogram of the template is shown on the right. The template contains part of the inter-syllable interval and the first 20 ms of the target syllable, so the end of the template (detection time) is approximately in the middle of the 40-ms long syllable.

Performance of the system was checked by comparing the results of automatic detections of the system with the manual identification of the target song syllables carried out by off-line examination of the spectrograms. Out of 659 target syllables, 610 were correctly detected and 49 were missed. There were zero false positives. Thus, the system shows robust performance with the real-time syllable recognition task; over 92% of the target syllables were correctly identified.

This demonstrates that the system is capable of real-time detection of target syllables in the song. Note that the syllables occurring after the target syllables in **Figure 2** are frequency sweeps that overlap with the template's frequencies. The system discriminates them from the target syllables because they have a different frequency profile. Such discrimination is an advantage of the spectrogram-based detection; this would not be possible if only instantaneous frequencies were detected.

Additionally, we tested the system on the detection of syllables in the song of a zebra finch—another bird species. We used our dataset of zebra finch songs with known syllable sequences obtained in a previous study (Kozhevnikov and Fee, 2007). Zebra finch songs were played back through the speaker, and the results of the real-time detection by our DAF system were compared to the known occurrences of the target syllable.

A small subset of songs (10 songs) was used as a test set: the threshold value for the syllable detection was adjusted to optimize the percentage of correctly detected syllables in this small test set. After this, the threshold kept was fixed, and the performance of the system was tested on the whole dataset (about 100 songs). Out of 756 target syllables in the dataset, 728 were correctly detected, 28 were missed; there were 4 false positives. The system correctly detected over 96% of the target syllables in the dataset; the probability of a false positive detection was less than 1%.

EFFECTS OF AUDITORY FEEDBACK ON THE TIMING OF THE BIRDSONG

Auditory feedback has been shown to have immediate effects on some animal vocalizations. For Bengalese finches, DAF has been shown to affect the timing of song syllables. DAF played after the song syllable increases the time interval between that syllable and the next syllable in the song (Sakata and Brainard, 2006). We tested whether our feedback system is effective in causing real-time changes to the Bengalese finch song. The system was programmed to detect one of the song syllables and, once the syllable was detected, to play back the same song syllable with a probability of 0.05. This ensured that the feedback was sufficiently sparse so almost in all cases there was only one playback during each song. The feedback and control trials were randomly interleaved. This simplified the analysis of the syllable timing and eliminated any confounding effects from playbacks being too close to one another. The delay between the syllable sung by the bird and the syllable playback was 40 ms.

The playback causes some pickup on the input channel, which can cause difficulties in precise determination of the timing of the syllable that is occurring during the playback. Therefore, the time interval between the target syllable and the following syllable (which is partially overlapped with playback) was computed as one half of the difference between the detection time of the target syllable and the detection time of the second syllable after the target syllable. The same procedure was performed in control trials to ensure consistency in data analysis. Since the distributions of time intervals may not be Gaussian, we use a non-parametric statistical test—two-way Kolmogorov–Smirnov test—to assess the statistical significance of DAF effects on the song timing.

Figure 3 shows the distributions of the time intervals between the target syllable and the following syllable when the feedback is present (blue histogram) and when there is no feedback (red histogram). The widths of the distributions are due to the natural variability of the song timing. In the presence of feedback, the time intervals between the syllables become longer. Without DAF, the mean interval is 74.8 ms ($N = 637$ syllables); in the presence of DAF, the mean interval is 75.7 ms ($N = 97$ syllables). Although the change of the mean duration is small compared to the widths of the distributions, the effect is highly statistically significant ($p = 0.001$, two-way Kolmogorov–Smirnov test). The observed lengthening of the time interval between the song syllables is consistent with previous observations (Sakata and Brainard, 2006). Thus, our acoustic feedback has an immediate effect on the song: DAF immediately and reversibly affects song timing.

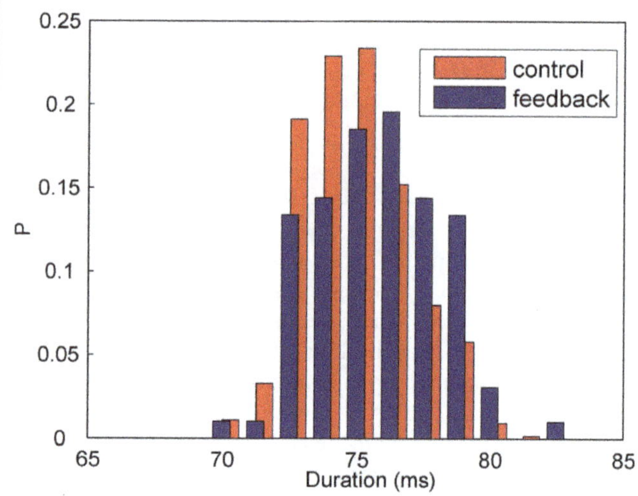

FIGURE 3 | DAF increases the duration of the time interval between Bengalese finch song syllables. Shown above are the histograms of the time intervals between two subsequent syllables in the song in the presence of DAF (blue) and without DAF (red). The means are: $\Delta t_{mean} = 74.8$ ms (control, $N = 637$ syllables) and $\Delta t_{mean} = 75.7$ ms (feedback, $N = 97$ syllables), the difference is statistically significant ($p = 0.001$, two-way Kolmogorov–Smirnov test).

LONG-TERM EFFECTS OF DAF ON ACOUSTIC STRUCTURE OF THE SONG

DAF has been shown to cause long-term changes to animal vocalizations. For songbirds, prolonged repeated presentation of DAF can cause gradual change of the song (Leonardo and Konishi, 1999; Warren et al., 2011). We tested out system on the task of causing long-term changes of the frequency of one of the song syllables.

The system is programmed to detect the fundamental frequency of one of the song syllables. After the target song syllable is detected, the temporal profile of the pitch (defined as the largest peak in the FFT of the latest 256 points) was computed. The lowest value in the pitch profile in the time window between 3 and 12 ms after the detection time was taken to be the pitch of the syllable. The feedback (white noise) is conditional on the detected pitch of the song syllable. For example, the feedback can be generated if the detected syllable pitch is smaller than a threshold value. Continuous exposure to such feedback has been shown to cause the bird to gradually shift the mean pitch of the syllable so that the feedback is generated less often—the bird adapts its song to avoid hearing DAF (Warren et al., 2011).

We tested whether such conditional DAF could shift the mean syllable pitch in both directions. **Figure 4** shows the long-term effects of DAF which is conditional on the syllable pitch. During days 1–6, the feedback was played back if the pitch was less than 3530 Hz; during days 7–12, the feedback was played back if the pitch was greater than 3530 Hz; during days 13–18, the feedback was played back if the pitch was less than 3510 Hz.

Our feedback is effective in causing gradual changes in the syllable pitch. Playing back DAF when the frequency is lower than the threshold value causes an upward drift of the mean pitch (days 1–6 and 13–18). Presenting feedback when the pitch is higher than the threshold causes a downward drift in pitch (days 7–12). This shows that the system is suitable for studies of long-term effects of DAF on animal vocalizations.

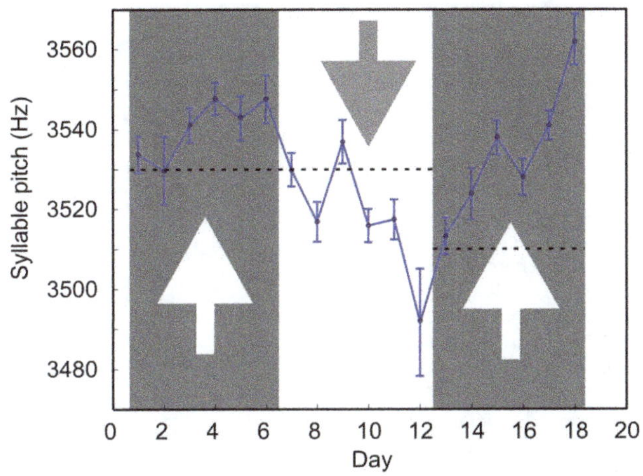

FIGURE 4 | Prolonged exposure of the bird to DAF causes gradual changes in the song. The mean pitch of one of the target song syllable was manipulated by feedback conditional on pitch. Each datapoint is the pitch of the target syllable averaged over all the renditions of the target syllable sung by the bird on a given day. The number of renditions varies from day to day (mean = 208, min = 126, max = 288). Error bars are s.e.m. Dashed lines are the values of the threshold. Arrows indicate the direction in which the syllable frequency was expected to change in response to DAF. Larger error bars on day 12 are mostly due to the smallest number of target syllable renditions ($n = 126$) sung on that day.

DISCUSSION

The described real-time acoustic feedback system is a versatile tool for studies of the effects of auditory feedback on ongoing animal vocalization. The advantage of the system is the flexibility of the processing than can be realized. The circular buffer allows real-time acquisition of arbitrary-length segments of the most recent data without affecting the timing of data acquisition. In addition, having a separate FFT buffer facilitates real-time spectral processing of acquired signals. This feature enables a very quick creation of the spectrograms of long (tens or even hundreds of milliseconds) segments of signals at a high rate (the spectrogram is updated every 1 ms).

This capability is very useful for the detection of complex vocal signals. Often, it is not just a certain frequency that needs to be detected, but rather a certain spectrogram pattern, like multiple frequencies or the frequency sweeps frequently seen in birdsong syllables. Since the same frequency can occur in many syllables, it is the whole pattern of the spectrogram that allows real-time detection of the syllable. Our system is very well-suited for rapid spectrogram-based detection of acoustic elements.

The performance of the system will vary depending on the type of animal vocalization and the nature of the acoustic element being detected for two main reasons. First, there is always a natural variability in the acoustic structure of a vocal element, and the degree of this variability may be different for different vocal elements; this will affect the reliability of detection. For example, a birdsong syllable can possess a more or less stereotyped spectrogram; the detection will be easier for a more stereotypical song syllable. Second, a given vocal element can be more or less similar in its acoustic structure to other vocal elements; reliable detection of a target vocal element will be easier if it is spectrally more dissimilar to other vocal elements. To achieve optimum performance, adjustments to the threshold or detection algorithm may be needed; thus, it is important to have a highly customizable system.

It is worth mentioning that, when the song syllables are detected, data processing is not a time-limiting step, and significantly more complex processing can be done without decreasing the A/D rate. We tested the system with longer templates (60 and 100 ms); they did not affect performance. We also tested the simultaneous detection of two templates, so that, every 1 ms, the system computed the correlation coefficient of the sound spectrogram with two template spectrograms, and that also did not affect the A/D rate. For a template 60 ms long, the computation of the correlation coefficient takes 16 μs; this time scales linearly with the length of the template. The computation of the FFT (to fill the column in the spectrogram buffer) takes 7–8 μs. FFT and correlation coefficient computations are the slowest signal processing steps; all other steps combined take less than 1 μs. Thus—If the spectrogram update rate is kept at 1 ms—the system should be capable of simultaneously detecting of over 10 different song syllables. Therefore, fairly complex real-time analysis and detection of multiple vocal elements can be done without compromising the speed of the system.

The system is usually used with 1 output channel and 2 input channels (one input channel for acoustic input and one channel for recording the actual output of the A/D card). It is possible to increase the number of input channels. This way, one could use the data recording capability of the system to collect physiological data (e.g., EEG or neural) during acoustic feedback experiments. However, the process limiting the speed of the system appears to be reading the data from the A/D card and sending the data to the D/A. Thus, increasing the number of channels will slow the system down and decrease the A/D rate. We tested the performance of the system with 3 input channels and 1 output channel. To achieve stable operation, the A/D rate had to be decreased to 20 kHz. Despite this decrease, this is an acceptable rate for many experiments where acoustic and electrophysiological data have to be collected.

Finally, the real-time processing capabilities of the system could be used for neural feedback experiments. The spectrogram-based signal processing capability can be useful for the detection of neural oscillations. The output can be used for targeted microstimulation. The described auditory feedback system is a flexible low-cost tool for behavioral neuroscience research.

ACKNOWLEDGMENTS

The authors wish to acknowledge Ryan Wendt for his contribution to the initial stages of the acoustic system development and Jonathan Bettencourt and John White for their expert advice on RTXI capabilities and installation. This work was supported by NSF Grant 0827731 and the NSF Research Experience for Undergraduates program at the Pennsylvania State University.

REFERENCES

Andalman, A. S., and Fee, M. S. (2009). A basal ganglia-forebrain circuit in the songbird biases motor output to avoid vocal errors. *Proc. Natl. Acad. Sci. U.S.A.* 106, 12518–12523.

Brainard, M. S., and Doupe, A. J. (2000). Auditory feedback in learning and maintenance of vocal behaviour. *Nat. Rev. Neurosci.* 1, 31–40.

Cynx, J., and Von Rad, U. (2001). Immediate and transitory effects of delayed auditory feedback on bird song production. *Anim. Behav.* 62, 305–312.

Honda, E., and Okanoya, K. (1999). Acoustical and syntactical comparisons between songs of the white-backed munia *(Lonchura striata)* and its domesticated strain, the Bengalese finch *(Lonchura striata var. domestica)*. *Zoolog. Sci.* 16, 319–326.

Houde, J. F., and Jordan, M. I. (1998). Sensorimotor adaptation in speech production. *Science* 279, 1213–1216.

Kao, M. H., Doupe, A. J., and Brainard, M. S. (2005). Contributions of an avian basal ganglia – forebrain circuit to real-time modulation of song. *Nature* 433, 638–643.

Keller, G. B., and Hahnloser, R. H. R. (2009). Neural processing of auditory feedback during vocal practice in a songbird. *Nature* 457, 187–190.

Konishi, M. (1965). The role of auditory feedback in the control of vocalizations in the white-crowned sparrow. *Z. Tierpsychol.* 22, 770–783.

Kozhevnikov, A. A., and Fee, M. S. (2007). Singing-related activity of identified HVC neurons in the Zebra Finch. *J. Neurophysiol.* 97, 4271–4283.

Lee, B. S. (1950). Effects of delayed speech feedback. *J. Acoust. Soc. Am.* 22, 824–826.

Leonardo, A., and Fee, M. S. (2005). Ensemble coding of vocal control in birdsong. *J. Neurosci.* 25, 652–661.

Leonardo, A., and Konishi, M. (1999). Decrystallization of adult birdsong by perturbation of auditory feedback. *Nature* 399, 466–470.

Lin, R. J., Bettencourt, J., White, J. A., Christini, D. J., and Butera, R. J. (2010). "Real-time experiment interface for biological control applications," in *2010 Annual International Conference of the IEEE Engineering in Medicine and Biology Society (EMBC)* (Buenos Aires, Argentina), 4160–4163.

Okanoya, K., and Yamaguchi, A. (1997). Adult Bengalese finches (Lonchura striata var. domestica) require real-time auditory feedback to produce normal song syntax. *J. Neurobiol.* 33, 343–356.

Sakata, J. T., and Brainard, M. S. (2006). Real-time contributions of auditory feedback to avian vocal motor control. *J. Neurosci.* 26, 9619–9628.

Tchernichovski, O., Nottebohm, F., Ho, C. E., Pesaran, B., and Mitra, P. P. (2000). A procedure for an automated measurement of song similarity. *Anim. Behav.* 59, 1167–1176.

Tschida, K., and Mooney, R. (2012). The role of auditory feedback in vocal learning and maintenance. *Curr. Opin. Neurobiol.* 22, 320–327.

Warren, T. L., Tumer, E. C., Charlesworth, J. D., and Brainard, M. S. (2011). Mechanisms and time course of vocal learning and consolidation in the adult songbird. *J. Neurophysiol.* 106, 1806–1821.

Woolley, S. M. N., and Rubel, E. W. (1997). Bengalese finches *Lonchura striata domestica* depend upon auditory feedback for the maintenance of adult song. *J. Neurosci.* 17, 6380–6390.

7

Decreased Hering–Breuer input-output entrainment in a mouse model of Rett syndrome

Rishi R. Dhingra[1,2], Yenan Zhu[2,3], Frank J. Jacono[1,4], David M. Katz[2], Roberto F. Galán[2,3] and Thomas E. Dick[1]*

[1] *Division of Pulmonary, Critical Care and Sleep Medicine, Department of Medicine, Case Western Reserve University, Cleveland, OH, USA*
[2] *Department of Neurosciences, Case Western Reserve University, Cleveland, OH, USA*
[3] *Systems Biology and Bioinformatics Program, Case Western Reserve University, Cleveland, OH, USA*
[4] *Louis Stokes Veterans Affairs Medical Center, Case Western Reserve University, Cleveland, OH, USA*

Edited by:
Ahmed El Hady, Max Planck Institute for Dynamics and Self Organization, Germany

Reviewed by:
Mathias Dutschmann, Florey Neuroscience Institutes, Australia
Donald R. McCrimmon, Northwestern University Feinberg School of Medicine, USA
Angelina Y. Fong, Macquarie University, Australia

Correspondence:
Thomas E. Dick, Division of Pulmonary, Critical Care and Sleep Medicine, Department of Medicine, Case Western Reserve University, 10900 Euclid Avenue, Cleveland, OH 44106, USA.
e-mail: thomas.dick@cwru.edu

Rett syndrome, a severe X-linked neurodevelopmental disorder caused by mutations in the gene encoding methyl-CpG-binding protein 2 (*Mecp2*), is associated with a highly irregular respiratory pattern including severe upper-airway dysfunction. Recent work suggests that hyperexcitability of the Hering–Breuer reflex (HBR) pathway contributes to respiratory dysrhythmia in *Mecp2* mutant mice. To assess how enhanced HBR input impacts respiratory entrainment by sensory afferents in closed-loop *in vivo*-like conditions, we investigated the input (vagal stimulus trains) – output (phrenic bursting) entrainment *via* the HBR in wild-type and MeCP2-deficient mice. Using the *in situ* perfused brainstem preparation, which maintains an intact pontomedullary axis capable of generating an *in vivo*-like respiratory rhythm in the absence of the HBR, we mimicked the HBR feedback input by stimulating the vagus nerve (at threshold current, 0.5 ms pulse duration, 75 Hz pulse frequency, 100 ms train duration) at an inter-burst frequency matching that of the intrinsic oscillation of the inspiratory motor output of each preparation. Using this approach, we observed significant input-output entrainment in wild-type mice as measured by the maximum of the cross-correlation function, the peak of the instantaneous relative phase distribution, and the mutual information of the instantaneous phases. This entrainment was associated with a reduction in inspiratory duration during feedback stimulation. In contrast, the strength of input-output entrainment was significantly weaker in *Mecp2*$^{-/+}$ mice. However, *Mecp2*$^{-/+}$ mice also had a reduced inspiratory duration during stimulation, indicating that reflex behavior in the HBR pathway was intact. Together, these observations suggest that the respiratory network compensates for enhanced sensitivity of HBR inputs by reducing HBR input-output entrainment.

Keywords: closed-loop, entrainment, vagus, Hering–Breuer reflex, *Mecp2*

INTRODUCTION

Rett syndrome is caused by loss of MeCP2 function and is associated with an increase in respiratory pattern irregularity characterized by periods of forceful breathing (hyperventilation), breathing pauses, and abnormal cardiorespiratory coupling, as well as increased mean respiratory frequency (Weese-Mayer et al., 2006; Katz et al., 2012). MeCP2-deficient mice have a similar irregular breathing phenotype including increased mean respiratory frequency, increased variability in frequency, and increased frequency of apneas of both central and obstructive types (Katz et al., 2009; Voituron et al., 2010). The intrinsic neuronal mechanisms associated with these breathing alterations include widespread hyperexcitability in several respiratory areas of the brainstem including the nucleus tractus solitarius (nTS, Kline et al., 2010; Kron et al., 2012), Kölliker–Fuse nuclei (KFn, Stettner et al., 2007), locus coeruleus (Taneja et al., 2009), and ventrolateral medulla (Medrihan et al., 2008). Accordingly, therapies targeted at reducing neuronal hyperexcitability are effective in reducing the frequency of central apnea in mice (Abdala et al., 2010).

At the network level, MeCP2-deficiency leads to exaggerated post-inspiratory (PI) activity in vagal nerve recordings whose efferent fibers innervate the upper-airway (Stettner et al., 2007). The PI motor pattern is controlled by peripheral and pontine drives (See **Figure 1A**). Activation of pulmonary stretch receptor (PSR) inputs, located in the airways and lungs, send feedback encoding lung volume to the respiratory network via the vagal nerves to inhibit inspiration and facilitate expiration [the Hering–Breuer reflex (HBR); Kubin et al., 2006]. Neurons in the nTS, called pump cells, receive these vagal inputs and relay the information to medullary PI neurons as well as to the KFn causing robust inhibition of inspiration and prolongation of expiration (Berger, 1977; Ezure and Tanaka, 1996; Ezure et al., 1998, 2002). The dorsolateral pontine drive for the PI motor pattern was identified in studies in which blockade of NMDAergic transmission in the KFn after transection of the vagal nerves eliminates the inspiratory off-switch and leads to an apneustic breathing pattern (Fung et al., 1994; Ling et al., 1994). Moreover, pump cell projections to the dl pons may gate an excitatory efference copy of central pattern generator

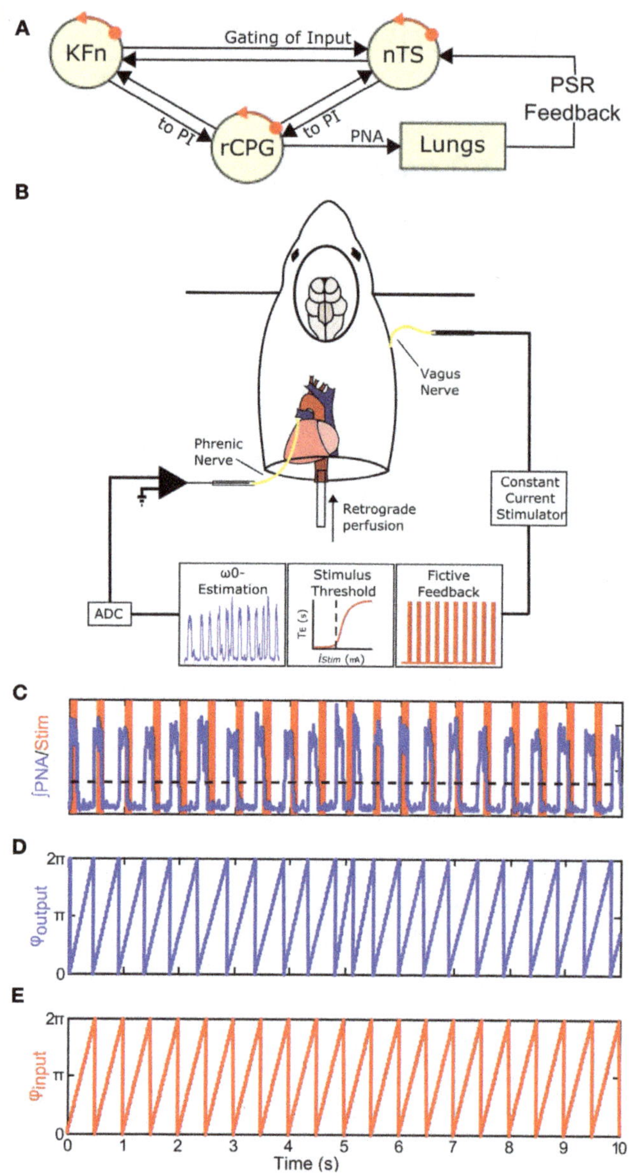

FIGURE 1 | Closing the Hering–Breuer mechanosensory feedback loop in the *in situ* arterially perfused preparation. (A) Schematic of the closed-loop *in vivo* respiratory rhythm generating network. *rCPG*, respiratory CPG; *PSR*, pulmonary stretch receptor; *nTS*, nuclei of the solitary tract; *KFn*, Kölliker–Fuse nuclei. **(B)** To mimic Hering–Breuer reflex (HBR) feedback, we first estimated the intrinsic oscillation frequency, ω_0, from an epoch of integrated phrenic nerve activity (PNA). Second, we estimated the minimum threshold to evoke the inspiratory inhibitory HBR by applying 10 s stimulus trains (20 Hz, 0.5 ms pulse-width) of increasing stimulus intensities to the contralateral vagus nerve. Once these two parameters were determined from each experimental preparation, we generated a fictive feedback input that consisted of a 2-min stimulus of rhythmic 100 ms trains (75 Hz, 0.5 ms pulse-width) whose inter-burst frequency matched ω_0 with pulse amplitude just above the threshold for resetting. **(C)** A representative tracing of fictive feedback input (*shaded bars*) and PNA output (*trace*) from a wild-type mouse. The dashed line indicates the threshold used for *post hoc* event detection. **(D,E)** To analyze (*Continued*)

FIGURE 1 | Continued
entrainment between the input and output, onset times for the two signals were extracted and used to generate the instantaneous phase time series, $\varphi_{output}(t)$ **(D)** and $\varphi_{input}(t)$ **(E)**. $\varphi(t)$ increases linearly from 0 to 2π between events and represents the movement of each oscillator around its limit-cycle.

(CPG) output from late-inspiratory neurons of the pre-Bötzinger complex (Cohen and Shaw, 2004; Dick et al., 2008). Thus in the absence of vagal afferent activity, the central representation of the "pattern" is disinhibited in the pons and dl pontine activity can drive PI activity. Thereby, this circuit motif allows the network to generate a PI rhythm in the absence of closed-loop feedback control.

In MeCP2-deficient mice, because both the nTS and the KFn appear functionally hyperexcitable, it is unclear whether the excessive PI activity and the resultant respiratory pattern dysrhythmia are due to a peripheral PI mechanism involving the nTS or a pontine PI mechanism involving the KFn. To disentangle this issue, we simulate the closed-loop behavior of the network by re-introducing rhythmic vagal feedback *in situ* and measuring the ability of the wild-type versus MeCP2-deficient networks to entrain to a threshold-amplitude periodic vagal input. Entrainment to rhythmic inputs is a fundamental property of any oscillator that occurs when the weak external forcing causes the oscillator to adjust its periods to become phase-locked with the imposed rhythm. In the entrained regime, the ratio between the intrinsic oscillation frequency and the imposed forcing takes on rational values. From the phase approximation model, we know that the existence of stable coupled dynamics between the oscillator and the rhythmic forcing depends on (1) the difference in frequency between the intrinsic oscillation frequency and that of the rhythmic input and (2) the strength of the coupling. In humans and cats, respiration readily entrains to HBR inputs during mechanical ventilation (Petrillo and Glass, 1984; Graves et al., 1986). In rats, respiration can also be entrained directly by rhythmically stimulating vagal afferent nerve endings (Dutschmann et al., 2009).

In this report, we test the hypothesis that increased respiratory pattern irregularity in *Mecp2*$^{-/+}$ mice is associated with an enhancement of respiratory entrainment by HBR inputs. While the strengthening of the coupling at the level of the nTS in MeCP2-deficient mice predicts an increase in entrainment between the CPG and the vagal input, we observed that *Mecp2*$^{-/+}$ mice display reduced input-output entrainment consistent with a dysfunctional pontine PI mechanism that causes respiratory dysrhythmia in these mice. However, the peripheral HBR pathway is still functional because inspiratory duration decreased during rhythmic vagal stimulation.

MATERIALS AND METHODS

Experimental protocols were approved by the Case Western Reserve University Institutional Animal Care and Use Committee and were performed with strict adherence to all American Association for Accreditation of Laboratory Animal Care International (AAALAC), National Institutes of Health and National Research Council guidelines.

Experiments were performed in adult (10–12 week postnatal age), female $Mecp2^{tm1.1Jae}$ mice maintained on a mixed background (129Sv, C57BL/6, Balb/c; $n = 6$ wild-type, $n = 5$ $Mecp2^{-/+}$; Chen et al., 2001; Guy et al., 2001). We utilized heterozygous female mice because they more closely model the human condition in which the mutation is lethal in males and results in somatic mosaicism in females due to the stochastic nature of X-chromosome inactivation. Female $Mecp2^{tm1.1Jae}$ heterozygotes show respiratory pattern irregularities like their null male littermates albeit at a later developmental time (Schmid et al., 2012). Further, a recent consortium on developing translational therapies for Rett syndrome has highlighted the importance of validating preclinical findings in heterozygous female *Mecp2* mutants (Katz et al., 2012).

To close the vagal mechanosensory feedback loop (**Figure 1B**), we stimulated the vagus nerve in the arterially perfused *in situ* preparation (*in situ* preparation), which is devoid of peripheral feedbacks, but maintains both an intact pontomedullary respiratory CPG and intact peripheral sensory nerve inputs (Paton, 1996). Briefly, mice were deeply anesthetized with isoflurane (1.5-3%, Piramal Healthcare, Andhra Pradesh, India). Once the mouse failed to respond to a noxious paw pinch, it was transected below the diaphragm and transferred into an ice-cold artificial cerebrospinal fluid (aCSF) bath for precollicular decerebration, cerebellectomy, and dissection of phrenic and vagal nerves. The preparation was then transferred to a recording chamber. The descending aorta was cannulated and perfused with aCSF (125 mM NaCl, 3 mM KCl, 1.25 mM KH_2PO_4, 2.5 mM $CaCl_2$, 1.25 mM $MgSO_4$, 25 mM $NaHCO_3$, 10 mM D-glucose) containing 1.25% Ficoll (31°C) using a peristaltic pump (Watson and Marlow 505S, Cornwall, UK). The perfusate was continuously bubbled with a gas mixture containing 94% O_2/6% CO_2. Because of the small size of the descending aorta, we were not able to measure perfusion pressure accurately. Adequate perfusion of the brainstem was maintained with flows between 17 and 20 ml/min. Within minutes of cannulation, respiratory movements resumed. If the respiratory activities were initially disorganized, then a single bolus of NaCN (0.1 ml, 0.03% w/v) was delivered to stimulate the peripheral chemoreceptors and restore the eupneic-like patterning of respiratory motor output. Vasopressin was not administered during these experiments.

NERVE RECORDINGS

Phrenic (PNA) and vagal (VNA) nerve activities were used as an index of fictive respiratory motor output. The distal end of either nerve was recorded via suction electrodes, filtered (0.003–3 kHz) and amplified (5–20 K; Grass P511, West Warwick, RI, USA), digitized (Power 1401, CED, Cambridge, UK), and stored (10 kHz sampling frequency) on a computer using Spike2 acquisition software (CED, Cambridge, UK).

EXPERIMENTAL PROTOCOL

After the tuned respiratory rhythm stabilized (15–20 min), baseline activity was recorded for at least 5 min to assess differences in respiratory patterning between the genotypes and to measure the intrinsic oscillation frequency of each preparation for determining the burst frequency of fictive vagal feedback. Next, the threshold amplitude for evoking the HBR was determined by measuring the threshold for an expiratory prolongation response to a constant train of vagal stimulation (20 Hz, 10 s train duration, 0.5 ms pulse duration). The threshold amplitude was defined as the stimulus current necessary to evoke an expiratory prolongation of at least 1.5 × the baseline expiratory duration. Having determined feedback burst frequency and pulse amplitude parameters, custom scripts written in MATLAB were used to generate rhythmic event trains (75 Hz, 100 ms train duration, 0.5 ms pulse duration) whose inter-burst frequency was matched to the intrinsic PNA burst frequency (~75–200 breaths/min). Burst stimulation was used because afferent discharge of slowly adapting PSRs are characterized by sinusoidal ramps in impulse frequency *in vivo* (Widdicombe, 1954; Luck, 1970). As these vagal PSR fibers are large and myelinated (Düring et al., 1974), the pulse duration was chosen to preferentially activate myelinated fibers.

Fictive feedback stimulation trials (2 min duration) were separated by at least 1 min of baseline activity and were repeated until the decay of the preparation caused the intrinsic oscillation frequency to drift by more than 30% from baseline which typically occurred 1.5–5 h after the resumption of PNA. During fictive feedback stimulation trials, custom Spike2 scripts transformed the MATLAB-generated event time series into a TTL output to deliver the fictive feedback to the preparation. Importantly, the fictive feedback was not triggered by the PNA. Instead, the rhythmic feedback was started irrespective of the current phase of the respiratory CPG. Nonetheless, the respiratory CPG quickly entrained the ongoing respiratory oscillation within a few cycles in wild-type mice (**Figure 4A**, *left panels*).

DATA ANALYSIS

Phrenic nerve activities onset and offset times were derived from a threshold crossing algorithm and visually inspected for artifacts (**Figures 1C–E**). Respiratory period, phase durations, variability, and apnea index were calculated from the recorded baseline epoch ($n = 6$ wild-type; 5 $Mecp2^{-/+}$). Apneas were defined as respiratory cycles with duration more than 1.5 times the mean period. The Wilcoxon signed rank test was used to determine the significance of HBR-induced reduction in Ti (**Figure 3**).

To test our hypothesis that increased pattern irregularity in MeCP2-deficient mice is associated with alterations in the ability of the CPG to entrain to afferent feedback inputs, we characterized the input-output entrainment generated by fictive vagal feedback in $Mecp2^{-/+}$ mice ($n = 11$ trials) versus wild-type littermates ($n = 22$ trials) using the cross-correlogram and several statistical measures derived from the instantaneous phase time series including the relative phase histogram, the instantaneous phase coherence, the synchronization index, and the mutual information of the instantaneous phases.

The normalized cross-correlogram, or transfer function, was computed using standard routines available in the MATLAB Signal Processing Toolbox. For computation of the cross-correlogram, the input signal was represented by a square-wave function with a pulse-width equal to the train duration. Before computing the cross-correlogram, both input and output signals were scaled between 0 and 1 and DC-removed. The maximum of the cross-correlogram was used as an index of the strength of input-output coupling.

The instantaneous phase time series was determined from onset times of the phrenic or input signals, t_k. The instantaneous phase, $\varphi(t)$, which is assumed to grow linearly in time within each cycle, was defined according to the following equation:

$$\varphi(t) = 2\pi \frac{t - t_k}{t_k - t_{k+1}} + 2\pi, \quad t_k < t < t_{k+1} \tag{1}$$

where t_k is the time of the k-th event, and t_{k+1} is the time of the next event.

From the instantaneous phase time series', the instantaneous relative phase difference time series, $\varphi_{\text{output}} - \varphi_{\text{input}}$, was computed. Histograms of the instantaneous relative phase were computed using 21 bins over the range 0–2π and scaled by the number of samples to determine the probability of a given instantaneous relative phase. The deviation from a uniform distribution was determined using the Rayleigh test for circular uniformity. The maximum of the instantaneous relative phase histogram was used as a measure of input-output coupling.

To define the regions in the instantaneous relative phase time series that were associated with strong input-output entrainment, we computed the phase coherence of the relative phases. The phase coherence is a windowed statistic that measures the squared magnitude of the mean phase angle:

$$\gamma(t) = \left\| \frac{1}{N} \sum_{i=t-w}^{t} e^{i[\varphi_{\text{output}} - \varphi_{\text{input}}]} \right\|^2 \tag{2}$$

The phase coherence was computed with a 3s window. The phase coherence yields a value between 0 and 1. Values near zero are not phase-locked, whereas values closer to 1 indicate the presence of phase-locking. To measure the latency to entrainment, the duration of entrainment and number of phase slips, we used a phase coherence threshold of 0.9.

The synchronization index, or phase-locking value, also maps the circular distribution of relative instantaneous phase onto the unit circle. The magnitude of the synchronization index is proportional to the degree of input-output entrainment. The synchronization index is computed via the following equation:

$$\gamma_{(n,m)} = \left| \left\langle e^{i[n\varphi_{\text{output}} - m\varphi_{\text{input}}]} \right\rangle \right| \tag{3}$$

for any *n:m* coupling. In the present study, the input oscillation frequency was chosen such that only 1:1 coupling was observed.

Mutual information is a measure of statistical dependence in a pair of time series. We used mutual information of the instantaneous phases in combination with surrogate data testing to quantify input-output entrainment and to allow for a statistical determination of the significance of the observed phase-locking. The mutual information index is defined according to the following equation:

$$I(\varphi_{\text{input}}, \varphi_{\text{output}}) = H(\varphi_{\text{input}}) + H(\varphi_{\text{output}}) - H(\varphi_{\text{input}} | \varphi_{\text{output}}) \tag{4}$$

where $H(\varphi_X)$ is the entropy of time series φ_X computed from the individual probability histogram, and $H(\varphi_X|\varphi_Y)$ is the conditional entropy of time series φ_X and φ_Y computed from the joint probability histogram. The entropy of either distribution is computed according to:

$$H(\varphi_X) = -\sum_{k=1}^{L} P(\varphi_X(k)) \ln P(\varphi_X(k)) \tag{5}$$

where L is the number of bins in the histogram and $P(\varphi_X(k))$ is the probability of observing φ_X in bin k. Note that because the mutual information index is sensitive to the number of bins L, we consistently used 50 bins in the generation of all histograms to allow for comparisons across experiments.

To determine the significance of the observed input-output coupling, a surrogate data testing scheme was needed to represent the null hypothesis of independent pairs of oscillatory activity. To generate bootstrapped distributions of the null hypothesis, we randomized the inter-event intervals of both the input and output before computing the instantaneous phases (500 surrogates/trial). The mutual information of these surrogate time series' was then computed to generate the bootstrapped mutual information histogram. The observed mutual information value of the coupling was considered significant if it fell above the 99% confidence interval of the bootstrap distribution. This criteria served as the basis for the identification of intermediate and severe *Mecp2*$^{-/+}$ entrainment defects discussed in **Figures 4** and **5**.

All data were expressed as mean ± SEM. Unless stated otherwise, we applied one-way repeated measures ANOVA to determine the significance of the results. If significant, we used a Bonferroni *post hoc* test to determine specific differences.

RESULTS

Representative traces of PNA from wild-type and *Mecp2*$^{-/+}$ baseline breathing patterns are shown in **Figure 2A**. The duration of the respiratory period was not significantly different between genotypes (**Figure 2B**), but the variability of the respiratory period [CV(Ttot)] was greater in *Mecp2*$^{-/+}$ than wild-type mice (*Mecp2*$^{-/+}$, 0.23 ± 0.02 versus wild-type, 0.09 ± 0.01; $p < 0.001$; **Figure 2C**). The irregularity of the pattern was characterized by a higher frequency of spontaneous apnea in *Mecp2*$^{-/+}$ versus wild-type mice (*Mecp2*$^{-/+}$, 3.7 ± 0.4 apneas/min versus wild-type, 0 ± 0 apneas/min; $p < 0.001$; **Figure 2D**). The intrinsic respiratory oscillation in *Mecp2*$^{-/+}$ mice had strong vagal efferent activity (*data not shown*) consistent with patterns reported previously (Stettner et al., 2007; Abdala et al., 2010).

During rhythmic vagal nerve stimulation (**Figure 3A**), inspiratory duration (Ti) decreased in both wild-type and *Mecp2*$^{-/+}$ mice as indicated by the pair-wise deviation from the line of identity (wild-type: baseline, 0.20 ± 0.01 s versus stimulation, 0.13 ± 0.001 s, $p = 5 \times 10^{-7}$; *Mecp2*$^{-/+}$: baseline, 0.15 ± 0.01 s versus stimulation, 0.10 ± 0.01 s, $p = 5 \times 10^{-4}$; **Figure 3B**) consistent with the role of this peripheral sensory modality in the inspiratory off-switching mechanism. Further, the reduction in Ti induced by vagal stimulation tended to be smaller in *Mecp2*$^{-/+}$

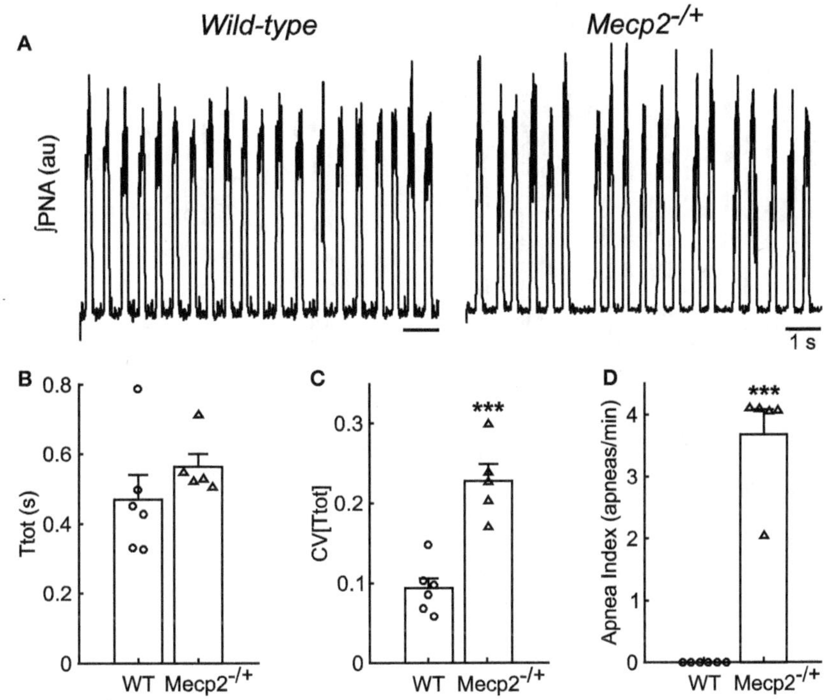

FIGURE 2 | *Mecp2$^{-/+}$* mice have increased respiratory pattern variability *in situ*. **(A)** Representative traces of ∫PNA during baseline recordings show the presence of spontaneous apneas in *Mecp2$^{-/+}$*, but not wild-type mice. **(B)** Respiratory period does not differ between wild-type and *Mecp2$^{-/+}$* mice *in situ*. **(C)** *Mecp2$^{-/+}$* mice have increased variability in the respiratory period. **(D)** *Mecp2$^{-/+}$* mice have an increased frequency of spontaneous apnea. ***$p < 0.001$.

versus wild-type mice, though this difference was not significant (*Mecp2$^{-/+}$*, $-5.0 \pm 1.0\%$ versus wild-type, $-7.1 \pm 0.1\%$, $p = 0.065$; **Figure 3C**).

To test our hypothesis, we analyzed the input-output phase-locking between rhythmic vagal stimulation and the central respiratory oscillation (**Figures 4** and **5**). To characterize the significance of input-output coupling in individual trials, we relied on the mutual information index applied in conjunction with a bootstrapping approach wherein surrogate time series were generated via shuffling the inter-burst intervals (**Figures 4D,E** and **5A–G**; See Materials and Methods). As expected, wild-type mice had significant input-output entrainment in all trials (19/19 trials). By contrast, entrainment varied in *Mecp2$^{-/+}$* mice: a severe group (6/11 trials) had a complete loss of input-output coupling; and an intermediate group (5/11 trials) had weak, but still significant input-output phase-locking (**Figure 4**). To fully characterize the changes in input-output coupling, we analyzed the relative phase difference time series (**Figures 4A,B**), the input-output cross-correlogram (**Figure 4C**), and the mutual information of the instantaneous phases (**Figures 4D,E**).

Representative traces of the relative phase time series during closed-loop stimulation are presented in **Figure 4A** (*top panels*). Entrainment between input and output is observed as epochs with a slope near 0, whereas sharp spikes in the time series are indicative of phase slips (**Figure 4A**). To characterize the duration and latency to input-output phase-locking, we measured the phase coherence, or mean phase angle on the unit circle, using a sliding windowed algorithm (**Figure 4A**, *bottom panels*). Phase-locked epochs within the trial were indicated by contiguous time regions where the phase coherence was >0.9 (**Figure 4A**, *shaded regions in top panels, horizontal lines in bottom panels*). *Mecp2$^{-/+}$* mice had a strong tendency toward greater latency to input-output phase-locking from the beginning of a stimulation trial relative to wild-type mice (*Mecp2$^{-/+}$*, 11.3 ± 3.3 s versus wild-type, 3.7 ± 1.4 s, $p = 0.07$). Further, severe *Mecp2$^{-/+}$* mice had a significantly greater latency to phase-locking compared to intermediate or wild-type mice (severe, 18.2 ± 3.9 s versus wild-type, 3.7 ± 1.4 s, $p < 0.001$, versus intermediate, 3.0 ± 2.1 s, $p < 0.01$, **Figure 5A**). Wild-type mice had longer durations of stable entrainment relative to *Mecp2$^{-/+}$* mice (wild-type, 7.8 ± 0.8 s versus *Mecp2$^{-/+}$*, 4.5 ± 0.4 s, $p < 0.01$, versus severe, 3.7 ± 0.3 s, $p < 0.05$, **Figure 5B**). Compared to the severe group, intermediate *Mecp2$^{-/+}$* mice had a tendency for longer durations of entrainment, but this was not significant. Further, *Mecp2$^{-/+}$* mice also showed a mild tendency for an increased number of phase slips during stimulation trials relative to wild-type mice (*Mecp2$^{-/+}$*, 37.5 ± 6.9 slips/trial versus wild-type, 24.9 ± 5.4 slips/trial, $p = 0.37$, **Figure 4C**). Finally, the severe *Mecp2$^{-/+}$* group had fewer bouts of input-output phase-locking (3/6 trials), whereas the intermediate *Mecp2$^{-/+}$* group consistently showed short bouts of input-output phase-locking (5/5 trials).

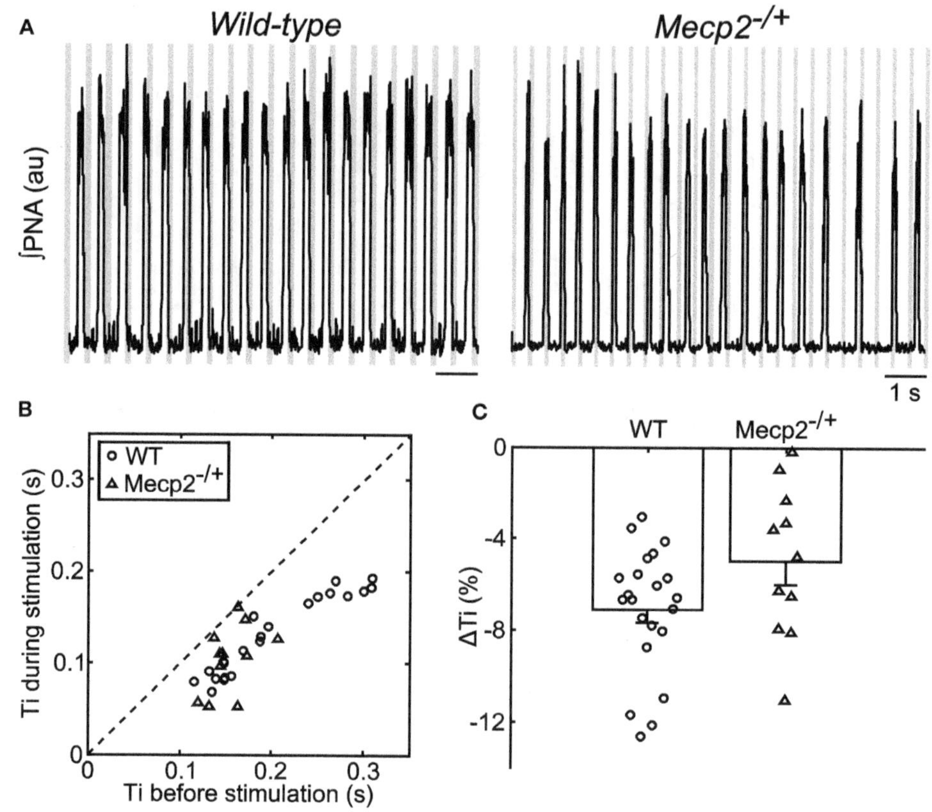

FIGURE 3 | Hering–Breuer feedback stimulation decreases inspiratory phase duration of the respiratory pattern in wild-type and *Mecp2*$^{-/+}$ mice. (A) Representative traces of ∫PNA (traces) during rhythmic vagal stimulation. Gray bars indicate the fictive feedback stimulation. **(B)** Rhythmic stimulation significantly decreases inspiratory duration in both wild-type and *Mecp2*$^{-/+}$ mice (wild-type, $p = 4.8 \times 10^{-7}$; *Mecp2*$^{-/+}$, $p = 9.8 \times 10^{-4}$). **(C)** HBR-dependent reduction in inspiratory duration tends to be smaller in *Mecp2*$^{-/+}$ versus wild-type mice ($p = 0.065$).

Representative relative phase histograms are shown in **Figure 4B**. A preferred relative phase between the vagal input and phrenic output was observed in both wild-type and the intermediate *Mecp2*$^{-/+}$ group, but not the severe *Mecp2*$^{-/+}$ group, which had a more uniform circular distribution of relative phases during rhythmic stimulation trials. However, all distributions had a measurable directionality as indicated by the Rayleigh test for deviance from circular uniformity indicative of a functional HBR. For the group, the maximum of the relative phase histogram and the synchronization index – the mean resultant vector of the relative phase time series – were both greater in wild-type relative to *Mecp2*$^{-/+}$ mice [Max (Rel. Phase Hist.): wild-type, 0.66 ± 0.05 versus *Mecp2*$^{-/+}$, 0.48 ± 0.08, $p < 0.05$, wild-type versus severe, 0.28 ± 0.02, $p < 0.001$, severe versus intermediate, 0.71 ± 0.10, $p < 0.01$, **Figure 5D**; and synchronization index: wild-type, 0.67 ± 0.04 versus *Mecp2*$^{-/+}$, 0.44 ± 0.09, $p < 0.05$, wild-type versus severe, 0.19 ± 0.03, $p < 0.001$, severe versus intermediate, 0.72 ± 0.08, $p < 0.001$, **Figure 5F**].

We also computed the transfer function of the system during rhythmic feedback stimulation as a measure of input-output phase-locking (**Figure 4C**). Cross-correlograms were periodic with the successive peaks and troughs decaying monotonically with increasing lag. While the qualitative structure of the functions was not changed between wild-type and *Mecp2*$^{-/+}$ mice, the peak of the transfer function decreased in *Mecp2*$^{-/+}$ mice [Max (Cross-correlation): *Mecp2*$^{-/+}$, 0.23 ± 0.05 versus wild-type, 0.50 ± 0.04, $p < 0.001$]. Wild-type and intermediate mice also significantly differed from the severe group [Max (Cross-correlation): wild-type, 0.23 ± 0.05 versus severe, 0.11 ± 0.01, $p < 0.001$, severe versus intermediate, 0.38 ± 0.05, $p < 0.05$, **Figure 5E**].

Finally, we characterized the joint probability distribution functions of the instantaneous input- and output-phases by computing their mutual information, which quantifies the general dependence between the phase of the input and the phase of the output. To determine the significance of the observed entrainment, we performed bootstrap analyses by shuffling the inter-event intervals and re-computing the mutual information of the instantaneous phases. Phase-locking, characterized by clear banding in the joint probability distribution function, was observed in the wild-type and intermediate *Mecp2*$^{-/+}$ group (**Figure 4D**, left and center panels respectively), whereas the uniform joint probability distribution function of the severe *Mecp2*$^{-/+}$ group (**Figure 4D**, right panel) reflected the drifting of the instantaneous phases. Representative bootstrapped mutual information histograms were roughly Gaussian, though bounded >0 because of the rarity of obtaining a perfectly uniform joint probability distribution (**Figure 4E**).

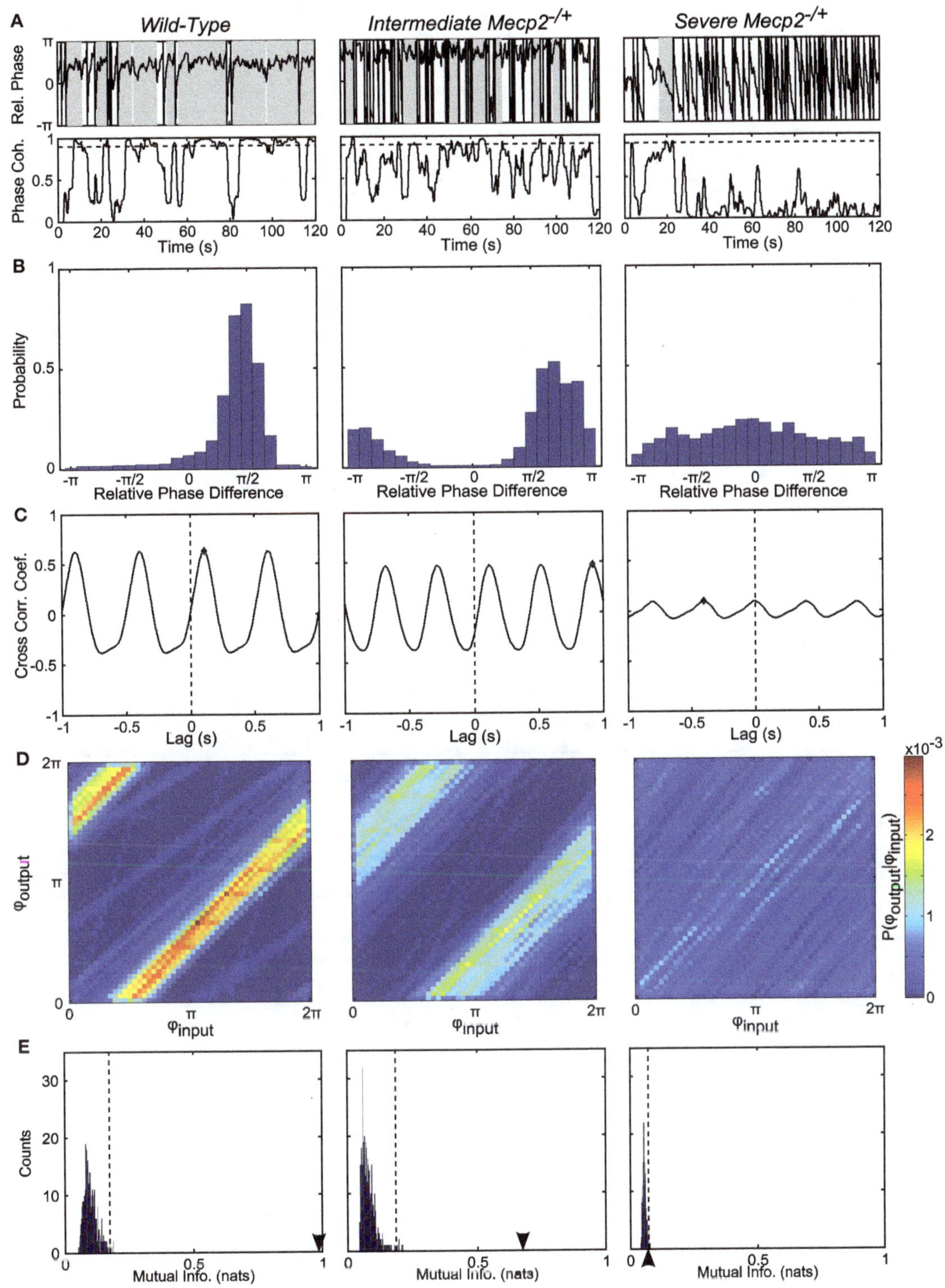

FIGURE 4 | Representative analyses show reduced phase-locking in *Mecp2*$^{-/+}$ compared to wild-type mice. (A) From the instantaneous phase time series, φ_{output} and φ_{input}, we computed the relative instantaneous phase difference time series, $\varphi_{output} - \varphi_{input}$ (*top panels*). Regions with near zero slope are indicative of input-output entrainment, which was more frequently observed in wild-type relative to *Mecp2*$^{-/+}$ mice. Phase coherence (*bottom panels*) is a windowed measure that captures the strength of input-output entrainment. A threshold of 0.9 (*dashed line in bottom panels*) was used to determine windows with significant input-output phase-locking (*shaded regions in top panels*). *Mecp2*$^{-/+}$ mice had increased latency to and reduced duration of entrainment relative to wild-type mice. **(B)** Representative histograms of the instantaneous phase difference are shown for a wild-type (left panel) and *Mecp2*$^{-/+}$ mice (*middle and right panels*). In all cases, even the severe *Mecp2*$^{-/+}$ mice, the distribution was significantly different from a uniform circular distribution as determined by the Rayleigh test for circular non-uniformity. **(C)** Representative cross-correlograms are shown for a wild-type (left panel), intermediate *Mecp2*$^{-/+}$ (middle panel), and severe

(*Continued*)

FIGURE 4 | Continued
Mecp2$^{-/+}$ (right panel) mice. The maximum of the cross-correlogram was reduced in *Mecp2*$^{-/+}$ versus wild-type mice. **(D)** Representative joint probability histograms of the instantaneous input- and output-phases depict the strength of input-output entrainment in the intensity of banding. Entrainment was strong in wild-type and intermediate *Mecp2*$^{-/+}$ preparations, but was abolished in severe *Mecp2*$^{-/+}$ mice. **(E)** The significance of the observed input-output entrainment was determined by generating bootstrap distributions of the mutual information of the instantaneous phases. Surrogate instantaneous phase time series were generated by shuffling the input- and output-inter-event intervals before determining the phase. The observed value of the mutual information is indicated by the arrowheads on the abscissa. The upper-bound of the 99% confidence interval is indicated by dashed vertical lines. Wild-type and intermediate *Mecp2*$^{-/+}$ mice always showed significant input-output entrainment, whereas severe *Mecp2*$^{-/+}$ mice did not have significant input-output entrainment.

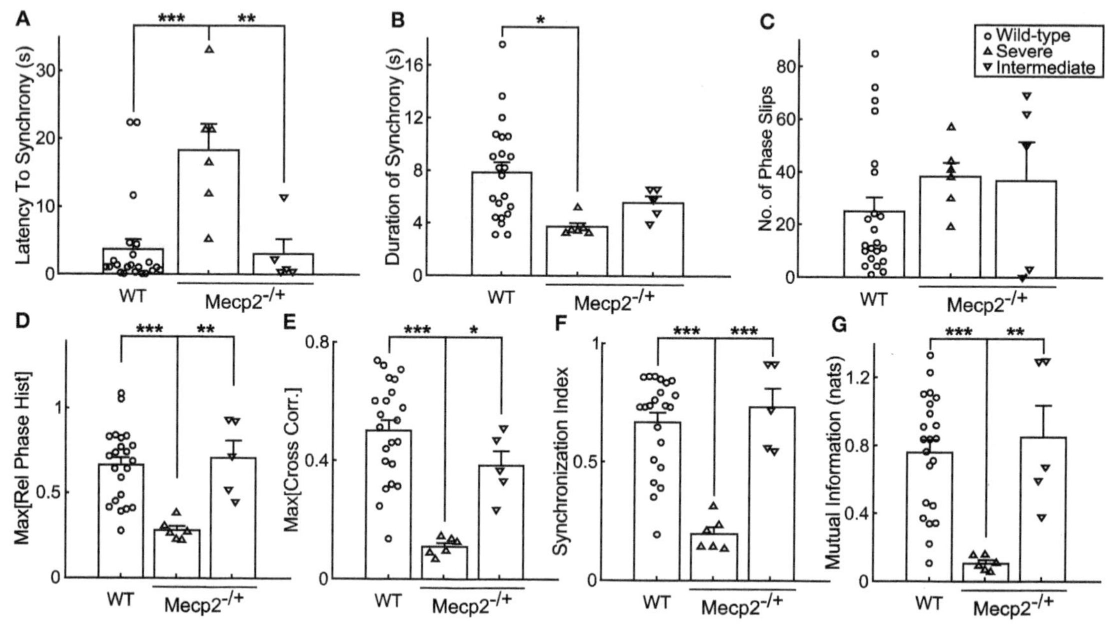

FIGURE 5 | *Mecp2*$^{-/+}$ mice show reductions in input-output phase-locking across multiple entrainment measures. **(A)** Severe *Mecp2*$^{-/+}$ mice had significantly increased latency to input-output entrainment from the start of rhythmic stimulation compared to both wild-type and intermediate *Mecp2*$^{-/+}$ mice. **(B)** Severe *Mecp2*$^{-/+}$ mice had significantly shorter bouts of input-output phase-locking compared to wild-type mice. **(C)** Severe and intermediate *Mecp2*$^{-/+}$ mice had a mild tendency for increased phase slips. **(D)** Relative to wild-type and intermediate mice, the maximum of the phase histogram was significantly less in severe *Mecp2*$^{-/+}$ mice. **(E)** The maximum of the cross-correlation function was significantly reduced in severe *Mecp2*$^{-/+}$ compared to wild-type and intermediate *Mecp2*$^{-/+}$ mice. **(F)** For the group, severe *Mecp2*$^{-/+}$ mice had a significantly lower synchronization index relative to both wild-type and intermediate *Mecp2*$^{-/+}$ mice. **(G)** Analysis of the mutual information of the instantaneous phases also revealed significantly weaker input-output entrainment in severe *Mecp2*$^{-/+}$ compared to wild-type and intermediate *Mecp2*$^{-/+}$ mice. $^{*}p < 0.05$, $^{**}p < 0.01$, $^{***}p < 0.001$.

The input-output entrainment was considered significant if the observed mutual information was greater than the 99% confidence interval of the bootstrap distribution. Five of 11 *Mecp2*$^{-/+}$ had significant entrainment according to the bootstrap results and were thereby classified as the intermediate *Mecp2*$^{-/+}$ phenotype. For the group, the mutual information of the instantaneous phases was greater in wild-type relative to *Mecp2*$^{-/+}$ mice (mutual information: wild-type, 0.76 ± 0.07 versus *Mecp2*$^{-/+}$, 0.44 ± 0.14, $p < 0.05$). Severe mice also had significantly weaker entrainment as measured by the mutual information of the instantaneous phases compared to both wild-type and intermediate mice (severe, 0.11 ± 0.02 versus wild-type, 0.76 ± 0.07, $p < 0.001$, versus intermediate, 0.85 ± 0.19, $p < 0.01$, **Figure 5G**).

DISCUSSION

Imposing rhythmic vagal feedback stimulation in the *in situ* preparation decreased Ti and evoked robust bouts of input-output phase-locking in wild-type mice. Contrary to our hypothesis, *Mecp2*$^{-/+}$ mice had significantly weaker input-output phase-locking though the decrease in Ti during vagal feedback stimulation suggested that the HBR was still intact. Using mutual information with bootstrapped surrogate distributions to evaluate significant input-output entrainment, *Mecp2*$^{-/+}$ mice were separated into intermediate and severe entrainment phenotypes consistent with the mosaic expression of MeCP2. Severe *Mecp2*$^{-/+}$ mice completely lost input-output entrainment, where as intermediate *Mecp2*$^{-/+}$ mice had significant input-output entrainment, but was weaker relative to wild-type mice. Together, our findings identify a compensatory adaptation of the MeCP2-deficient respiratory network that decouples the respiratory rhythm from vagal feedback inputs.

TECHNICAL CONSIDERATIONS

In the present study, we assessed the ability of the isolated adult brainstem respiratory network to entrain to rhythmic vagal stimulation as a model of the *in vivo* closed-loop condition. As noted in the introduction, the presence of stable entrainment depends on two factors: (1) the frequency difference between the oscillators, e.g., the weakly coupled oscillator network that comprises the respiratory rhythm generator, and the periodic input, e.g., the rhythmic vagal stimulation; and (2) the strength of the coupling between the oscillator and the input. We controlled for frequency differences by tuning the fictive vagal feedback frequency to that of each preparation. Thus, even though the *Mecp2*$^{-/+}$ mice used in this study had a slightly increased period *in situ*, this did not prevent stable entrainment because they received a suitably slower fictive feedback input. Similarly, we controlled for differences in the strength of coupling stimulating the vagus nerve at the threshold for evoking HBR-like responses. Additionally, for the purpose of investigating closed-loop control of respiratory behavior, the utilization of the*in situ* preparation was critical because it maintains an intact pontomedullary axis, spares sensory afferent, and motoneuronal efferent pathways, and produces an *in vivo*-like respiratory rhythm allowing re-introduction of fictive vagal feedback without confounding changes in chemosensory and baroreceptor afferent pathways (Paton, 1996). Further, the absence of anesthesia was particularly important for investigating the MeCP2-deficient breathing phenotype as breathing arrhythmias in these mice are reduced by anesthetics (Viemari et al., 2005; Abdala et al., 2010).

A key caveat of our study is that fictive feedback was delivered by stimulating whole vagal nerve bundles which contain fibers from three types of pulmonary receptors: slowly adapting receptor (SAR) fibers, rapidly adapting receptor fibers, and C-fibers. In rats, SAR and RAR fibers can be stimulated preferentially because they are thick and myelinated. Accordingly, a short pulse duration and a low stimulus current were chosen to activate myelinated rather than unmyelinated fibers. Moreover, vagal stimulation, unlike lung inflation, has been shown to activate PI output recorded from the pharyngeal branch of the vagus (Hayashi and McCrimmon, 1996). However, in this study, the authors observed similar effects on inspiratory and expiratory phase durations when comparing vagal stimulation- and lung inflation-induced HBRs suggesting that functional effects of vagal stimulation and lung inflation on network output are similar enough to warrant such comparison. Moreover, these authors went on to use this same paradigm of vagal stimulation to identify neurons in the ventrolateral medulla whose activities are modulated in a paucisynaptic fashion to mediate the HBR (Hayashi et al., 1996). Similarly, in the present study and others, we observe HBR-like responses to vagal stimulation consistent with those reported for lung inflation (Karczewski et al., 1980; Budzinska et al., 1981; Siniaia et al., 2000; Dutschmann et al., 2009). Moreover, the respiratory network readily entrains to rhythmic vagal stimulation in rats (Dutschmann et al., 2009) as well as our fictive feedback trials in wild-type mice. However, from the present findings, we can conclude only that the vagal feedback entrainment behavior is lost in the MeCP2-deficient respiratory network without further experiments to dissect the mechanistic basis for the loss of functional connectivity between input and output.

RELEVANCE TO RESPIRATORY ABNORMALITIES IN RETT SYNDROME

Given previous findings of hyperexcitablity in TS-nTS synapses and exaggerated HBR-like responses to vagal stimulation, we hypothesized that entrainment between peripheral feedbacks and the respiratory rhythm should be enhanced in MeCP2-deficient mice (Stettner et al., 2007; Kline et al., 2010; Song et al., 2011). Instead, by using rhythmic vagal stimulation, we observed a reduction in input-output entrainment suggesting that despite the exaggerated HBR responses, observed during vagal stimulation with continuous trains, vagal feedback appears to be filtered by a compensatory adaptation of the network such that rhythmic inputs above the threshold for eliciting phase resetting have little consistent effect on the respiratory rhythm. Previous findings support a role for dysfunctional postnatal maturation of the KFn in the loss of phase-locking with afferent feedbacks. As mentioned earlier, the KFn is a key determinant of the PI motor pattern because local blockade of NMDAergic transmission results in apneusis (Fung et al., 1994; Ling et al., 1994; Dutschmann and Herbert, 2006). Moreover, the KFn has reciprocal connectivity with the vl NTS such that the KFn can gate the influence of peripheral inputs on the respiratory rhythm (Herbert et al., 1990; Ezure et al., 2002; Dutschmann and Dick, 2012). Dutschmann et al. (2009) demonstrated that after postnatal maturation, repeated trials of vagal stimulation leads to an anticipatory transition to from inspiration to expiration that precedes the arrival of vagal stimuli. This learning process also depended on NMDAergic transmission, which has been shown to mature postnatally with a similar developmental time course (Kron et al., 2008). In MeCP2-deficient mice, glutamate microinjection in the KFn results in an exaggerated PI apnea (Stettner et al., 2007). Moreover, the response to constant vagal stimulation shows a loss of habituation and desensitization (Stettner et al., 2007; Song et al., 2011), which have previously been shown to depend on the KFn (Siniaia et al., 2000). These data lead to the speculation that ponto-vagal interactions may be the critical factor mediating the irregular breathing pattern in *Mecp2*$^{-/+}$ mice.

Alternatively, the noise in the respiratory network is likely a critical factor in preventing stable coupling between the network and its peripheral feedbacks in MeCP2-deficient mice. From the phase approximation model, we know that noise reduces the parameter space associated with stable phase-locked dynamics between an oscillator and a rhythmic forcing. Thus, if the respiratory rhythm generator itself is more variable, this would prevent stable entrainment with the dynamics of the periphery. Accordingly, variability in the respiratory rhythm recorded from MeCP2-deficient mice is present in the absence of peripheral feedbacks: both in the isolated CPG *in vitro* (Viemari et al., 2005), as well as *in situ* where the network is intact, but functionally isolated from peripheral feedback (Stettner et al., 2007; Abdala et al., 2010).

PHASE SYNCHRONIZATION MEASURES FOR INVESTIGATING CLOSED-LOOP RESPIRATORY BEHAVIOR

Over the past decade, several reports have explored the restoration of rhythmic vagal feedback in reduced preparations. Mellen and Feldman (2000) first re-introduced phasic lung inflation in the *en bloc* preparation which was modified to maintain the lungs and vagal nerve pathways. Though they established that the medullary components were sufficient to evoke the HBR mechanism as evidenced by a reduction in inspiratory duration, their preparation did not include pontine components that also modulate the PI motor pattern. Utilization of the *in situ* preparation overcomes this limitation and confirmed that phasic lung inflation reduces inspiratory duration and increases respiratory frequency (Harris and St-John, 2005). Importantly, these earlier approaches utilized closed-loop stimulation wherein lung inflation was triggered by the onset of PNA. Interactions between the respiratory rhythm and rhythmic HBR feedback inputs are also apparent when the stimulation is not coupled with the motor output as in the present study. As mentioned above, Dutschmann et al. (2009) used this latter approach to demonstrate that the pontine control of PI activity is subject to postnatal maturation and depends on NMDAergic transmission in the KFn. However, in this report, only cycle-triggered averaging was used to demonstrate the presence of functional input-output entrainment. Our approach extends this and earlier methodologies by introducing robust measures of phase synchronization that are necessary to evaluate entrainment. In the present study, the use of surrogate data sets in concert with mutual information of the instantaneous phases as a test statistic permitted assessment of significant phase-locking between the rhythmic input and respiratory motor output in individual stimulation trials. Additionally, the use of instantaneous relative phase and phase coherence allowed us to identify bouts of entrainment within individual stimulation trials. Applying our improved methodology to MeCP2-deficient mice revealed intermediate and severe decrements in input-output entrainment that were not recognized previously. In the future, our approach could be extended with a data-driven modeling approach based on the generic phase oscillator model by incorporating multiple central field recordings within the pontomedullary respiratory column to understand changes in the directionality of coupling within the respiratory network during HBR feedback stimulation (Zhu et al., 2013).

On a more general level, the findings of this study raise the possibility that the respiratory rhythm is tuned to the dynamics of the periphery. In locomotor CPGs, central oscillations are coupled to the dynamics of the limb at the a frequency between the intrinsic frequencies of the neural oscillator and of the physical limb system (Hatsopoulos, 1996; Chiel and Beer, 1997). A hallmark of this phenomenon, resonance tuning of a CPG, is that the frequency of the instrinsic oscillation is reduced in the absence of feedback (Pearson et al., 1983). Mathematically, considering the most general model of phase-coupled oscillators, this property is a consequence of the fact that the coupling between oscillators is both weak and additive with respect to the intrinsic oscillation frequency. While researchers have not previously considered resonance tuning in the context of respiration, the intrinsic respiratory oscillation frequency is reduced after removal of PSR (Stella, 1938; Dhingra et al., 2011) or peripheral chemoreceptor (Eldridge, 1974; Miller and Tenney, 1975; Hayashi et al., 1983) afferent inputs in cats and rodents. Further investigation of whether resonant tuning of respiratory dynamics may be critical for rhythmogenesis is warranted because the presence of excitatory feedback changes membrane current dynamics underlying phase switching in models of feedback-coupled locomotor CPGs (Spardy et al., 2011). Even though CPGs are defined by their ability to transform a constant drive into a rhythmic output without sensory feedback, in the intact animal, output rhythms are modulated continuously in a closed-loop fashion by peripheral afferent oscillations that, contrary to the assertions of the last decades, may be central to the rhythm generating mechanism.

ACKNOWLEDGMENTS

This work was supported by National Institutes of Health Grants HL-080318 (Thomas E. Dick), HL-42131 (David M. Katz), T32 HL-007913 (Rishi R. Dhingra), The Mt. Sinai Health Care Foundation (Roberto F. Galán) and Award I01BX000873 from the Biomedical Laboratory Research and Development Service of the VA Office of Research and Development (Frank J. Jacono). We also wish to thank Dr. Richard Romaniuk and Dr. Miriam Kron for their insightful comments on the manuscript.

REFERENCES

Abdala, A. P. L., Dutschmann, M., Bissonnette, J. M., and Paton, J. F. R. (2010). Correction of respiratory disorders in a mouse model of rett syndrome. *Proc. Natl. Acad. Sci. U.S.A.* 107, 18208–18213.

Berger, A. J. (1977). Dorsal respiratory group neurons in the medulla of cat: spinal projections, responses to lung inflation and superior laryngeal nerve stimulation. *Brain Res.* 135, 231–254.

Budzinska, K., Gøowicki, K., and Romaniuk, J. R. (1981). Short-latency phrenic response to electrical vagal stimulation in rabbits. *Acta Neurobiol. Exp. (Wars)* 41, 87–94.

Chen, R. Z., Akbarian, S., Tudor, M., and Jaenisch, R. (2001). Deficiency of methyl-CpG binding protein-2 in CNS neurons results in a Rett-like phenotype in mice. *Nat. Genet.* 27, 327–331.

Chiel, H. J., and Beer, R. D. (1997). The brain has a body: adaptive behavior emerges from interactions of nervous system, body and environment. *Trends Neurosci.* 20, 553–557.

Cohen, M. I., and Shaw, C.-F. (2004). Role in the inspiratory off-switch of vagal inputs to rostral pontine inspiratory-modulated neurons. *Respir. Physiol. Neurobiol.* 143, 127–140.

Dhingra, R. R., Jacono, F. J., Fishman, M., Loparo, K. A., Rybak, I. A., and Dick, T. E. (2011). Vagal-dependent nonlinear variability in the respiratory pattern of anesthetized, spontaneously breathing rats. *J. Appl. Physiol.* 111, 272–284.

Dick, T. E., Shannon, R., Lindsey, B. G., Nuding, S. C., Segers, L. S., Baekey, D. M., et al. (2008). Pontine respiratory-modulated activity before and after vagotomy in decerebrate cats. *J. Physiol. (Lond.)* 586, 4265–4282.

Düring, M., Andres, K. H., and Iravani, J. (1974). The fine structure of the pulmonary stretch receptor in the rat. *Anat. Embryol.* 143, 215–222.

Dutschmann, M., and Dick, T. E. (2012). Pontine mechanisms of respiratory control. *Compr. Physiol.* 2, 2443–2469.

Dutschmann, M., and Herbert, H. (2006). The Kölliker–Fuse nucleus gates the postinspiratory phase of the respiratory cycle to control inspiratory off-switch and upper airway resistance in rat. *Eur. J. Neurosci.* 24, 1071–1084.

Dutschmann, M., Mörschel, M., Rybak, I. A., and Dick, T. E. (2009). Learning to breathe: control of the inspiratory-expiratory phase transition shifts from sensory- to central-dominated during postnatal development in rats. *J. Physiol. (Lond.)* 587, 4931–4948.

Eldridge, F. L. (1974). Central neural respiratory stimulatory effect of active respiration. *J. Appl. Physiol.* 37, 723–735.

Ezure, K., and Tanaka, I. (1996). Pump neurons of the nucleus of the solitary tract project widely to the medulla. *Neurosci. Lett.* 215, 123–126.

Ezure, K., Tanaka, I., and Miyazaki, M. (1998). Pontine projections of pulmonary slowly adapting receptor relay neurons in the cat. *Neuroreport* 9, 411–414.

Ezure, K., Tanaka, I., Saito, Y., and Otake, K. (2002). Axonal projections of pulmonary slowly adapting receptor relay neurons in the rat. *J. Comp. Neurol.* 446, 81–94.

Fung, M. L., Wang, W., and St John, W. M. (1994). Involvement of pontile NMDA receptors in inspiratory termination in rat. *Respir. Physiol.* 96, 177–188.

Graves, C., Glass, L., Laporta, D., Meloche, R., and Grassino, A. (1986). Respiratory phase locking during mechanical ventilation in anesthetized human subjects. *Am. J. Physiol.* 250, R902–R909.

Guy, J., Hendrich, B., Holmes, M., Martin, J. E., and Bird, A. (2001). A mouse mecp2-null mutation causes neurological symptoms that mimic Rett syndrome. *Nat. Genet.* 27, 322–326.

Harris, M. B., and St-John, W. M. (2005). Phasic pulmonary stretch receptor feedback modulates both eupnea and gasping in an in situ rat preparation. *Am. J. Physiol. Regul. Integr. Comp. Physiol.* 289, R450–R455.

Hatsopoulos, N. G. (1996). Coupling the neural and physical dynamics in rhythmic movements. *Neural. Comput.* 8, 567–581.

Hayashi, F., Coles, S. K., and McCrimmon, D. R. (1996). Respiratory neurons mediating the Breuer–Hering reflex prolongation of expiration in rat. *J. Neurosci.* 16, 6526–6536.

Hayashi, F., and McCrimmon, D. R. (1996). Respiratory motor responses to cranial nerve afferent stimulation in rats. *Am. J. Physiol. Regul. Integr. Comp. Physiol.* 271, R1054–R1062.

Hayashi, F., Yoshida, A., Fukuda, Y., and Honda, Y. (1983). The ventilatory response to hypoxia in the anesthetized rat. *Pflugers Arch.* 396, 121–127.

Herbert, H., Moga, M. M., and Saper, C. B. (1990). Connections of the parabrachial nucleus with the nucleus of the solitary tract and the medullary reticular formation in the rat. *J. Comp. Neurol.* 293, 540–580.

Karczewski, W. A., Naslonska, E., and Romaniuk, J. R. (1980). Respiratory responses to stimulation of afferent vagal fibres in rabbits. *Acta Neurobiol. Exp. (Wars)* 40, 543–562.

Katz, D. M., Berger-Sweeney, J. E., Eubanks, J. H., Justice, M. J., Neul, J. L., Pozzo-Miller, L., et al. (2012). Preclinical research in Rett syndrome: setting the foundation for translational success. *Dis. Model Mech.* 5, 733–745.

Katz, D. M., Dutschmann, M., Ramirez, J.-M., and Hilaire, G. (2009). Breathing disorders in Rett syndrome: progressive neurochemical dysfunction in the respiratory network after birth. *Respir. Physiol. Neurobiol.* 168, 101–108.

Kline, D. D., Ogier, M., Kunze, D. L., and Katz, D. M. (2010). Exogenous brain-derived neurotrophic factor rescues synaptic dysfunction in Mecp2-null mice. *J. Neurosci.* 30, 5303–5310.

Kron, M., Howell, C. J., Adams, I. T., Ransbottom, M., Christian, D., Ogier, M., et al. (2012). Brain activity mapping in Mecp2 mutant mice reveals functional deficits in forebrain circuits including key nodes in the default mode network, that are reversed with ketamine treatment. *J. Neurosci.* 32, 13860–13872.

Kron, M., Reuter, J., Gerhardt, E., Manzke, T., Zhang, W., and Dutschmann, M. (2008). Emergence of brain-derived neurotrophic factor-induced postsynaptic potentiation of NMDA currents during the postnatal maturation of the Kolliker-Fuse nucleus of rat. *J. Physiol. (Lond.)* 586, 2331–2343.

Kubin, L., Alheid, G. F., Zuperku, E. J., and McCrimmon, D. R. (2006). Central pathways of pulmonary and lower airway vagal afferents. *J. Appl. Physiol.* 101, 618–627.

Ling, L., Karius, D. R., and Speck, D. F. (1994). Role of N-methyl-D-aspartate receptors in the pontine pneumotaxic mechanism in the cat. *J. Appl. Physiol.* 76, 1138–1143.

Luck, J. C. (1970). Afferent vagal fibres with an expiratory discharge in the rabbit. *J. Physiol. (Lond.)* 211, 63–71.

Medrihan, L., Tantalaki, E., Aramuni, G., Sargsyan, V., Dudanova, I., Missler, M., et al. (2008). Early defects of GABAergic synapses in the brain stem of a MeCP2 mouse model of Rett syndrome. *J. Neurophysiol.* 99, 112–121.

Mellen, N. M., and Feldman, J. L. (2000). Phasic lung inflation shortens inspiration and respiratory period in the lung-attached neonate rat brain stem spinal cord. *J. Neurophysiol.* 83, 3165–3168.

Miller, M. J., and Tenney, S. M. (1975). Hyperoxic hyperventilation in carotid-deafferented cats. *Respir. Physiol.* 23, 23–30.

Paton, J. F. (1996). A working heart-brainstem preparation of the mouse. *J. Neurosci. Methods* 65, 63–68.

Pearson, K. G., Reye, D. N., and Robertson, R. M. (1983). Phase-dependent influences of wing stretch receptors on flight rhythm in the locust. *J. Neurophysiol.* 49, 1168–1181.

Petrillo, G. A., and Glass, L. (1984). A theory for phase locking of respiration in cats to a mechanical ventilator. *Am. J. Physiol. Regul. Integr. Comp. Physiol.* 246, R311–R320.

Schmid, D. A., Yang, T., Ogier, M., Adams, I., Mirakhur, Y., Wang, Q., et al. (2012). A TrkB small molecule partial agonist rescues TrkB phosphorylation deficits and improves respiratory function in a mouse model of Rett syndrome. *J. Neurosci.* 32, 1803–1810.

Siniaia, M. S., Young, D. L., and Poon, C.-S. (2000). Habituation and desensitization of the Hering–Breuer reflex in rat. *J. Physiol. (Lond.)* 523, 479–491.

Song, G., Tin, C., Giacometti, E., and Poon, C.-S. (2011). Habituation without NMDA receptor-dependent desensitization of Hering–Breuer apnea reflex in a mecp2 mutant mouse model of Rett syndrome. *Front. Integr. Neurosci.* 5:6. doi:10.3389/fnint.2011.00006

Spardy, L. E., Markin, S. N., Shevtsova, N. A., Prilutsky, B. I., Rybak, I. A., and Rubin, J. E. (2011). A dynamical systems analysis of afferent control in a neuromechanical model of locomotion: I. Rhythm generation. *J. Neural Eng.* 8, 065003.

Stella, G. (1938). On the mechanism of production, and the physiological significance of "apneusis." *J. Physiol. (Lond.)* 93, 10–23.

Stettner, G. M., Huppke, P., Brendel, C., Richter, D. W., Gärtner, J., and Dutschmann, M. (2007). Breathing dysfunctions associated with impaired control of postinspiratory activity in Mecp2-/y knockout mice. *J. Physiol. (Lond.)* 579, 863–876.

Taneja, P., Ogier, M., Brooks-Harris, G., Schmid, D. A., Katz, D. M., and Nelson, S. B. (2009). Pathophysiology of locus ceruleus neurons in a mouse model of Rett syndrome. *J. Neurosci.* 29, 12187–12195.

Viemari, J.-C., Roux, J.-C., Tryba, A. K., Saywell, V., Burnet, H., Peña, F., et al. (2005). Mecp2 deficiency disrupts norepinephrine and respiratory systems in mice. *J. Neurosci.* 25, 11521–11530.

Voituron, N., Menuet, C., Dutschmann, M., and Hilaire, G. (2010). Physiological definition of upper airway obstructions in mouse model for Rett syndrome. *Respir. Physiol. Neurobiol.* 173, 146–156.

Weese-Mayer, D. E., Lieske, S. P., Boothby, C. M., Kenny, A. S., Bennett, H. L., Silvestri, J. M., et al. (2006). Autonomic nervous system dysregulation: breathing and heart rate perturbation during wakefulness in young girls with Rett syndrome. *Pediatr. Res.* 60, 443–449.

Widdicombe, J. G. (1954). The site of pulmonary stretch receptors in the cat. *J. Physiol. (Lond.)* 125, 336–351.

Zhu, Y., Hsieh, Y.-H., Dhingra, R. R., Dick, T. E., Jacono, F. J., and Galán, R. F. (2013). Quantifying interactions between real oscillators with information theory and phase models: application to cardiorespiratory coupling. *Phys. Rev.* E87, 022709.

8

Coupling BCI and cortical stimulation for brain-state-dependent stimulation: methods for spectral estimation in the presence of stimulation after-effects

Armin Walter[1]*, Ander R. Murguialday[2,3], Wolfgang Rosenstiel[1], Niels Birbaumer[2,4] and Martin Bogdan[1,5]

[1] Department of Computer Engineering, Wilhelm-Schickard-Institute, Eberhard Karls Universität Tübingen, Tübingen, Germany
[2] Institute of Medical Psychology and Behavioural Neurobiology, University Hospital Tübingen, Tübingen, Germany
[3] Health Technologies Department, TECNALIA, San Sebastian, Spain
[4] Ospedale San Camillo, IRCCS, Venice, Italy
[5] Department of Computer Engineering, University of Leipzig, Leipzig, Germany

Edited by:
Ahmed El Hady, Max Planck Institute for Dynamics and Self Organization, Germany

Reviewed by:
Yang Dan, University of California, USA
Pratik Y. Chhatbar, Medical University of South Carolina, USA

***Correspondence:**
Armin Walter, Department of Computer Engineering, Wilhelm-Schickard-Institute, Eberhard Karls Universität Tübingen, Sand 14, 72076 Tübingen, Germany.
e-mail: armin.walter@uni-tuebingen.de

Brain-state-dependent stimulation (BSDS) combines brain-computer interfaces (BCIs) and cortical stimulation into one paradigm that allows the online decoding for example of movement intention from brain signals while simultaneously applying stimulation. If the BCI decoding is performed by spectral features, stimulation after-effects such as artefacts and evoked activity present a challenge for a successful implementation of BSDS because they can impair the detection of targeted brain states. Therefore, efficient and robust methods are needed to minimize the influence of the stimulation-induced effects on spectral estimation without violating the real-time constraints of the BCI. In this work, we compared four methods for spectral estimation with autoregressive (AR) models in the presence of pulsed cortical stimulation. Using combined EEG-TMS (electroencephalography-transcranial magnetic stimulation) as well as combined electrocorticography (ECoG) and epidural electrical stimulation, three patients performed a motor task using a sensorimotor-rhythm BCI. Three stimulation paradigms were varied between sessions: (1) no stimulation, (2) single stimulation pulses applied independently (open-loop), or (3) coupled to the BCI output (closed-loop) such that stimulation was given only while an intention to move was detected using neural data. We found that removing the stimulation after-effects by linear interpolation can introduce a bias in the estimation of the spectral power of the sensorimotor rhythm, leading to an overestimation of decoding performance in the closed-loop setting. We propose the use of the Burg algorithm for segmented data to deal with stimulation after-effects. This work shows that the combination of BCIs controlled with spectral features and cortical stimulation in a closed-loop fashion is possible when the influence of stimulation after-effects on spectral estimation is minimized.

Keywords: brain-computer interfaces, cortical stimulation, spectral estimation, brain-state-dependent stimulation, autoregressive models

1. INTRODUCTION

Cortical stimulation is being used to study cortical function, e.g., (Matsumoto et al., 2007). In clinical settings, it is employed for surgical planning (Lefaucheur and de Andrade, 2009) and therapy (Tsubokawa et al., 1991). Furthermore, preliminary studies on the use of cortical stimulation for stroke rehabilitation which used stimulation together with physiotherapy in order to modulate cortical excitability have been conducted (Brown et al., 2008; Levy et al., 2008). Taking the current brain activity of the patient into account when selecting stimulation parameters has been proposed as a possible improvement (Plow et al., 2009). Such an activity-dependent stimulation paradigm has been used by Jackson et al. (2006), who were able to show that cortical microstimulation associated in time with brain activity during a motor task can induce neural reorganization lasting for several days after stimulation in primates.

The effects of transcranial magnetic stimulation (TMS) as well depend on brain states of the stimulated person (Mitchell et al., 2007). Recently, Bergmann et al. (2012) applied TMS coupled to electroencephalography (EEG) to investigate the dependency of stimulation effects on the phase of slow EEG oscillations during sleep. In general, such activity-dependent or brain-state-dependent stimulation (BSDS) paradigms allow to investigate cortical networks at specific activation levels, making BSDS a potentially useful tool in cognitive neuroscience (Jensen et al., 2011) as well as in clinical studies improving consistency of the stimulation effects (Plow et al., 2009).

For effective BSDS, reliable decoding of the brain-state from the ongoing brain activity is necessary. Over the last decades in the field of brain-computer interfaces (BCIs) several different strategies were investigated (Birbaumer et al., 1999; Birbaumer and Cohen, 2007). Especially in the case of movement-related brain states during active or imagined limb movements, spectral power has been shown to be useful for their decoding. In particular, event-related (de-) synchronization of sensorimotor rhythms is an informative measure for discriminating movement and resting states (Wolpaw et al., 2002). Therefore, if one wants to combine BSDS with a movement task, one has to minimize the interference of the stimulation on the estimation of the spectral features to detect the brain-state properly.

The stimulation effects involve problems with spectral estimation caused by the stimulation artefact and the evoked neural activity. A stimulation pulse evokes an artefact in the signal (**Figure 1A**) with an amplitude in the range of several hundred millivolts or even volts, thus often exceeding the dynamic range of the amplifier (Veniero et al., 2009). In the vicinity of stimulation, evoked potentials are recorded (**Figure 1B**) which can reach amplitudes of several hundred microvolts (Matsumoto et al., 2007). Thus, if an analyzed window contains a stimulation pulse, the estimation of the spectrum of this window is difficult, because it is not stationary. This is evident in **Figure 1C**, showing that each stimulation pulse results in strong jumps in the estimated spectral power. Waiting long enough after the pulse is one solution. This approach results in non-continuous brain-state decoding with waiting periods after a stimulus of at least several hundred milliseconds. It dictates a longer inter-stimulus interval (ISI), because a robust

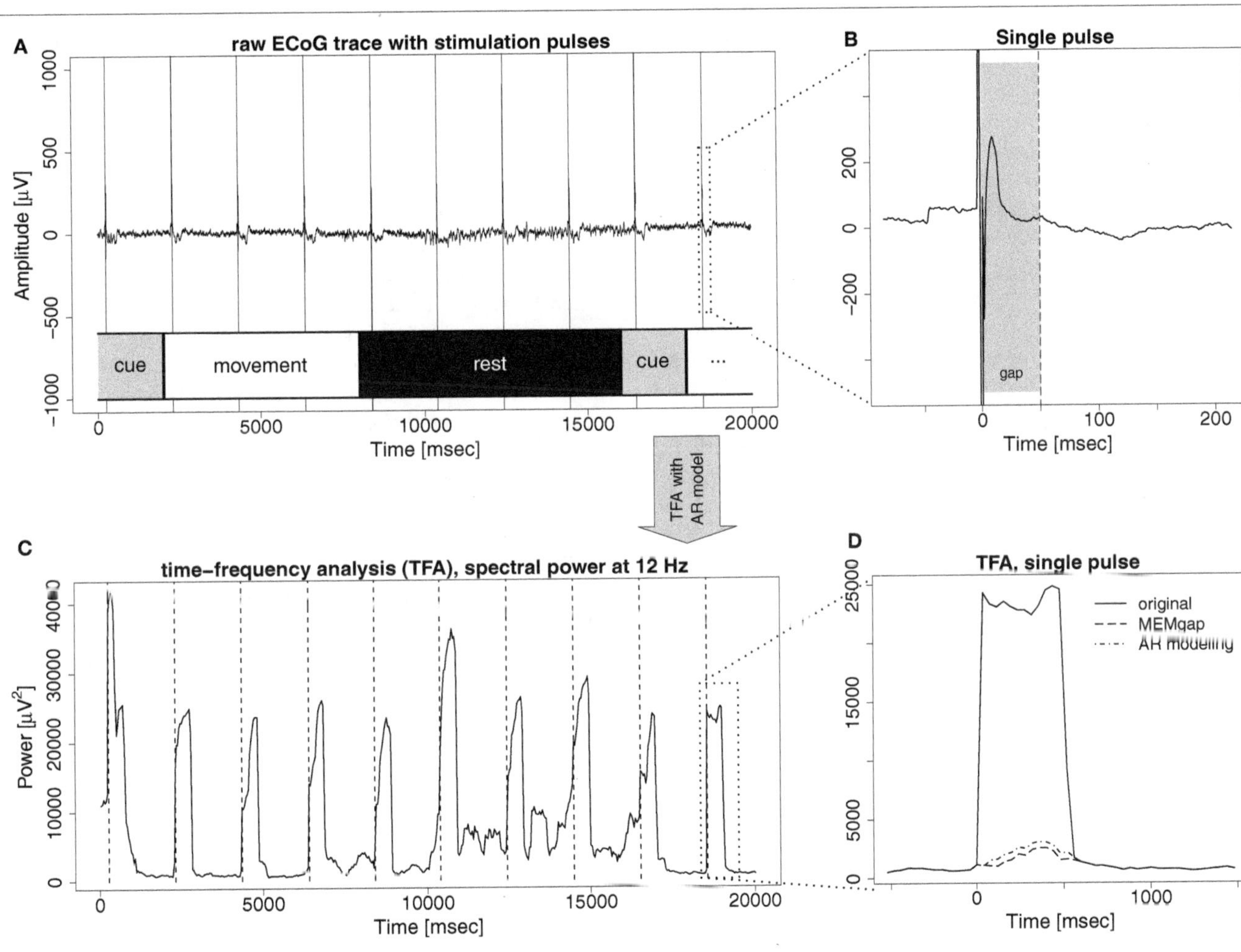

FIGURE 1 | The effect of stimulation pulses on time-frequency analysis (TFA) with AR models. (A) Example trace of ECoG data with intermittent stimulation pulses. Each pulse is visible as a sharp, strong artefact in the signal. The lower part of the illustrates the phases of the trial over the course of the recording: *cue*: an auditory cue, *movement*: patient attempts to move the hand, and *rest*: patient relaxes. **(B)** A zoom on the last stimulation pulse visible in **(A)**, also displaying an evoked potential, peaking 13 ms after the pulse. If the gray-shaded area up to the dashed line is defined as a gap, both the stimulation artefact and the strongest evoked components are covered. **(C)** Time-course of the power at 12 Hz of the signal displayed in **(A)**, resulting from a time-frequency analysis with auto-regressive models (order 16) when a window of 500 ms is shifted in 40 ms steps over the data. Hence, a single stimulation pulse distorts the spectrum for the next 500 ms because it remains in the data window. **(D)** Zoom on the region of the last stimulation pulse. Power at 12 Hz without stimulus processing (solid line) and when the gap is defined as in **(B)** and either MEMgap (dashed line) or AR modeling with order 16 (dashed-and-dotted line) are applied to deal with it.

estimate of the brain-state is needed before the next pulse can be applied.

If small ISIs and/or continuous decoding of the brain-state is necessary, methods that enable spectral estimation of data containing stimulation after-effects are mandatory. One potential solution for this, which has been used mainly in offline studies (no BSDS), is to separate the stimulation effects from the signal, as for example in Litvak et al. (2007). This places restrictions on the recording setup, such as the need for an amplifier with high dynamic range to cover the entire amplitude of the artefact and it is unclear whether such a procedure can be performed online without resulting in residual artefacts which would still lead to distortions of the spectrum. We present in this paper another solution suitable for online BSDS: we ignore the short segment of data dominated by the after-effects of stimulation when estimating the spectrum, leaving us with the challenge to estimate the spectrum when portions of the data are missing from a continuous data flow. We term such an excluded data segment a *gap*. In online experiments, using either signals synchronized with the stimulator or a peak detection algorithm, one can mark a sample before the stimulation pulse as the beginning of the gap. The number of following samples marked as belonging to the gap (i.e., the *gap size*) should be chosen in advance such that the gap, ideally, encloses just the stimulation artefact, and the largest evoked components. The dashed line and the dashed-and-dotted line in **Figure 1D** show the results of two approaches introduced in this work to extract the spectral power when the artefacts are masked by the gap shown in **Figure 1B**. They are much closer to the power before and after the stimulus, compared to the power without any processing of the stimulus (solid line).

In this paper we compare different online brain-state decoding methods on their suitability to perform spectral estimation using autoregressive (AR) models on data containing stimulation pulses and gaps. We consider here only stimulation paradigms with pulsed stimuli and restrict ourselves to data acquired with EEG or electrocorticography (ECoG) and stimulation performed using TMS or epidural electrodes. First, we introduce the methods for spectral estimation in the presence of gaps and investigate the effects of parameter estimates such as AR model order and gap size on the resulting spectrum. We present results from a simulation study in which gaps are artificially inserted into a BCI data set recorded without stimulation. We then show the different results of the algorithms on short data segments of two BCI training experiments, one with simultaneous TMS and one with simultaneous epidural electrical stimulation to illustrate the effects of cortical stimulation on spectral estimation and the results of correcting stimulation after-effects. Finally, we investigate the separability of intended hand movement and rest for different experimental paradigms (no stimulation, open-loop, or closed-loop stimulation) using non-invasive and invasive data during BCI experiments in three chronic stroke patients.

2. METHODS

2.1. PARTICIPANTS

Data was recorded from three chronic stroke patients (**Table 1**) suffering from paresis of the left hand. None of the patients was able to produce voluntary finger movements with the left hand. All procedures were approved by the local ethics committee of the medical faculty of the university hospital in Tübingen. Each stroke patient was implanted with 16 epidural platinum iridium disk electrodes (Resume II, Medtronic, Fridley, USA) with a contact diameter of 4 mm placed over the ipsilesional S1, M1, and pre-motor cortex on four strips with an inter-electrode center-to-center distance of 10 mm. They were arranged in a 4 × 4 grid-like pattern (**Figure 2**). During pre-surgical evaluation, all subjects completed the task described below with combined EEG-TMS (*non-invasive case*) and repeated the same task after the surgery using electrical epidural stimulation and recordings from the implanted electrodes (*invasive case*). The BCI and stimulation experiments were conducted during a period of 4 weeks following the implantation.

2.2. TASK

The patient was facing a 19″ monitor. The left upper limb of the patient was fixed using two straps, one at the forearm and one around the wrist and magnets fixed the fingertips to the actuators

Table 1 | Patient characteristics.

Patient	Age (y)	Sex	Months lapsed since injury	Paralysis	Infarct side	Lesion	Affected area
P1	56	M	80	Left	Right subcortical and cortical	Basal ganglia hemorrhage	Putamen, internal capsule, insula, opercular part of inferior frontal gyrus
P2	52	M	159	Left	Right subcortical and cortical	MCA territory infarct (frontal)	Frontal lobe including motor cortex (M1), parietal lobe including somatosensory cortex (S1)
P3	63	F	71	Left	Right subcortical and cortical	Basal ganglia hemorrhage	Head of striate body, lentiform nucleus, thalamus, whole internal capsule, insula, frontal lobe

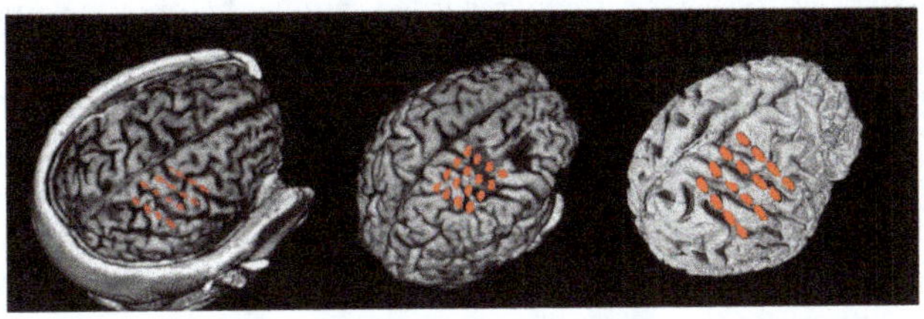

FIGURE 2 | ECoG electrode positions from overlay of MRI and post-surgical CT for the three patients. From left to right: P1–P3.

of a mechatronic hand orthosis (Tyromotion Amadeo HTS, Graz, Austria). This device was controlled by a BCI and moved the fingers of the paralyzed hand between an opened and a closed position. The range of the movement was adjusted in each session (Ramos-Murguialday et al., 2012) because it was limited by the spasticity of the patient. Each trial of the task consisted of three phases: preparation (2 s), feedback (6 s), and rest (8 s). During preparation, the subject received an auditory cue ("Left Hand") but was instructed to wait with the execution until the next auditory command ("Go!") was given at the start of the feedback phase. During the feedback phase starting with a closed position of the left hand, the patient had to try to open the left hand until the end of the feedback phase. At that point, another auditory cue ("Relax!") was given. During the rest period, the left hand of the patient was returned to its original closed position (2–3 s) and the patient was instructed to relax. An experimental session was divided into a 4–16 runs, each of these consisting of 11 trials. Runs with clear non-stimulation-related artefacts (e.g., amplifier saturation) on the analyzed channels were excluded from further analysis, resulting in a minimum of three runs per session for analysis and an average of 8.7 ± 4.3.

2.3. ELECTROPHYSIOLOGICAL RECORDING

Both EEG and ECoG were recorded with monopolar 32-channel amplifiers (BrainAmp MR plus, BrainProducts, Munich, Germany) with a sampling rate of 1000 Hz. The data was acquired in a packet-wise fashion, where the recording computer received every 40 ms one packet of data consisting of 40 samples per channel. The same behavior was modeled in our simulations of an online BCI. A high-pass filter with a cutoff frequency at 0.16 Hz and a low-pass filter with a cutoff frequency at 1000 Hz were applied. We recorded 32 channels of EEG in the standard 10–10 system, referenced to FCz, using circular Ag-AgCl electrodes. ECoG data was referenced to an electrode at the medio-frontal corner of the electrode grid over pre-motor cortex. Signal acquisition, signal processing and control of the orthosis and (if present in the experiment) the TMS or electrical stimulator were performed using the general-purpose BCI framework BCI2000 (http://www.bci2000.org) (Schalk et al., 2004) extended with custom-developed features for the control of these devices.

2.4. STIMULATION

We applied stimulation in the non-invasive case over the hotspot for *extensor digitorum communis* (EDC) activity, identified by a standard mapping paradigm (Wassermann et al., 2008). TMS was applied with a figure-of-eight coil (NeXstim, Helsinki, Finland) with single biphasic pulses (sinusoidal coil current, positive phase first, pulse width 280 μs) and an intensity of 110% of the resting motor threshold. The ISI of successive pulses was set to 3 s.

For epidural electrical stimulation we used single biphasic anodal square-wave pulses with a length of 500 μs. Stimulation intensity was selected individually per patient and session and chosen to reliably evoke MEPs on the paretic upper limb of the patient. The minimum ISI was set to 2 s in most experiments except when stimulation was applied coupled with the BCI output. In this case, a minimum ISI of 500 ms was chosen. The pulses were applied using a constant current stimulator (STG4008, Multichannel systems, Reutlingen, Germany) with the anode as the epidural electrode that evoked the strongest MEPs on the left upper limb and the cathode being a 50×90 mm adhesive electrode placed on the left clavicle of the patient. The current source of the stimulator was switched off 2 s after the last stimulation pulse if no other pulse was triggered before due to a software error, leading to a small but visible step in the recorded signal (**Figure 1B**).

2.5. AUTOREGRESSIVE (AR) MODELS

A popular choice for spectral estimation in BCI research is to use an AR model for which the coefficients are estimated with the maximum entropy method (Krusienski et al., 2006; McFarland and Wolpaw, 2008). An AR model can be viewed as a linear predictor of the signal samples $x(t_k)$, defined as:

$$x(t_k) = \sum_{i=1}^{p} c_i x(t_{k-i}) + e$$

where p is the order of the model and e a sample of a white noise process. If one uses a continuous window of length N with $N \gg p$ consisting of samples $x(t_0)$ to $x(t_{N-1})$, one could solve the following equations with a least-squares procedure to get the coefficients c_i:

$$x(t_k) = \sum_{i=1}^{p} c_i x(t_{k-i}) \quad (1)$$

$$x(t_{k-p}) = \sum_{i=1}^{p} c_i x(t_{k-p+i}) \text{ for all } k = p, \ldots, N-1$$

However, the resulting coefficients do not guarantee a stable AR model (de Waele and Broersen, 2000). Burg proposed a recursive algorithm for the solution of this system that provides stable models with less variance compared to least squares solutions and the Yule-Walker algorithm (Kay and Marple, 1981; de Waele and Broersen, 2000). The Burg algorithm computes the AR coefficients in p steps by evaluating in the i-th step the residuals of forward and backward prediction of the samples using the coefficients obtained in the $(i-1)$-th step. It is described in Appendix 1.1 in more detail. Spectral estimation with AR models is briefly introduced in Appendix 1.2.

The Burg algorithm requires that the input data is sampled continuously without gaps, a condition which is shared by most of the other algorithms for AR model estimation. Therefore, we need to either fill or remove the gaps before applying one of these algorithms to our data or modify the AR model estimation algorithms to be usable for data with gaps.

2.6. SPECTRAL ESTIMATION IN THE PRESENCE OF GAPS

This section contains a short description of the different algorithms we compare in this paper that deal with the pre-processing of data containing gaps for spectral estimation with AR models. The input for these algorithms are a segment of data and a vector that contains for each sample in the segment either a 1 (sample belongs to a gap, it has to be excluded from spectral estimation) or a 0 (sample is "clean").

Four methods for dealing with gaps in the data are described below: (1) *linear interpolation*, (2) *AR modeling* which fill the gap with generated data, (3) the *joining of data segments* that removes the gap, and (4) a *modified Burg algorithm for segmented data*. After application of the methods (1)–(3), the standard Burg algorithm is used to estimate the AR model and the spectrum.

2.6.1. Linear interpolation

We can bridge gaps in the data by linear interpolation between the last sample before and the first sample after the gap:

$$\hat{x}(t_{g+k}) = x(t_{g-1}) + \frac{k+1}{l+1} \cdot \left(x(t_{g+l}) - x(t_{g-1})\right),\ 0 \leq k \leq l-1 \tag{2}$$

where x are the signal samples recorded at times t_i, l is the length of the gap in samples and t_{g-1} is the index of the last sample before the gap.

While this might work for offline analysis of a data set, in the case of online analysis during a BCI experiment, in which data is received in a sample- or packet-wise system, one might have not yet received the first clean sample after the gap when trying to produce an estimate for $x(t_{g+k})$ within the gap. We used a simple approach to solve this problem which consists of filling the gap with the value of the last sample before the gap ($\hat{x}(t_{g+k}) = x(t_{g-1})$) as long as we have not received the packet containing the end of the gap and using linear interpolation for the rest of the gap otherwise. We term this approach *on-line compatible linear interpolation*.

2.6.2. AR modeling

As a somewhat more sophisticated technique compared to linear interpolation, we generated data from an AR model to fill the gap. For this we used the coefficients c_i of the AR model estimated for the data window directly before the gap to predict the missing samples $\hat{x}$:

$$\hat{x}(t_{g+k}) = \sum_{i=1}^{p} c_i x'(t_{g+k-i}) + \sigma \cdot e(t_{g+k}),\ 0 \leq k \leq l-1, \tag{3}$$

$$x'(t_{g+j}) = \begin{cases} x(t_{g+j}) & \text{if } j < 0 \\ \hat{x}(t_{g+j}) & \text{otherwise} \end{cases}$$

x' can refer to either actually recorded samples before the gap or estimated samples by the AR procedure. σ is the standard deviation of the white noise component in the estimated AR model and $e(t)$ one value of a white noise process. While this approach has the property to generate data for the gap consistent with the previously measured data, one might prefer to use a mixture of AR modeling and linear interpolation for the online case. This would avoid jumps in the data when merging generated data within the gap with new samples acquired after the gap. These jumps occur for all AR model orders we have tested in our simulations (see Appendix 1.4 for details). We have used this combination here by performing AR extrapolation when information about the first sample after the gap was not available and using linear interpolation otherwise. The signal was received in packets with a length of 40 ms and for each packet, one of three actions were taken: (1) if a packet contained the start and the end of a gap, then linear interpolation was used to fill the gap. (2) If it contained only the start or if the whole packet was part of the gap, then the AR model was used as a linear predictor to fill the gap. (3) If it contained only the end of the gap, then the last sample of the last packet and the first sample after the gap were connected by linear interpolation.

2.6.3. Joining two segments

If one chooses to ignore the information of the gap altogether when estimating the model, one might consider simply joining the two segments around the gap, therefore sacrificing information about the timing in the vicinity of the gap. In practice, this means that we update the data window only with those samples from a newly acquired data packet that do not belong to a gap. In order to keep the window size for spectral estimation constant, this has the consequence that older samples are used to compute the spectrum with this method compared to the other algorithms.

2.6.4. Burg algorithm for segments (MEMgap)

For standard algorithms that compute the AR coefficients, the samples within the data window need to be continuous. We can make the least-squares estimation of the AR coefficients compatible with data containing gaps by eliminating all equations from (Equation 1) that contain samples from within a gap and then solving the rest of the equations for the coefficients c_i. As the Burg algorithm (see Appendix 1.1) yields more stable AR models than the least-squares estimation, we modified it to work with gaps based on the Burg algorithm for segmented data proposed in de Waele and Broersen (2000). This was achieved by limiting the computation of forward and backward prediction errors in each step of the algorithm to those samples that are far enough away from a gap. In the remainder of this paper, this algorithm is called MEMgap (Maximum Entropy Method for data with gaps) for brevity. A detailed description of the algorithm is given in Appendix 1.3.

2.7. SIMULATIONS ON CLEAN DATA

To study empirically the influence of gaps on the estimated spectrum, we performed simulations on 12 data sets that were recorded without stimulation by artificially inserting gaps, then applying the methods described above to estimate the spectrum. The results of the different methods were compared with a reference time-frequency analysis obtained when using the original data set without gaps. Each data set has a length of 182 s. These data sets, each containing 11 trials, were recorded with ECoG in patient P1 in one experimental session. For clarity reasons, we restrict ourselves to one channel (an electrode over right M1). For spectral computation we kept the length of the window constant at 500 ms and the update rate at 25 Hz = 40 samples. We estimated the power at frequencies between 5 and 99 Hz in 2 Hz increments and varied for each method the gap size (0–100 ms in steps of 5 ms) and the model order (values: 16, 32, and 64). We computed the normalized bias, root mean squared error (RMSE) and variance (var) of the stimulus processing algorithms as follows:

$$\mathrm{bias}(f) = \frac{\frac{1}{n}\sum_i (P(f,i) - P_0(f,i))}{\overline{P_0(f)}}$$

$$\mathrm{RMSE}(f) = \frac{\sqrt{\frac{1}{n}\sum_i (P(f,i) - P_0(f,i))^2}}{\overline{P_0(f)}}$$

$$\mathrm{var}(f) = \mathrm{Var}\left(\frac{P(f) - P_0(f)}{\overline{P_0(f)}}\right)$$

$P(f,i)$ is the spectral power of data window i for frequency bin f, $P_0(f,i)$ is the power of the original data window without gaps and $\overline{P_0(f)}$ is the average power of the full original recording without gaps for frequency bin f. n is the number of data windows that are affected by gaps (i.e., data windows where $P(f,i) - P_0(f,i)$ is not zero). var(f) is the variance of the difference between the power values of the original data and the power values of the data with gaps for all data windows affected by gaps and frequency bin f, divided by the average power for frequency bin f in the data set without gaps. For example, a normalized bias of −0.1 means that the estimated power after application of the stimulus processing algorithm is on average 10% smaller than the power of the original data set if a gap is present.

The statistical evaluation of the spectral bias results in the simulations was performed as follows: we obtained the bias for each data set, resulting in 12 values, and performed a non-parametric Wilcoxon signed-rank test for zero median. If the p-value for this test was below 0.01, we regarded the bias as significant.

3. RESULTS

First we show results of simulated gaps on data without stimulation to assess the influence of gaps and the stimulation-processing algorithms on the estimated spectrum. Then we illustrate the influence of real single TMS and epidural stimulation pulses on the spectrum if they are left untreated and how the methods of this paper deal with their after-effects. Finally, we apply the algorithms to data sets of BCI experiments with open-loop or closed-loop stimulation and investigate the effect of each method on the discrimination between the brain states during intended movements and rest.

3.1. GAP SIZE

Figures 3A–C show the influence of gap sizes between 5 and 100 ms on the error in spectral estimation for three particular frequencies (9, 21, and 81 Hz) and a model order of 32. We find that the RMSE increases with the gap size for all methods. This happens, because the information of the samples that are excluded by the gap is missing for the AR estimation, leading to a greater deviation from the AR coefficients without gaps for increasing gap size. The linear interpolation methods exhibit a negative bias and the AR-prediction shows positive bias (**Figures 3D–F** and **5**). The negative bias of the linear interpolation methods occurs because a section of the data window is reduced to a straight line which has a power of almost 0 for higher frequencies, leading to a decrease in the estimated power for these frequencies. This effect increases with greater gaps. AR modeling can lead to jumps in the data, because the extrapolated signal from the start of the gap is not necessarily connected to the actual recorded signal at the end of the gap. Such jumps result in higher estimated power across all frequencies and thus a positive bias. For longer gaps this bias increases because the potential deviation from the true values after the gap (the jumps) becomes larger. The mixture of linear interpolation and AR prediction is in general closer to 0 than the other two, but the sign of its bias depends on data packet size and gap size. The joining and MEMgap algorithms exhibit a bias close to zero, but the RMSE is smaller for MEMgap than for joining. The variance (**Figures 3G–I**) also scales with gap size but there are strong differences between the methods visible, with MEMgap and the linear interpolation methods having the lowest variance.

3.2. MODEL ORDER

Variations of the model order have the largest effect on the AR modeling and the MEMgap algorithm. While AR modeling exhibits a significant positive bias at 21 Hz for gaps longer than 60 ms at a model order of 16 (**Figure 4D**), it is not significantly biased for a model order of 32 and 64 (**Figures 4E,F**). As shown in section 3.3 and **Figure 5**, this is due to the frequency-dependency of the bias for AR modeling which has a global minimum around 20 Hz for model order 32 and 64. For MEMgap we find no significant bias for all model orders (**Figures 4D–F**) and that the absolute error of the power estimation, captured by the normalized RMSE, as well as the variance, increases rapidly with increasing model orders (**Figures 4A–C,G–I**). This is probably due to the lower number of samples fully available for AR estimation with MEMgap compared to the standard Burg algorithm: for MEMgap, forward or backward prediction errors can not be calculated for up to $2p$ samples around each gap, where p is the model order. Higher values of p only increase this difference, leaving MEMgap with less and less samples for AR estimation, thus probably leading to greater errors. In general, MEMgap has the lowest RMSE for orders 16 and 32 and gaps longer than 30 ms and the lowest RMSE of all methods with a bias close to 0 at an order of 64.

3.3. FREQUENCY

In **Figure 3**, we show the results for low and high frequencies with 9 and 81 Hz as parts of the μ and high γ bands, respectively, in

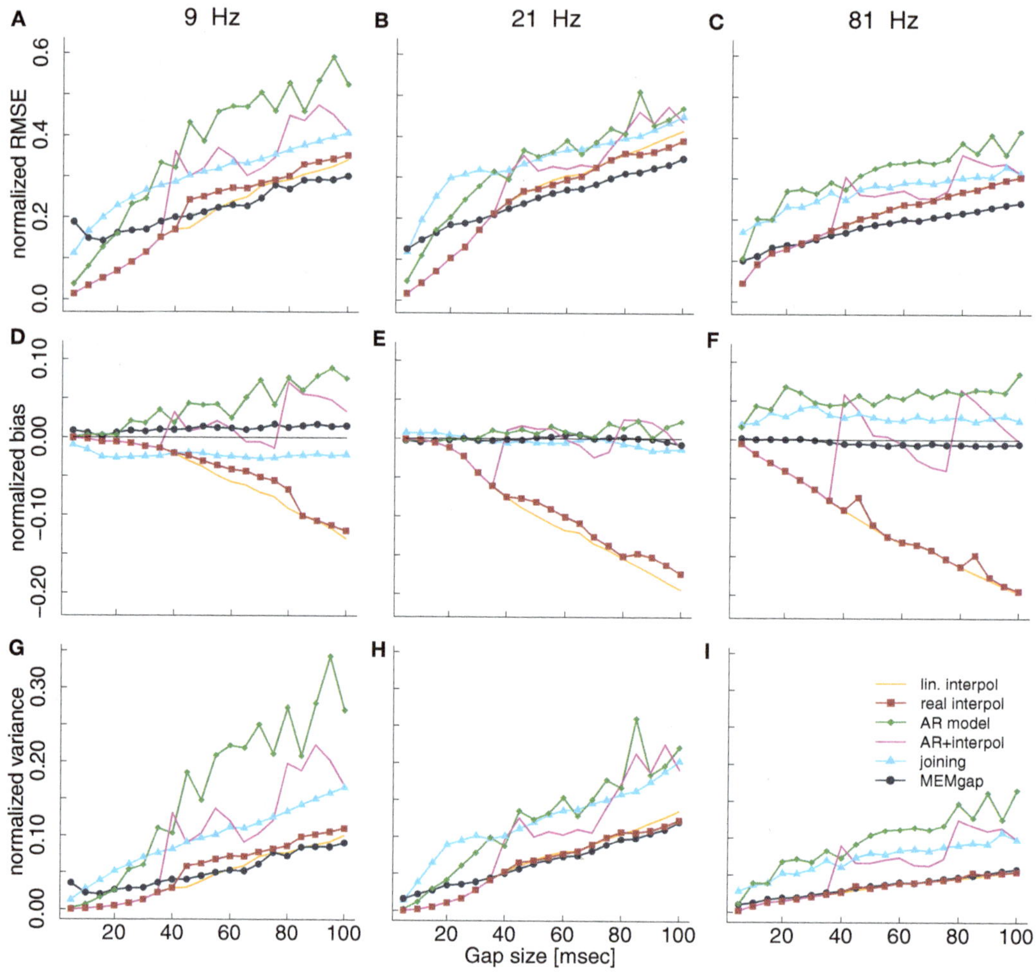

FIGURE 3 | Normalized RMSE, bias, and variance of the spectral power estimation for the frequency bin at 9 Hz (A,D,G), 21 Hz (B,E,H), and 81 Hz (C,F,I) for a model order of 32. The colored lines illustrate the course of the normalized RMSE in **(A–C)**, the normalized estimation bias in **(D–F)**, and the normalized variance in **(G–I)** relative to the gap size for the different algorithms. The thin black line in **(D–F)** denotes an ideal estimation bias of 0.

addition to the "intermediate" frequency of 21 Hz as part of the β-band. For 81 Hz, the linear interpolation methods already show a significant negative bias for gaps of 5 ms, whereas for 9 Hz this only becomes significant for gaps greater than 35 ms. This is easily understandable considering that one cycle of a 9 Hz oscillation lasts for more than 100 ms, therefore linear interpolation over a gap of 10–20 ms would be fairly consistent with the real shape of the undisturbed signal. The bias of MEMgap is not significant for any frequency (**Figures 3D–F**). The joining method on the other hand exhibits a negative bias for 9 Hz and gaps smaller than 40 ms and a significant positive bias for 81 Hz. For 21 Hz, The bias is significant only for gaps smaller than 10 ms. In terms of RMSE and variance (**Figures 3A–C,G–I**), MEMgap always displays the lowest values for gap sizes greater than 50 ms.

The results in **Figures 3D–F**, especially for AR modeling and joining, suggest that the bias might be frequency-dependent. In **Figure 5**, the bias is shown relative to the frequency bin for model orders of 16, 32, and 64 for a gap size of 100 ms where it should be most pronounced. We find that for the joining method, the bias is negative, although non-significant, for frequencies lower than 25 Hz and positive otherwise (significant for most frequencies >60 Hz). For AR modeling, the bias is in general positive (significantly for all frequencies for model order 16 and above 55 Hz for 32) and increases with frequency, has a minimum around 20 Hz for a model order of 32 and 64 and is also increased for lower frequencies. For linear interpolation, there is a bias close to −0.2, indicating a reduction in power of about 20%, for frequencies higher than 20 Hz. This value can be explained with the fact that 20% (100 ms of a 500 ms window) of the data had to be filled by linear interpolation which removes the high-frequency content. MEMgap exhibits no significant bias across all frequencies and model orders, except for very low frequencies and high model orders where all methods show a positive bias. Although the bias for the mixture of AR modeling and interpolation is also not significant for most frequencies above 10 Hz and higher model orders, this is due to the interaction between gap size and packet size for this particular method. As seen in **Figures 3D** or **F**, for example, a gap size of 80 would lead to a positive bias.

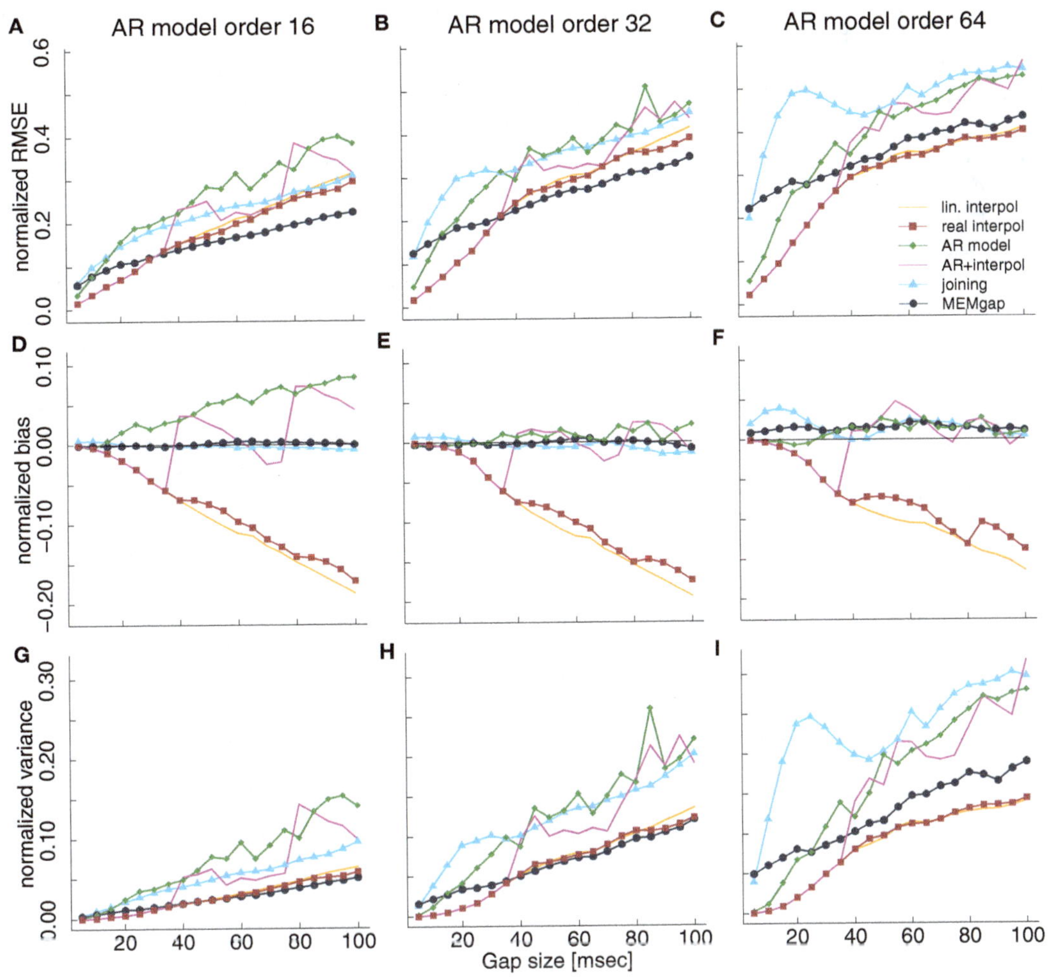

FIGURE 4 | Normalized RMSE, bias, and variance of the spectral power estimation for a model order of 16 (A,D,G), 32 (B,E,H), and 64 (C,F,I) for the frequency bin at 21 Hz. The colored lines illustrate the course of the normalized RMSE in **(A–C)**, the normalized estimation bias in **(D–F)**, and the normalized variance in **(G–I)** relative to the gap size for the different algorithms. The thin black line in **(D–F)** denotes an ideal estimation bias of 0.

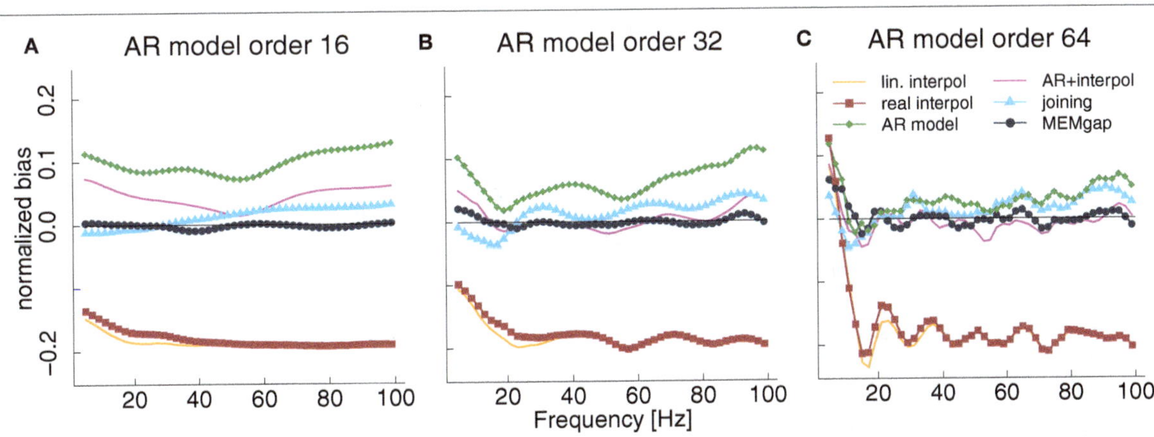

FIGURE 5 | Normalized bias for a gap size of 100 ms and an AR model order of 16 (A), 32 (B), and 64 (C) as a fraction of the power of the original signal. The thin solid line always indicates a bias of 0.

3.4. APPLICATION ON DATA WITH STIMULATION

In our experiments, we received the data in packets with a length of 40 ms. This leads to the jumps seen in the bias relative to the gap size for the combination of AR modeling and linear interpolation (e.g., **Figure 3F**, magenta line) as either linear interpolation of AR modeling dominate the outcome. The packet length might be different for other recordings, so we excluded this method from the rest of the experiments, as the conclusions would be very specific for our setup. Further experiments are needed to investigate the influence of this specific parameter. As the simulation results of the two versions of linear interpolation did not differ much, we restricted ourselves to four of the six methods for the remainder of the paper: online-compatible linear interpolation, AR modeling, joining, and MEMgap.

A model order of 16 was chosen for spectral estimation and AR extrapolation as this section is mostly illustrative in nature and serves the purpose to study whether the results from the simulations are transferable to data with actual stimulation. In terms of the estimation bias, we found the clearest effects for a model order of 16: a negative bias for linear interpolation and a positive bias for AR modeling. The latter bias was not present for higher model orders around the studied frequency bin of 21 Hz.

Figure 6 illustrates the effect of epidural stimulation on the recorded ECoG activity, the evoked activity after stimulation and their influence on spectral estimation for one representative stimulation pulse. **Figure 6A** shows the raw trace of data with a single pulse of electrical epidural stimulation occurring at time point 0. **Figure 6B** displays a zoom on the first 100 ms after the pulse. The stimulation artefact itself is contained within the first 10 ms after the pulse. After that, one can find evoked activity with its peak occurring 13 ms after the pulse and an amplitude of 240 μV. This is much higher than the short-term amplitude fluctuations found in our ECoG data without stimulation.

Figure 6C demonstrates the importance of adjusting the length of the gap to the actual stimulation effects on the signal. Applying a gap of 10 ms to the data might be enough to cover the stimulation artefact itself, but the spectrum then still shows a clear positive bias due to the influence of the evoked activity. The results for short gap sizes are very similar to those without any gap. Only gaps greater than 20 ms cover the extent of the artefact and the initial evoked activity, leading to power values that are similar to those obtained for data windows without the stimulation event (windows 16–26). There is no clear difference in the outcome of the gaps greater than 20 ms.

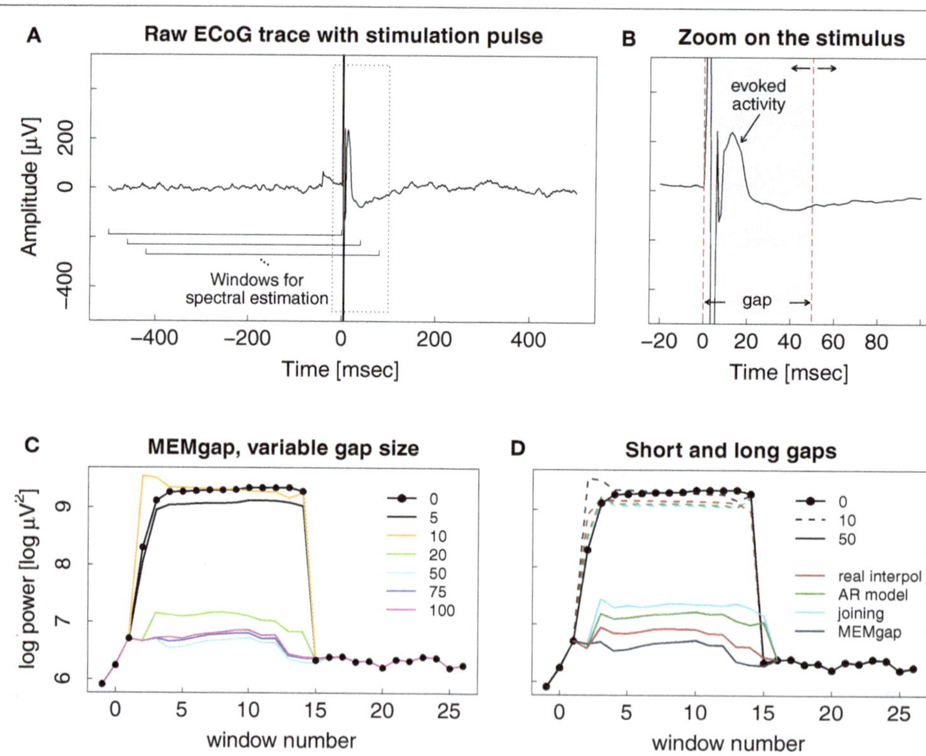

FIGURE 6 | Example ECoG trace of an epidural stimulation event. **(A)** One second of data with the stimulation at time point 0. The brackets show the moving window used for spectral analysis. **(B)** Zoomed version of the left plot, showing the evoked activity and the stimulation artefact in greater detail. Dashed lines show the start and end markings of the gap, here with a length of 50 ms. The end point of the gap can be varied in time. **(C)** Output of the spectral estimation using MEMgap for gap sizes of 5, 10, 20, 50, 75, and 100 ms and the frequency bin centered at 21 Hz. The logarithm of the estimated power is shown because of the large differences between the power at a gap size of 0 and 50 and above. Window numbers correspond to the brackets shown in **(A)**, where the first one is 1, the second one (shifted by 40 ms) is 2 and so on. The computation of windows −1, 0, and 15–26 used data that is outside the margins of **(A)**. **(D)** Comparison of linear interpolation (red), AR modeling (green), joining (blue), and MEMgap (gray) with gap sizes of 10 (dashed) and 50 (solid) applied on the data in **(A)**. The solid black line with circles in **(C)** and **(D)** shows the result of spectral estimation without processing of the stimulation after-effect (gap size = 0).

In **Figure 6D**, linear interpolation, joining the data segments, MEMgap, and AR modeling are compared when applied to the stimulation event both for short and long gaps. All methods perform poorly for a gap size of 10 ms, but there are differences for 50 ms. Applying joining and AR modeling results in higher power values than linear interpolation and MEMgap with a clear difference in estimated power between the windows with and without stimulation. Assuming perfect exclusion of all stimulus-related effects, we expect that the power does not differ strongly between e.g., window 15 (which includes a small portion of the gap) and window 16 (without the gap), therefore the result of MEMgap and linear interpolation is more realistic than the output of the other methods. At least for the AR modeling method, the increased estimate of the power compared to, for example, linear interpolation is consistent with the positive bias shown in **Figure 3B**. A reason for the positive bias of the joining method for this example data set might be that drifts of the signal after a stimulation on epidural electrodes are common. If we take a data segment with post-stimulus drifts, exclude the gap and join the data before and after the gap into one window, it will contain a sharp discontinuity and have a comparatively high spectral power. With linear interpolation, the discontinuity will be less severe and have a smaller impact on the signal power. For MEMgap it does not play a role as data before and after the gap is always separated during estimation of the AR coefficients.

Stimulation artefacts and evoked activity are found for combined EEG and TMS in a similar way as for stimulation over implanted electrodes with the strength of the evoked activity depending on the distance to the stimulation site. We illustrate this in **Figure 7** with the result of a TMS pulse on the activity recorded on a distant EEG channel. There is no strong evoked potential visible after the stimulation, therefore, as is evident in **Figures 7C,D**, a short window of 10 ms is already sufficient to cover the artefact and to produce an estimation of spectral power that is similar in value compared to that resulting for data windows long after the stimulation when using either linear interpolation, joining or MEMgap to correct for the gap.

3.5. INFLUENCE ON DECODING PERFORMANCE

The stimulation-processing algorithm can bias the estimated spectrum, or will at least produce deviations from the original spectral power without gaps. This poses the question, how strongly these errors influence the actual brain-state decoding during a BCI experiment. For example, if the bias of linear interpolation toward underestimation of the signal power directly influences, how well we can differentiate data packets obtained during a movement from those recorded during rest, then this algorithm is not suitable for BSDS because it might induce a bias in the subject's performance in an online experiment.

To investigate this, we used data sets with different stimulation paradigms and recording methods (EEG and ECoG) to assess the influence of the algorithms and gap size on the decoding abilities of a BCI system. The patients always performed the

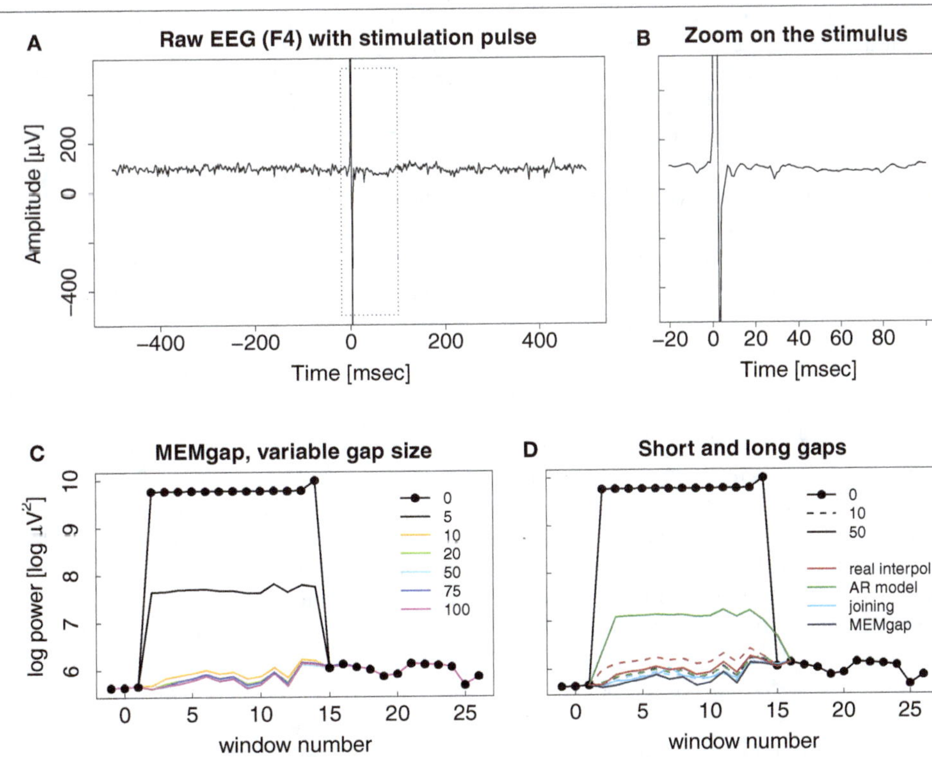

FIGURE 7 | Example trace of a TMS pulse applied over EEG channel (C4) but recorded on a distant channel (F4). (A–D) Same as in **Figure 6**. Note the missing evoked activity in **(A)** and **(B)** after the pulse.

same cued attempted hand movements but we varied the stimulation paradigm between no stimulation, stimulation with fixed ISI and stimulation coupled to the output of the BCI (i.e., BSDS). In the last paradigm, the stimulation pulses were only applied while the BCI detected an intention to move from modulations of the power in the β-band and therefore moved the orthosis. If stimulation was used, stimulation artefacts were identified online with a peak detector if the voltage of two consecutive samples differed by more than 1 mV. The start of the gap was set 2 ms before this artefact and the gap size was adjusted for each patient and session depending on the length of the evoked activity as determined by several test stimuli applied before the start of the session. This resulted typically in a gap length between 30 and 70 ms. Stimulus processing was performed during recording with the online-compatible linear interpolation method.

In the offline analysis, we applied the four methods: joining, linear interpolation, AR modeling, and MEMgap on these data sets and varied the gap size between 0, 10, 50, and 100. We simulated the two different stimulation conditions on the data without stimulation by varying, in which phases of the trial gaps are placed: in the uncoupled condition the whole trial was valid, so the placement of gaps was independent of the activity and brainstate of the patient. For the coupled condition only time points within the movement phase were used as gaps, thus simulating a BSDS paradigm. In both cases the ISI was fixed at 2 s.

After applying the respective stimulation processing algorithm, we computed the spectral power between 16 and 22 Hz on channels located over the right motor cortex. For EEG measurements we used FC4, C4, and CP4 as defined by the 10–10 system (Society, 2006), whereas for ECoG measurements the electrodes were selected individually per patient based on the results of a screening session. We used a window size of 500 ms and a model order of 16 for spectral estimation. These were the same parameters, channels and frequencies that had been used during the online feedback experiments in which the data was recorded. Furthermore, our simulations showed a positive estimation bias for AR modeling at 16–22 Hz only for a model order of 16, not for 32 or 64. Thus, we only used an order of 16 for the simulations on data without stimulation. In order to investigate, whether higher model orders have a substantial effect on the processing of real stimuli, we used model orders of 16, 32, and 64 on the data with open-loop and closed-loop stimulation. For each run (consisting of 11 trials), we calculated the area under the ROC curve (AUC) for the sum of the logarithm of the power values within each data window in the movement phase versus those in the rest phase. We used this as a measure of the separability of these phases on a single-packet level. Taken together from all three patients, we analyzed 87 runs of EEG recordings without stimulation, 24 runs with uncoupled EEG-TMS, 131 ECoG runs without stimuli, 51 runs of ECoG with uncoupled, and 82 runs of ECoG with coupled stimulation. For each recording and stimulation condition, algorithm and gap size, this resulted in a distribution of AUC scores, one per run.

The conditions without stimulation allowed us to test for the bias and absolute error introduced by the gaps into the AUC scores. Thus, we computed the pair-wise differences between the AUC scores of a gap size of 0 and those of all combinations of algorithms and gap size for these conditions. Using Kruskal–Wallis tests, Bonferroni-corrected for multiple comparisons, we tested which algorithm leads to the smallest absolute differences in AUC scores. We also applied Wilcoxon signed rank tests to assess, whether the median of the differences deviates significantly from 0, indicating a systematic bias in the AUC scores. As there is no "true" reference distribution of the AUC scores possible for data with stimulation, we used Bonferroni-corrected non-parametric Friedman tests which account for possible effects of using the same sessions in all conditions to test whether gap sizes greater than 0 lead to different AUC scores compared to a gap size of 0 and to test whether there is a difference between the algorithms at a certain gap size.

Figure 8 shows data without any actual stimulation, so ideally the difference in AUC scores between a gap size of 0 and of 100 should be zero for all runs. In **Figures 8A,B**, stimuli were simulated throughout the trial, thus independent of the task or the output of the BCI. Session-wise comparison of the AUC values with Friedman tests for each gap size show significant differences between MEMgap and the other algorithms only for long gaps. There is a slight decrease in the average AUC value for all algorithms for a gap size of 100 compared to 0 and MEMgap and joining yield significantly smaller absolute differences in AUC scores compared to AR modeling and interpolation ($p < 0.000001$). In **Figures 8C,D**, the stimuli were simulated only throughout the movement phase. We find a significant decrease in AUC values for AR modeling and a significant increase for linear interpolation. This means that linear interpolation artificially "improves" the decoding power. As shown in the simulation studies, linear interpolation of large gaps leads to a decrease of the power between 16 and 22 Hz (negative bias) which increases the event-related desynchronization effect of sensorimotor rhythms during attempted movements (Wolpaw et al., 2002). The MEMgap method shows a significantly smaller deviation of the AUC values at gap sizes of 50 and 100 from the AUC values without gaps than all the other methods ($p < 0.000001$). In contrast to the other algorithms, the median of the AUC differences after MEMgap never differs significantly from 0 for the BSDS condition, except for the ECoG data set with a gap size of 100 ($p = 0.005$). The other algorithms differ significantly from MEMgap in almost all cases of the coupled conditions.

Patients in the data sets shown in **Figures 9A,B** were stimulated independent of the task. We show only a model order of 16, because the results for an order of 32 and 64 are very similar. It is evident from gap sizes of 0 and 10 that untreated stimulation after-effects are detrimental for decoding. Online decoding will be more successful if enough samples are excluded after a stimulus (in these examples: a gap size of 50 ms seems to work well, although this varies between patients). Using Friedman tests for session-wise comparison of the AUC scores, significant differences of the algorithms are found, although the mean absolute differences are very small (≤ 0.01). In case of the uncoupled ECoG condition, AUC scores with untreated stimulation after-effects are significantly lower than AUC scores for gap sizes of 50 and 100, independent of the applied algorithm ($p < 0.01$). This effect is due to residual stimulation after-effects for small or absent gaps that lead to a very high power of data windows that contain

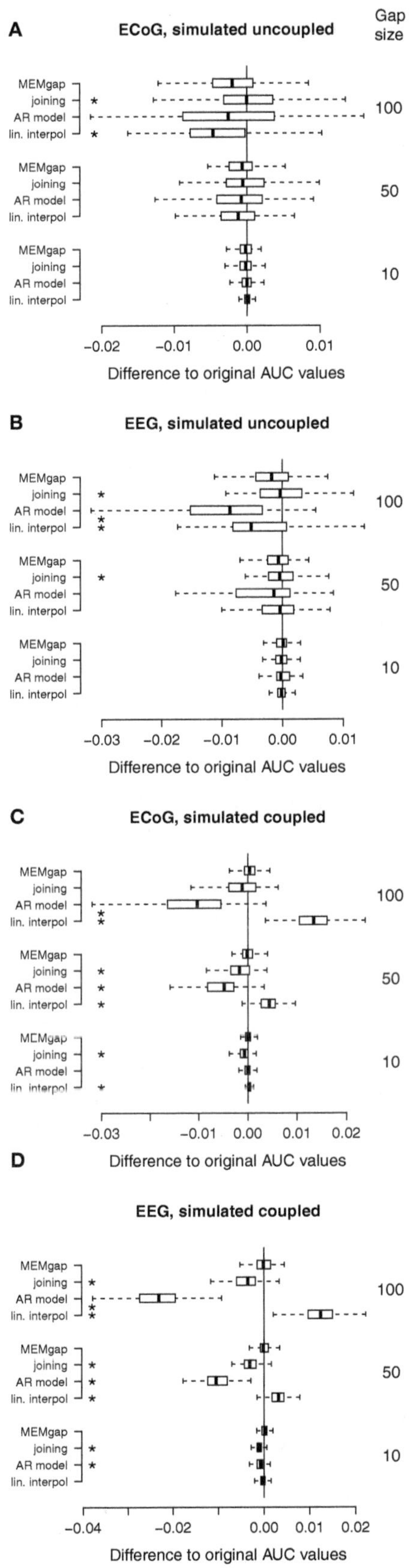

FIGURE 8 | Continued

FIGURE 8 | Distributions of the differences between AUC values without gaps and AUC values of gap sizes of 10, 50, and 100 for data sets without stimulation. A deviation from 0 indicates an over- or under-estimation of class separability. **(A)** ECoG and **(B)** EEG data with gaps simulated throughout the whole trial (*uncoupled* condition). **(C,D)** AUC values computed on the same data sets as in **(A)** and **(B)**, respectively, but with gaps simulated only within the movement phase (*coupled* condition, BSDS). Boxes cover the range between the lower and upper quartile of AUC differences with the median depicted as a black line. The whiskers extend to the most extreme data point which is no more than 1.5 times the interquartile range away from the box. *AUC scores differ significantly from MEMgap for this gap size ($p < 0.05$, Friedman test, Bonferroni-corrected).

electrical or magnetic pulses. In particular such data windows in the movement phase will be classified incorrectly. If the strong after-effects are removed by longer gaps, the classifier is more likely to produce a correct result which is reflected in the increased AUC score for gaps of at least 50 ms.

Finally, in **Figure 9C**, stimulation was given only during the movement phase. The average AUC value for a gap size of 0 is smaller than 0.5, indicating a higher power during movement than during rest, as opposed to the expected event-related desynchronization. This is due to the task-dependent existence of the stimulation effects: the large stimulation after-effects that occur only during the movement phase lead to a very high spectral power of this phase. Thus, the spectral power of the movement phase is very well separable from the power of the rest phase for a gap size of 0. For a gap size of 10, there is a large variability in the AUC scores. This is because for one of the three patients, a gap of 10 ms was not sufficient to cover all artefact-related jumps in the recording, resulting in AUC scores lower than 0.5. If the after-effects are dealt with by using a gap size of 50, the relationship between the power during rest and feedback reverses and resembles the expected ERD/ERS pattern. For a gap size of 100, we find in **Figure 9C** that the largest average AUC value is reached for linear interpolation and the smallest one for AR modeling, both differing significantly from the AUC values for MEMgap ($p < 0.000001$). This relationship is found for all tested model orders, where joining and AR modeling are on average worse than MEMgap by more than 0.02 and 0.05, respectively, while linear interpolation yields higher scores by at least 0.01. This is consistent with the simulation results in **Figures 8C,D** indicating an artificial over- and under-estimation of class separability by these methods. It supports the hypothesis that MEMgap is probably best suited to deal with large gaps in the data, especially for BSDS, because based on the simulation studies the deviation from the true AUC value is significantly smaller than for the other methods.

4. DISCUSSION

One challenge when trying to combine online brain-state decoding from spectral data and direct cortical stimulation is that the after-effects of stimulation such as artefacts (Taylor et al., 2008) or evoked activity (Matsumoto et al., 2007) can have a much higher amplitude than the background brain signals. Therefore, estimation of the brain-state from a segment of data has been unreliable,

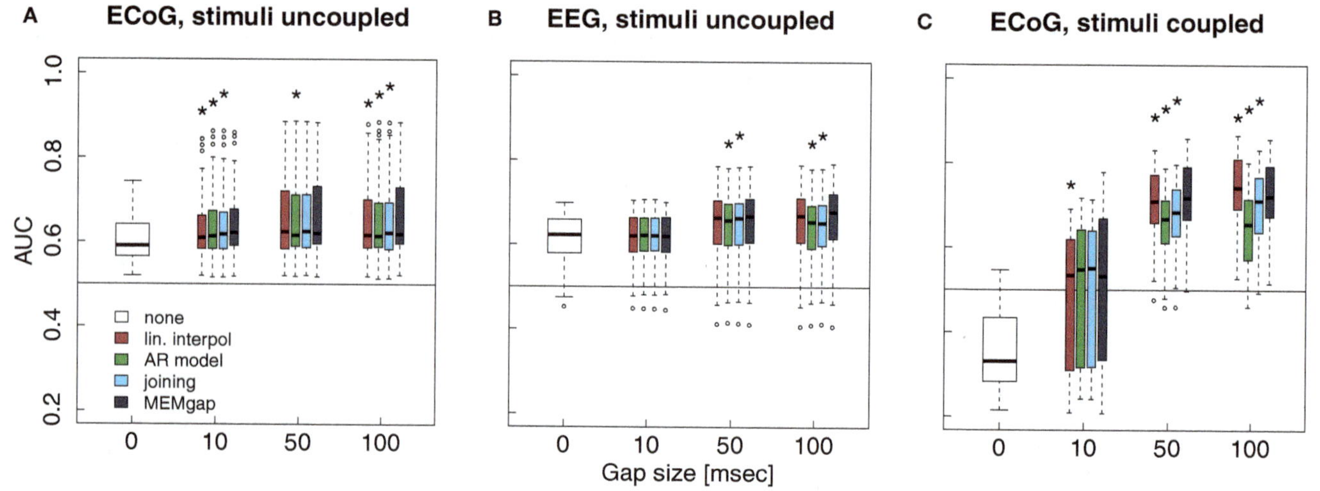

FIGURE 9 | Influence of the stimulation processing algorithm and gap size on the separability between intended movement and rest for experiments with stimulation. No processing of the stimulation after-effects was conducted for a gap size of 0. For gap sizes of 10, 50, and 100, AUC values were calculated after application of the four algorithms (boxes from left to right) *real interpol, AR model, joining,* and *MEMgap*. A baseline AUC value of 0.5 is shown as a solid line, because this is the chance level for a purely random classifier (Fawcett, 2006). **(A)** Average AUC values for the separation of movement and rest from experiments with epidural stimulation and ECoG recordings. Stimulation pulses were given throughout the whole trial with a fixed ISI of 2 s and the gap size was varied between 0, 10, 50, and 100. **(B)** Same as **(A)**, but for TMS-EEG data with an ISI of 3 s. **(C)** Average AUC values for ECoG data sets where stimulation pulses were triggered only if the BCI system detected an intention to move within the movement phase (BSDS). Boxes are defined as in **Figure 8**, open circles depict AUC values outside the range of the boxplot whiskers. *AUC scores for this algorithm and gap size differ significantly from MEMgap ($p < 0.05$, Friedman test, Bonferroni-corrected).

if such stimulation after-effects are contained in this segment. This leaves us with three options: we can (1) use only data segments for decoding that are free of any after-effects, (2) attempt to separate stimulation after-effects from background brain activity, e.g., by fitting a template of the expected shape of the effects to the recording, or (3) isolate the portions of the data segment that are "contaminated" by stimulation effects and use only the "clean" parts for decoding.

In earlier studies combining TMS and EEG without BSDS (i.e., without the necessity to perform real-time brain-state-decoding from the EEG), options (1) and (2) have been used. In such studies, either a fixed length window around the stimulus was removed offline (Fuggetta et al., 2006), a decomposition into artefact-free and contaminated data was attempted in post-processing (Litvak et al., 2007; Morbidi et al., 2007; Erez et al., 2010) or a sample-and-hold circuit was used during recording to fix the amplifier output at a constant level during the pulse (Ilmoniemi et al., 1997). The latter method is especially helpful for amplifiers that recover from TMS pulses only after a delay of several hundred milliseconds (Ilmoniemi and Kičić, 2010), although some current amplifiers are able to keep this delay lower than 10 ms (Veniero et al., 2009). The drawback of the sample-and-hold approach is that information on the brain signal directly after the pulse is invariably lost and that the signal contains gaps.

Option (1) has also been used by Bergmann et al. (2012) in their study on EEG-guided TMS, making a waiting period of several seconds between stimulation pulses necessary. If the brain-state is decoded from spectral features and for example 500 ms of data is needed to estimate these features robustly, one has to wait for 500 ms plus the expected duration of the stimulation after-effects for making the first estimate of the brain-state after a stimulation pulse. This duration is therefore also the absolute minimum ISI in this scenario. Removal of the after-effects by template subtraction is only possible, if several constraints are met: the full amplitude range of the stimulation effects has to be within the dynamic range of the amplifier, as portions of the data in which the amplifier is in saturation can not be recovered with this method, resulting in the necessity to correct for gaps in the signal as in option (3). If the recorded effects are not sufficiently stable, attempting to remove them will lead to residuals in the signal. Like the original after-effects, these residuals can have a detrimental effect on the quality of the estimated spectrum and, thus, the decoding process. The employed removal algorithms need to be suitable for an online BCI, so they need to work on a single-trial level and therefore should not be too computationally demanding.

We have chosen approach (3) for this work, the deliberate introduction of gaps into the signal covering the strongest after-effects of stimulation and correcting for these gaps during spectral estimation. This allows continuous decoding without influence of the stimulation after-effects, as long as the duration of the after-effects is estimated properly. To apply this approach, methods are needed that do not depend on continuous data segments for brain-state decoding and can deal with gaps in the data.

In our experiments, we analyzed the spectral power in the μ- and/or β-band to detect the patient's intention to move the paralyzed hand. We compared different approaches (linear interpolation, AR modeling, joining of data segments, and the Burg algorithm adapted for segmented data) on their ability to estimate the spectrum with gaps in the data. To this end, we used an ECoG BCI training data set and analyzed the normalized RMSE, bias and variance of the difference between the estimated spectrum with and without gaps. The RMSE increased with the gap size, although the slope of the error increase was smaller for MEMgap and joining than for algorithms that fill the gap with artificial data (linear interpolation and AR modeling). We found a clear systematic negative bias for linear interpolation and a systematic positive bias for AR modeling. We studied the frequency range between 16 and 22 Hz in most detail, where the bias of AR modeling was only apparent for a model order of 16, but a clear bias of AR modeling can be found for other frequencies at higher model orders, making this method also potentially unreliable. The joining method produces a bias close to 0 around a frequency of 20 Hz, but can lead to a positive bias for higher frequencies, whereas the MEMgap method always results in a bias close to 0. For gaps smaller than 40 ms, linear interpolation typically has the smallest absolute deviation from the true power values while MEMgap outperforms the other methods for longer gaps.

As our simulations show, the RMSE for linear interpolation is smaller than for MEMgap, thus at first glance making linear interpolation superior to MEMgap for large model orders and/or small gaps. However, in the context of a continuous BCI decoding for BSDS, the negative bias exhibited by the linear interpolation methods will bias the output of the BCI in favor of ERD, thus distorting the real performance of the participant to some extent if stimulation is coupled to the detected brain-state. We therefore think that MEMgap is most suited for BSDS as it is superior or at least equal to the other methods in terms of RMSE and variance, does not introduce a systematic bias and outperforms the other methods in minimizing the stimulation after-effects in our BCI paradigm.

Whether this approach of identifying and ignoring the segments of data dominated by stimulation after-effects is feasible in any given experimental setting depends on the duration of stimulation-evoked potentials after the pulse. As we showed here in the simulation studies, if the strongest evoked activity is contained within the first 50–100 ms after the pulse, then a decoding approach using MEMgap is feasible. If no strong evoked activity is observed, e.g., in the case of a remote recording location as illustrated in **Figure 7**, then a short gap of 10 ms covering the stimulus artefact together with linear interpolation or MEMgap would be sufficient. In Ferreri et al. (2011), evoked EEG activity following single pulse TMS was found for up to 300 ms after the pulse with amplitude fluctuations of less than 20 μV for late components. Although we do not expect that such small potentials would have a large impact on the estimated spectrum, especially compared to the stimulation artefact itself or early evoked activity, for every experiment of BSDS with continuous decoding, the size and shape of the evoked activity should be carefully studied to get a proper estimate of the duration of strong after-effects. As was shown by Casarotto et al. (2010), the after-effects depend on a number of parameters, such as stimulation intensity, location and (in the case of TMS) coil orientation. If gaps longer than the 100 ms tested here are necessary to cover all stimulation-related activity, one should either wait long enough until all effects have ceased before making the next brain-state decoding attempt, or increase the size of the data window on which the spectrum is estimated to ensure that it contains enough clean samples to compute a valid estimate.

In conclusion, we have shown that the application of cortical stimulation coupled to the output of an online brain-state decoder based on spectral features is feasible as long as the employed algorithms remove both the stimulation artefact and large early components of evoked activity and allow spectral estimation on non-continuous data. Especially if closed-loop BSDS is used, algorithms that do not introduce a strong bias into the estimated spectrum such as MEMgap are to be preferred over biased methods like linear interpolation to ensure a reliable decoding of the brain-state. In general, the methods investigated here are not restricted to applications with cortical stimulation but can be employed whenever spectral estimation has to be performed on non-continuous data sets with missing blocks of samples.

ACKNOWLEDGMENTS

This work was funded by the European Research Council (ERC) grant 227632 "BCCI– A Bidirectional Cortical Communication Interface" and the Reinhardt-Koselleck Award of the Deutsche Forschungsgemeinschaft (DFG). We thank Alireza Gharabaghi, Maria Teresa Leão, Georgios Naros, Alexandros Viziotis, and Martin Spüler for insightful discussions and their help in data acquisition and the two reviewers for helpful comments on the manuscript.

REFERENCES

Bergmann, T. O., Mölle, M., Schmidt, M. A., Lindner, C., Marshall, L., Born, J., et al. (2012). EEG-guided transcranial magnetic stimulation reveals rapid shifts in motor cortical excitability during the human sleep slow oscillation. *J. Neurosci.* 32, 243–253.

Birbaumer, N., and Cohen, L. G. (2007). Brain-computer interfaces: communication and restoration of movement in paralysis. *J. Physiol.* 579(Pt 3), 621–636.

Birbaumer, N., Ghanayim, N., Hinterberger, T., Iversen, I., Kotchoubey, B., Kübler, A., et al. (1999). A spelling device for the paralysed. *Nature* 398, 297–298.

Brown, J. A., Lutsep, H. L., Weinand, M., and Cramer, S. C. (2008). Motor cortex stimulation for the enhancement of recovery from stroke: a prospective, multicenter safety study. *Neurosurgery* 62(Suppl. 2), 853–862.

Casarotto, S., Romero Lauro, L. J., Bellina, V., Casali, A. G., Rosanova, M., Pigorini, A., et al. (2010). EEG responses to TMS are sensitive to changes in the perturbation parameters and repeatable over time. *PLoS ONE* 5:e10281. doi: 10.1371/journal.pone.0010281

de Waele, S., and Broersen, P. (2000). The Burg algorithm for segments. *IEEE Trans. Signal Process.* 48, 2876–2880.

Erez, Y., Tischler, H., Moran, A., and Bar-Gad, I. (2010). Generalized framework for stimulus artifact removal. *J. Neurosci. Methods* 191, 45–59.

Fawcett, T. (2006). An introduction to ROC analysis. *Pattern Recogn. Lett.* 27, 861–874.

Ferreri, F., Pasqualetti, P., Määttä, S., Ponzo, D., Ferrarelli, F., Tononi, G., et al. (2011). Human brain connectivity during single and paired pulse transcranial magnetic stimulation. *Neuroimage* 54, 90–102.

Fuggetta, G., Pavone, E., Walsh, V., Kiss, M., and Eimer, M. (2006). Cortico-cortical interactions in spatial attention: a combined ERP/TMS study. *J. Neurophysiol.* 95, 3277.

Ilmoniemi, R., and Kičić, D. (2010). Methodology for combined TMS and EEG. *Brain Topogr.* 22, 233–248.

Ilmoniemi, R. J., Virtanen, J., Ruohonen, J., Karhu, J., Aronen, H. J., Näätänen, R., et al. (1997).

Neuronal responses to magnetic stimulation reveal cortical reactivity and connectivity. *Neuroreport* 8, 3537–3540.

Jackson, A., Mavoori, J., and Fetz, E. E. (2006). Long-term motor cortex plasticity induced by an electronic neural implant. *Nature* 444, 56–60.

Jensen, O., Bahramisharif, A., Oostenveld, R., Klanke, S., Hadjipapas, A., Okazaki, Y. O., et al. (2011). Using brain-computer interfaces and brain-state dependent stimulation as tools in cognitive neuroscience. *Front. Psychology* 2:100. doi: 10.3389/fpsyg.2011.00100

Kay, S., and Marple, S. (1981). Spectrum analysis–A modern perspective. *Proc. IEEE* 69, 1380–1419.

Krusienski, D. J., McFarland, D. J., and Wolpaw, J. R. (2006). "An evaluation of autoregressive spectral estimation model order for brain-computer interface applications," in *Proceedings of the 28th Annual International Conference of the IEEE Engineering in Medicine and Biology Society EMBS '06, Vol. 1*, (New York, NY), 1323–1326.

Lefaucheur, J.-P., and de Andrade, D. C. (2009). Intraoperative neurophysiologic mapping of the central cortical region for epidural electrode placement in the treatment of neuropathic pain by motor cortex stimulation. *Brain Stimul.* 2, 138–148.

Levy, R., Ruland, S., Weinand, M., Lowry, D., Dafer, R., and Bakay, R. (2008). Cortical stimulation for the rehabilitation of patients with hemiparetic stroke: a multicenter feasibility study of safety and efficacy. *J. Neurosurg.* 108, 707–714.

Litvak, V., Komssi, S., Scherg, M., Hoechstetter, K., Classen, J., Zaaroor, M., et al. (2007). Artifact correction and source analysis of early electroencephalographic responses evoked by transcranial magnetic stimulation over primary motor cortex. *Neuroimage* 37, 56–70.

Matsumoto, R., Nair, D. R., LaPresto, E., Bingaman, W., Shibasaki, H., and Lüders, H. O. (2007). Functional connectivity in human cortical motor system: a cortico-cortical evoked potential study. *Brain* 130(Pt 1), 181–197.

McFarland, D. J., and Wolpaw, J. R. (2008). Sensorimotor rhythm-based brain-computer interface (BCI): model order selection for autoregressive spectral analysis. *J. Neural Eng.* 5, 155–162.

Mitchell, W. K., Baker, M. M. R., and Baker, S. S. N. (2007). Muscle responses to transcranial stimulation in man depend on background oscillatory activity. *J. Physiol.* 583(Pt 2), 567–579.

Morbidi, F., Garulli, A., Prattichizzo, D., Rizzo, C., Manganotti, P., and Rossi, S. (2007). Off-line removal of TMS-induced artifacts on human electroencephalography by Kalman filter. *J. Neurosci. Methods* 162, 293–302.

Pardey, J., Roberts, S., and Tarassenko, L. (1996). A review of parametric modelling techniques for EEG analysis. *Med. Eng. Phys.* 18, 2–11.

Plow, E. B., Carey, J. R., Nudo, R. J., and Pascual-Leone, A. (2009). Invasive cortical stimulation to promote recovery of function after stroke: a critical appraisal. *Stroke* 40, 1926–1931.

Ramos-Murguialday, A., Schürholz, M., Caggiano, V., Wildgruber, M., Caria, A., Hammer, E. M., et al. (2012). Proprioceptive feedback and brain computer interface (BCI) based neuroprostheses. *PLoS ONE* 7:e47048. doi: 10.1371/journal.pone.0047048

Schalk, G., McFarland, D. J., Hinterberger, T., Birbaumer, N., and Wolpaw, J. R. (2004). BCI2000: a general-purpose brain-computer interface (BCI) system. *IEEE Trans. Biomed. Eng.* 51, 1034–1043.

Society, A. C. N. (2006). Guideline 5: guidelines for standard electrode position nomenclature. *J. Clin. Neurophysiol.* 23, 107–110.

Taylor, P., Walsh, V., and Eimer, M. (2008). Combining TMS and EEG to study cognitive function and cortico-cortico interactions. *Behav. Brain Res.* 191, 141–147.

Tsubokawa, T., Katayama, Y., Yamamoto, T., Hirayama, T., and Koyama, S. (1991). Chronic motor cortex stimulation for the treatment of central pain. *Acta Neurochir. Suppl.* 52, 137–139.

Veniero, D., Bortoletto, M., and Miniussi, C. (2009). TMS-EEG co-registration: on TMS-induced artifact. *Clin. Neurophysiol.* 120, 1392–1399.

Wassermann, E., Epstein, C., and Ziemann, U. (2008). *Oxford Handbook of Transcranial Stimulation (Oxford Handbooks).* New York, NY: Oxford University Press.

Wolpaw, J. R., Birbaumer, N., McFarland, D. J., Pfurtscheller, G., and Vaughan, T. M. (2002). Brain-computer interfaces for communication and control. *Clin. Neurophysiol.* 113, 767–791.

1. APPENDIX

1.1. THE BURG ALGORITHM

The Burg algorithm is used for the estimation of the coefficients c_i of an autoregressive (AR) model

$$x(t_p) = \sum_{i=1}^{p} c_i x(t_{p-i}) + e$$

with order p for samples $x(t_k), 0 \leq k < N$, e a sample from a white noise sequence. The algorithm needs p recursive steps and in each step j, the coefficients $c_{j,i}$ for an autoregressive model of order j are computed by the following procedure:

An initial estimation of the power of the white noise component in the AR model is obtained by

$$P_0 = \frac{1}{N} \sum_{k=0}^{N-1} |x(t_k)|^2.$$

Each new coefficient $c_{i,i}$ is computed by minimizing the forward and backward prediction errors

$$f_{p,k} = x(t_k) - \sum_{i=1}^{p} c_{p,i}\, x(t_{k-i}) \qquad \text{with } k = p, \ldots, N-1$$

$$b_{p,k} = x(t_{k-p}) - \sum_{i=1}^{p} c_{p,i}\, x(t_{k-p+i}) \qquad \text{with } k = p, \ldots, N-1$$

with the formula

$$c_{i,i} = \frac{-2 \sum_{k \in I_i} f_{i-1,k} \cdot b_{i-1,k-2}}{\sum_{k \in I_i} \left(|f_{i-1,k}|^2 + |b_{i-1,k-1}|^2 \right)}, \quad I_i = \{i+1, \ldots, N-1\}. \tag{A1}$$

Each previously computed coefficient $c_{i-1,k}$ is then adjusted by

$$c_{i,k} = c_{i-1,k} + c_{i,i} \cdot c_{i-1,i-k}$$

and we update the power estimation to

$$P_i = (1 - |c_{i,i}|^2) \cdot P_{i-1}$$

and the forward and backward prediction errors:

$$f_{i,k} = f_{i-1,k} + c_{i,i} \cdot b_{i-1,k-1}$$
$$b_{i,k} = b_{i-1,k-1} + c_{i,i} \cdot f_{i-1,k}\,.$$

After p steps, this results in the AR coefficients $c_i = c_{i,p}$, $i = 1, \ldots, p$.

1.2. ESTIMATING THE SPECTRUM FROM AN AR MODEL

An AR model can be interpreted as an all-pole infinite-impulse-response filter with order p and coefficients c_i which is applied to a white noise process with a power of P_p (Pardey et al., 1996). Thus, after finding the p autoregressive coefficients c_i, one can estimate the spectrum by evaluating the transfer function $H(z) = \sqrt{P_p}\left(1 - \sum_{k=1}^{p} c_k z^k\right)^{-1}$ of the filter to find power values

$$P(\omega) = \frac{P_p}{|1 - \sum_{k=1}^{p} c_k e^{-jk\omega}|^2}$$

at (normalized) frequencies ω.

1.3. THE MEMgap ALGORITHM

If one assumes that a sequence g of length N exists and that $g(n) = 1$ only if the corresponding sample $x(t_n)$ is part of a gap in the data and 0 otherwise then we just have to make sure that none of the samples $x(t_n)$ with $g(n) = 1$ influence the estimation of the model coefficients. The Burg algorithm computes the AR coefficients for order p in p steps, yielding in the i-th step the coefficients of an AR model with order i. If we use in the i-th step only those samples fully for computation of the AR coefficients that are at least $i + 1$ time steps away from a sample with $g(n) = 1$, we achieve the desired effect. To be more precise, the coefficients are computed by evaluating forward and backward prediction errors (see Appendix 1.1). In the MEMgap algorithm, forward prediction errors are only computed for samples that are at least $i + 1$ time steps after a gap, backward prediction errors only for those at least $i + 1$ time steps before a gap. Formally, this is done by modifying I_i in Equation (A1) to the set

$$\begin{aligned} I_i = &\{k \mid g(k) = 0 \wedge i < k < N \wedge \\ &(k - n < 0 \vee k - n > i)\ \forall n \text{ with } g(n) = 1\}. \end{aligned}$$

This set can also be computed iteratively in each step of the Burg algorithm as $I_i = I_{i-1} \cap I'_{i-1}$, where I'_{i-1} is the set I_{i-1} with each entry incremented by 1 and $I_0 = \{k \mid g(k) = 0 \wedge 0 < k < N\}$. This resembles a "forbidden zone" that initially contains only the gaps but grows in each step of the algorithm by one sample. The estimation of the white noise power P_0 has to be calculated only with samples outside of gaps: $P_0 = \frac{1}{|I_0|} \sum_{k \in I_0} |x(t_k)|^2$. The rest of the algorithm works as the standard Burg algorithm described in Appendix 1.1.

Obviously, this method can only work if the continuous segments between gaps are long enough. Therefore, there needs to be at least one segment of samples with a length that is at least equal to the model order p in order to make an estimation of the spectrum with this method. In practice, it is preferable if the number of samples in such a segment is several times higher than the model order in order to reduce the bias and variance of the estimator. If there are n_s segments of clean data with a length greater than p and the total number of samples in these segments equals M, then only $M - 2n_s p$ forward and backward prediction errors are available in the p-th step of the MEMgap algorithm, although all M samples are evaluated to compute these errors. This means that even if the total number of samples within gaps might be the same, one can expect that the variance of the spectral estimation will be smaller if there are only a few large gaps in the data compared to having many small gaps because less samples contribute fully in the second case. According to de Waele and Broersen (2000), the same holds for the estimation bias which is inversely proportional to the number of available samples.

1.4. AR MODELING INDUCES JUMPS IN THE SIGNAL

The approach to fill the gap with samples that were extrapolated by an AR model fitted to the data before the gap can be problematic, if the extrapolation diverges strongly from the measured data. When actually measured samples are added to the data buffer after the gap, there can be a large amplitude difference between the last (extrapolated) sample within the gap and the first measured sample after the gap (**Figure A1A**). Such a "jump" in the signal results in high power across all frequencies, thus distorting the spectrum. To assess the influence of the model order and the gap size on the jumps, we ran simulations on the data from the ECoG recordings without stimulation used in **Figure 8A**: in total, 11266 stimuli were simulated on 397 minutes of data, the gap size was varied between 0 and 100 ms in steps of 5 ms and model orders 16, 32, and 64 were tested.

We applied AR modeling to deal with the gaps and measured the jump as the absolute voltage difference between the last sample generated by the AR model at the end of the gap and the first sample after the gap. The results are shown in **Figure A1B**. For comparison, the average absolute voltage difference between neighboring samples of the original ECoG data without any gaps or stimuli is $1.68 \pm 0.43\,\mu V$ (mean ± std).

We found that for all model orders, the average height of the jump increases sharply up to a gap size of 10, yielding $12.35 \pm 5.0\,\mu V$ for order 16, $11.82 \pm 4.43\,\mu V$ for 32 and $11.29 \pm 4.37\,\mu V$ for 64. For further increasing gap size, the average jump height increases more slowly for higher model orders than for lower ones. For a gap size of 100 ms we find average jump heights of $28.08 \pm 14.94\,\mu V$ for order 16, $23.45 \pm 12.51\,\mu V$ for 32 and $20.23 \pm 11.94\,\mu V$ for 64. Thus, while the jump height at the end of the gap is significantly smaller for a model order of 64 compared to 32 and 16 (gap size = 100, paired Wilcoxon signed rank tests, both $p < 10^{-17}$), it is still vastly higher than the average sample-to-sample difference for ongoing ECoG activity. Therefore, we cannot conclude that higher model orders prevent jumps after the gap.

Furthermore, if the gaps are used to cover the effects of real stimulation, there has to be a jump at the end if the gap is filled by AR modeling and evoked activity is present. AR modeling attempts to extrapolate the pre-stimulus signal which almost certainly differs in its time course from the stimulation-evoked activity, therefore extrapolation can not work perfectly, regardless of the model order.

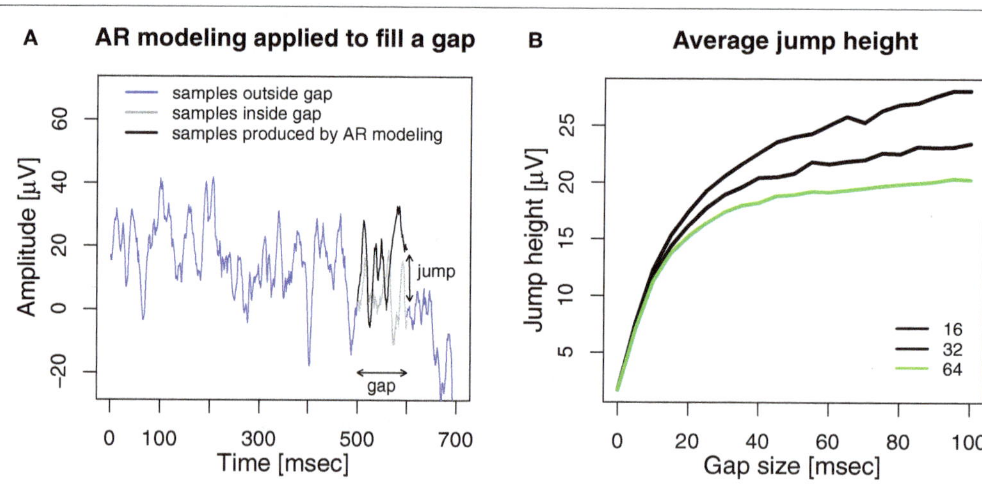

FIGURE A1 | (A) An example, how AR modeling fills a gap in the signal. A gap is introduced into an ECoG signal (blue) between 500 and 600 ms. An AR model of order 32 is estimated from the 500 ms before the gap and applied as a linear predictor to generate 100 samples to fill the gap (red). The original ECoG samples within the gap are shown in gray. The voltage difference between the last sample generated for the gap and the first ECoG sample after the gap is the jump height. **(B)** Average jump height after filling the gap with AR modeling for model orders 16 (black), 32 (red), and 64 (green).

9

Toward a self-wired active reconstruction of the hippocampal trisynaptic loop: DG-CA3

Gregory J. Brewer[1,2*†], Michael D. Boehler[1], Stathis Leondopulos[1,3], Liangbin Pan[3], Sankaraleengam Alagapan[3], Thomas B. DeMarse[3] and Bruce C. Wheeler[3]

[1] *Department of Medical Microbiology, Immunology and Cell Biology, Southern Illinois University School of Medicine, Springfield, IL, USA*
[2] *Department of Neurology, Southern Illinois University School of Medicine, Springfield, IL, USA*
[3] *Pruitt Family Department of Biomedical Engineering, University of Florida, Gainesville, FL, USA*

Edited by:
Ahmed El Hady, Max Planck Institute for Dynamics and Self Organization, Germany

Reviewed by:
Ulrich Egert, University of Freiburg, Germany
Inah Lee, Seoul National University, South Korea

****Correspondence:***
Gregory J. Brewer, Department of Medical Microbiology, Immunology and Cell Biology, Southern Illinois University School of Medicine, PO Box 19626, Springfield, IL 62794-9626, USA
e-mail: gbrewer@siumed.edu

The mammalian hippocampus functions to encode and retrieve memories by transiently changing synaptic strengths, yet encoding in individual subregions for transmission between regions remains poorly understood. Toward the goal of better understanding the coding in the trisynaptic pathway from the dentate gyrus (DG) to the CA3 and CA1, we report a novel microfabricated device that divides a micro-electrode array into two compartments of separate hippocampal network subregions connected by axons that grow through $3 \times 10 \times 400\,\mu m$ tunnels. Gene expression by qPCR demonstrated selective enrichment of separate DG, CA3, and CA1 subregions. Reconnection of DG to CA3 altered burst dynamics associated with marked enrichment of GAD67 in DG and GFAP in CA3. Surprisingly, DG axon spike propagation was preferentially unidirectional to the CA3 region at 0.5 m/s with little reverse transmission. Therefore, select hippocampal subregions intrinsically self-wire in anatomically appropriate patterns and maintain their distinct subregion phenotype without external inputs.

Keywords: multielectrode array, dentate gyrus, GAD67, burst, GFAP

INTRODUCTION

The mammalian hippocampus crucially encodes the formation of long-term episodic memories and spatial navigation, yet the staged encoding mechanisms remain elusive. While we know molecular details of many types of synapses in the major regions of the hippocampus important to learning and memory at the single neuron level, we don't know if these regions self-wire into the anatomically accurate network or require external electrical or chemical inputs. Further, brain functional studies are saddled with a tradeoff between high-spatial resolution (e.g., MRI, fMRI, EEG, EcoG) vs. high-temporal resolution (e.g., *in vivo* electrode arrays, single cell patch clamp). To bridge this gap, our strategy employs *in vitro* culture in an attempt to recapitulate entire *in vivo* brain regions in culture. Today a wide variety of cell types from various areas of the brain can easily be explanted, cultured *in vitro*, and studied in detail. While *in vitro* technology does provide exquisite temporal and spatial access it too has significant shortcomings. A key hurdle toward reconstructing brain areas *in vitro* has been the difficulty controlling the structural connectivity among cells to begin to recapitulate the *in vivo* architecture. The connections in the hippocampal formation of the brain uniquely propagate forward excitatory communication from one region to the next with the CA3 region distinctive for recurrent collateral excitation. We begin to create a functional tri-synaptic network of the hippocampal formation from the entorhinal cortex (EC) to the dentate gyrus (DG) to the CA3 to the CA1 (Cajal, 1968; Amaral and Lavenex, 2006). Other aspects of hippocampal anatomy not modeled here are the connections from the EC through the perforant path to the CA3 in a feed-forward fashion. In addition, the hippocampus receives modulatory inputs from the amygdala and basal forebrain. Output from the CA1 proceeds through the subiculum and returns to the EC to complete the loop. With smaller numbers of electrodes placed in the rat brain, others have monitored activity from each hippocampal region in behaving animals to describe specific patterns of activity for each region (Rolls and Kesner, 2006; Leutgeb et al., 2007), suggesting staged encoding, but we lack information about the inputs necessary to evoke these patterns and their network relationships.

To achieve these staged connections, we combine microfabrication (MEMS) technology to channel connections between cultured subregions of the hippocampus on a multi-electrode array to simultaneously monitor activity (**Figure 1**). Inspired by Campenot (1977, 1987), the MEMS device creates compartments in which we separately place cells from each major area of the hippocampus (EC, DG, CA3, CA1) connected by micro-scale tunnels through which axons can pass between the wells to define neuronal communication pathways between each well (Taylor et al., 2005; Dworak and Wheeler, 2009; Pan et al., 2011; Kanagasabapathi et al., 2012). Due to the defined geometry of the hippocampus, the cells can be dissociated from micro-dissected subregions of DG, CA3, CA1, and EC (Mattson et al., 1989; Baranes et al., 1996; Zhao et al., 2001; Lein et al., 2004). Cells

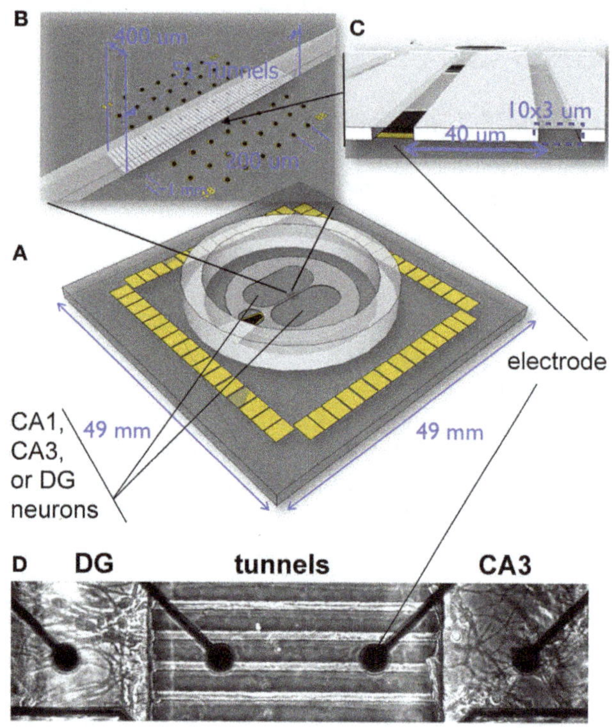

FIGURE 1 | Experimental system for reconstruction of hippocampal sub-regional circuits on multi-electrode array. (A) Dual culture chamber on microelectrode array separated by microtunnels. Note ground electrode on lower left for common culture medium, **(B)** 51 tunnels of 400 um length aligned to the 8 columns of electrodes. **(C)** Fifty-one tunnels of 3 × 10 um cross section were separated by 40 um with alignment over one pair of dark electrodes shown. **(D)** Phase contrast imaging of live neurons shows how the tunnels promoted selective growth of axons from one compartment into another.

are loaded into the compartments after the device is placed over an array of extracellular electrodes (microelectrode array or MEA) to measure neural activity in each subnetwork as well as communication between the subnetworks through the tunnels (Morefield et al., 2000; Czarnecki et al., 2012; Downes et al., 2012; Kanagasabapathi et al., 2012; Dranias et al., 2013).

Here we reconstructed paired components of the tri-synaptic pathway, with a focus on the DG to CA3 connection to determine: (1) whether specific subregions of the hippocampus be reproducibly dissected as evidenced by region-restricted gene expression? (2) Will these regions maintain and establish their original identity in a uniform culture environment when removed from external hormonal gradients and input activity? (3) Given that CA3 development precedes DG *in vivo* (Bayer, 1980), is the natural axonal polarity of DG>CA3 intrinsically controlled by the neurons or does *in vivo* recapitulation of connectivity require external cues? (4) Do the dynamics of neural activity differentiate between each area *in vitro* and to what extent are they similar to activity patterns seen *in vivo*? We addressed the above issues by quantitative PCR of region-restricted gene expression, by evaluation of distinct spike and burst dynamics in each sub-region compartment and by establishing the polarity of directional communication between sub-regions, whether random or anatomically accurate from the DG to the CA3. Surprisingly, intrinsic capabilities of the DG neurons promote axon extension toward the CA3 neurons, with limited back propagation.

RESULTS

In order to reconstruct subregions of the rat hippocampus, we microscopically dissected these regions from postnatal day 4 rats. At this time, the CA3 and CA1 are well-developed and the dentate granule and hilar region (DG) have nearly completed neurogenesis (Bayer, 1980). Single cell suspensions from each region were plated into separate compartments of a microfabricated PDMS device, positioned over a 60 electrode microarray (**Figure 1**). Cells were plated at physiological density ratios of 100 for DG to 33 for CA3 or 41 for CA1. Between the two compartments was a 400 um barrier perforated by a series of 51 narrow channels that excluded cell somata, but promoted growth of axons along the length of the tunnels (Taylor et al., 2005; Dworak and Wheeler, 2009; Berdichevsky et al., 2010; Pan et al., 2011; Kanagasabapathi et al., 2012; Wang et al., 2012). For quality control of the dissection and to determine whether the microdissected DG, CA1, and CA3 regions maintain their *in vivo* identity in culture, we performed qPCR on the neurons that developed in the compartments for 3 weeks. We selected several genes based on their demonstrated enrichment in specific regions of the adult hippocampus (Lein et al., 2004). When standard, uniform cultures from a single subregion were assessed from glass slips without tunnel devices, the adult animal enriched gene expression was replicated with detection of specific transcripts for each region DG, CA1, and CA3 cultured in the common culture medium (**Figure 2A**). But would the subregion types of expression be maintained across the microtunnel devices? **Figure 2B** shows that the same subregion-enriched gene expression is maintained between compartments with the same subregion in each compartment as well as in devices with different subregions on each side (**Figures 2C–E**). These results indicate the fidelity of the dissection and culture process as well as the ability of these hippocampal subregions to maintain their specific identities in the absence of external vascular, hormonal, or electrical instruction.

We examined network spike and burst dynamics with the goal of decoding communication between hippocampal subregions. We recorded from paired compartments of DG and CA3 neurons as a model of this part of the brain anatomy. As controls, we recorded activity from networks comprised of either DG on both sides or CA3 neurons on both sides of tunnel-connected compartments or in random single compartment models. Regardless of configuration, 80% of electrodes were active with an average spike rate around 12 Hz in the NbAct4 medium (data not shown). However, burst dynamics differed between hippocampal subregions. The spike rate outside of bursts for DG increased with anatomically correct tunnel connection to CA3 neurons, while CA3 neurons showed the opposite trend (**Figure 3A**). **Figure 3B** shows that about 60% of spikes occurred within bursts in DG networks, regardless of configuration, while only 45% of spikes occurred in bursts in the CA3 networks apposed in tunnels. The average duration of each burst (**Figure 3C**) showed trends that

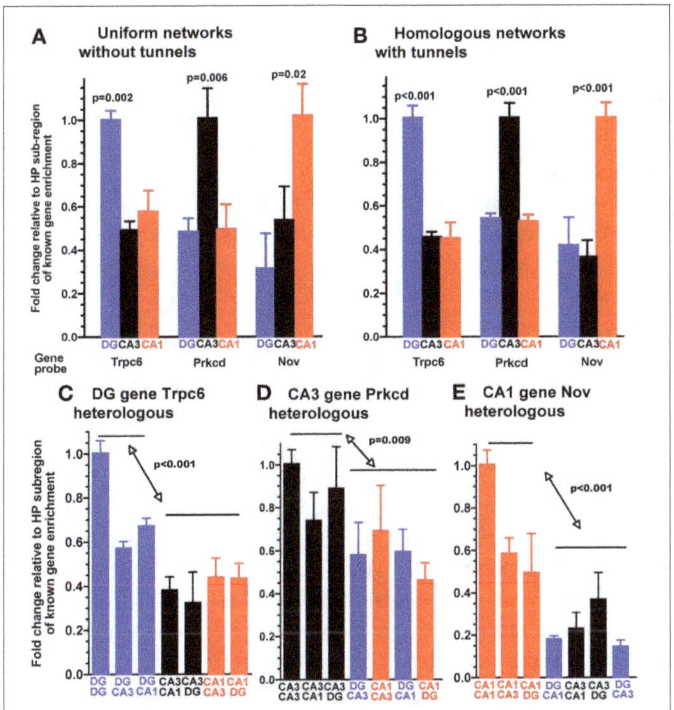

FIGURE 2 | Expression of region-enriched genes in sub-compartments phenocopies selective expression in the adult hippocampus as measured by qPCR. Specific genes probed for expression after 3 weeks in **(A)** the indicated homogeneous random cultures without tunnel devices. Note enrichment of Trpc6 in the DG cultures, Prkcd in the CA3 cultures, and Nov in the CA1 cultures. **(B)** The same hippocampal subregions plated into each of two compartments of the tunnel device. Note same enrichment profile in the tunnel device as in the random cultures. **(C)** Enriched expression of the DG gene Trpc6 whenever DG neurons are present in heterologous combinations of hippocampal subregions cultured between tunnels, normalized to DG cultured on both sides of the tunnels. **(D)** Enriched expression of the CA3 gene Prkcd when CA3 neurons are present in heterologous combinations of hippocampal sub-regions cultured between tunnels, normalized to CA3 cultured on both sides of the tunnels. **(E)** Enriched expression of the CA1 gene Nov when CA1 neurons are present in heterologous combinations of hippocampal sub-regions cultured between tunnels, normalized to CA1 cultured on both sides of the tunnels. Note the similar expression of each region-specific gene to neurons of that region in combination with heterologous regions, while the other 4 combinations without this region express lower levels of this marker mRNA ($n = 3$ separate cultures).

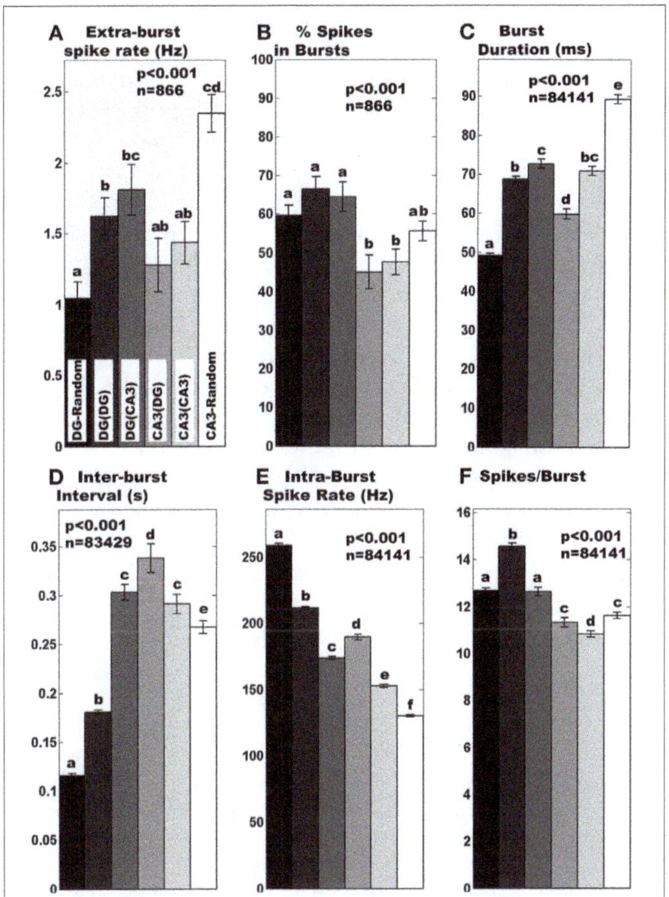

FIGURE 3 | Region-specific burst dynamics. Normal distribution statistics indicate **(A)** mean extra-burst spike rate differs (i) in tunnels compared to corresponding random cultures and (ii) is higher for DG than CA3 apposed across tunnels. **(B)** Percent spikes in bursts are generally higher for any DG culture than any CA3 culture. Log normal distribution statistics apply to **(C–F)**. **(C)** Burst duration was longer for DG than CA3 when they were apposed. For random cultures without tunnel devices, DG burst durations are much lower than CA3 random cultures. **(D)** Inter-burst intervals are lengthened by 50% in DG apposed to CA3 compared to DG self-apposed across tunnels and 300% compared to DG in random networks. Similarly, inter-burst times are longer for CA3 apposed to DG than CA3 apposed to itself or random CA3 cultures. **(E)** Intra-burst spike rates are shortened by 20% in DG apposed to CA3 compared to DG self-apposed across tunnels but longer in the reverse direction. **(F)** Spikes per burst decreased by 14% in DG apposed to CA3 compared to DG self-apposed across tunnels and even less in the reverse direction. In all cases n displayed is total degrees of freedom from burst or non-burst segments from 3 min recordings of networks of 4 random DG, 4 random CA3, 8 DG(DG), 8 CA3(CA3), 5 DG(CA3), and 5 CA3(DG). Different letters above bars indicate significant differences (a shared letter indicates a non-significant comparison) by *post-hoc* Tukey multiple-comparison analysis after significant ANOVA, $p < 0.05$, normal distribution statistics.

mirrored the extra-burst spike rate, with DG apposed to CA3 showing longer burst durations while CA3 bursts were shorter. The larger changes in inter-burst interval (**Figure 3D**) showed a co-modulation upon anatomical connection with increased intervals for the DG and CA3 apposed configuration. Intraburst spike rate (**Figure 3E**) and spikes per burst (**Figure 3F**) also differed with configuration.

In vivo, granule cells in DG uni-directionally synapse with pyramidal cells in CA3 with no back-propagation of connections from CA3 to DG. In our preparation, cells from DG and CA3 were plated simultaneously in apposing compartments that would permit connectivity in either direction. If axonal polarity of DG → CA3 is intrinsically controlled by the neurons (i.e., self-wire) in the absence of other external cues found *in vivo*, then polarity of connectivity from DG-CA3 should be maintained *in vitro* and could also account for the distinct burst dynamics of DG apposed to CA3. Previously, we showed that selective axon polarity from one side to the other, as opposed to bi-directional axon crossing, could be achieved in cortical neurons across tunnels by plating and culture of one side of a device followed after 1 week by plating and culture on the opposite side (Dworak et al., 2010; Pan et al., 2011). Here we tested whether intrinsic DG neuron properties would mimic *in vivo* conditions and preferentially cross the tunnels to innervate the CA3 neurons in the other compartment when both compartments were plated on the same day, with fewer axons crossing from CA3 to DG (reverse direction). This axon polarity could be measured in our devices by the direction of the time delay between spikes detected on the two microelectrodes embedded in the tunnels as shown in **Figure 4Ai** where a 0.48 ms delay from the DG side to the CA3 side over the 0.2 mm distance indicates a forward conduction velocity of 0.42 m/s. In contrast, when CA3 was connected to CA3 (or DG-DG), **Figure 4Aii** shows a 0.40 ms delay in the opposite direction, implying a reverse speed of 0.50 m/s that was evident in about half the spikes in these configurations. Individual tunnels were examined to determine whether axon conduction velocity was directionally polarized or whether evidence of multiple spike heights and shapes suggested several axons in a tunnel. Statistics based on all spike pairs above

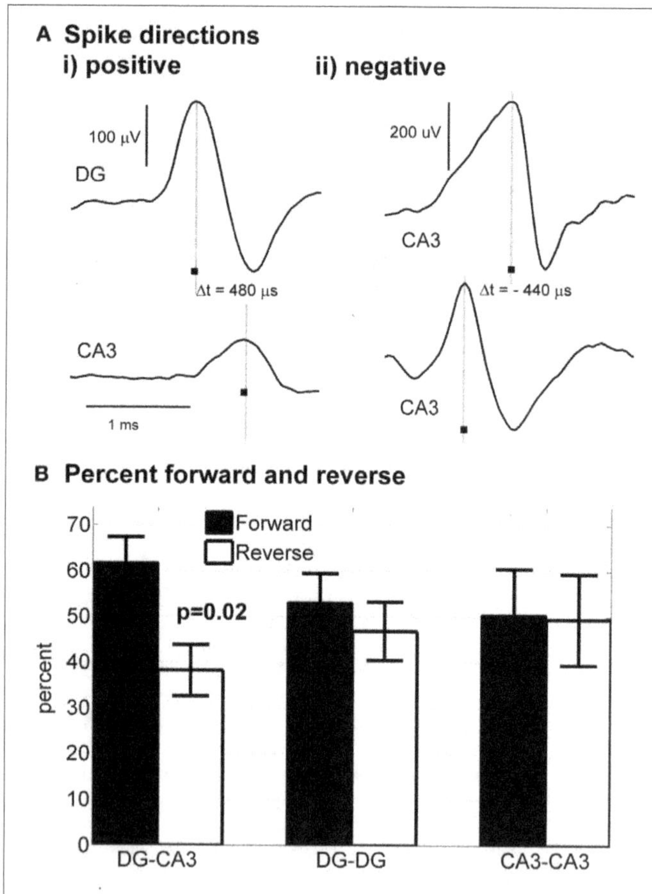

FIGURE 4 | Native polarity established from DG to CA3. Delay times of spikes traveling in axons in tunnels were determined from the difference in spike times at two tunnel electrodes separated by 200 µm. **(Ai)** Example of spike travelling from DG to CA3 with a 480 µs delay indicating a velocity of 0.42 m/s. **(ii)** Example of spike propagation from the top to the bottom compartment (arbitrarily designated reverse direction for CA3-CA3). **(B)** Statistical analysis of directional propagation indicates 62% of tunnels spontaneously connect axons with anatomical accuracy from DG-CA3, while homologous regions across tunnels fail to show polarity (Wilcoxin non-parametric test).

a high positive threshold indicated 81% unidirectional axon conduction from DG to CA3 at a mean velocity of 0.54 ± 0.02 m/s (SD., $n = 9167$ spike pairs). Other positive conduction velocities were DG:DG 0.47 ± 0.02 ($n = 2615$) and CA3:CA3 0.51 ± 0.01 ($n = 1343$) m/s, all within the range for the hippocampus *in vivo* (Patolsky et al., 2006).

Closer examination on a tunnel by tunnel basis revealed a more complicated situation. In 3 tunnels on one array, >99% of the spikes propagated from DG to CA3. In other tunnels, examination of the waveforms for negative directions from CA3 back to DG indicated multiple roughly simultaneous spikes, likely the spikes from two or more axons, whose sum was detected by the electrode as a shift in the peak within the 2 ms detection window. We never observed a tunnel with only back propagation, suggesting that these events are rare and supporting the conclusion that axons from DG neurons preferentially connect to CA3. For all the DG-CA3 tunnels with measurable spike pairs ($n = 26$ tunnels), more than >60% of the spikes propagated from the DG to CA3 direction (**Figure 4B**). This polarity contrasts with the nearly equal directional distributions of DG-DG and CA3-CA3.

Differences in GABAergic neuron and astroglia content could also affect burst dynamics. Transfection of networks with a Lenti virus carrying a GFP reporter driven by the inhibitory neuron GAD67 promoter was used to evaluate neurons expressing the GABA synthetic enzyme GAD67. **Figure 5** shows higher GAD$^+$ inhibitory neuron density in heterologous sub-region connections in DG compared to CA3 (**Figures 5A,B**) and higher GAD$^+$ inhibitory neurons/nucleus in homologous sub-region connection in DG compared to CA3 (**Figures 5C,D**). Quantitation of GAD67 neurons relative to nuclei (**Figure 5G**) showed a 5-fold increase in GAD$^+$ neuron density in DG over CA3 for heterologous and a 3-fold increase in the homologous configuration. The dissected DG region which includes the hilus contains a higher percentage of GAD67 expressing neurons than CA3 (Harvey and Boksa, 2011) that could contribute to a stronger inhibitory drive to enable a higher percentage of spikes in bursts (**Figure 3B**) and a longer burst duration (**Figure 3C**) for DG than CA3. The same mechanism could also contribute to the longer inter-burst intervals in DG apposed to CA3 (**Figure 3D**) and offer more opportunity for higher extra-burst spike rates. Some of these GAD67 neurons sent axons across the tunnels (not shown), better seen with GAD65 immunoreactivity (**Figure 5I**), as a feed-forward inhibitory component (Cabezas et al., 2012).

By increasing glutamate uptake, higher astroglial density could also affect burst dynamics (Boehler et al., 2007). A nuclear count of more than 2-fold above the plating density for CA3 apposed to DG (**Figure 5H**) suggested proliferation of astroglia. **Figures 5E,F** show that GFAP stain for astroglia are indeed more activated in the CA3 side than the DG side.

DISCUSSION

Here we reconstructed rat hippocampal sub-regions in pairs connected by axon-conducting tunnels to demonstrate intrinsic retention of *in vivo* behavior in the absence of external electrical and hormonal stimuli. The subregions maintained their physiological distinctions based on qPCR expression of

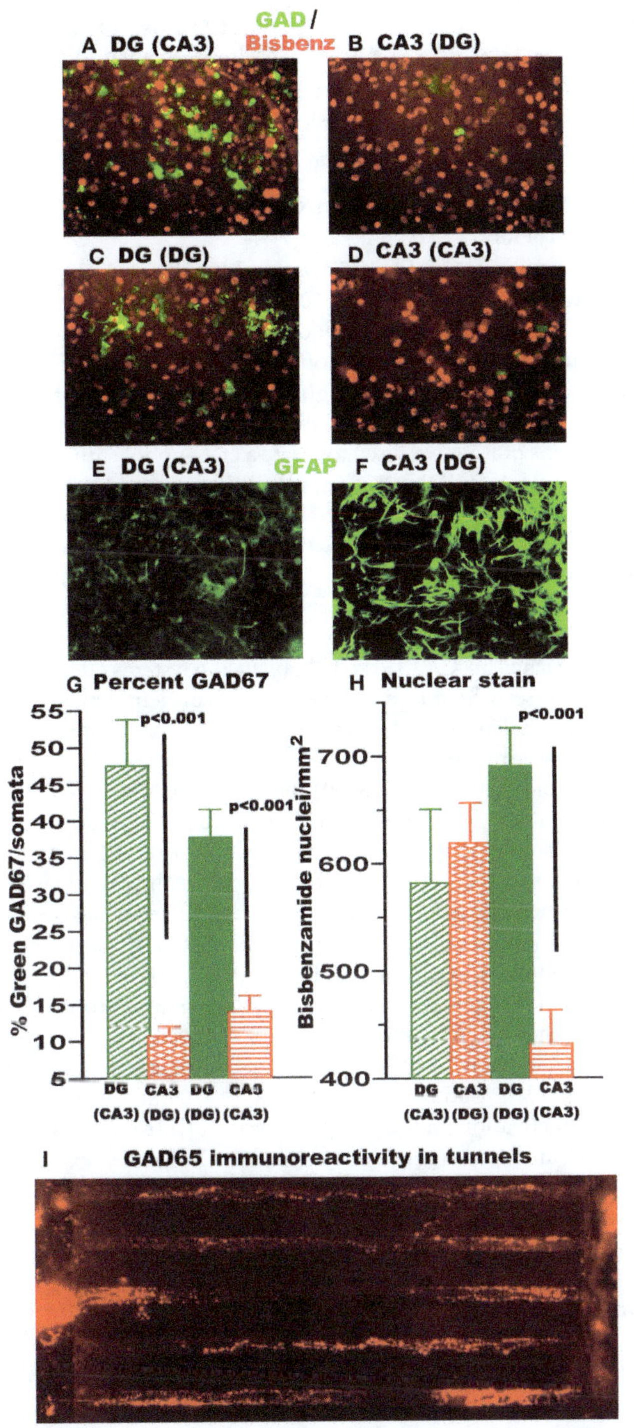

FIGURE 5 | DG networks contain 3–5x more GABAergic (GAD67-GFP) neurons than CA3 networks while CA3 has more astroglia. Some GAD$^+$ neurons traverse the tunnels. **(A–D)** Green is GAD67-GFP expression 11 days after infection with Lenti-virus with GAD-67 promoter fused to GFP. Red is pseudocolored for blue bisbenzamide labeled nuclei. **(E,F)** GFAP immunostain in DG or CA3 compartments. **(G)** Nuclei per somata from bisbenzamide stain for DNA. Note red vertical striped CA3 apposed to DG is 50% higher than CA3 by itself. **(H)** Percent GAD67 labeled neurons per nuclei. (N = 6 20x fields from each of 2 networks). **(I)** GAD65 immunolabeled axons traverse tunnels.

subregion-enriched genes, distinct spike dynamics, GABAergic neurons, astroglia, and preferential wiring direction.

Our observations on spike and burst dynamics are consistent with a synchronously connected network; neither DG nor CA3 operates as an independent oscillating/bursting center. Isolated DG neurons in the network burst at a higher rate than CA3 neurons, suggestive of regions preprogrammed to drive faster bursting DG onto slower bursting CA3, but operating in constrained fashion with predominantly forward connectivity from DG to CA3, but sufficient recurrent GABA-ergic innervation in DG and astroglia (Boehler et al., 2007) in CA3 to modulate the dynamic behavior. Further, the higher extra burst spike rate, slightly longer burst duration and GABAergic neuron density in DG provide extra drive from DG to CA3, establishing the background readiness of CA3 to be receptive to other inputs for learning or information fusion.

A key hurdle toward reconstructing brain areas *in vitro* has been the difficulty controlling the structural connectivity among cells to reflect, or even begin to adequately recapitulate the *in vivo* architecture in an *in vitro* model. A variety of novel *in vitro* technologies address this difficult problem. These technologies have been targeted toward modifying the surface chemistry to provide guidance cues that promote preferential attachment and growth (Boehler et al., 2012), using microfluidics (Morin et al., 2006), or alternatively, to capitalize on the intrinsic neuronal property to follow topographical features in their environment such as pillars (Dowell-Mesfin et al., 2004), ridges (Curtis and Wilkinson, 1997), or gradients (Hattori et al., 2010). The tunnel approach used in this paper confirms the intrinsic ability of *ex vivo* neurons to reconnect in an *in vivo* order (Czarnecki et al., 2012; Downes et al., 2012; Kanagasabapathi et al., 2012; Dranias et al., 2013).

Our model is a greatly reduced analogue of the *in vivo* circuit due to its anatomical incompleteness as a two-dimensional network. It fails to include modulatory cholinergic, noradrenergic, seratonergic, or dopaminergic inputs. It certainly lacks hormonal fluctuations and efficient removal of waste metabolites. With extracellular electrodes, we only monitor the net effects of thousands of synapses as individual action potentials per neuron.

Advantages of this model include direct stimulation and monitoring of electrical activity on time scales of milliseconds to weeks, pharmacologic access and most importantly, the ability to monitor inputs, axon communication, and outputs of the hippocampal region. The hippocampus is well-known for its different levels of information processing, but the details of the coding remain elusive. Our model has the potential to decode the information from the easily monitored spiking dynamics between hippocampal subregions. This technology will enable determination of the network integration of stimulation-dependent plasticity and how subregion-specific information patterns are reliably transmitted but differentially processed within each hippocampal subregion.

MATERIALS AND METHODS

MICROFABRICATION OF TWO-COMPARTMENT TUNNEL DEVICES

A multilayered mold made of photoresist SU-8 was fabricated on a silicon wafer. The first layer of the mold was made for the micro-tunnel structure. Briefly SU-8 2002 (Microchem, Inc.) was spun on a 4-inch silicon wafer at a nominal thickness of 3 μm, baked, exposed with the first mask, baked again, and developed. The second thicker layer of the mold was made for the well-structure. SU-8 2050 was spun on at a nominal thickness of 120 μm and then baked. The second mask was aligned to marks on the silicon wafer and then the second SU-8 film was exposed, baked again and developed. This mold was slowly filled with PDMS silicone rubber [polydimethylsiloxane; Sylgard 184 (Dow-Corning, Midland, Michigan) 10:1 ratio of pre-polymer (base)/cross-linker (curing agent)]. Once the PDMS spread over the entire wafer, it was heated for 2 h at 70°C for curing or in later devices, 10 h at 70°C. Two wells for culture and another smaller circular well for a reference electrode were formed on the peeled PDMS with a punch. Finally, a circular PDMS ring was placed around the entire device to form a chamber for holding cell culture media.

DISSECTION OF RAT HIPPOCAMPAL SUBREGIONS

The SIUSM LACUC approved these experiments as conforming to the Laboratory and Animal Use Guidelines of the NIH. To obtain neurons for electrical and genetic analysis, hippocampal sub-regions were isolated from anesthetized 4-day-old Sprague–Dawley rat pups as described (Mattson et al., 1989; Baranes et al., 1996; Zhao et al., 2001; Lein et al., 2004). The entire hippocampus was dissected away from the overlying neocortex of each brain hemisphere and removed as an intact structure for further sub-region dissection. The boundaries of the DG could be seen in the dissected hippocampus. Briefly, the CA1 or top portion of Ammon's horn was isolated at the natural division of the hippocampal fissure separating CA1 and DG-CA3. Using DG rostral and ventral ends as anchors, cuts were first made along the DG-CA1 boundary until the CA1 was separated and isolated. The CA3 sub-region (bottom remainder of Ammon's horn) was then dissected away from the DG following the clearly visible boundaries.

NEURON CULTURE

Hippocampal sub-region cells were plated at 1000 cells/mm^2 for DG, 330 cells/mm^2 for CA3, and 410 cells/mm^2 for CA1 on poly-D lysine coated MEAs or glass cover-slips with attached PDMS micro-tunnels in NbActiv4™ medium (Brewer et al., 2008) (BrainBits, Springfield, IL). Poly-D-lysine (Sigma SLBB8061V) was dissolved at 37°C for 1 h in sterile water before application to the devices at 100 μg/mL and incubation overnight at room temperature. The PDMS tunnels served to connect axons from the separated source sub-region to the target sub-region. Sub-region cultures were plated at a ratio respective to their anatomical density *in vivo* (final ratios DG-CA3 3:1, CA3-CA1 1:1.25) (Braitenberg, 1981). **Figure 1** depicts tunnel dimensions in relation to MEA dimensions. Briefly, the dimensions of 51 tunnels were 400 μm long, 10 μm wide, and 3 μm height with spacing 40 μm apart allowing for the coverage of seven electrode pairs in the middle of the MEA. Twenty-two electrodes were left uncovered in each of the top (target) and bottom (source) wells of the MEA (well area = 6.28 mm^2). Homologous cultures connected with tunnels were plated at a 1:1 ratio. Homologous random cultures were plated on 15 mm glass slips (Assistant Brand, Carolina Biologicals). Source cultures were plated first on the bottom half of the MEA and incubated for 15–30 min before adding target cultures. Cultures were incubated at 37°C, 5% CO_2, 9% O_2 and saturating humidity (Thermo-Forma, Columbus, OH). Every 4–5 days, one-half of the culture medium was removed and replaced with the same volume of fresh medium up until the day of recording.

HIPPOCAMPAL SUB-REGION RNA EXTRACTION AND DETECTION THROUGH qPCR

RNA was extracted from 3 week old cultures using 20 μL (device compartments) or 100 μL (random) Trizol (Life Technologies #15596-026) applied directly to glass cover-slips or tunnel wells. After addition of 20% volume chloroform and 5% glycogen (final 250 ug/mL), samples were centrifuged and precipitated according to the manufacturer. Five hundred nanograms of RNA was used to create a cDNA pool with the High Capacity RNA-to-cDNA Kit (Applied Biosystems #4387406) per instructions. Hundred nanograms of cDNA was used in a 20 μL multiplex Taqman reaction using primers known to be enriched in specific hippocampal sub-regions (Lein et al., 2004): Transient receptor potential cation channel 6 enriched in DG (Trpc6, Applied BioSystems 00677559); Protein kinase C delta enriched in CA3 (Prkcd, Applied BioSystems #00440891), family of serine and threonine specific protein kinases activated by calcium and secondary messenger diacylglycerol; Nephroblastoma overexpressed gene enriched in CA1 (Nov, Applied BioSystems #00578390), family of CCN secreted extracellular matrix associated signaling proteins; and polymerase (RNA) II (DNA directed) polypeptide A (POLR2a, Applied BioSystems #4448489) as the internal standard reference. POLR2a was chosen as the internal standard reference over the more conventional housekeeping gene GAPDH because the lower level of expression (Alan Brain Atlas) is more appropriate for other low expression genes. qPCR reactions were run with a 2× master mix (Applied Biosystems #4369016) in a StepOne Plus PCR system (Applied Biosystems) at the manufacturer's recommended optimized conditions of 10 min at 95°C for enzyme activation followed by 40 cycles of (15 s denaturation at 95°C and 1 min anneal/extend at 60°C). Primer expression was normalized to POLR2A with fold change differences determined using the $2^{\Delta\Delta Ct}$ method. Graphed results show fold changes in the hippocampal sub-region gene probe expression relative to the hippocampal sub-region of known gene enrichment.

MULTI-ELECTRODE ARRAYS AND RECORDING

MEA's from Multichannel Systems (MCS, Reutlingen, Germany) consisted of 60 TiN_3 electrodes with diameters of 30 μm and spacing of 200 μm, one of which served as ground. The spontaneous activity on the MEA's was measured using an MCS 1100× amplifier at 25 kHz sampling with a hardware filter of 1–3000 Hz at 37°C under continuous flow of hydrated, sterile 5% CO_2, 9% O_2, balance N_2 (custom made, AGA, Springfield, IL). A Teflon membrane (ALA Scientific, Westbury, NY) was used to reduce evaporation and chances of contamination. MCRack software was used to record 3 week old cultures for 3 min of spontaneous activity.

SPIKE ACTIVITY ANALYSIS

Offline data analysis was performed using a modification of SpyCode V2.0 software (Bologna et al., 2010) including custom MATLAB scripts (The Mathworks, Natick, MA). After filtering the data with at 300 Hz high pass, spikes were identified as peak-to-peak amplitudes that exceeded 9 times the minimum root-mean-square of 200 ms contiguous windows. A dead-time or refractory period of 1 ms was assumed after each detected spike. Bursts were defined as 4 or more spikes with no greater than a 50 ms inter-spike interval.

Delay times of spikes within tunnels were used to determine directionality. Due to larger amplitudes in tunnels, thresholds were determined on a per-electrode basis as visually selected asymptotic minima of the continuous voltage distribution. Furthermore, the time stamp of any *spike event* was chosen as the time of occurrence of the voltage maximum within any such event. A histogram of delay times between spike pairs was constructed within the limits of ±280–600 μs, conforming to the known range of axonal conduction delays (Patolsky et al., 2006) and limited in resolution by the 40 μs sampling period. The histograms showed distinct peaks, each indicating the high precision in delay time that is consistent with an action potential propagating on a single axon past a pair of electrodes.

GAD67 GFP REPORTER FOR GABAergic NEURONS

At 7 DIV, a fluorescent GAD67 lenti-virus reporter (System Biosciences #SR10023VA-1, 10 μg/ml) diluted in 8 μg/ml protamine sulfate for better adsorption (Sigma# P4020) was added to DG and CA3 sub-cultures with PDMS micro-tunnels on glass cover-slips. Cultures were incubated in NbActiv4 medium for two more weeks before imaging. At 3 weeks, cultures were switched from NbActiv4 medium to Hibernate Low Fluorescence—Glucose (BrainBits #112012) and bisbenzamide was added to stain cell nuclei for 2 min (final concentration 300 ng/ml, diluted in PBS, Sigma #B2261). Cultures were rinsed two times in Hibernate LF—glucose before being imaged. Images were taken through an Olympus 20×/0.45 objective, and recorded with a Retiga Exi CCD camera (QImaging, Surrey, BC, Canada). Image Pro$^+$ software was used in digital analysis and display of the immunostain and nuclear stain. After flattening backgrounds, a constant density segmentation threshold was set for cell counts.

GFAP OR GAD65 IMMUNOSTAINS FOR ASTROGLIA OR GABAergic NEURONS

For immunostains, DG and CA3 sub-cultures with PDMS micro-tunnels were plated as described previously on glass cover-slips and cultured for 3 weeks, then fixed in 4% paraformaldehyde for 10 min. Cells were permeabilized and weakly antigenic sites blocked in 5% normal goat serum and 0.5% Triton X-100 in PBS. Conjugate mouse anti-GFAP/Alexa Fluor 488 (Molecular Probes #A21294) was diluted 1:500 in 5% NGS and 0.05 TX-100. Cells for incubated for 90 min at 22°C, then rinsed four times in PBS. Other antibodies were mouse anti-GAD65 1:250 (Sigma #G1166) with secondary Alexafluor 588 conjugated goat anti-mouse 1:1000 (Molecular Probes #11031). Nuclei of cells were stained for 2 min with bisbenzamide (final concentration 300 ng/ml, diluted in PBS, Sigma #B2261). Slips were rinsed two final times, imaged through an Olympus 20×/0.45 objective, and recorded with a Retiga Exi CCD camera (QImaging, Surrey, BC, Canada).

STATISTICS

Statistical differences were determined by Student's t-test with $p < 0.05$ considered significant for two-way comparisons of data normally distributed. Log-normal adjustments were made when appropriate. *Post-hoc* Tukey adjustments for multiple-comparisons are reported after significant ANOVA. Statistical differences of spike times were determined by the Wilcoxon test with significance at $p < 0.05$ (Hollander and Wolfe, 1999).

ACKNOWLEDGMENTS

This work was supported by a grant from NIH, R01 NS052233.

REFERENCES

Amaral, D. G., and Lavenex, P. (2006). "Hippocampal neuroanatomy," in *The Hippocampus Book*, eds P. Andersen, R. Morris, D. Amaral, T. Bliss, and J. O'Keefe (New York, NY: Oxford University Press), 37–114.

Baranes, D., Lopez-Garcia, J. C., Chen, M., Bailey, C. H., and Kandel, E. R. (1996). Reconstitution of the hippocampal mossy fiber and associational-commissural pathways in a novel dissociated cell culture system. *Proc. Natl. Acad. Sci. U.S.A.* 93, 4706–4711. doi: 10.1073/pnas.93.10.4706

Bayer, S. A. (1980). Development of the hippocampal region in the rat. I. Neurogenesis examined with 3H-thymidine autoradiography. *J. Comp. Neurol.* 190, 87–114. doi: 10.1002/cne.901900107

Berdichevsky, Y., Staley, K. J., and Yarmush, M. L. (2010). Building and manipulating neural pathways with microfluidics. *Lab Chip* 10, 999–1004. doi: 10.1039/b922365g

Boehler, M. D., Leondopulos, S. S., Wheeler, B. C., and Brewer, G. J. (2012). Hippocampal networks on reliable patterned substrates. *J. Neurosci. Methods* 203, 344–353. doi: 10.1016/j.jneumeth.2011.09.020

Boehler, M. D., Wheeler, B. C., and Brewer, G. J. (2007). Added astroglia promote greater synapse density and higher activity in neuronal networks. *Neuron Glia Biol.* 3, 127–140. doi: 10.1017/S1740925X07000440

Bologna, L. L., Pasquale, V., Garofalo, M., Gandolfo, M., Baljon, P. L., Maccione, A., et al. (2010). Investigating neuronal activity by SPYCODE multi-channel data analyzer. *Neural Netw.* 23, 685–697. doi: 10.1016/j.neunet.2010.05.002

Braitenberg, V. (1981). "Anatomical basis for divergence, and intergration in the cerebral cortex," in *Advances in Physiological Sciences*, eds E. Grastyban and P. Molnbar (Elmsford, NY: Pergamon Press), 411–419.

Brewer, G. J., Boehler, M. D., Jones, T. T., and Wheeler, B. C. (2008). NbActiv4 medium improvement to Neurobasal/B27 increases neuron synapse densities and network spike rates on multielectrode arrays. *J. Neurosci. Methods* 170, 181–187. doi: 10.1016/j.jneumeth.2008.01.009

Cabezas, C., Irinopoulou, T., Gauvain, G., and Poncer, J. C. (2012). Presynaptic but not postsynaptic GABA signaling at unitary mossy fiber synapses. *J. Neurosci.* 332, 11835–11840. doi: 10.1523/JNEUROSCI.5543-11.2012

Cajal, R. Y. (1968). *The Structure of Ammon's Horn*. Springfield, IL: C. C. Thomas.

Campenot, R. B. (1977). Local control of neurite development by nerve growth factor. *Proc. Natl. Acad. Sci. U.S.A.* 74, 4516–4519. doi: 10.1073/pnas.74.10.4516

Campenot, R. B. (1987). Local control of neurite sprouting in cultured sympathetic neurons by nerve growth factor. *Brain Res.* 465, 293–301.

Curtis, A., and Wilkinson, C. (1997). Topographical control of cells. *Biomaterials* 18, 1573–1583. doi: 10.1016/S0142-9612(97)00144-0

Czarnecki, A., Tscherter, A., and Streit, J. (2012). Network activity and spike discharge oscillations in cortical slice cultures from neonatal rat.

Eur. J. Neurosci. 35, 375–388. doi: 10.1111/j.1460-9568.2011.07966.x

Dowell-Mesfin, N. M., Abdul-Karim, M. A., Turner, A. M., Schanz, S., Craighead, H. G., Roysam, B., et al. (2004). Topographically modified surfaces affect orientation and growth of hippocampal neurons. *J. Neural Eng.* 1, 78–90. doi: 10.1088/1741-2560/1/2/003

Downes, J. H., Hammond, M. W., Xydas, D., Spencer, M. C., Becerra, V. M., Warwick, K., et al. (2012). Emergence of a small-world functional network in cultured neurons. *Plos Comput. Biol.* 8:e1002522. doi: 10.1371/journal.pcbi.1002522

Dranias, M. R., Ju, H., Rajaram, E., and Vandongen, A. M. (2013). Short-term memory in networks of dissociated cortical neurons. *J. Neurosci.* 33, 1940–1953. doi: 10.1523/JNEUROSCI.2718-12.2013

Dworak, B., Varghese, K., Pan, L., Brewer, G. J., Wheeler, B. C. (2010). "Creating unidirectional neural networks on a chip," in *7th International Meeting on Substrate-Integrated Microelectrode Arrays* (Reutlingen).

Dworak, B. J., and Wheeler, B. C. (2009). Novel MEA platform with PDMS microtunnels enables the detection of action potential propagation from isolated axons in culture. *Lab Chip* 9, 404–410. doi: 10.1039/b806689b

Harvey, L., and Boksa, P. (2011). A stereological comparison of GAD67 and reelin expression in the hippocampal stratum oriens of offspring from two mouse models of maternal inflammation during pregnancy. *Neuropharmacology* 62, 1767–1776. doi: 10.1016/j.neuropharm.2011.11.022

Hattori, S., Suzurikawa, J., Kanzaki, R., Jimbo, Y., Hamaguchi, T., Takahashi, H., et al. (2010). Direction control of information transfer between neuronal populations with asymmetric three-dimensional microstructure. *Electron. Commun. Jpn.* 93, 17–25. doi: 10.1002/ecj.10240

Hollander, M., and Wolfe, D. A. (1999). *Nonparametric Statistical Methods.* Hoboken, NJ: John Wiley and Sons.

Kanagasabapathi, T. T., Massobrio, P., Barone, R. A., Tedesco, M., Martinoia, S., Wadman, W. J., et al. (2012). Functional connectivity and dynamics of cortical-thalamic networks co-cultured in a dual compartment device. *J. Neural Eng.* 9, 036010. doi: 10.1088/1741-2560/9/3/036010

Lein, E. S., Zhao, X., and Gage, F. H. (2004). Defining a molecular atlas of the hippocampus using DNA microarrays and high-throughput in situ hybridization. *J. Neurosci.* 24, 3879–3889. doi: 10.1523/JNEUROSCI.4710-03.2004

Leutgeb, J. K., Leutgeb, S., Moser, M. B., and Moser, E. I. (2007). Pattern separation in the dentate gyrus and CA3 of the hippocampus. *Science* 315, 961–966. doi: 10.1126/science.1135801

Mattson, M. P., Guthrie, P. B., and Kater, S. B. (1989). Intrinsic factors in the selective vulnerability of hippocampal pyramidal neurons. *Prog. Clin. Biol. Res.* 317, 333–351.

Morefield, S. I., Keefer, E. W., Chapman, K. D., and Gross, G. W. (2000). Drug evaluations using neuronal networks cultured on microelectrode arrays. *Biosens. Bioelectron.* 15, 383–396. doi: 10.1016/S0956-5663(00)00095-6

Morin, F., Nishimura, N., Griscom, L., Lepioufle, B., Fujita, H., Takamura, Y., et al. (2006). Constraining the connectivity of neuronal networks cultured on microelectrode arrays with microfluidic techniques: a step towards neuron-based functional chips. *Biosens. Bioelectron.* 21, 1093–1100. doi: 10.1016/j.bios.2005.04.020

Pan, L., Alagapan, S., Franca, E., Brewer, G. J., and Wheeler, B. C. (2011). Propagation of action potential activity in a predefined microtunnel neural network. *J. Neural Eng.* 8, 046031. doi: 10.1088/1741-2560/8/4/046031

Patolsky, F., Timko, B. P., Yu, G., Fang, Y., Greytak, A. B., Zheng, G., et al. (2006). Detection, stimulation, and inhibition of neuronal signals with high-density nanowire transistor arrays. *Science* 313, 1100–1104. doi: 10.1126/science.1128640

Rolls, E. T., and Kesner, R. P. (2006). A computational theory of hippocampal function, and empirical tests of the theory. *Prog. Neurobiol.* 79, 1–48. doi: 10.1016/j.pneurobio.2006.04.005

Taylor, A. M., Blurton-Jones, M., Rhee, S. W., Cribbs, D. H., Cotman, C. W., and Jeon, N. L. (2005). A microfluidic culture platform for CNS axonal injury, regeneration and transport. *Nat. Methods* 2, 599–605. doi: 10.1038/nmeth777

Wang, L., Riss, M., Buitrago, J. O., and Claverol-Tinture, E. (2012). Biophysics of microchannel-enabled neuron-electrode interfaces. *J. Neural Eng.* 9, 026010. doi: 10.1088/1741-2560/9/2/026010

Zhao, X., Lein, E. S., He, A., Smith, S. C., Aston, C., and Gage, F. H. (2001). Transcriptional profiling reveals strict boundaries between hippocampal subregions. *J. Comp. Neurol.* 441, 187–196. doi: 10.1002/cne.1406

10

In vitro large-scale experimental and theoretical studies for the realization of bi-directional brain-prostheses

Paolo Bonifazi[1†], Francesco Difato[2†], Paolo Massobrio[3†], Gian L. Breschi[2], Valentina Pasquale[2], Timothée Levi[4], Miri Goldin[1], Yannick Bornat[4], Mariateresa Tedesco[3], Marta Bisio[2], Sivan Kanner[5], Ronit Galron[5], Jacopo Tessadori[2], Stefano Taverna[2] and Michela Chiappalone[2]*

[1] School of Physics and Astronomy, Tel Aviv University, Tel Aviv, Israel
[2] Department of Neuroscience and Brain Technologies, Istituto Italiano di Tecnologia, Genova, Italy
[3] Department of Informatics, Bioengineering, Robotics and System Engineering, University of Genova, Genova, Italy
[4] IMS laboratory, UMR CNRS 5218, University of Bordeaux, Talence, France
[5] Department of Neurobiology, George S. Wise Faculty of Life Sciences, Sagol School of Neuroscience, Tel Aviv University, Tel-Aviv, Israel

Edited by:
Ahmed El Hady, Max Planck Institute for Dynamics and Self Organization, Germany

Reviewed by:
Suguru N. Kudoh, Kwansei Gakuin University, Japan
Hsin Chen, National Tsing-Hua University, Taiwan
Jason G. Fleischer, The Neurosciences Institute, USA
Pavel M. Itskov, Champalimaud Foundation, Portugal

***Correspondence:**
Michela Chiappalone, Department of Neuroscience and Brain Technologies, Istituto Italiano di Tecnologia, Via Morego 30, Genova, 16163, Italy.
e-mail: michela.chiappalone@iit.it

† These authors have contributed equally to this work.

Brain-machine interfaces (BMI) were born to control "actions from thoughts" in order to recover motor capability of patients with impaired functional connectivity between the central and peripheral nervous system. The final goal of our studies is the development of a new proof-of-concept BMI—a neuromorphic chip for brain repair—to reproduce the functional organization of a damaged part of the central nervous system. To reach this ambitious goal, we implemented a multidisciplinary "bottom-up" approach in which *in vitro* networks are the paradigm for the development of an *in silico* model to be incorporated into a neuromorphic device. In this paper we present the overall strategy and focus on the different building blocks of our studies: (i) the experimental characterization and modeling of "finite size networks" which represent the smallest and most general self-organized circuits capable of generating spontaneous collective dynamics; (ii) the induction of lesions in neuronal networks and the whole brain preparation with special attention on the impact on the functional organization of the circuits; (iii) the first production of a neuromorphic chip able to implement a real-time model of neuronal networks. A dynamical characterization of the finite size circuits with single cell resolution is provided. A neural network model based on Izhikevich neurons was able to replicate the experimental observations. Changes in the dynamics of the neuronal circuits induced by optical and ischemic lesions are presented respectively for *in vitro* neuronal networks and for a whole brain preparation. Finally the implementation of a neuromorphic chip reproducing the network dynamics in quasi-real time (10 ns precision) is presented.

Keywords: ***In vitro* modular networks, whole brain, lesioned circuits, *in silico* neuronal circuit, hardware spiking neural network**

INTRODUCTION

Millions of people worldwide are affected by neurological disorders that disrupt connections between brain and body, causing paralysis, or impair cognitive capabilities. This number is likely to increase in coming years, yet current assistive technology is still limited. Over the last decade Brain-Machine Interfaces (BMIs) and neuro-prostheses (Nicolelis, 2003; Hochberg et al., 2006, 2012; Nicolelis and Lebedev, 2009) have been the object of extensive research and offer the promise of treatment for such disabilities. These devices could profoundly improve the quality of life for affected individuals, and could have a more widespread impact on society.

Neural interfaces have mainly been devoted to restoring motor function that is lost due to injuries at the level of the spinal cord (Collinger et al., 2013), or to recover sensorial capacities, e.g., artificial retinal or cochlear implants (Chader et al., 2009). However, recent interest has also focused on neural prostheses for restoring cognitive functions. For example, a hippocampal prosthesis for improving memory function in behaving rats was recently presented (Berger et al., 2011, 2012), and the same group has also tested a device in primate prefrontal cortex aimed at restoring impaired cognitive functions (Hampson et al., 2012; Opris et al., 2012).

The realization of such prostheses implies that we know how to interact with neuronal cell assemblies, taking into account the intrinsic spontaneous activation of neuronal networks and understanding how to drive them into a desired state in order to produce a specific behavior. The long-term goal of replacing damaged brain areas with artificial devices requires neural network-like prosthetics or models that could be fed with recorded electrophysiological patterns and that could provide a substitute output to recover the desired functions. While ultimately this approach must be tested and applied *in vivo*, important insights could be gained using *in vitro* systems of increasing architectural complexity, which can be more easily and thoroughly accessed, monitored, manipulated, and modeled than *in vivo* systems (at least at present).

The final goal of the studies presented in this paper is to develop a test-bed for the development of a new generation of neuro-prostheses capable of restoring lost communication between neuronal circuits. These studies constitute the object of the European project BRAIN BOW (www.brainbowproject.eu). Healthy and lesioned *in vitro* neuronal circuits are characterized in parallel to the development of *in silico* neuronal networks, with the goal of establishing bi-directional communication to mimic or bypass an injured neuronal network. In order to develop an experimental and computational platform for the prototyping of neuro-prostheses, we followed a bottom-up approach using *in vitro* biological neuronal systems with increasing structural complexity. Our approach takes advantage of the unique features of *in vitro* neuronal cultures, which represent a powerful experimental model to investigate the inherent properties of neuronal cell assemblies as a complement to artificial computational models. We use engineered networks of increasing structural complexity, from isolated finite-size networks up to interacting assemblies, as a model of intercommunicating neuronal circuitries. Moreover, we scaled our studies up to the isolated whole guinea-pig brain (IWB), to translate to an *in vivo* model.

In this paper we present the overall multidisciplinary strategy and preliminary results on the different building blocks of the project. The structure-function relationship of "finite size circuits" was characterized with single cell resolution by combining calcium imaging and immunocytochemistry. Similarly to what previously observed in isolated neuronal clusters (Shein-Idelson et al., 2010), we found that the frequency of synchronous network events increased with circuit size. This result was reproduced by *in silico* neural network models based on Izhikevich neurons with scale-free connectivity. The feasibility of controlled network lesions was explored by optically transecting cell processes and monitoring the subsequent change in functional network connectivity. In addition, in a whole brain preparation, a focal ischemic lesion in the hippocampus was demonstrated to cause an interruption of the limbic olfactory pathway. Finally, a neural network hardware model with arbitrary connectivity based on Izhikevich neurons, working at nanosecond time scale, is presented. These experimental and computational platforms represent a starting point for restoring functional closed-loop communication in a neuronal network with lesioned circuitries.

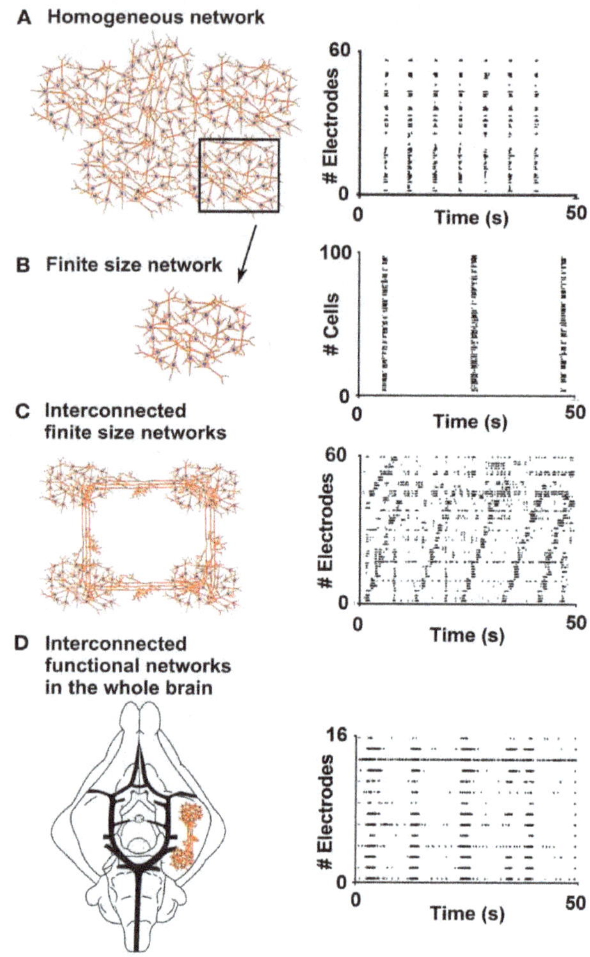

FIGURE 1 | From finite size networks up to the whole brain: a bottom-up approach. (A) Sketch of a homogeneous network composed of about 1000 neurons (left panel) and the typical raster plot of its electrophysiological activity, recorded by using 60 electrodes of a Micro Electrode Array (MEA) chip (right panel). The black box highlights a sub-region of the homogeneous network, which can be described as a finite size network (black arrow pointing to panel **B**). **(B)** Sketch of a finite size network used in the framework of this paper, composed of about 100 neurons (left panel), and its raster plot, obtained by calcium imaging recording (right panel). **(C)** Scheme of interconnected finite size networks, each composed of about 100 neurons (left panel), and the raster plot of the electrophysiological activity recorded by a MEA (right panel). **(D)** Sketch of the *in-vitro* whole brain of a guinea pig composed by interconnected functional networks (left panel), and raster plot of the spontaneous periodic events recorded by an array of 16 electrodes (right panel).

MATERIALS AND METHODS

EXPERIMENTAL MODELS

The repertoire of activity patterns exhibited by an *in vitro* neural network is strongly dependent on the complexity of its geometry (Shein-Idelson et al., 2011). While homogeneous networks (**Figure 1A**) tend to display highly stereotyped bursts which spread to most of the connected cells (Kamioka et al., 1996; Van Pelt et al., 2004; Chiappalone et al., 2006; Eytan and Marom, 2006), networks composed of smaller sub-networks with sparse connections (**Figure 1C**) usually present non-repetitive patterns of sparse spiking and local bursts (Macis et al., 2007; Shein-Idelson et al., 2010). The first cellular model proposed in this work is that of finite size network (**Figure 1B**), namely an isolated neuronal circuit consisting of a small number of neurons (dozens to a few hundreds) that is still able to spontaneously produce bursts similar to those observed in larger homogeneous networks (cf. section "Results"). Characterization of activity within these assemblies could allow their use as building blocks for larger, more complex structures of interconnecting sub-networks. At the other end of the complexity spectrum we set the isolated whole brain of a guinea pig (**Figure 1D**). This model is used to investigate the properties of one complex functional neuronal assembly (the olfactory tract, see below) embedded in an intact brain (cf. section "Results").

Finite size networks: patterning, cell culture, and calcium imaging

The procedure adopted for the preparation of "finite size networks" is in accordance with the NIH standards for care and use of laboratory animals and was approved by the Tel-Aviv University Animal Care and Use Committee.

Cultures were prepared as described in Herzog et al. (2011). After the fourth day *in vitro*, the growth medium was enriched with 0.5% Pen-Strep (Biological Industries Beit Haemek), 2% B-27 (Gibco), and 0.75% glutamax (Biological Industries Beit Haemek). Cells were plated at a density of 750 cells/mm^2 on a 23 mm square glass coverslip previously glued on a 35 mm petri dish. Coverslips were coated with spots of poly-D-lysine (PDL, Sigma), and petri dishes were homogenously coated with PDL. The cells attaching homogeneously on the free surface of the petri dish (i.e., not covered by the glass coverslip) functioned as a "supporting network" (Kleinfeld et al., 1988). PDL spots were created using either manual drop deposition or polydimethylsiloxane (PDMS) stencils. For manual drop deposition, an Eppendorf pipette with a tip of 10 μl capacity was used. The spots were created by touching the tip filled with 2 μl PDL on the coverslip surface and then drying the coverslips at 37°C for 30 min.

When PDMS stencils were used, the procedure to create PDL spots was based on a soft lithography process, as described in Sorkin et al. (2006). Briefly, an SU8-2075 (Micro Chem) mould on a silicon wafer with a feature thickness of approximately 200 μm was used to shape the PDMS. The feature was composed of squares of 700 μm × 700 μm separated by at least 1 mm, in order to obtain isolated neuronal islands. The size of the square was chosen to fit the field of view of a 10× objective in the calcium imaging setup described in detail below and in Herzog et al. (2011). Once the PDMS substrate was shaped and dried on the silicon wafer, the PDMS stencils were detached and placed directly on the glass coverslips. Drops of the PDL solution were dripped onto the PDMS stencil until the features were completely covered. After mild vacuum degassing for 15 min, the excess PDL solution was removed and the sample was dried at 37°C for 30 min. The PDMS stencil was removed before cell plating.

Calcium imaging of the patterned neuronal networks grown on coverslips was performed in buffered-ACSF solution (containing, in mM, 10 HEPES, 4 KCl, 1.5 $CaCl_2$, 0.75 $MgCl_2$, 139 NaCl, 10 D-glucose, adjusted with sucrose to an osmolarity of 325 mOsm, and with NaOH to a pH of 7.4). In order to load the cells with the calcium-sensitive dye, cultures were incubated for 30 min in 1 ml ACSF supplemented with 1 μl of 10% pluronic acid F-127 (Biotium 59000) and 1 μl Oregon-Green BAPTA-I AM (Invitrogen 06807) previously diluted with 7.6 μl anhydrous-DMSO. Following incubation, cultures were washed with ACSF and recorded at 37°C. In order to avoid artifacts due to evaporation and pH change, the ACSF was replaced every 20 min during the recording session.

Calcium-fluorescence images were acquired with an EMCCD camera (Andor Ixon-885) mounted on an upright Olympus microscope (BX51WI) using a 10× water-immersion objective (Olympus, NA 0.4). Fluorescent excitation was provided via a 120 W mercury lamp (EXFO X-Cite 120PC) coupled to the microscope optical axis with a dichroic mirror, and equipped with an emission filter matching the dye spectrum (Chroma T495LP). Images were acquired at 59 fps in 2 × 2 binning mode using Andor software data-acquisition card (SOLIS) installed on a personal computer.

Immunocytochemical staining

At the end of calcium-imaging experiments, cultures were washed twice with PBS, then fixed with 4% PFA (15 min) and left in PBS for not more than 5 days before staining. For immunocytochemical staining, fixed cultures were washed three times with PBS (10 min each) and then incubated with 1% Triton ×100 in PBS for 30 min. Cultures were blocked with 2% BSA, 10% normal serum and 0.5% Triton × 100 in PBS for 2 h at room temperature. The cultures were incubated overnight with the first primary antibody (GAD67, 1:250, Millipore, MAB5406) in blocking solution at 4°C. The next day cultures were incubated with the second primary antibody (MAP2, 1:500, Chemicon, AB5622) overnight at 4°C. Cultures were then washed three times with TBS and incubated with the secondary antibodies in 2% BSA, 2 mM $CaCl_2$ in TBS for 1 h at room temperature. After being washed three times with TBS the cultures were mounted with aqueous mounting medium containing DAPI (vector).

In vitro whole brain

Young adult Hartley guinea pigs (150–300 g, Charles River) were used for IWB recordings. All procedures were approved by the Italian Department of Health and were conducted in accordance to FELASA guidelines and Italian and European directives (DL 116/92 and 2010/63/EU). Animals were anesthetized with sodium thiopental (125 mg/kg, i.p.) and transcardially perfused with a cold (4°C), oxygenated (95% O_2, 5% CO_2) saline solution composed of 126 mM NaCl, 3 mM KCl, 1.2 mM KH_2PO_4, 1.3 mM $MgSO_4$, 2.4 mM $CaCl_2$, 26 mM $NaHCO_3$, 15 mM glucose, 2.1 mM HEPES, and 3% dextran (MW 70,000). The pH of the solution was corrected to 7.1 with 1N HCl. After assessing the absence of nociceptive and ocular reflexes, the brain was gently dissected out of the skull, transferred to a recording chamber, and perfused at 7 ml/min with the above solution (pH = 7.3, 15°C) via a peristaltic pump (Minipulse II, Gilson, France) through a cannula inserted in the basilar artery (**Figure 5**). Prior to recording, the temperature of the preparation was gradually increased to 32°C (0.2°C/min) (Llinas et al., 1981; Muhlethaler et al., 1993; De Curtis et al., 1998). In order to induce an ischemic insult in the hippocampal formation, a silk thread was positioned under the left rostral and caudal posterior cerebral arteries [r- and c-PCA, see Librizzi et al. (1999)] and a loose knot was prepared around the vessels. The flow was interrupted by pulling the thread ends to tighten the knot (**Figure 5**) (Pastori et al., 2007).

READ-OUT SYSTEMS

Optical manipulation and recording system for in vitro neural networks

The optical system combined a laser dissector with a microscope for simultaneous fluorescence and bright field imaging during electrophysiological recording of neural network activity, as previously described (Difato et al., 2011a).

The light source used to perform calcium fluorescence imaging was composed of TTL modulable laser diodes (TECBL-15 G-473-TTL-FC, World Star Tech. Inc., USA) coupled to the microscope (BX51, Olympus, Italy) through a circle top-hat engineered diffuser (ED1-C20-MD, Thorlabs, Optoprim, Italy) to remove laser speckles. A pair of UV doublets (Thorlabs, Optoprim, Italy) coupled the laser light to the microscope objective (60×, 0.9 NA water dipping). The laser light was focused on the back focal plane of the microscope objective to produce a homogenous wide field illumination on the sample. A light emitting diode at 590 nm wavelength served as the bright field illumination source (M590L2, Thorlabs, Optoprim, Italy). The wavelength of the diode was chosen to avoid interference with the emission spectra of the fluorochrome (Fluo4-AM, Invitrogen) used to label the sample. A dichroic mirror separated the light coming from the sample (green and red portion of light spectra) onto two cameras. Green emission light was deviated on CCD1 (V887ECSUVB EMCCD, Andor, Lot Oriel, Italy) acquiring the calcium fluctuations due to network activity, and the red portion of the light spectra was deviated on CCD2 (Pilot PIA1000-48GM, Basler, Advanced Technologies, Italy) to perform bright-field imaging. The CCDs image acquisitions and light sources were synchronized with a TTL signal coming from a D/A board (PCI-6529, National Instruments, Italy). The use of TTL-modulable light sources for fluorescence and bright field imaging allowed a precisely timed illumination of the sample, thereby reducing phototoxicity and facilitating long term calcium imaging of neural networks. Bright-field images were acquired at 1 Hz to detect network topography before and after laser dissection of network connections. Cells were previously incubated for 10 min with 5 μm Fluo-4 AM (Invitrogen, Italy). To monitor the neural network activity before and after laser induced network lesions, calcium imaging was performed at 60 Hz (light exposure of 3 ms each frame, at an average power at the sample of 60 μW).

Cells were kept under the microscope at 35°C using a Peltier device (QE1 resistive heating with TC-344B dual channel heater controller, Warner Instruments, Italy). For neuronal cultures plated on Petri dishes, pH and humidity were controlled by aerating a custom-designed polydimethylsiloxane (PDMS) sleeve, which integrated the objective for optical access, with humidified carbogen (95% O_2, 5% CO_2).

A pulsed, sub-nanosecond UV Nd:YAG laser at 355 nm (PowerChip nano-Pulse UV laser PNV-001525-040, Teem Photonics, Italy) served as the source for performing laser microdissection experiments. The diaphragm of the epi-illuminator was substituted by a narrow-band laser mirror, which reflects 355 nm laser light while passing all other wavelengths coming from the laser diodes used for fluorescence microscopy (DM6, TLM1-350-45-P, CVI, Italy), thus allowing fluorescence imaging and laser dissection to be performed simultaneously. Damage to neural network was inflicted with laser pulse repetition rate settled at 100 Hz, and an average power at the sample of about 4 μW.

Electrophysiological system for the in vitro whole brain

Extra- and intracellular recordings were performed simultaneously in piriform and medial entorhinal cortex (PC and m-ERC). To test the viability of the preparation throughout the experiment, we monitored evoked local field potentials (LFPs) in PC and m-ERC in response to the electrical stimulation (0.5–3 mA, 0.3 ms) of the lateral olfactory tract (LOT) using custom-made bipolar electrodes made of twisted, insulated silver wires. Intracellular recordings were performed with sharp micropipettes filled with 3M potassium acetate (input resistance 70–110 MΩ) and attached to an electronically controlled micromanipulator (Sutter Instruments, Novato, CA, USA). Signals were amplified by an intracellular amplifier (IR-283A Cygnus Technology, PA, USA). Field potentials were recorded using glass pipette filled with 0.9% NaCl (resistance 2–5 mΩ) or microwire arrays (Tucker-Davis Technologies, Alachua, FL, USA) featuring 16 tungsten planar recording wires (filament diameter 50 μm, tip angle 45°), each separated by 250 μm (impedance 30–40 KΩ). The extracellular signals were acquired using a PBX3 preamplifier (Plexon, Dallas, TX, USA) configured to separately process spikes (150 Hz–8 KHz bandwidth) and local field potentials (0.7–300 Hz).

Data were digitized at 25 kHz using a PCI-6071E A/D board (National Instruments, Austin, TX, USA) and stored on the hard drive of a personal computer. Recordings were performed using ELPHO software developed by Dr. Vadym Gnatkovsky at the C. Besta Neurological Institute (Milan, Italy).

COMPUTATIONAL MODEL

In the following sections we will present the computational model used to mimic the dynamics expressed by finite size networks (cf. section "Experimental Models").

Neuron model

The neuron model used for the finite size networks is based on the Izhikevich equations (Izhikevich, 2003). The dynamics of this model depend on four parameters that, correctly chosen, reproduce the spiking behavior and voltage traces of specific types of cortical neurons. From a mathematical point of view, the model is described by a two-dimensional system of ordinary differential equations.

$$\frac{dv}{dt} = 0.04v^2 + 5v + 140 - u + I_{syn} + I_{noise} \tag{1}$$

$$\frac{du}{dt} = a(bv - u) \tag{2}$$

with the after-spike resetting conditions:

$$\text{if } v \geq 40\,\text{mV} \rightarrow \begin{cases} v \leftarrow c \\ u \leftarrow u + d \end{cases} \tag{3}$$

In Equations (1–3), v is the membrane potential of the neuron, u is a membrane recovery variable which takes into account the activation of K^+ and inactivation of Na^+ channels; I_{syn} describes the synaptic input from other neurons; I_{noise} is a current source generator introduced to model the spontaneous subthreshold electrophysiological activity of the neurons. Practically, we introduced a stochastic source of noise (modeled according to an Ornstein-Uhlenbeck process) to each neuron described as follows:

$$dI_{\text{noise}} = -\frac{I_{\text{noise}}}{\tau_I}dt + \frac{m_I}{\tau_I}dt + s_1\sqrt{\frac{2dt}{\tau_I}}\xi_t \tag{4}$$

In Equation (4) the quantity ξ_t is a white noise with zero mean and unitary variance. In this way, I_{noise} is Gauss-distributed at any time t and, after a transient of magnitude τ_I (correlation length), converges to a process with a mean equals to m_I and standard deviation s_I. For the simulation, we set $\tau_I = 1$ ms, $m_I = 25$ pA, and $s_I = 9$ pA.

Among the possible firing patterns generated by the neuron model of Equations (1, 2), we implemented the family of regular spiking (RS) and the family of fast spiking neurons (FS) in percentage of 75% and 25%, respectively, in agreement with the experimental findings (cf. section "Finite Size Network Dynamics"). Mathematically, the four aforementioned parameters were set as follows:

$$a = \begin{bmatrix} 0.02 \\ 0.02 + 0.08r_i \end{bmatrix} \quad b = \begin{bmatrix} 0.2 \\ 0.25 - 0.05r_i \end{bmatrix}$$
$$c = \begin{bmatrix} -65 + 15r_i^2 \\ -65 \end{bmatrix} \quad d = \begin{bmatrix} 8 - 6r_i^2 \\ 2 \end{bmatrix} \tag{5}$$

In Equation (5), the first row is relative to the excitatory, while the second one to the inhibitory neurons. r_i is a random variable which spans from 0 to 1, and i the neuron index. r_i was added in order to introduce a further variability in the neuron dynamics: for example, a neuron exhibits classic RS behavior if $r_i = 0$, and bursting behavior if $r_i = 1$.

Finite size network model

Graph theory was used to represent the network connectivity. All graphs are defined by nodes which represent the neurons, and edges which model the morphological connections among the neurons. The structure of the graph is described by the adjacency matrix, a square matrix of size equal to the number of nodes N with binary entries. If the element $a_{ij} = 1$, a connection between the node j to i is present, otherwise $a_{ij} = 0$ means no connection. All the auto-connections are avoided ($a_{ii} = 0, \forall$ i). Then, the value 1 of the non-zero a_{ij} elements has been replaced to mimic different synaptic strengths. Synaptic weights were chosen randomly from a normal distribution with a mean value and standard deviation equal to 10 and 3.5, respectively.

To model the synaptic transmission we chose the approach of the pulse-coupled neural networks: practically, the firing of the j-th neuron causes an instantaneous change in the membrane potential of the neuron i-th by means of the weight s_{ij}.

Among the possible graphs, following the experimental findings regarding the functional connectivity of such confined neuronal assemblies (cf. section "Finite Size Network Dynamics"), we implemented neuronal networks with a scale-free (SF) connectivity (Barabasi and Albert, 1999). Briefly, in SF networks the degree distribution follows a power law: if m is the number of edges incident to a node, i.e., the degree, the power law distribution is given by Dorogovtsev and Mendes (2002):

$$P(m) = m^{-\gamma} \tag{6}$$

where γ is the characteristic exponent. This law suggests that most nodes have just a few connections and other, named *hubs*, have a very high number of links. To build a SF network, we made use of the algorithm described in Batagelj and Brandes (2005), particularly efficient in terms of computation when dealing with large-scale networks. Nodes are added successively. For each node, m edges are generated. The endpoints are selected from the nodes whose edges have already been created, with a bias toward high degree nodes.

In order to mimic the experimental conditions of the confined assemblies described in section "Finite Size Network Dynamics," in section "Simulation Results" we presented the results regarding the ongoing activity of networks made up of 90, 100, 120, 150, 240, 320, and 520 neurons.

DATA ANALYSIS AND STATISTICS

Analysis of network dynamics based on calcium fluorescence imaging

Custom software running in MATLAB (Crépel et al., 2007; Bonifazi et al., 2009) was used for the automatic identification of the cells loaded with the calcium indicator and for the extraction of their fluorescence signals as a function of time (time resolution 59 Hz). To detect the calcium events (i.e., the onset and offset of neuronal firing) from the fluorescent trace F_{ij} of the neurons ($1 \leq i \leq M$, M number of neurons; $1 \leq j \leq N$, N number of frames) we calculated the first derivative of the fluorescent signal ($\Delta F_{ij} = F_{ij+1} - F_{ij}$) and we integrated ΔF_{ij} in overlapping sliding time windows of 1 s ($I_{ij'} = \Sigma_{j' \leq n \leq j'+59} \Delta F_{nj}$; $1 \leq j' \leq N - 59$). A Gaussian fit centered at zero was used to extract the standard deviation σ_i of the noise of the processed signal I_{ij}. Signal transients exceeding the threshold of $3\sigma_i$ for at least 5 consecutive points were considered as calcium events. The onset and the offset of these calcium events were determined using a four-parameter sigmoidal equation as described in Takano et al. (2012). The estimated onset and offset times were fixed respectively to the 5% and the 95% of the sigmoidal plateau.

The reconstruction of the functional connectivity of the network was based on pair-wise correlation analysis of the onset time series extracted from the calcium imaging data, as described in Bonifazi et al. (2009). Briefly, when the firing onset of cell j preceded in a repetitive way the firing onset of cell k, a functional connection directed from j to k was established. In order to reveal these temporal correlations, the post-stimulus time histogram of cell k centered on the firing onsets of cell j was calculated within a maximal time lag of 500 ms. Both the Student's t-test and the Kolmogorov-Smirnov test with a level of confidence of 5% were used to exclude the possibility that the poststimulus time distribution could be a Gaussian distribution with zero mean or a uniform distribution, respectively. In this way, we excluded cases where the activation of two neurons was completely uncorrelated (uniform distribution) or synchronous (Gaussian centered at zero).

The cross correlation between firing onsets time series of individual neurons was used to estimate the average correlation and average time of activation of each neuron relative to all others, similarly to what described in Bonifazi et al. (2009) and Marissal et al. (2012). Briefly, the cross correlation between the time series of neurons a and b was calculated as follows:

$$CC_{ab}(\tau) = \frac{\sum\limits_{0<t<T} (a_{t+\tau} - <a>) \cdot (b_t - <b>)}{\sigma_a \cdot \sigma_b} \quad (7)$$

where σ_a and σ_b are the standard deviation of the time series, t is the sampling time, T the duration of the entire movie and $|\tau| \leq 1$ s.

The maximum cross-correlation value (CC_{ab}^{max}) and the time lag of its occurrence (τ_{ab}^{max}) were used to calculate, respectively, the average correlation and average time of activation of neuron i to the following formulas $\langle CC_i^{max} \rangle = \frac{1}{n} \sum_{j \neq i} CC_{ij}^{max}$ and $\langle \tau_i^{max} \rangle = \frac{1}{n} \sum_{j \neq i} \tau_{ij}^{max}$ where n is the number of neurons displaying a positive cross-correlation with neuron I.

Processing of electrophysiological signals from the IWB

Raw data acquired by the ELPHO software were loaded into MATLAB (Mathworks Inc., Natick, MA, USA) for off-line processing. First, raw traces were band-pass filtered to select either multi-unit activity (MUA, 800 Hz–3 KHz) or local field potentials (LFP, 1–300 Hz). Stimulation artifacts were suppressed using an off-line MATLAB implementation of the SALPA algorithm (Wagenaar and Potter, 2002). Highly noisy channels were visually excluded from the analysis. Then, MUA raw data were spike-detected by means of the PTSD algorithm (Maccione et al., 2009) (peak lifetime period = 2 ms; refractory period = 1 ms; threshold = ±8 times the estimated noise standard deviation). The result of the spike-detection procedure consists of a series of point processes (i.e., spike trains), one for each recording channel (Bologna et al., 2010).

We evaluated the network-wide evoked response by computing the Peri Stimulus Time Histogram (PSTH; Perkel et al., 1967) for each recording channel of the array and for the full array [time bin = 4 ms, time window = (−100 ms, +400 ms) relative to the stimulus onset]. We also measured the intensity of the response as the average number of evoked spikes in a 200-ms time window following each stimulus. The final dataset comprised 4 recordings in control brains (duration ~300 s, 10–20 paired pulses delivered to the LOT at 0.05 Hz, inter-pulse interval 200 ms) and 3 recordings before and after the induction of focal ischemia (same stimulation protocol).

RESULTS

FINITE SIZE NETWORK DYNAMICS

Spontaneous synchronizations in finite size networks

To build an experimental model for the study of physiological and impaired communications between neuronal assemblies we grew finite size neuronal networks, i.e., networks composed of neuronal assemblies spatially separated by hundreds of micrometers and interconnected through long neuritis. As a first step, we focused on the properties of single modules, i.e., the structural and dynamical properties of isolated and spatially confined neuronal circuits (**Figure 2**). Isolated neuronal circuits located within an 800 × 800 μ m spot were obtained by plating the cells on glass cover slips previously coated with a geometrically defined molecular adhesive layer (PDL). The individual cell populations varied between a few dozen up to a few hundred neurons. Similar to homogenous and clustered cultures (Chiappalone et al., 2006; Shein-Idelson et al., 2010), finite size circuits displayed spontaneous synchronized events after 2 weeks in culture (**Figure 2**, panel B1) occurring with a frequency linearly correlated with the number of cells present in the circuit (Pearson correlation 0.88, **Figure 2C1**). Likewise, depending on the density of the plating and on the vicinity to the supporting network, finite size circuits organized into monolayers or in three-dimensional clusters, with a higher propensity of clustering at increased plating density or at larger distances from the supporting network (data not shown). We used calcium imaging of monolayer neuronal circuits (performed with a 10× objective) in combination with immunocytochemical staining to map the functional and structural properties of all the neurons in the circuits with single-cell resolution. GABAergic cells could be specifically identified (**Figure 2A3**), allowing us to investigate their specific involvement in spontaneous synchronization processes, similar to the work of Bonifazi et al. (2009) in developing hippocampal networks.

A pair-wise analysis based on the cross-correlation between the firing onsets time series of pairs of neurons (see section "Materials and Methods") was used to estimate the average correlation and average time of activation of each neuron relative to all others (Bonifazi et al., 2009; Marissal et al., 2012). In all the circuits analyzed ($n = 4$) the time correlation graph presented a bimodal distribution (**Figure 2C2**), indicating that network events synchronized first the population of neurons plotted on the left side of the graph (i.e., with a time lag < 0), whereas neurons on the right (i.e., with a time lag > 0) were activated next. In addition, the presence of highly correlated early activated GABAergic neurons was observed (red points within the violet circle in **Figure 2C2**). Interestingly, the existence of a characteristic, early-activated neuronal population within the network synchronizations has been already documented in developing hippocampal circuits (Bonifazi et al., 2009) even in absence of GABAergic transmission (Marissal et al., 2012). Notably, in the presence of GABAergic transmission it has been shown that early-activated GABAergic neurons can play the role of hub cells in orchestrating network dynamics (Bonifazi et al., 2009). The similarity between these previous observations and the results presented here suggest that cortical circuits share common innate features in their functional organization.

Effect of laser ablation on functional connectivity

To monitor the synaptic re-organization of lesioned neuronal circuits with single cell resolution, we reconstructed the functional connectivity of a neuronal subset of a larger neuronal network 20 min before and after laser-induced ablations (see section "Materials and Methods").

Two micro-lesions (lesion 1 and lesion 2) were induced next to the center of the field of view, using an average laser power

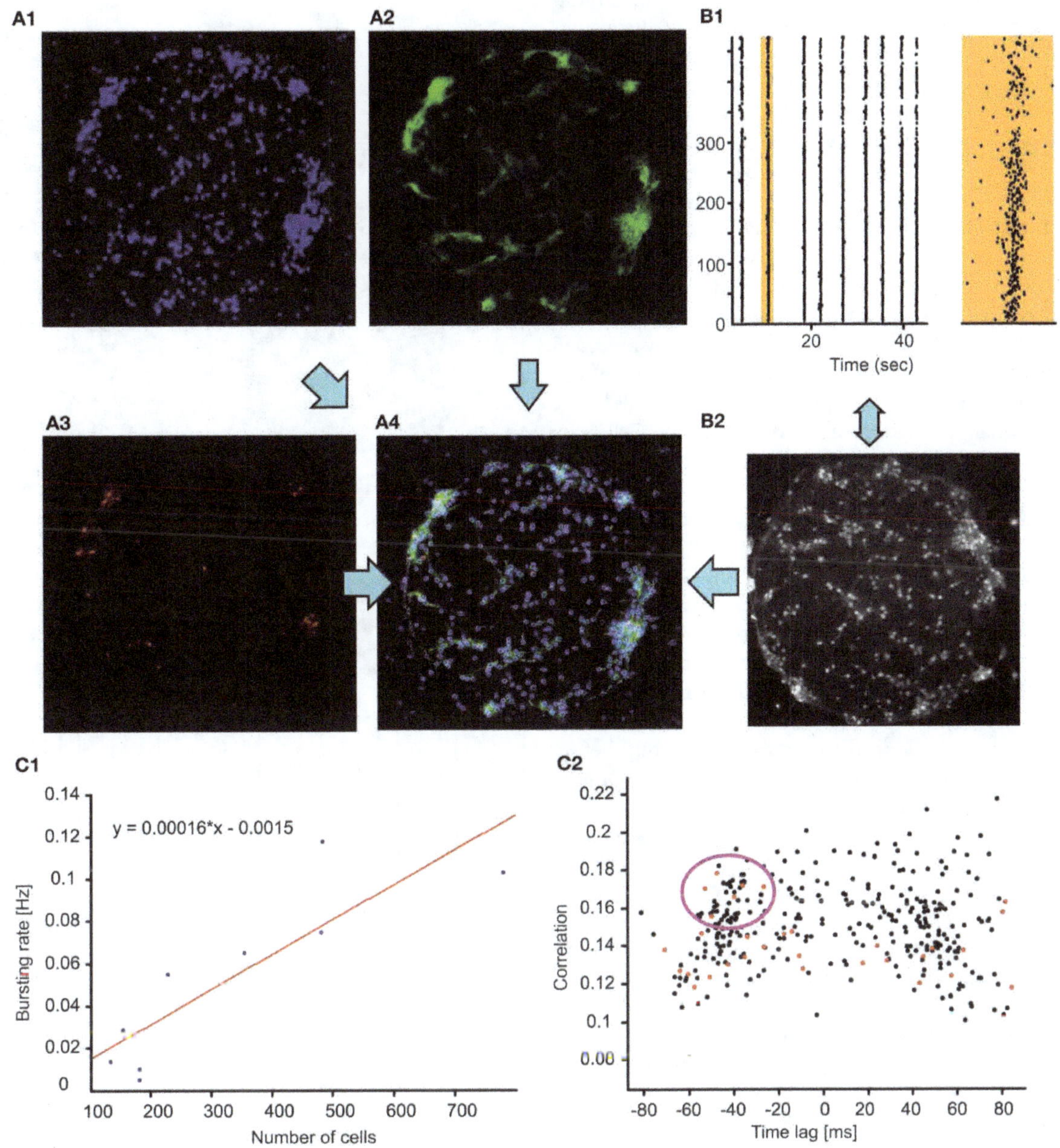

FIGURE 2 | Structure *vs.* function relations in neocortical finite circuits. **(A)** Immunocytochemical staining revealing cellular nuclei (blue, DAPI, **A1**), neuronal cells (green, MAPs, **A2**), GABAergic neurons (red, GAD67, **A3**). In panel **(A4)**, the contours of the cells monitored through calcium imaging (white) are superimposed to the merged immunocytochemical pictures. **(B)** Monitoring the dynamics of the neuronal circuit through calcium imaging. Raster plot (**B1** left plot) of the activity of the circuit (shown in panel **A**) displaying stereotyped spontaneous network synchronizations (broken vertical lines). The activity of a representative network synchronization (marked in orange) is shown with higher temporal resolution on the right orange plot (bottom scale bar 0.5 s). The cells loaded with the calcium indicator OGB are shown in the panel **(B2)** (objective magnification 10×, field of view 800 × 800 μm). **(C1)** Frequency of spontaneous synchronizations as a function of circuits' population size (blue dots, $n = 9$). The cell number was estimated by counting the cellular nuclei stained with DAPI. The result of the linear fit with least-squares regression (Pearson correlation coefficient 0.88) is represented by the red line and by the equation. **(C2)** Time lag—correlation graph for the circuit shown in **(A)** plotting for each imaged neuron the average correlation and average time of activation relative to all other cells (see section "Materials and Methods"). Red dots indicate GABAergic cells. The violet circle highlight GABAergic cells reliably activated at the synchronization build up possibly playing a key role in the orchestration of network synchrony similarly to what previously documented for the developing hippocampal circuits (Bonifazi et al., 2009).

at the sample of 4 μW and 5 μW, respectively. The second lesion was performed at higher power to obtain a more pronounced alteration of the network. Indeed, this lesion produced a strong intracellular calcium increase in several cells, and a calcium "shockwave" started to propagate through the network. After a few minutes, only directly ablated cells displayed a saturated calcium fluorescence signal, while the other neurons recovered a relatively low basal calcium level and presented spontaneous activity (cf. **Figure A1**). The frequency of occurrence of spontaneous network synchronizations was not affected by the lesions (**Figure 3**, 4th and 5th rows) with no significantly statistical difference between the inter-burst interval distribution before and after lesion (student *t*-test, $p > 0.05$). However, the number of cells recruited within the network events in the imaged field (i.e., close to the location of the lesion) decreased by 31 ± 10% (student *t*-test, $p < 0.05$).

Based on the calcium dynamics of the cells imaged in a circular field of 244 μm diameter (**Figure 3**), we reconstructed the functional connectivity of the neuronal population through a pair-wise analysis of the onset of firing (see section "Materials and Methods"). Briefly, if the activation of cell i reliably preceded the activation of cell j (i.e., over several repetitions with statistical significance, see section "Materials and Methods"), we inferred a functional connection directed from i to j. Cell pairs that were synchronously activated or not displaying any activation order were not included in the directed functional connectivity reconstruction (see section "Materials and Methods"). **Figure 3** (1st row) shows the location of ten neurons with the highest number of functional INPUT (violet) and OUTPUT (yellow) connections before and after the lesions. Interestingly, after the lesions, top rank INPUT and OUTPUT neurons segregated into spatially distinct regions. Top rank OUTPUT neurons relocated in the bottom right region while top rank INPUT neurons remained in the rest of the circuit. In addition, just one out of the ten neurons for each group belonged to the top rank group before and after the lesion. The relocation of the functional connections (drawn for clarity just for the five best ranked neurons) can additionally be observed in **Figure 3** (2nd and 3rd row).

In vitro WHOLE BRAIN

We also characterized the activity of an *ex vivo* experimental model (i.e., the isolated brain of a guinea pig, **Figure 4**) before and after a lesion induced by a focal ischemia.

Network response to LOT stimulation in the m-ERC

Electrical stimulation of the LOT induced a polysynaptic response in the m-ERC mediated by the interposed activation of the hippocampus (Biella and De Curtis, 2000; Gnatkovsky and De Curtis, 2006) (**Figure 4**). The intracellular correlate of the LOT-evoked delayed response in neurons of m-ERC superficial layers was characterized by an early $GABA_A$ receptor- mediated inhibitory postsynaptic potential (IPSP; latency from LOT stimulation: 51 ± 1 ms, $n = 12$), followed by a relatively slow (duration 409 ± 36 ms) NMDA-dependent depolarizing component which often reached threshold for spike firing. Conversely, pyramidal cells in deeper layers responded to LOT stimulation with an early excitatory postsynaptic potential (EPSP) occurring 15 ± 1 ms after the population spike recorded in the dentate gyrus (DG, **Figure 4**). The EPSP often crossed the threshold for action potential firing and was followed by a relatively slow inhibitory potential mediated by $GABA_B$ receptors (Gnatkovsky and De Curtis, 2006). The early inhibition of the superficial principal cells is presumably due to a feed-forward mechanism sustained by interneurons recorded in layers II/III (i.e., basket and chandelier cells; Canto et al., 2008). In **Figure 4** the firing of an interneuron

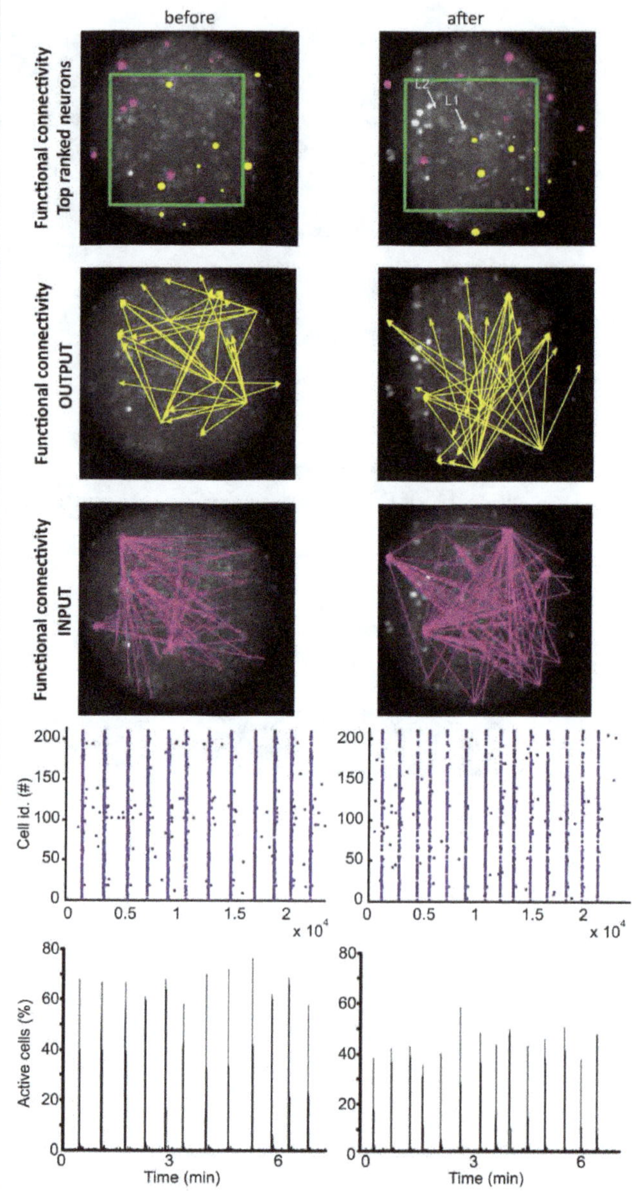

FIGURE 3 | Directed functional connectivity before (left) and after (right) lesion. The number of OUTPUT and INPUT functional connections has been calculated for all the imaged neurons based on the temporal correlation between the firing onsets of the neurons (see section "Materials and Methods"). The ten top ranked cells, i.e., the cells with the largest number of functional OUTPUT (yellow) and INPUT connections (pink), are represented in the top row. For graphic clarity, the connectivity graphs shown in the 2nd and 3rd rows (respectively INPUT and OUTPUT connections) include only the five top ranked cells. The data refers to a homogenous neuronal network where functional hub cells (i.e., neurons with a very large number of functional connections) were not identified. The fluorescent images show the cells loaded with the calcium indicator Fluo4 (see section "Materials and Methods"). The locations of the two lesions (L1 and L2) are marked by the white arrows. The green rectangle highlights the region shown in **Figure A1**. The field of view is a circular region of 244 μm diameter. The raster plot (representing the firing onsets) and the fraction of activated cells are shown respectively in the 4th and 5th row.

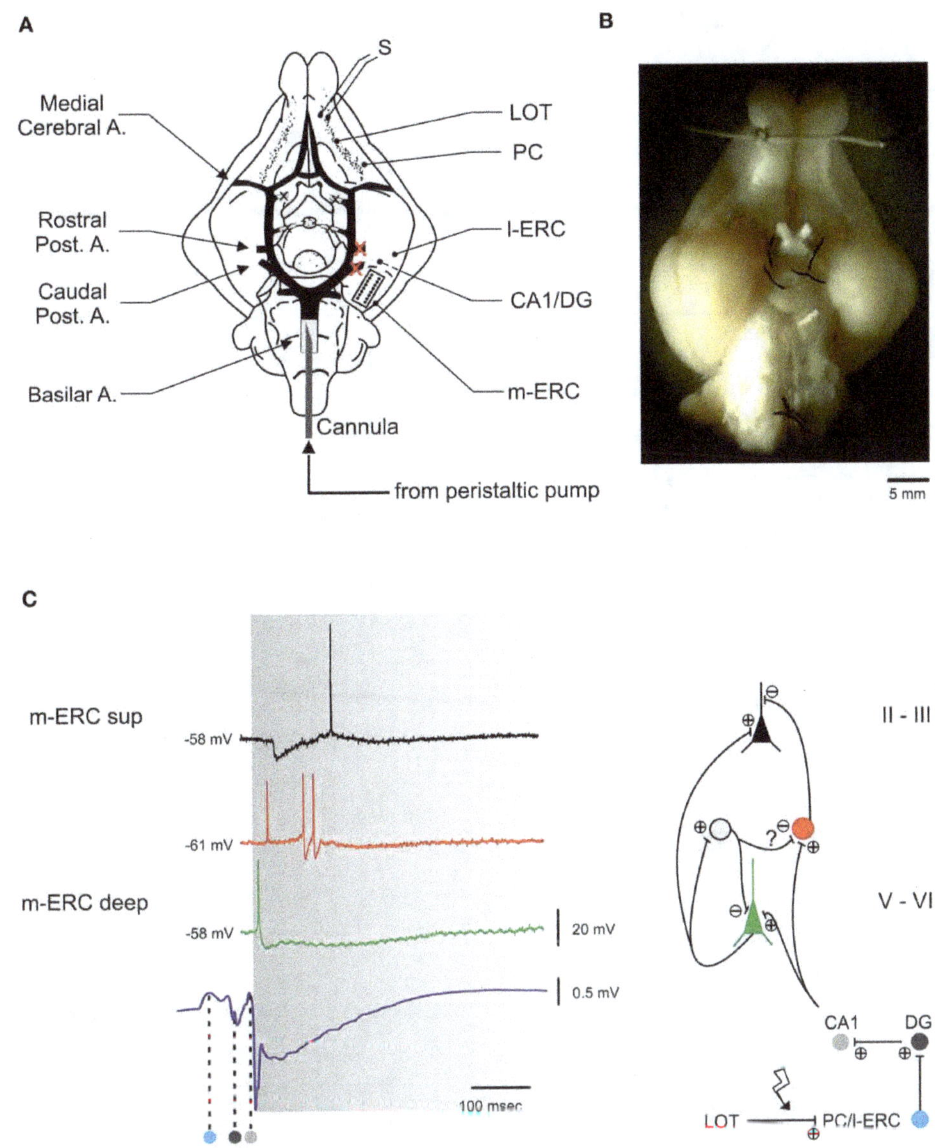

FIGURE 4 | The guinea pig isolated whole brain (IWB). (A) Schematic view of IWB observed from its ventral surface. The circle of Willis with its principal branching arteries is highlighted in black. The whole brain is perfused by means of a peristaltic pump that delivers ACSF to the brain through a polyethylene cannula inserted into the basilar artery. The two vessels that are occluded to induce the hippocampal ischemia are marked by red crosses. In the same hemisphere a microelectrode array (MEA) is positioned in the center of the m-ERC (delimited by dotted line). S, stimulating electrode; LOT, lateral olfactory tract; PC, piriform cortex; I-ERC, lateral entorhinal cortex; DG, dentate gyrus; m-ERC, medial entorhinal cortex. **(B)** Stereomicroscope photograph of the isolated brain positioned in the perfusion chamber. **(C)** Electrical responses to LOT stimulation recorded in the m-ERC. Left, intracellularly recorded voltage traces from a superficial pyramidal cell lying at 200–300 μm from pial surface (black trace), a GABAergic interneuron (400–500 μm, red trace), and a deep pyramidal cell (600–1000 μm, green trace). Note the correspondence between the early firing of an action potential in the interneuron and an IPSP (asterisk) recorded in the superficial pyramidal cell. The bottom trace is an extracellularly recorded field potential (LFP) characterized by a volume conducted component propagating from the rostral part of the LOT-activated synaptic pathway (PC and I-ERC) and subsequently invading the hippocampal structure (DG and CA1, dark and light gray spots, respectively). The left margin of the gray area is aligned to the first component of the m-ERC LFP. Right, simplified scheme of the polysynaptic neuronal circuitry within the m-ERC, based on the evoked response pattern and delay analysis of the neuronal response to LOT stimulation. The gray cell represents a putative interneuron mediating a feedback GABAergic inhibition onto a deep pyramidal cell and a feed-forward inhibition onto another interneuron.

corresponds to the early IPSP measured in the pyramidal cells in the same layer.

Spiking responses to paired-pulse LOT stimulation (interpulse interval 200 ms) were recorded by 16-channel MEAs implanted in the superficial layers of the m-ERC (200–500 μm from pial surface; **Figure 5A**). **Figure 5B** shows the peri-stimulus raster plots of two selected channels (19 and 24, experiment #1) in response to each of the two LOT stimulations for a selected

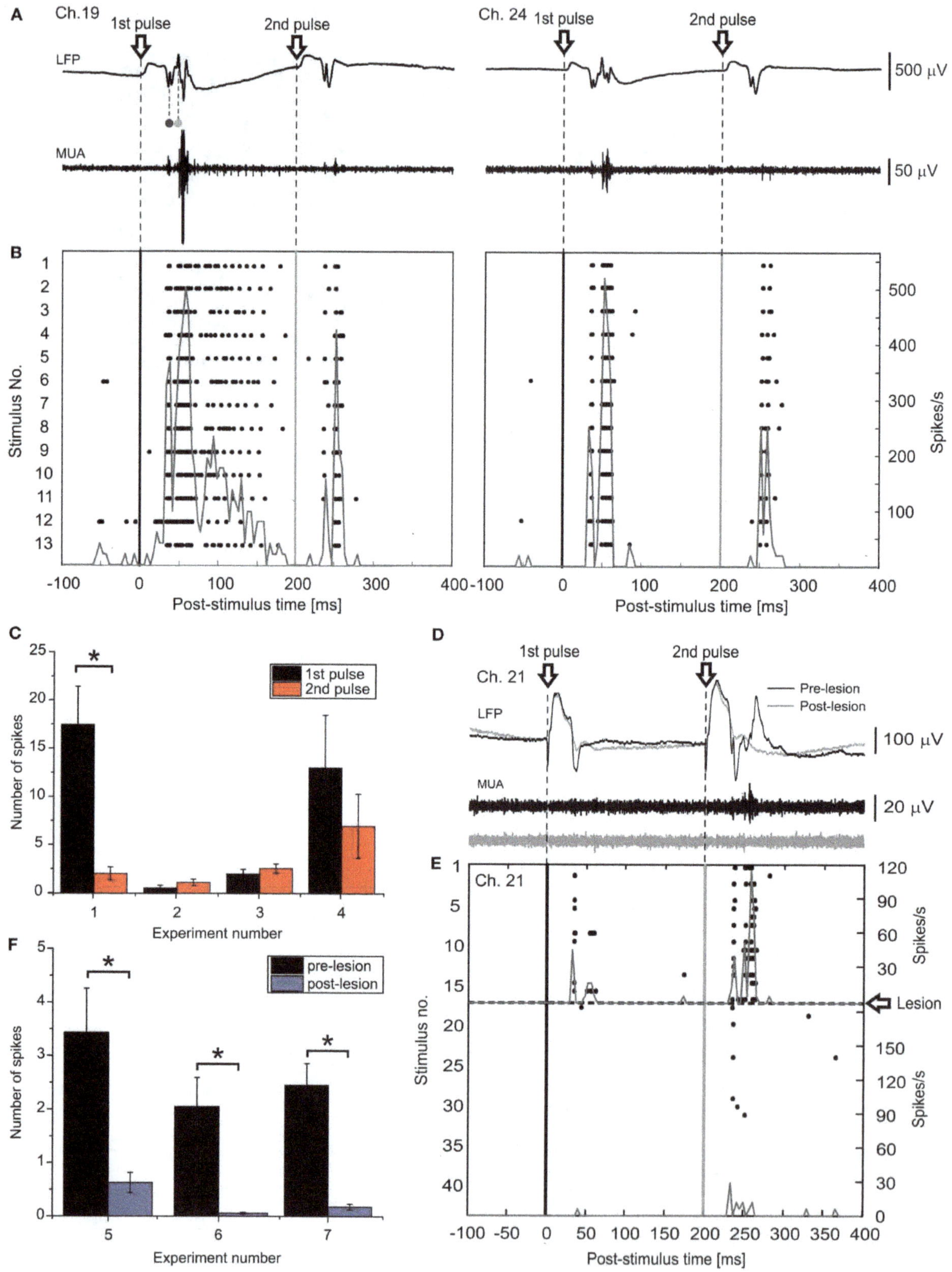

FIGURE 5 | LOT-evoked m-ERC network activity is abolished after ischemic lesioning of the hippocampus. (A) Local field potentials (LFP) and multi-unit activity (MUA) raw traces from two selected electrodes (19 and 24, experiment #1) recorded in response to an individual paired-pulse stimulus (ISI 200 ms) delivered to the LOT. The volume-conducted components originating in DG and CA1 are indicated by the dark gray and light gray dots, respectively. **(B)** Peri-stimulus raster plots for the same two representative

(Continued)

FIGURE 5 | Continued
electrodes. The corresponding PSTHs are superimposed (bin size = 4 ms). **(C)** Summary plot of mean number of evoked spikes (mean ± S.E.M.) after 1st and 2nd pulse for all four experiments. $^*p < 0.05$, Mann–Whitney *U*-test. **(D)** LFP and MUA raw traces of one selected electrode recorded in response to a paired-pulse stimulus either before (black trace) or after (gray trace) an ischemic lesion of the hippocampus. **(E)** Peri-stimulus raster plot for the same representative electrode, before and after the lesion. The corresponding PSTHs are superimposed (bin size = 4 ms). **(F)** Summary plot of mean number of evoked spikes by a paired pulse stimulus delivered to the LOT (mean ± S.E.M.) either before or after the ischemic lesion of the hippocampus for all analyzed experiments. $^*p < 0.05$, Mann–Whitney *U*-test.

experiment. An earlier phase, which we observed in almost all active recording channels, was characterized by two relatively sharp peaks: the first corresponding to the far-field response originating in the hippocampus and the other corresponding to the initial phase of the m-ERC response (**Figure 4**). This was followed by a late, long-lasting but less reliable component (cf. channels 19 and 24). The histogram in **Figure 5C** displays the number of spikes (mean ± S.E.M.) evoked by the 1st and the 2nd pulse for all experiments (control condition) as a measure of response intensity. In 2 out of 4 experiments (#1, #4) we observed a stronger activation after the 1st rather than 2nd pulse, whereas in the other 2 experiments (#2, #3) responses to the 2nd pulse were slightly stronger than to the 1st pulse (no significant statistical difference). However, one must consider that first evoked responses in experiments #1 and #4 were on average more intense, probably reflecting a relatively high probability of excitatory neurotransmitter release upon the first pulse. This would nearly deplete the available pool of synaptic glutamatergic vesicles, leading to a paired-pulse depression of the postsynaptic response.

Cutting the olfactory pathway: hippocampal focal ischemia

Occlusion of the posterior left cerebral arteries abruptly reduced ACSF perfusion of the hippocampus, resulting in a block of the propagation of the synaptic activity toward the entorhinal cortex (**Figure 4**). About 5 min after the ischemic insult, LOT stimulation failed to evoke any response (**Figure 5**). Stimulus-triggered raster plots and the corresponding pre- and post-lesion PSTH are shown in **Figure 5E**. The bar graph in **Figure 5F** summarizes the total number of spikes evoked by a paired-pulse stimulus before and after the ischemic lesion. A significant reduction of the response intensity caused by the lesion was observed in all three analyzed experiments.

SIMULATION RESULTS

In this section, we report the results of simulations in which we modeled the effects changing the number of neurons in confined networks. Each simulation lasted 10 min, sampled at 10 kHz. Networks were simulated in MATLAB (The Mathworks, Natik, US). Peak trains were stored and then processed by using SpyCode software (Bologna et al., 2010), conveniently adapted to manage large-scale networks.

Dynamics of finite size networks

We simulated the ongoing activity of neuronal networks made up a 90, 100, 120, 150, 240, 320, and 520 neurons. The choice of these networks sizes followed from the experimental findings described in section "Finite Size Network Dynamics" (assuming a neuron/glia ratio equal to 2:1). In addition, 25% of such neurons were considered inhibitory (Isaacson and Scanziani, 2011) and were modeled as FS neurons (cf. section "Computational Model").

Model neurons were connected following a scale-free (SF) topology. **Figure 6A** shows the degree distribution of the simulated SF networks. For all SF networks, the degree distribution was fitted by a power law and the corresponding exponent lay between −1.04 (network made up of 90 neurons) and −1.34 (networks made up of 520 neurons).

The simulated networks displayed spontaneous synchronized events (network bursts) independently of their size (**Figure 6B**). However, the frequency of occurrence of those synchronized events varied in a linear manner with respect to the number of cells present in the circuit (Pearson correlation 0.96, **Figure 6C**). To facilitate comparison with **Figure 2C1**, the *x*-axis of **Figure 6C** reports the total cell number (neurons + glia), although the number of neurons effectively simulated is indicated near the blue dots. The results of the simulation were fit well with the experimental data, as confirmed by the slope of the linear fit (0.00015 vs. 0.00016). An interesting finding was that the simulated networks tended to show a higher proportion of random spiking activity and less bursting than normally observed in actual finite-size neuronal networks. This is consistent with other experimental results of interconnected finite-size networks previously reported in the literature (Macis et al., 2007).

HARDWARE SET-UP FOR A BRAIN PROSTHESIS

The hardware set-up that will be used to interface the biological component (either the neuronal culture or the *in vitro* whole brain) is a Spiking Neural Network (SNN) system. This SNN implements biologically realistic neural network models, spanning from the electrophysiological properties of one single neuron up to network plasticity rules. As already discussed in the modeling section, the choice of Izhikevich neuron model is relevant because (1) it is biologically realistic, and (2) it operates in biological real time. By real-time, we mean that computation results are provided within a firmly controlled delay (10 ns precision), which is lower than the sampling period (100 μs to 1 ms). Among these modules, the computation-critical task is the implementation of a SNN model, which represents the prosthesis itself, and the analysis of biological signals to produce events from the recorded activity.

The digital Izhikevich neurons and detection system are implemented as a configurable digital integrated circuit (field-programmable gate array, FPGA) using the VHDL language. We implement Regular Spiking (RS) neurons (excitatory) and Fast Spiking (FS) interneurons (inhibitory) similar to those found in cell culture (**Figures 2, 3** and **6**). The hardware models follow the Izhikevich equations with parameters corresponding to RS activity ($a = 0.02$, $b = 0.2$, $c = -65$, and $d = 8$). In **Figure 7A1**

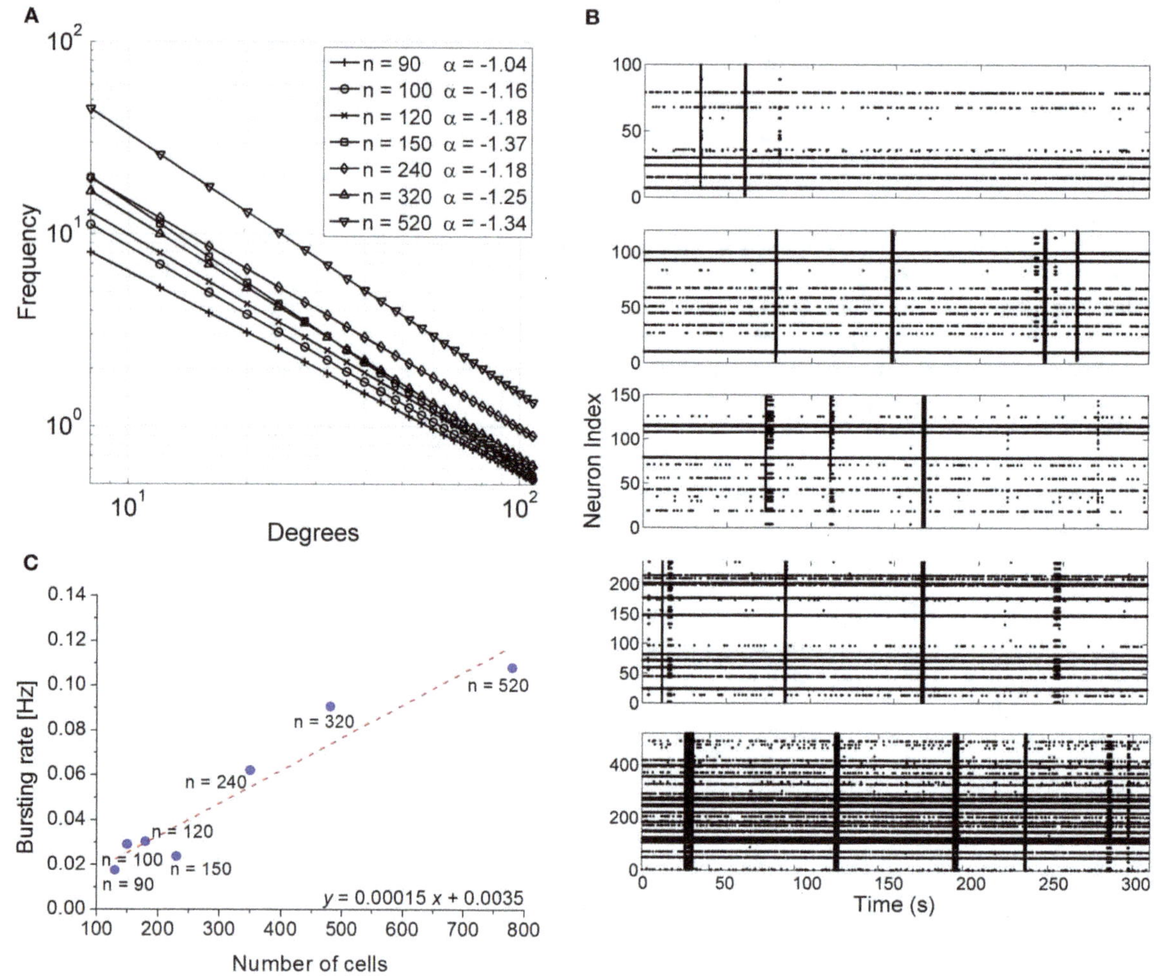

FIGURE 6 | Simulation results. (A) Degree distribution of the 7 scale-free networks. **(B)** Raster plots showing 300 s of spontaneous activity of simulated confined networks. Each raster is relative to a different network size. From top to bottom networks with 100, 120, 150, 240, 520 neurons can be observed.. IFR profiles was evaluated over simulations lasting 600 s (bin size = 100 ms). **(C)** Bursting rate frequency as a function of network population size. The number of neurons of the simulated networks was reported near the blue dots. The *x*-axis reports the total number of cells (glia + neurons) in order to make easier a comparison with **Figure 2C1**. The result of the linear fit with least-squares regression (Pearson correlation coefficient 0.96) is represented by the red-dotted line and by the fitting equation.

we describe the choice of the topology (Cassidy and Andreou, 2008) to implement the Izhikevich equations. We implement a neuron on FPGA board Xilinx Virtex 5 XC5VLX50. This neuron uses really few resources (only 2% of the FPGA) and works in real-time. In **Figure 7A2** we compare the behavior f(I) of biological RS neurons and one RS neuron implemented into the FPGA.

Concerning the SNN, our goal was to implement a model using 80 neurons (FS and RS) with high connectivity capacity (e.g., 6400 synapses). Network structure is fully configurable, and synapses are excitatory or inhibitory conductances which provide current depending on the postsynaptic membrane voltage. Delays are also implemented to provide good accuracy on timing. The network is defined into the RAM of the digital board where lie all characteristics of all neurons and synaptic connections in the network. A synaptic connection is defined by a synaptic weight and the address of the neuron linked by this synapse. Added with complementary functions like loopback stimulation and monitoring, this system will be able to perform cross-platform neural computation.

The detection of neural electrophysiological activity is done by a reconfigurable acquisition based on wavelet detection circuit for *in vitro* biological signals. Our strategy for real-time spike detection is to implement a pre-processor, which emphasizes spikes shapes and attenuates out-of-band noise. This pre-processor provides two outputs corresponding to different wavelet detail levels. The first one is essentially composed of out-of-band noise used to determine a threshold level adapted to the signal amplitude. The second output is compared to the threshold to discriminate spike events. The pre-processing algorithm is the Stationary Wavelet Transform (SWT). The detection system computes in real-time the SWT, the adaptive threshold and the

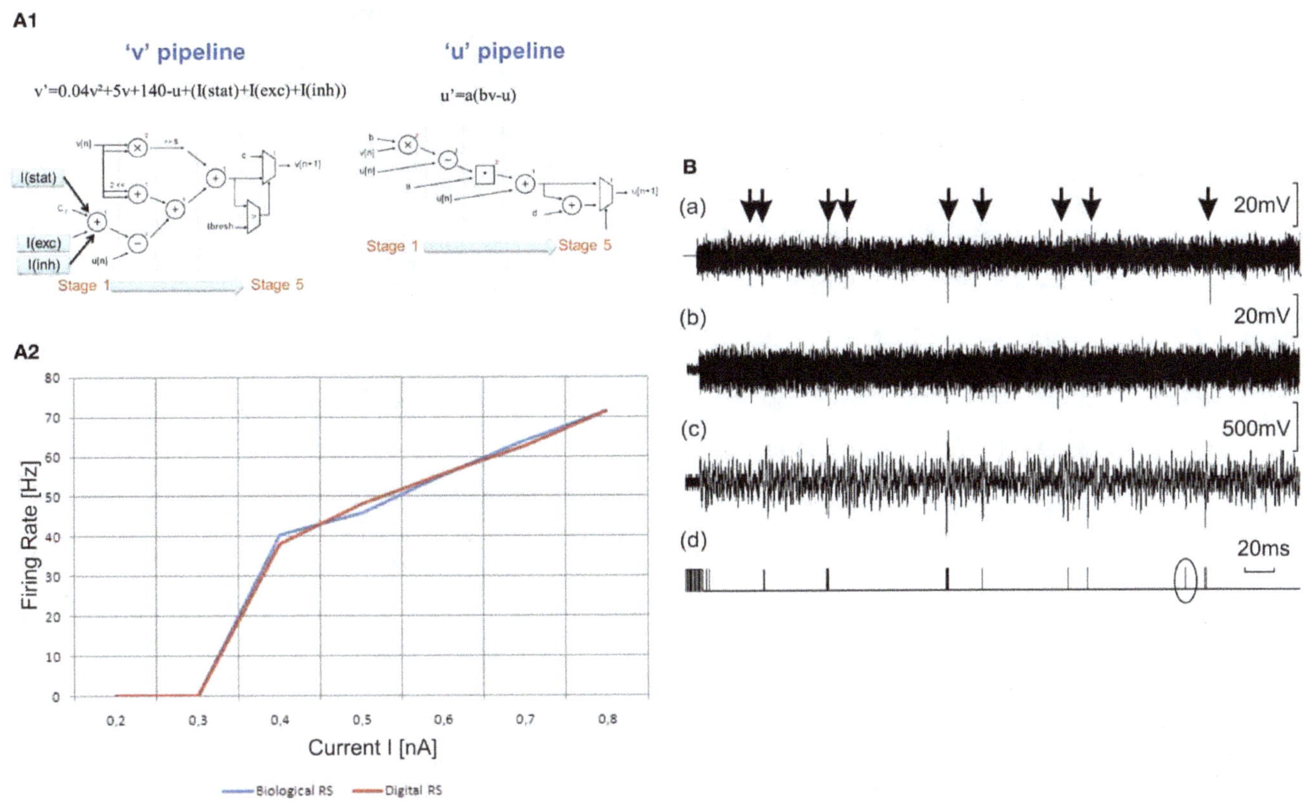

FIGURE 7 | Hardware elements for the neuro-prosthesis. (A1) Choice of the topology. To implement the two equations of Izhikevich model, two topology of pipeline are chosen (Cassidy and Andreou, 2008). There are five stages of computing for each equation. The I(stat), I(exc), and I(inh) currents describe the synaptic contribution. **(A2)** Hw-based model. Comparison of f(I) curves between biological Regular Spiking (RS) neuron and digital one. The biological curves are intracellular recordings of regular-spiking neurons in ferret visual cortex *in vitro*. The neuromorphic board gives the same results in term of frequency of the neuron *vs.* the stimulation current. **(B)** Outputs of the detection system to be implemented in the closed-loop set-up of the brain prosthesis. *First row—(a).* Raw electrophysiological signal. *Second row—(b).* The same signal with added Gaussian white noise to reduce Signal to Noise Ratio. This step was added to stress the capability of the system to detect action potentials in difficult conditions. *Third row—(c).* Output of the stationary wavelet decomposition preprocessing module. We used a Haar mother wavelet with 16 bits fixed point computation. The output signal is the sixth level detail output of the decomposition tree. *Fourth row—(d).* Binary output of the detection module. This output is the result of a threshold applied to the signal in (c). The threshold is computed from the standard deviation of the first level detail output of the wavelet decomposition tree. The emphasized detected spike is a false positive. This shows that the signal *(b)* represents the limit of signals that can be reliably processed by our system. These signals were first recorded then input to the system with a waveform generator.

comparison. This method proved to be very efficient to extract action potential of excitable cells from very noisy signals (Raoux et al., 2012). **Figure 7B** shows the performance of the method on a single channel setup. Action potentials are emphasized by arrows on the signal A. We added significant noise [signal (b)] and then sent the signal to the detector that provides outputs (c) and (d).

To summarize, all modules (i.e., Izhikevich neuron, neural network specifications, detection and stimulation modules) will be implemented into the FPGA. This modular system will be used as a cross-platform neural computation unit. Microelectrode arrays will be used to record and electrically stimulate living neural networks, with a specific emphasis on stimulation localization. Dedicated integrated electronics will be designed to implement the communication channels between the living and the artificial networks. The biological signals (from living to artificial) will be processed by using on-line spike detection algorithms and a rate-based decoding (Rieke et al., 1997; Novellino et al., 2007; Tessadori et al., 2012), while the firing rate of an artificial neuronal sub-network will be translated into the stimulation frequency for the biological network (from artificial to living), thus following a similar rate-based strategy. The system including the artificial and living neural networks will form a closed loop with a regulated feedback (cf. next Section).

A BI-DIRECTIONAL NEURO-PROSTHESIS

The knowledge that we gained through the various studies presented here will contribute to the final realization of a bi-directional communication between *in vitro* and *in silico* models of interconnected cell assemblies. By studying the dynamics of *in vitro* networks (see **Figures 2, 3**), we will create a computational model (see **Figure 6**) exhibiting the same I/O function of its biological counterpart (**Figure 8**, panel A). Through this approach we also plan to further our knowledge about the

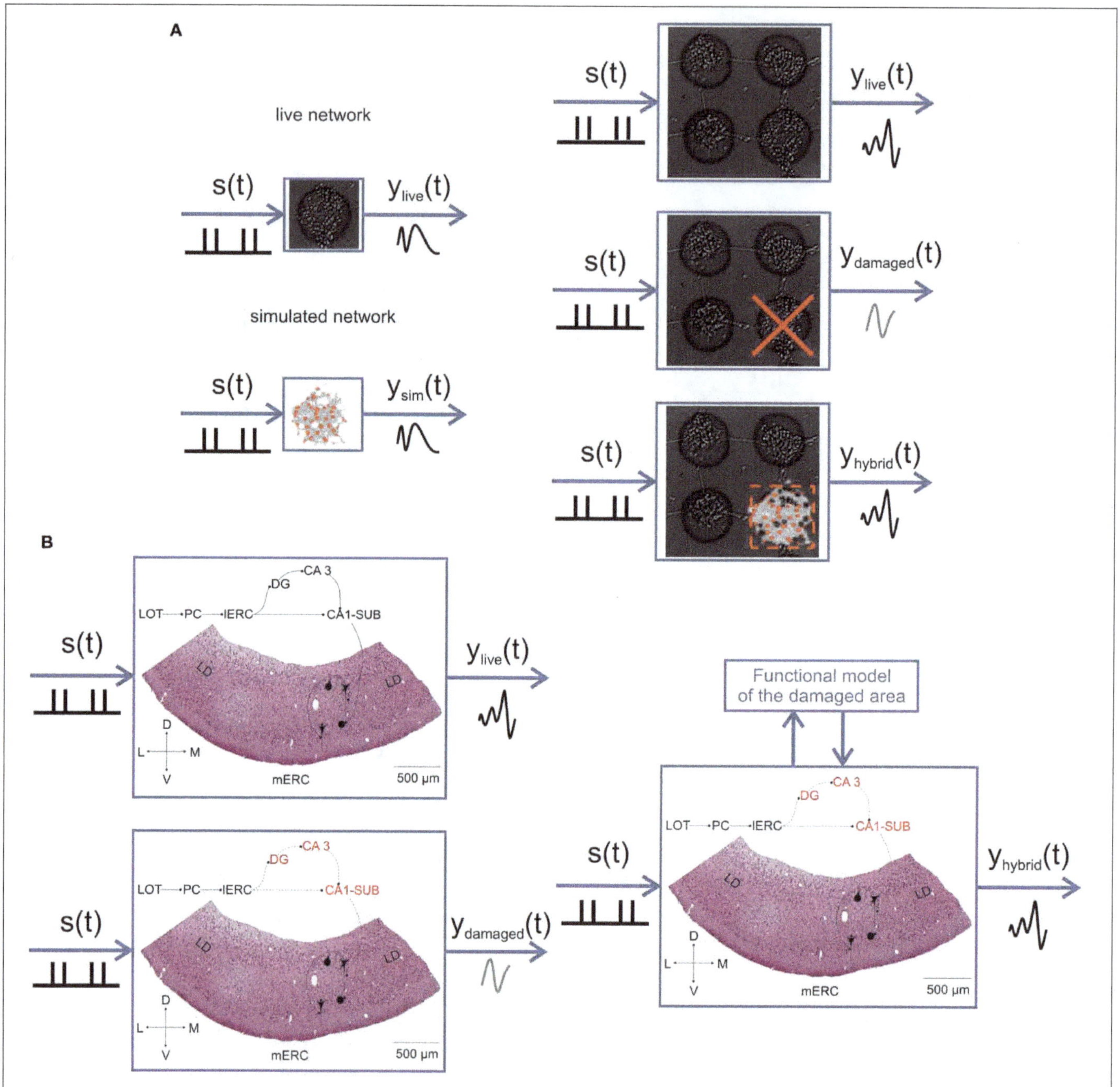

FIGURE 8 | *In vitro* neuro-prostheses. Sketch illustrating the main approach of the BRAIN BOW project. First, we will characterize the I/O function of simple finite-size networks and reproduce it by means of a computational model (**A**, left). Second, we will use more complex modular networks and replace one sub-network module with our computational model of the finite-size network, in order to replicate the function of the intact system (**A**, right). Finally, the same conceptual approach will be adopted to recover the function of the olfactory-limbic circuit after an ischemic lesion of the hippocampus **(B)**. The bidirectional interaction with a model reproducing the function of the damaged area will allow restoring the original I/O pattern. $s(t)$: stimulus function; $y_{live}(t)$: response function of a healthy preparation; $y_{sim}(t)$: response function of the neuronal network model; $y_{damaged}(t)$: response function after lesion in the IWB; $y_{hybrid}(t)$: response function of the hybrid system resulting from the combination of biological and artificial components. In panel **(B)**, the hippocampal areas targeted by the ischemic lesion are marked in red.

interplay between structural connectivity and dynamics in neuronal networks. Once we have realized and tested our model, we will bi-directionally integrate it into a biological network made up of few interconnected sub-networks in replacement of one of these that has been previously lesioned (**Figure 8A**, right panel).

The same conceptual approach will be applied to the olfactory-limbic pathway in the IWB (**Figure 8**, panel B). After a thorough characterization of spontaneous activity patterns (e.g., spontaneous periodic events, which strikingly resemble the ones shown by primary cortical cultures; see **Figure 1**) and LOT-evoked responses generated in the m-ERC (see **Figure 8**), we will include such information into a realistic computational model. We will then induce an ischemic lesion of the hippocampus and realize a functional model able to reproduce the same transfer function of the damaged part in order to restore the original pathway. **Figure 8** summarizes this approach, both for *in vitro* interconnected finite-size networks and for the guinea pig IWB.

The final step foreseen in the BRAIN BOW project is the hardware implementation of the signal processing algorithms and computational models to achieve our proof-of-concept neuroprosthesis based on a neuromorphic chip. **Figure 9** illustrates the closed-loop architecture that we plan to develop. Raw traces recorded by means of either planar or implanted MEAs (depending on the biological sample) will be fed into the artificial element and pre-processed online to extract multi-unit activity patterns (MUA). Spatio-temporal spiking patterns will then be translated by the "decoding" block into signals delivered to the neuronal network model. After elaboration, output patterns produced by the model will be finally translated by the "coding" block into a stimulation delivered to the neural element (**Figure 9**).

DISCUSSION

This paper presents a bottom-up, multidisciplinary approach toward the realization of a neural prosthesis capable of replacing lesioned neuronal circuitries. The final goal of the studies consists of developing a neuromorphic chip reproducing the function of a lesioned circuit without replicating its specific architecture or structural organization.

As a general model of a self-organized neuronal circuit, finite size neuronal circuits in culture are produced and studied in an isolated configuration to reveal innate (and therefore most general) features of intra-circuit organization (cf. **Figure 1**). Since finite size networks can spontaneously interconnect in a "multi-modular" network organization, they also represent an optimal experimental model to reveal innate inter-circuit communication properties (cf. **Figure 1**), as shown in previous studies (Macis et al., 2007; Raichman and Ben-Jacob, 2008; Shein-Idelson et al., 2010, 2011). The structural—functional configuration of the finite size circuits can be replicated by an *in silico* neuronal

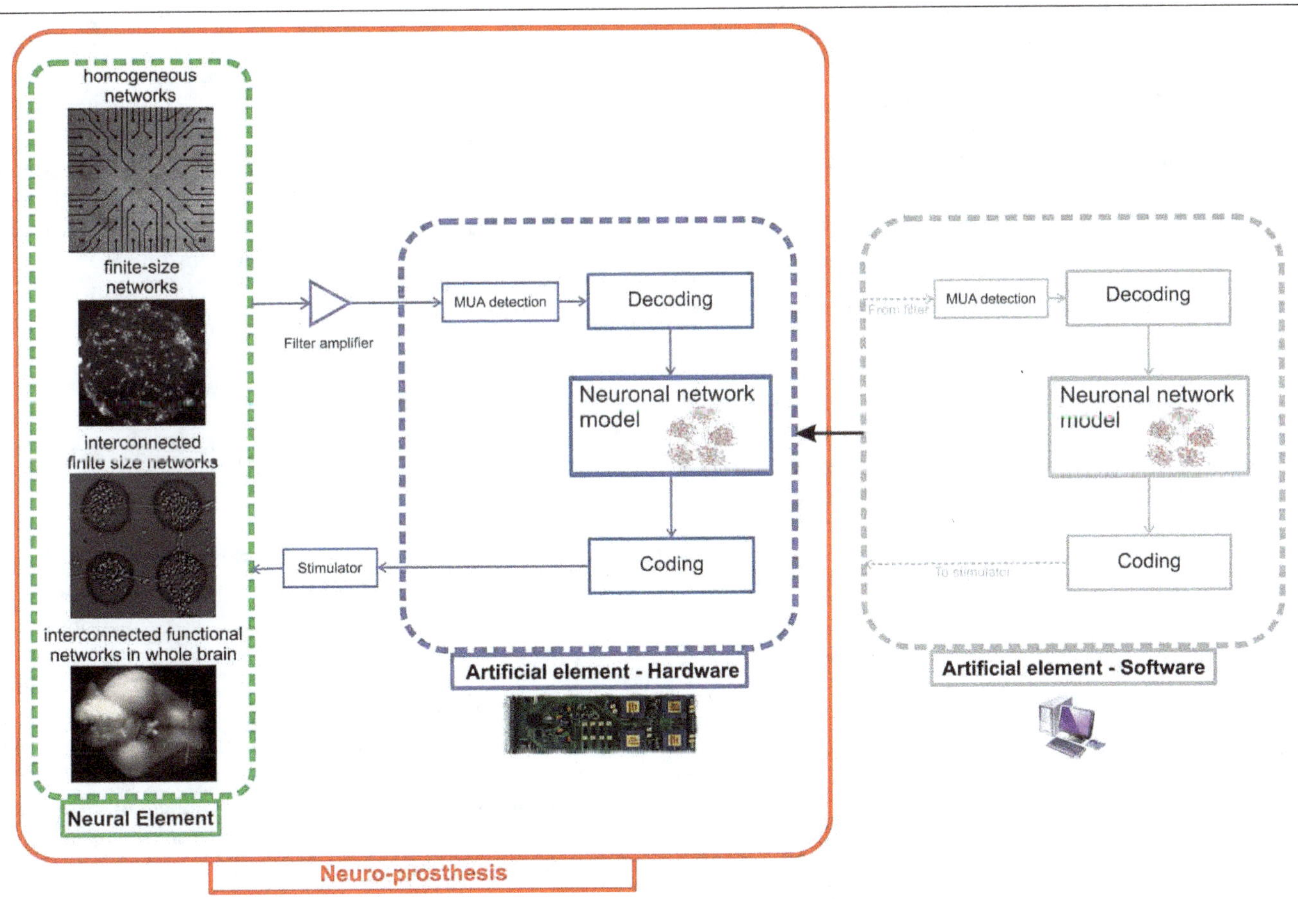

FIGURE 9 | Schematic representation of the closed-loop system to be implemented as a proof-of-concept neuro-prosthesis. Different *in vitro* neural models with increasing degrees of architectural complexity ("Neural element") will be interfaced to a hardware neuromorphic chip ("Artificial element—Hardware"), implementing both signal processing ("MUA detection") and modeling ("Neuronal network model") algorithms previously tested in software ("Artificial element—Software"). The communication between the neuronal network model and its biological counterpart is accomplished by the "Coding" and "Decoding" blocks.

network and then implemented on a neuromorphic prosthetic chip. The capability of the neuromorphic chip to replace the function of a lesioned circuit will be tested at increasing levels of network complexity from an *in vitro* modular network to an isolated whole brain system (IWB). In the attempt to present the overall scientific approach of the BRAIN BOW project (cf. section "Introduction" and "A Bi-Directional Neuro-Prosthesis"), this paper shows first results from the different level of investigation grounding the overall strategy.

FINITE SIZE CIRCUITS AND INNATE FUNCTIONAL ORGANIZATION OF CORTICAL CIRCUITS

As previously shown by Shein-Idelson et al. (2010), cultured cortical neuronal networks composed of at least a few dozen neurons are able to produce spontaneous collective dynamics known as network bursts, characterized by oscillatory activity in the gamma-theta range, and with the frequency of the bursts increasing with the number of neurons in the network. We confirmed these findings here using optical measurements on monolayer circuits (cf. **Figure 2**). By combining calcium imaging with immunocytochemistry, we have found that network events first recruit a characteristic population of neurons which includes GABAergic neurons. In particular, the time-lag correlation of the finite size cortical circuits is similar to what observed in developing hippocampal circuits (Bonifazi et al., 2009), in which a scale-free functional connectivity distribution was accompanied by the existence of GABAergic hub cells able to play a key role in the orchestration of the spontaneous network events. All together, these observations suggest that cortical neuronal circuits share a common innate functional organization which might include the existence of GABAergic hub cells.

MONITORING EFFECTS OF LESIONED NEURONAL CIRCUITS IN FINITE SIZE NETWORKS

After characterizing the spontaneous dynamics of the finite size networks we monitored how a focalized lesion can trigger functional reorganization in the neuronal circuit. We made controlled laser ablations of different intensities on our networks (e.g., targeting single modules, inter-connections between modules, single neuritis/cell bodies/cell assembly). After the lesions, the neuronal circuits continued to produce spontaneous networks events with no significant changes in the frequency of occurrence (**Figures 3** and **A1**). These were presumably generated out of the imaged field where the lesions were performed. The number of cells recruited during network events decreased either because they were directly lesioned by the laser ablation or because of a change in the local functional organization of the circuits (see the functional connectivity graphs of **Figure 4**). In a previous study by Maeda et al. (1995) the authors made a lesion in a homogeneous network over a MEA to study the origin of spontaneous network bursting. More recently, Difato et al. (2011a) reported controlled sequential ablation of single connections in a neuronal network, causing modulation of its activity without irreversibly damaging it. By combining MEA recording and calcium imaging the authors found changes in electrophysiological patterns in the network and identified the contribution of neuronal sub-populations to the network activity (Difato et al., 2011b). To the best of our knowledge, our study is the first to make a spatially defined micro-lesion at the single cell scale and to analyze the neuronal dynamics and connectivity by means of optical-only tools. This methodology, which can be extended to the use of genetically encoded calcium sensors, allows a more detailed and prolonged monitoring of the functional reorganization of the circuit over hours or days with the advantage, when compared to electrophysiological recordings, that the high spatial resolution (i.e., single cell) can be linked to morphological/structural cellular properties through *post-hoc* immunocytochemical characterizations. This could also facilitate testing of methods to promote functional circuit repair, such as pharmacological approaches.

SIMULATION RESULTS (SOFTWARE AND HARDWARE)

Given the similarity between the synchronization dynamics observed in developing hippocampal networks (Bonifazi et al., 2009) and in the finite circuits (**Figure 2**) with early activated GABAergic cells forecasting synchrony, we hypothesized a common innate structural-functional organization in neocortical and paleocortical circuits. Therefore, we used a scale-free topology (Barabasi and Albert, 1999) to model a neuronal network based on Izhikevich neurons (Izhikevich, 2003) (**Figure 6**). The proposed model was able to reproduce the empirical dependence between bursting rate and circuit size. However, the model predicted a richer repertoire of firing patterns (e.g., **Figure 6B**). Indeed, such patterns can be found in biological networks (Segev et al., 2002; Macis et al., 2007; Marconi et al., 2012). Thus our synthetic models (conveniently tuned and adapted) are able to reproduce the dynamics found in *in vitro* networks. Our results also demonstrate that the hardware element of the prosthesis (cf. section "Hardware Set-up for a Brain Prosthesis" and "A Bi-Directional Neuro-Prosthesis") can be constituted by a neuromorphic model (SNN) built on the same equations as the computational model (Izhikevich, 2003), since it reproduces similar firing rate distributions (**Figure 7**). Thus, the computational (software) model serves as a bridge between the biological networks and the hardware implementation.

COMPARISON TO PREVIOUS WORK AND PROSPECTIVE RESULTS

In the last decades, great efforts have been made to develop neuroprostheses to restore lost sensory or motor functions (Taylor et al., 2002; Chader et al., 2009; Collinger et al., 2013), but very few groups have focused on neuro-prostheses targeting lesions at the level of the CNS and aimed at recovering lost cognitive capabilities (Berger et al., 2011; Prueckl et al., 2011; Bamford et al., 2012; Hampson et al., 2012; Opris et al., 2012). Although our studies are limited to simplified *in vitro* models of cell assemblies, their final aim is to provide useful insights for the design of future cognitive prostheses. We believe that our approach would help us understand how we can influence/drive the dynamics of a neuronal assembly by interfacing it to an artificial network, implemented either in software or hardware. This is not the first attempt to realize an *in vitro* closed-loop system: previous studies have used a robotic actuator or a control algorithm aimed at clamping network activity to a desired level (Demarse et al., 2001; Martinoia et al., 2004; Wagenaar et al., 2005; Wallach et al., 2011). However, we seek to extend these approaches by replacing a real biological network with a simulated network, and hence by implementing bi-directional communication between biological and simulated networks. This research project builds on previously published results in the field of *in vitro* closed-loop electrophysiology (Arsiero et al., 2007). It can also be generalized to a more structured experimental model like the *in vitro* whole brain of a guinea pig, which lies between *in vivo* (as it retains the original tridimensional architecture) and *in vitro* (as it is disconnected from any sensory input/motor output). In contrast to other groups which have exclusively investigated *in vivo* brain prostheses (Prueckl et al., 2011; Bamford et al., 2012; Berger et al., 2012; Hampson et al., 2012; Opris et al., 2012), we are trying to exploit the unique advantages of *in vitro* electrophysiology—accessibility, visibility and control of physical and chemical conditions—to study neural information processing in neuronal assemblies, and to understand which parameters are relevant for effectively interfacing biological and artificial networks. In addition to informing the design of future *in vivo* approaches, our approach could also illuminate how network structure constrains and drives network dynamics.

ACKNOWLEDGMENTS

The research leading to these results has received funding from the European Union's Seventh Framework Programme (ICT-FET FP7/2007-2013, FET Young Explorers scheme) under grant agreement n. 284772 BRAIN BOW (www.brainbowproject.eu).

The authors wish to thank Dr. Marina Nanni and Claudia Chiabrera from NBT-IIT for technical assistance in cell culture preparation; Dr. Pieter Laurens Baljon for the MATLAB implementation of the SALPA algorithm; Prof. Marco de Curtis for helpful discussion about the *in vitro* guinea pig whole brain preparation and recording; Prof. Sergio Martinoia, Prof. Sylvie Renaud, Prof. Eshel Ben-Jacob, Prof. Ari Barzilai, and Prof. Yael Hanein for their support and for useful discussion.

The authors at TAU thank the help of Nitzan Herzog for calcium imaging set up, Mark Shein-Idelson for network patterning, Inna Brainis for cell culture and Moshe David-Pur for silicon wafer processing. Dr. Paolo Bonifazi is additionally supported by the Joint Italy—Israel Laboratory on Neuroscience.

REFERENCES

Arsiero, M., Luscher, H. R., and Giugliano, M. (2007). Real-time closed-loop electrophysiology: towards new frontiers in *in vitro* investigations in the neurosciences. *Arch. Ital. Biol.* 145, 193–209.

Bamford, S. A., Hogri, R., Giovannucci, A., Taub, A. H., Herreros, I., Verschure, P. F., et al. (2012). A VLSI field-programmable mixed signal array to perform neural signal processing and neural modeling in a prosthetic system. *IEEE Trans. Neural Syst. Rehabil. Eng.* 20, 455–467.

Barabasi, A.-L., and Albert, R. (1999). Emergence of scaling in random networks. *Science* 286, 509–512.

Batagelj, V., and Brandes, U. (2005). Efficient generation of large random networks. *Phys. Rev. E* 71, 036113.

Berger, T. W., Hampson, R. E., Song, D., Goonawardena, A., Marmarelis, V. Z., and Deadwyler, S. A. (2011). A cortical neural prosthesis for restoring and enhancing memory. *J. Neural Eng.* 8:046017. doi: 10.1088/1741-2560/8/4/046017

Berger, T. W., Song, D., Chan, R. H., Marmarelis, V. Z., Lacoss, J., Wills, J., et al. (2012). A hippocampal cognitive prosthesis: multi-input, multi-output nonlinear modeling and VLSI implementation. *IEEE Trans. Neural Syst. Rehabil. Eng.* 20, 198–211.

Biella, G., and De Curtis, M. (2000). Olfactory inputs activate the medial entorhinal cortex via the hippocampus. *J. Neurophysiol.* 83, 1924–1931.

Bologna, L. L., Pasquale, V., Garofalo, M., Gandolfo, M., Baljon, P. L., Maccione, A., et al. (2010). Investigating neuronal activity by SPYCODE multichannel data analyzer. *Neural Netw.* 23, 685–697.

Bonifazi, P., Goldin, M., Picardo, M. A., Jorquera, I., Cattani, A., Bianconi, G., et al. (2009). GABAergic hub neurons orchestrate synchrony in developing hippocampal networks. *Science* 326, 1419–1424.

Canto, C. B., Wouterlood, F. G., and Witter, M. P. (2008). What does the anatomical organization of the entorhinal cortex tell us? *Neural. Plast.* 2008:381243. doi: 10.1155/2008/381243

Cassidy, A., and Andreou, A. G. (2008). "Dynamical digital silicon neurons," in *Biomedical Circuits and Systems Conference, 2008. BioCAS (2008). IEEE* (Baltimore, MD).

Chader, G. J., Weiland, J., and Humayun, M. S. (2009). Artificial vision: needs, functioning, and testing of a retinal electronic prosthesis. *Prog. Brain Res.* 175, 317–332.

Chiappalone, M., Bove, M., Vato, A., Tedesco, M., and Martinoia, S. (2006). Dissociated cortical networks show spontaneously correlated activity patterns during *in vitro* development. *Brain Res.* 1093, 41–53.

Collinger, J. L., Wodlinger, B., Downey, J. E., Wang, W., Tyler-Kabara, E. C., Weber, D. J., et al. (2013). High-performance neuroprosthetic control by an individual with tetraplegia. *Lancet* 381, 557–564.

Crépel, V., Aronov, D., Jorquera, I., Represa, A., Ben-Ari, Y., and Cossart, R. (2007). A parturition-associated nonsynaptic coherent activity pattern in the developing hippocampus. *Neuron* 54, 105–120.

De Curtis, M., Biella, G., Buccellati, C., and Folco, G. (1998). Simultaneous investigation of the neuronal and vascular compartments in the guinea pig brain isolated *in vitro*. *Brain Res. Brain Res. Protoc.* 3, 221–228.

Demarse, T. B., Wagenaar, D. A., Blau, A. W., and Potter, S. M. (2001). The neurally controlled animat: biological brains acting with simulated bodies. *Auton. Robots* 11, 305–310.

Difato, F., Dal Maschio, M., Marconi, E., Ronzitti, G., Maccione, A., Fellin, T., et al. (2011a). Combined optical tweezers and laser dissector for controlled ablation of functional connections in neural networks. *J. Biomed. Opt.* 16:051306. doi: 10.1117/1.3560268

Difato, F., Schibalsky, L., Benfenati, F., and Blau, A. (2011b). Integration of optical manipulation and electrophysiological tools to modulate and record activity in neural networks. *Int. J. Optomechatronic.* 5, 191–216.

Dorogovtsev, S., and Mendes, J. (2002). Evolution of networks. *Adv. Phys.* 51, 1079–1187.

Eytan, D., and Marom, S. (2006). Dynamics and effective topology underlying synchronization in networks of cortical neurons. *J. Neurosci.* 26, 8465–8476.

Gnatkovsky, V., and De Curtis, M. (2006). Hippocampus-mediated activation of superficial and deep layer neurons in the medial entorhinal cortex of the isolated guinea pig brain. *J. Neurosci.* 26, 873–881.

Hampson, R. E., Gerhardt, G. A., Marmarelis, V., Song, D., Opris, I., Santos, L., et al. (2012). Facilitation and restoration of cognitive function in primate prefrontal cortex by a neuroprosthesis that utilizes minicolumn-specific neural firing. *J. Neural Eng.* 9:056012. doi: 10.1088/1741-2560/9/5/056012

Herzog, N., Shein-Idelson, M., and Hanein, Y. J. (2011). Optical validation of *in vitro* extra-cellular neuronal recordings. *J. Neural Eng.* 8:056008. doi: 10.1088/1741-2560/8/5/056008

Hochberg, L. R., Bacher, D., Jarosiewicz, B., Masse, N. Y., Simeral, J. D., Vogel, J., et al. (2012). Reach and grasp by people with tetraplegia using a neurally controlled robotic arm. *Nat. Methods* 485, 372–375.

Hochberg, L. R., Serruya, M. D., Friehs, G. M., Mukand, J. A., Saleh, M., Caplan, A. H., et al. (2006). Neuronal ensemble control of prosthetic devices by a human with tetraplegia. *Nature* 442, 164–171.

Isaacson, J. S., and Scanziani, M. (2011). How inhibition shapes cortical activity. *Neuron* 72, 231–243.

Izhikevich, E. M. (2003). Simple model of spiking neurons. *IEEE Trans. Neural Netw.* 6, 1569–1572.

Kamioka, H., Maeda, E., Jimbo, Y., Robinson, H. P., and Kawana,

A. (1996). Spontaneous periodic synchronized bursting during formation of mature patterns of connections in cortical cultures. *Neurosci. Lett.* 206, 109–112.

Kleinfeld, D., Kahler, K. H., and Hockberger, P. E. (1988). Controlled outgrowth of dissociated neurons on patterned substrates. *J. Neurosci.* 8, 4098–4120.

Librizzi, L., Biella, G., Cimino, C., and De Curtis, M. (1999). Arterial supply of limbic structures in the guinea pig. *J. Comp. Neurol.* 4, 674–682.

Llinas, R., Yarom, Y., and Sugimori, M. (1981). Isolated mammalian brain *in vitro*: new technique for analysis of electrical activity of neuronal circuit function. *Fed. Proc.* 40, 2240–2245.

Maccione, A., Gandolfo, M., Massobrio, P., Novellino, A., Martinoia, S., and Chiappalone, M. (2009). A novel algorithm for precise identification of spikes in extracellularly recorded neuronal signals. *J. Neurosci. Methods* 177, 241–249.

Macis, E., Tedesco, M., Massobrio, P., Raiteri, R., and Martinoia, S. (2007). An automated microdrop delivery system for neuronal network patterning on microelectrode arrays. *J. Neurosci. Methods* 161, 88–95.

Maeda, E., Robinson, H. P., and Kawana, A. (1995). The mechanisms of generation and propagation of synchronized bursting in developing networks of cortical neurons. *J. Neurosci.* 15, 6834–6845.

Marconi, E., Nieus, T., Maccione, A., Valente, P., Simi, A., Messa, M., et al. (2012). Emergent functional properties of neuronal networks with controlled topology. *PLoS ONE* 7:e34648. doi: 10.1371/journal.pone.0034648

Marissal, T., Bonifazi, P., Picardo, M. A., Nardou, R., Petit, L. F., Baude, A., et al. (2012). Pioneer glutamatergic cells develop into a morpho-functionally distinct population in the juvenile CA3 hippocampus. *Nat. Commun.* 3, 1316.

Martinoia, S., Sanguineti, V., Cozzi, L., Berdondini, L., Van Pelt, J., Tomas, J., et al. (2004). Towards an embodied *in-vitro* electrophysiology: the NeuroBIT project. *Neurocomputing* 58–60, 1065–1072.

Muhlethaler, M., De Curtis, M., Walton, K., and Llinas, R. (1993). The isolated and perfused brain of the guinea-pig *in vitro*. *Eur. J. Neurosci.* 5, 915–926.

Nicolelis, M. A. L. (2003). Brain-Machine interfaces to restore motor function and probe neural circuits. *Nat. Rev. Neurosci.* 4, 417–422.

Nicolelis, M. A. L., and Lebedev, M. A. (2009). Principles of neural ensemble physiology underlying the operation of brain-machine interfaces. *Nat. Rev. Neurosci.* 10, 530–540.

Novellino, A., D'Angelo, P., Cozzi, L., Chiappalone, M., Sanguineti, V., and Martinoia, S. (2007). Connecting neurons to a mobile robot: an *in vitro* bidirectional neural interface. *Comput. Intell. Neurosci.* 2007:12725. doi: 10.1155/2007/12725

Opris, I., Fuqua, J. L., Huettl, P. F., Gerhardt, G. A., Berger, T. W., Hampson, R. E., et al. (2012). Closing the loop in primate prefrontal cortex: inter-laminar processing. *Front. Neural Circuits* 6:88. doi: 10.3389/fncir.2012.00088

Pastori, C., Regondi, M. C., Librizzi, L., and De Curtis, M. (2007). Early excitability changes in a novel acute model of transient focal ischemia-reperfusion in the *in vitro* isolated guinea pig brain. *Exp. Neurol.* 204, 95–105.

Perkel, D. H., Gerstein, G. L., and Moore, G. P. (1967). Neuronal spike trains and stochastic point processes. I. The single spike train. *Biophys. J.* 7, 391–418.

Prueckl, R., Taub, A. H., Herreros, I., Hogri, R., Magal, A., Bamford, S. A., et al. (2011). "Behavioral rehabilitation of the eye closure reflex in senescent rats using a real-time biosignal acquisition system," in *Engineering in Medicine and Biology Society, EMBC (2011)*. (Boston, MA).

Raichman, N., and Ben-Jacob, E. (2008). Identifying repeating motifs in the activation of synchronized bursts in cultured neuronal networks. *J. Neurosci. Methods* 170, 96–110.

Raoux, M., Bornat, Y., Quotb, A., Catargi, B., Renaud, S., and Lang, J. (2012). Non-invasive long-term and real-time analysis of endocrine cells on micro-electrode arrays. *J. Physiol.* 590, 1085–1091.

Rieke, F., Warland, D., De Ruyter Van Steveninck, R., and Bialek, W. (1997). *Spikes: Exploring the Neural Code.* Cambridge, MA: The MIT Press.

Segev, R., Benveniste, M., Hulata, E., Cohen, N., and Palevski, A. (2002). Long term behavior of lithographically prepared *in vitro* neuronal networks. *Phys. Rev. Lett.* 88, 1181021–1118104.

Shein-Idelson, M., Ben-Jacob, E., and Hanein, Y. (2010). Innate synchronous oscillations in freely-organized small neuronal circuits. *PLoS ONE* 5:e14443. doi: 10.1371/journal.pone.0014443

Shein-Idelson, M., Ben-Jacob, E., and Hanein, Y. (2011). Engineered neuronal circuits: a new platform for studying the role of modular topology. *Front. Neuroeng.* 4:10. doi: 10.3389/fneng.2011.00010

Sorkin, R., Gabay, T., Blinder, P., Baranes, D., Ben-Jacob, E., and Hanein, Y. (2006). Compact self-wiring in cultured neural networks. *J. Neural Eng.* 3, 95–101.

Takano, H., Mccartney, M., Ortinski, P. I., Yue, C., Putt, M. E., and Coulter, D. A. (2012). Deterministic and stochastic neuronal contributions to distinct synchronous CA3 network bursts. *J. Neurosci.* 32, 4743–4754.

Taylor, D. M., Tillery, S. I., and Schwartz, A. B. (2002). Direct cortical control of 3D neuroprosthetic devices. *Science* 296, 1829–1832.

Tessadori, J., Bisio, M., Martinoia, S., and Chiappalone, M. (2012). Modular neuronal assemblies embodied in a closed-loop environment: toward future integration of brains and machines. *Front. Neural Circuits* 6:99. doi: 10.3389/fncir.2012.00099

Van Pelt, J., Wolters, P. S., Corner, M. A., Rutten, W. L., and Ramakers, G. J. (2004). Long-term characterization of firing dynamics of spontaneous bursts in cultured neural networks. *IEEE Trans. Biomed. Eng.* 51, 2051–2062.

Wagenaar, D. A., Madhavan, R., Pine, J., and Potter, S. M. (2005). Controlling bursting in cortical cultures with closed-loop multi-electrode stimulation. *J. Neurosci.* 25, 680–688.

Wagenaar, D. A., and Potter, S. M. (2002). Real-time multi-channel stimulus artifact suppression by local curve fitting. *J. Neurosci. Methods* 120, 113–120.

Wallach, A., Eytan, D., Gal, A., Zrenner, C., and Marom, S. (2011). Neuronal response clamp. *Front. Neuroeng.* 4:3. doi: 10.3389/fneng.2011.00003

APPENDIX

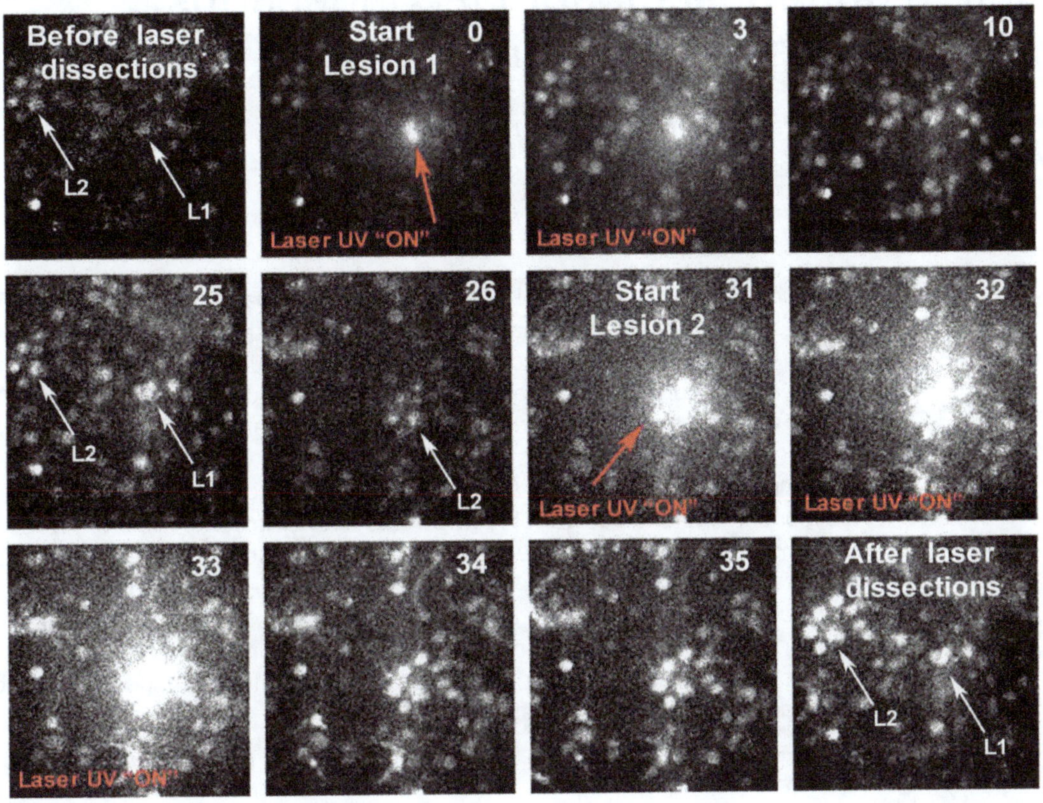

FIGURE A1 | Subpopulation of a neuronal network before and after laser induced lesions. The first panel, starting from the left upper corner, shows a subpopulation of a neuronal network loaded with Fuo4-AM. White arrows, depicted with L1 and L2, indicate the positions of the lesions inflicted to the network. The red arrows indicate the position of the UV laser focus spot. The average power delivered at the sample, during lesion one, is 4 μW, and during Lesion 2, is 5 μW. We delivered 300 UV light pulse for each lesion, at pulse-repetition rate of 100 Hz. At 25 s, after Lesion 1, the L2 position is centered onto the UV focus spot. The last panel shows the same field of view of the first one, after laser inflicted damages. The cells directly affected by the UV laser presented saturated calcium signal. Numbers indicate seconds. The field of view is 150 × 150 μm. Calcium imaging was acquired at 60 Hz.

11

Restoration of upper limb movement via artificial corticospinal and musculospinal connections in a monkey with spinal cord injury

Yukio Nishimura[1,2,3]*†, Steve I. Perlmutter[1,2] and Eberhard E. Fetz[1,2]*

[1] *Department of Physiology & Biophysics, University of Washington, Seattle, WA, USA*
[2] *Washington National Primate Research Center, University of Washington, Seattle, WA, USA*
[3] *Precursory Research for Embryonic Science and Technology, Japan Science and Technology Agency, Tokyo, Japan*

Edited by:
Steve M. Potter, Georgia Institute of Technology, USA

Reviewed by:
Liang Guo, Massachusetts Institute of Technology, USA
Abhishek Prasad, University of Miami, USA

****Correspondence:***
Yukio Nishimura, Department of Developmental Physiology, National Institute for Physiological Sciences, National Institutes of Natural Sciences, 38 Nishigonaka, Myoudaiji, Okazki, Aichi 444-858, Japan.
e-mail: yukio@nips.ac.jp;
Eberhard E. Fetz, Department of Physiology & Biophysics, University of Washington, 1705 NE Pacific Street, HSB G424, Box 357290, Seattle, WA 98195, USA.
e-mail: fetz@uw.edu

Functional loss of limb control in individuals with spinal cord injury or stroke can be caused by interruption of corticospinal pathways, although the neural circuits located above and below the lesion remain functional. An artificial neural connection that bridges the lost pathway and connects cortical to spinal circuits has potential to ameliorate the functional loss. We investigated the effects of introducing novel artificial neural connections in a paretic monkey that had a unilateral spinal cord lesion at the C2 level. The first application bridged the impaired spinal lesion. This allowed the monkey to drive the spinal stimulation through volitionally controlled power of high-gamma activity in either the premotor or motor cortex, and thereby to acquire a force-matching target. The second application created an artificial recurrent connection from a paretic agonist muscle to a spinal site, allowing muscle-controlled spinal stimulation to boost on-going activity in the muscle. These results suggest that artificial neural connections can compensate for interrupted descending pathways and promote volitional control of upper limb movement after damage of descending pathways such as spinal cord injury or stroke.

Keywords: brain–computer interface, artificial neural connection, hand, spinal cord injury, local field potential, muscle, spinal cord, monkey

INTRODUCTION

Functional loss of limb control in individuals with spinal cord injury or stroke can involve interruption of descending pathways to spinal networks, although the neural circuits located above and below the lesion retain their function. An artificial neural connection that bridges the lost pathway has potential to compensate for the functional loss. Recent studies showed that monkeys could use cortical activity to control functional electrical stimulation (FES) in muscles transiently paralyzed by nerve block (Moritz et al., 2008; Pohlmeyer et al., 2009; Ethier et al., 2012). However, restoring coordinated movement of paralyzed limbs with peripheral FES remains problematic (Popovic et al., 2002). Stimulation of peripheral nerve or muscle often evokes movement about only a single joint and recruits the largest, most fatigable motor units first. Spinal microstimulation offers an alternative method to produce coordinated movement and more natural recruitment of motor units (Mushahwar and Horch, 2000; Mushahwar et al., 2000; Mussa-Ivaldi and Bizzi, 2000; Saigal et al., 2004; Moritz et al., 2007). In anesthetized animals, current can be delivered to spinal sites to produce coordinated patterns of muscle contraction (Zimmermann et al., 2011).

Several studies have demonstrated that multichannel spike signals recorded with intracortical electrode arrays can be used to estimate arm movements (Kennedy et al., 2000; Wessberg et al., 2000; Serruya et al., 2002; Carmena et al., 2003; Choi et al., 2009; Vargas-Irwin et al., 2010) and muscle activity (Morrow and Miller, 2003; Santucci et al., 2005; Koike et al., 2006; Pohlmeyer et al., 2007; Schieber and Rivlis, 2007). Although recordings of cell assemblies by intracortical electrodes can provide a rich repertoire of signals, their limitations include signal deterioration due to glial scarring (Polikov et al., 2005), potential displacement from the recording site (Leuthardt et al., 2004) and invasive recording techniques. Chronically implanted electrode arrays typically lose the ability to record cell spikes after several years (Krüger et al., 2010; Simeral et al., 2011). Reliable spike recording is a challenge for the long durations required for clinical applications. Movement parameters can also be decoded from local field potentials (LFPs; Zhuang et al., 2010; Flint et al., 2012) and the electrocorticogram

(Schalk et al., 2007; Sanchez et al., 2008; Miller et al., 2009; Chao et al., 2010; Shin et al., 2012) in motor-related areas, potentially offering more stable signals that represent the activities of many neurons near the electrode. Thus, instead of relying on cell spikes recorded with intracortical electrodes, it is possible to use cortical field potentials, or muscle activity as a surrogate of cortical cell activity.

Here we describe a case study in which an awake monkey with spinal cord injury could volitionally control the paretic upper limb through artificial neural connections using LFPs in motor cortex or activity of muscles to trigger stimulation of a spinal site appropriate to restore goal-directed movement of the affected arm.

MATERIALS AND METHODS

Experiments were performed with a male *Macaca nemestrina* monkey (4 years old, weight 5.5 kg). The experiments were approved by the Institutional Animal Care and Use Committee (IACUC) at the University of Washington and all procedures conformed to the National Institutes of Health Guide for the Care and Use of Laboratory Animals.

SURGERIES

All implant surgeries were performed using sterile techniques while the animal was anesthetized using 1–1.5% sevoflurane. Dexamethasone, cephalexin, and ketoprofen were administered preoperatively and buprenorphine was given post-operatively.

Cortical implants

Silver electrode wires (0.1 mm diameter, ~50 kΩ at 1 kHz) were chronically implanted after making small incisions in the dura, in the digit, wrist and arm areas of primary motor cortex (M1) and the arm area of the dorsal aspect of premotor cortex (PMd) in the left hemisphere (contralateral to the spinal lesion, **Figure 1A**). The incisions of the dura mater were sutured closed. Small titanium-steel screws were attached to the skull as anchors. A stainless steel head-post was mounted on the skull for head fixation. The cortical electrodes and the head-post chamber were anchored to the screws with acrylic cement.

Surgery for EMG recording

Initially, electromyographic (EMG) activity was measured with electrodes surgically implanted in 16 arm and hand muscles, identified by anatomical features and by movements evoked by trains of low-intensity stimulation. Bipolar, multistranded stainless steel wires (Cooner Wire, Chatsworth, CA, USA) were sutured into each muscle and wires were routed subcutaneously to a connector on the animal's back. A jacket worn by the monkey prevented access to the back connector between recording sessions. After these electrodes were broken by the monkey, additional wires were implanted transcutaneously for subsequent EMG recordings.

Surgery for spinal implant and spinal cord lesion

We made two separate unilateral laminectomies on the right side in the same surgery to prepare to record the activity of spinal neurons during behavior. The laminae and dorsal spinous processes

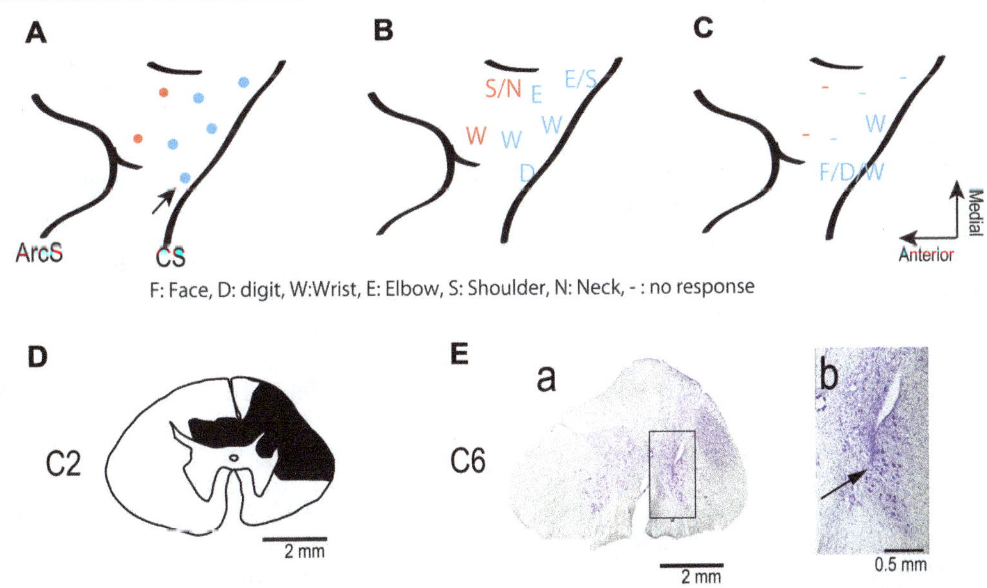

FIGURE 1 | (A) Electrode locations in the motor areas of the lateral aspect of the frontal lobe of the left (contralesional) hemisphere. Electrodes were placed in primary motor cortex (blue dots) and in dorsal premotor cortex (red dots). **(B,C)** Somatotopic map shows movements evoked from each site in frontal lobe before **(B)** and after **(C)** spinal cord injury. The pre-lesion maps were established by ICMS at movement threshold (20–120 μA). The post-lesion maps were established by ICMS at 450 μA on post-lesional day 14. The maps show the region between the central sulcus (CS: diagonal line to the right of each panel) and the arcuate sulcus (ArcS: curved line to the left). Arrow indicates site used in session illustrated in **Figure 3**. **(D)** Drawing of the C2 segments showing the extent of the spinal cord lesion (hatched in black). **(E)** Electrode location in spinal cord. **(a)** Electrodes were targeted at the ventral horn and intermediate zone of the spinal cord. **(b)** Higher magnification view of the location of an electrode tip (black arrow).

of the C2–C3 and C5–C7 vertebrae were removed. A chamber was implanted over the rostral laminectomy. Stimulus electrodes were implanted at the caudal site. After recovery from surgery the monkey exhibited an upper arm hemiparesis, including inability to control the digits independently, and the recordings were not performed. The deficit remained throughout the 3 months during which these experiments were performed. Post-mortem histology revealed that a spinal cord lesion was inadvertently created around C2 to C3 during surgery, perhaps due to a contusion on the spinal surface or hemorrhage (**Figure 1D**).

For the stimulus electrode, the dura mater and arachnoid under C5–C7 vertebrae were removed. Eleven polyurethane-coated, platinum–iridium wires (diameter 30 μm; impedance 200–600 kΩ at 1 kHz) were inserted 2.5–4 mm into the lower-cervical spinal cord targeting the ventral horn where hand motoneurons are located (Jenny and Inukai, 1983; Chiken et al., 2001). Penetration depth was determined by making a sharp bend in the microwire at the appropriate length. A second bend several mms more proximal provided strain relief and allowed the wires to float on the cord (Mushahwar et al., 2000). The microwires were bonded with cyanoacrylate glue to the spinal surface at each penetration point. The wires were routed into a silicone tube, which was glued with dental acrylic to bone screws placed in the lateral masses and T1 dorsal process, and routed through the skin to a connector. The spinal cord was covered with the subcutaneous fascia and gelfoam. The laminectomy was closed with acrylic cement. The skin and underlying soft tissue were then sutured closed.

TORQUE-TRACKING TASK

Prior to surgery the monkey had been trained to perform a torque-tracking task (Maier et al., 1998). The monkey controlled the one-dimensional position of a cursor on a video monitor with isometric flexion and extension wrist torques, and acquired targets displayed on the screen. The monkey was required to maintain torque within each target for 0.5–1.0 s to receive a juice reward. Targets remained on the screen until the hold criterion was met, followed by presentation of the next target, either immediately or after a variable reward period.

INTRACORTICAL MICROSTIMULATION

A few days after the cortical implant, movements evoked by intracortical microstimulation (ICMS) through the implanted electrodes with the monkey awake were documented by visual observation. Trains of 10 pulses of constant-current, biphasic square-wave pulses with 0.2-ms durations at 300 Hz evoked movements at thresholds of 20–120 μA (**Figure 1B**). The ICMS map was re-established 14 days after the spinal lesion with the monkey awake. After the spinal cord injury trains of ICMS at 450 μA were ineffective at most sites (**Figure 1C**).

SPINAL STIMULATION PROCEDURE

Intraspinal stimuli consisting of constant-current, biphasic square-wave pulses with 0.2-ms durations were delivered through the spinal microwires. In general, stimulation (10–700 μA) was delivered by a single electrode. The output effects evoked from each spinal site were documented with stimulus-triggered averages of rectified EMG (St-TA) during task performance. Current pulses were delivered at a low rate (10–20 Hz) to avoid temporal summation. Stimulus-evoked facilitation and suppression of EMG were identified as consistent features in the St-TAs above or below, respectively, 2 standard deviations (SD) of baseline. Baseline was defined as the interval from 30 to 0 ms preceding the trigger pulse. The mean percent increase (MPI) measured the average values between onset and offset of the feature minus baseline, divided by baseline. Based on post-stimulus effects in St-TAs, we chose a single electrode and current for the artificial neural connection paradigm.

BEHAVIORAL TASK WITH ARTIFICIAL NEURAL CONNECTION

Prior to establishing an artificial neural connection, the monkey learned to control a computer cursor with brain activity or muscle activity in separate operant conditioning sessions. Rack-mounted instrumentation was programmed to compile a running average (200 ms) of either EMG or rectified, high-gamma (90–160 Hz) LFP activity to create a continuous signal that controlled the one-dimensional position of a cursor on a video monitor. Targets that indicated high- or low-amplitude LFP or EMG were randomly presented on the screen. Targets remained on the screen until the monkey held the cursor within each target for 0.5–1.0 s to receive a juice reward.

After a few sessions of this preliminary task, an artificial connection to the spinal cord was established in subsequent sessions. Instead of directly controlling cursor position, LFP or EMG activity triggered spinal stimuli. Cursor position was now driven by isometric torque produced about the wrist. For each session, either flexion or extension torque controlled cursor position, depending on the torque produced by the spinal stimulation used in that session. The monkey learned to control LFP or EMG activity to acquire targets displayed on the monitor to receive a juice reward as described above (Maier et al., 1998). The direction of cursor movement was matched in all sessions; i.e., increases in LFP or EMG activity in preliminary sessions moved the cursor in the same direction as increases in torque during the sessions with an artificial connection.

ARTIFICIAL CORTICOSPINAL CONNECTION

In several preliminary sessions, the monkey controlled the cursor with high-frequency gamma (90–160 Hz) LFP activity recorded in either M1 or PMd. Then an artificial corticospinal connection (ACSC) was established using the same signal which had been used in the previous preliminary sessions to trigger trains of spinal stimulation to bridge the impaired corticospinal connection. Rack-mounted instrumentation was programmed to compile a running average of rectified LFP activity in the high-gamma band and to trigger delivery of intraspinal microstimulation at 300 Hz to a single electrode whenever the LFP exceeded a threshold determined by the experimenter. Prior to each session, we determined the background noise level of the high-gamma band signal and set the threshold so that no stimulation was delivered when the monkey was at rest. St-TAs of EMG guided the choice of a single electrode in the spinal cord, the stimulus current, and the position of the cursor on the screen for the artificial neural connection. A few sessions of ACSC were tested within a day, but different pairs of cortical and spinal sites were chosen.

ARTIFICIAL MUSCULOSPINAL CONNECTION

In several preliminary sessions, the monkey controlled the cursor with EMG activity recorded from a single forearm muscle. Even after the spinal cord lesion, the monkey could produce some muscle activity in the paretic hand. Then, an artificial musculospinal connection (AMSC) was established using the same EMG to trigger trains of spinal stimulation. Rack-mounted instrumentation was programmed to compile a running average of muscle activity and trigger a train of intraspinal microstimulation at 300 Hz during the time that EMG exceeded a threshold determined by the experimenter. Prior to each session, we determined the background noise level of the EMG signal and set the threshold so that no stimulation was delivered when the monkey was at rest. The stimulus-evoked EMG was insufficient to cross threshold, so the monkey could terminate stimulation by terminating his volitional EMG activity. Sessions of AMSC were tested on different days than ACSC. A few sessions of AMSC were tested within a day, but different pairs of muscles and spinal sites were chosen.

HISTOLOGICAL PROCEDURES

At the end of the experiments, the monkey was deeply anesthetized with an overdose of sodium pentobarbital (50–75 mg/kg, i.v.) and perfused transcardially with 0.1 M phosphate-buffered saline (PBS, pH 7.3), followed by 4% paraformaldehyde in 0.1 M PBS (pH 7.3). The spinal cord was removed immediately and saturated with fresh PBS containing, successively, 10, 20, and 30% sucrose. Serial sections 50 μm thick were cut on a freezing microtome. Sections processed for Nissl staining with 1% cresyl violet were used to assess the extent of the lesion and the location of electrode tracks.

STATISTICAL ANALYSIS

To determine the statistical difference of task performance between "artificial neural connection" and "catch" trials, we used the unpaired-*T* test. One-way analysis of variance (ANOVA) with repeated measures was performed to determine the significant differences in task performance among the M1, PMd, and M1 and PMd. *Post hoc* multiple comparisons were conducted using the Bonferroni test. Statistical significance level was set at $p < 0.05$. All pooled values are reported as mean ± SD.

RESULTS

EXTENT OF SPINAL LESION AND HISTOLOGIC EVIDENCE OF ELECTRODE LOCATION IN SPINAL CORD

Figure 1D shows the spinal cord section showing the maximum extent of the lesion located at the C2 level, as evidenced by gliosis. The dorsolateral region on the side ipsilateral to the lesion was severely deformed because of mechanical damage and degeneration of axons. The lesion area covered most of the right dorsolateral funiculus. The dorsal funiculi were partially damaged on both sides, but the ventrolateral funiculi were preserved on both sides. The lesion extended from the caudal part of C1 to most of C2. Thus, the lesion interrupted most of the corticospinal and rubrospinal tracts but preserved the reticulospinal tract and some ascending tracts.

We intended to position the electrode tips in the ventral horn and intermediate zone where motoneurons and premotoneuronal interneurons are located. We found two electrode tracks in the sections. **Figure 1E** shows one electrode track at the level of C6. The electrode tip was located in the ventral horn, as shown in **Figures 1E a,b**. The second recovered electrode was located in the medial intermediate zone.

FUNCTIONAL DEFICIT

The monkey's ability to independently control movement of digits, such as for precision grip, exhibited deficits shortly after the lesion and did not recover throughout the 3-month experimental period. Power grip recovered gradually 5–7 weeks after the lesion, consistent with a previous study (Alstermark et al., 2011).

The cortical somatotopic maps before and after lesion are shown in **Figures 1B,C**. Movements could be evoked from only two of five previously effective sites in M1, and only with higher currents than before the injury. The PMd was even more affected since no movements at all could be elicited from two previously effective sites after the lesion. Thus the extent and excitability of the upper limb representation in motor cortex decreased substantially after the spinal lesion, consistent with a previous study (Schmidlin et al., 2004).

SPINAL STIMULATION

To document the muscle responses evoked by intraspinal stimuli we compiled St-TAs of rectified EMG during performance of the wrist flexion and extension task. **Figure 2** shows the St-TAs for a spinal site located caudal to the lesion. Spinal stimulation below the lesion evoked facilitation or suppression effects in multiple muscles, as found for effects evoked from the intact spinal cord (Moritz et al., 2007). Furthermore, spinal stimulation activated synergistic muscle groups. For example, stimuli at the site in **Figure 2** strongly facilitated finger extensor muscles [e.g., extensor digitorum 4 and 5 (ED45) and extensor digitorum communis (EDC)] and suppressed antagonist flexor muscles. Facilitation or suppression effects were evoked in 45.6% of the 12–16 recorded muscles from all spinal sites. Based on the responses in St-TAs, we chose a single electrode and current for the artificial neural connection paradigm. For all electrodes, stimulus effects gradually deteriorated over 3 months, presumably due to electrode encapsulation by the physiological reaction (Mushahwar et al., 2000). Finally, the whole spinal implant including wire electrodes with dental acrylic and bone screws sloughed off the vertebrae after 3 months.

ARTIFICIAL CORTICOSPINAL CONNECTION

To bridge the spinal cord lesion, high-gamma LFP activity in either M1 or PMd was used to trigger trains of spinal stimulation (**Figure 3A**). **Figure 3B** shows a typical example of intraspinal stimulation controlled by the LFP signal recorded from the digit area of M1 (site identified by arrow in **Figure 1A**). During the period of FES (green bar), the monkey was able to trigger and stop stimulation volitionally, thereby repeatedly acquiring the targets. To document that the LFP-controlled intraspinal stimulation was necessary, the stimulation was briefly turned off during "catch trials" (white bar in **Figure 3B**) in five sessions. The monkey continued to make efforts to acquire the target in the catch trials, as evidenced by the above-chance increases in high-gamma

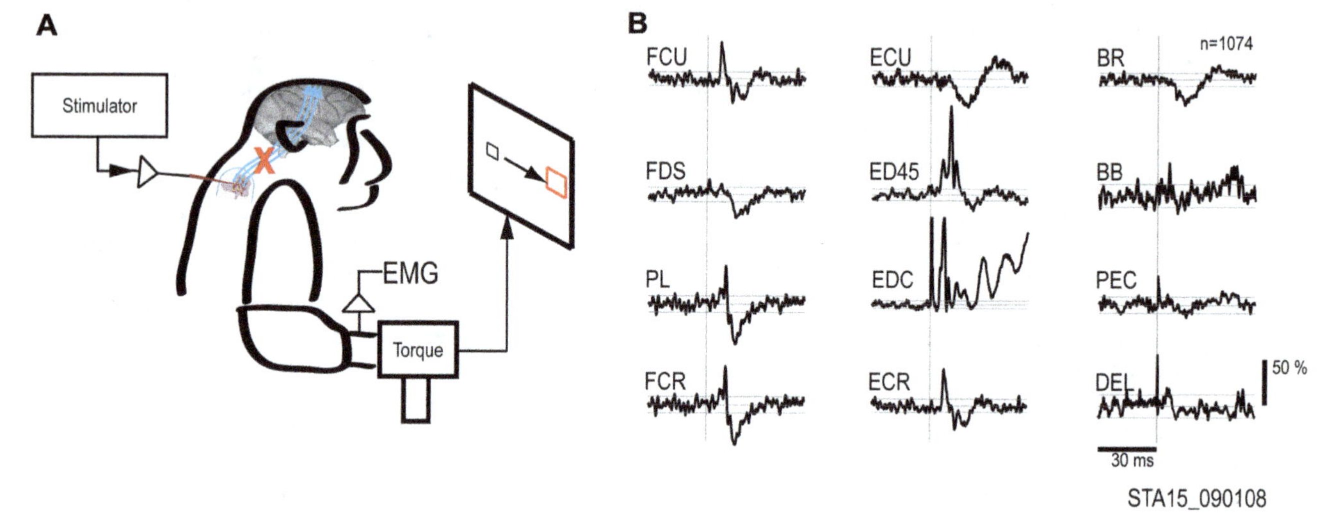

FIGURE 2 | Output effects evoked by intraspinal stimulation. (A) Electrical stimuli were delivered to a single intraspinal electrode while the monkey performed a two-dimensional wrist task, acquiring targets in wrist flexion and extension. **(B)** Muscle responses evoked by a single pulse at 90 μA. The vertical scale bar at right indicates mean percent increase (MPI) over baseline. EMGs were recorded from: flexor carpi ulnaris (FCU), flexor digitorum superficialis (FDS), palmaris longus (PL), flexor carpi radialis (FCR), extensor carpi ulnaris (ECU), extensor digitorum 4 and 5 (ED45), extensor digitorum communis (EDC), extensor carpi radialis (ECR), brachioradialis (BR), biceps brachii (BB), pectoralis (PEC), and deltoid (DEL).

activity, but did not succeed in acquiring the targets. We applied such LFP-controlled intraspinal stimulation in 12 different sessions (duration of sessions: 8–47 min; range of trial number within each session: 46–245 trials), using 11 different pairs of cortical and spinal sites, summarized in **Figure 4A**. The average task performance in LFP-controlled intraspinal stimulation trials was significantly higher than those in catch trials (compare green and black bars in **Figure 4A**). Task performance was comparable with LFP recorded from M1 and PMd (cf. blue and red bars in **Figure 4A**). Task performance using LFP from cortical sites from which movements could and could not be evoked after injury was similar. We also examined the task performance during the transition from the operant conditioning of LFP to ACSC. **Figure 4B** shows the time course of task performance in the operant conditioning session (before time zero in **Figure 4B**) and subsequent ACSC session (after time zero in **Figure 4B**) using LFP from the same cortical electrode. The monkey quickly learned after a few sessions to modulate the power of LFP to acquire targets. Switching from the operant control sessions to the ACSC session was very smooth. The task performance in the ACSC session was sustained at nearly the same level as in the operant conditioning session.

VOLITIONAL BOOSTING OF MUSCLE ACTIVITY BY AN ARTIFICIAL MUSCULOSPINAL CONNECTION

Although the spinal cord lesion produced a severe deficit in forearm movements, the monkey could still produce weak muscle activity. To investigate whether an artificial recurrent connection could boost the activity of a muscle, we used EMG of the paretic muscles to trigger spinal stimulation at a site that produced a contraction of the same muscle (**Figure 5A**). **Figure 5B** shows a typical example of the muscle-controlled intraspinal stimulation using EMG of the paretic extensor carpi ulnaris (ECU) wrist extensor muscle. As shown during the period of FES (green bar), the monkey was able to sustain the EMG burst and torque to acquire the target. During the catch trial, the monkey made a few unsuccessful attempts to produce wrist torque, as seen in the EMG and torque, but was unable to acquire the target. Thus, the muscle-controlled intraspinal stimulation effectively boosted on-going muscle activity of the paretic agonist. We applied similar muscle-controlled FES in 10 different sessions (duration of sessions: 12–33 min; range of trial number within each session: 42–180 trials), using five different pairs of muscle and spinal sites. The average task performance in muscle-controlled intraspinal stimulation trials was significantly higher than that in catch trials (compare green and black bars in **Figure 6A**). **Figure 6B** shows the time course of task performance in the session of operant conditioning of EMG activity and subsequent AMSC session using EMG from the same muscle. The task performance in AMSC sessions was sustained at nearly same level as with operant conditioning session.

DISCUSSION

This case report demonstrates that LFP- or EMG-controlled stimulation in a spinal site could be used to produce volitionally controlled functional wrist torque in a paretic monkey with a spinal cord lesion rostral to the stimulation site. The monkey could volitionally control brain and muscle activities to produce synergistic muscle responses with intraspinal stimulation caudal to the lesion. These results suggest that muscle- or LFP-controlled FES could compensate for the interrupted descending pathways and restore volitional control of functional movement in the upper limb after spinal cord injury or stroke.

The fact that stimulation in a spinal site caudal to a spinal cord lesion can evoke synergistic muscle responses suggests that activity-dependent spinal stimulation may be a promising target

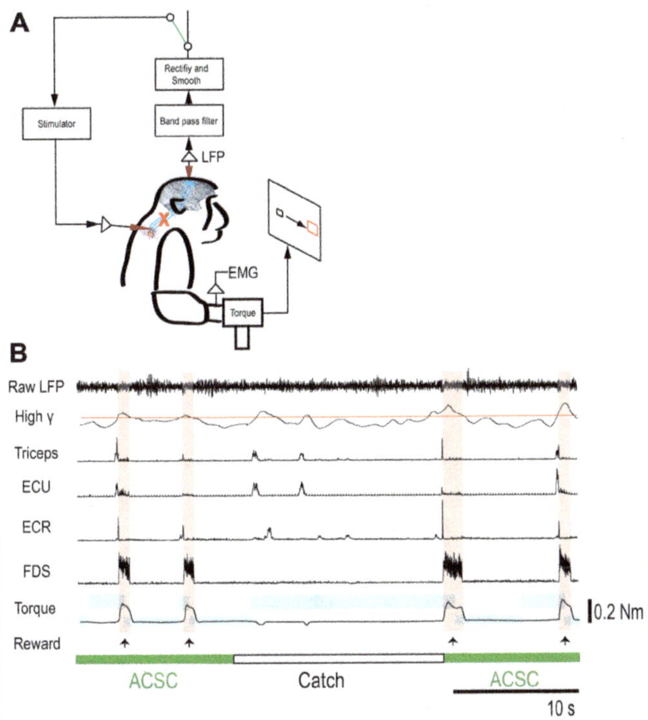

FIGURE 3 | Brain-controlled intraspinal stimulation below the lesion. **(A)** Schematic shows local field potential (LFP) in motor cortex gating trains of electrical stimulation (300 Hz) to a spinal site below the lesion. The switch in the recurrent loop was opened for catch trials. **(B)** Four successful trials with the artificial corticospinal connection (ACSC, green) and one catch trial (white). During the catch trial, the monkey made several unsuccessful attempts to produce wrist torque, as seen in the EMG and torque. The blue rectangles indicate duration and force range of target. The pink vertical bars indicate duration of electrical stimulation in the spinal site. The red line in second trace represents the threshold for spinal stimulation. From top, raw LFP in motor cortex, rectified and smoothed high-gamma LFP (90–160 Hz), EMG from four muscles (abbreviations as in **Figure 2**), and wrist torque. Arrows indicate times of successful task completion and reward.

for neuroprosthetics that can restore movements after spinal cord injury. In contrast to FES of muscles, spinal microwires are subject to less mechanical fatigue than wires implanted peripherally and require lower stimulus currents to evoke movements. Intraspinal stimulation also produces more natural, graded recruitment of motor units than muscle or nerve stimulation (Mushahwar and Horch, 1998). We found that spinal stimulation caudal to the lesion evoked facilitation or suppression effects in multiple muscles. Intraspinal stimulation is known to activate many afferent fibers of passage (Gaunt et al., 2006), and probably excites motoneurons transsynaptically by activating a sufficient number of their inputs, such as propriospinal, corticospinal, and/or afferent axons. Fibers of passage have lower activation thresholds than cell bodies and are thus recruited at lower stimulus currents (Gustafsson and Jankowska, 1976). Afferent axons directly excite synergist muscles and inhibit antagonist muscles via inhibitory spinal interneurons. Since we used a single signal, derived from either cerebral cortex or muscle, to control stimulation, the degree of movement control demonstrated here remains limited. Extending this strategy to control more natural and complex movements would require additional input signals and output spinal sites. Compared with FES in muscle, the activation of functional muscle synergies from single intraspinal sites could significantly reduce the number of implanted electrodes as well as the number of independent control signals required from a neuroprosthetic system.

Task performance with LFP recorded in M1 was comparable with performance using LFP from PMd or EMG from muscle. Furthermore, LFP from any cortical site could control spinal stimulation-evoked wrist movements, regardless of whether stimulation of the cortical site evoked wrist movements or not (cf. **Figure 1C**). Previous biofeedback studies have shown that cells in motor (Fetz and Baker, 1973; Fetz and Finocchio, 1975; Moritz et al., 2008) or somatosensory (Moritz and Fetz, 2011) cortex with no discernable relation to muscles can be volitionally modulated after brief practice sessions. We used a similar operant conditioning paradigm with biofeedback for eliciting cortical LFP or EMG to trigger spinal stimuli. The level of performance in the operant

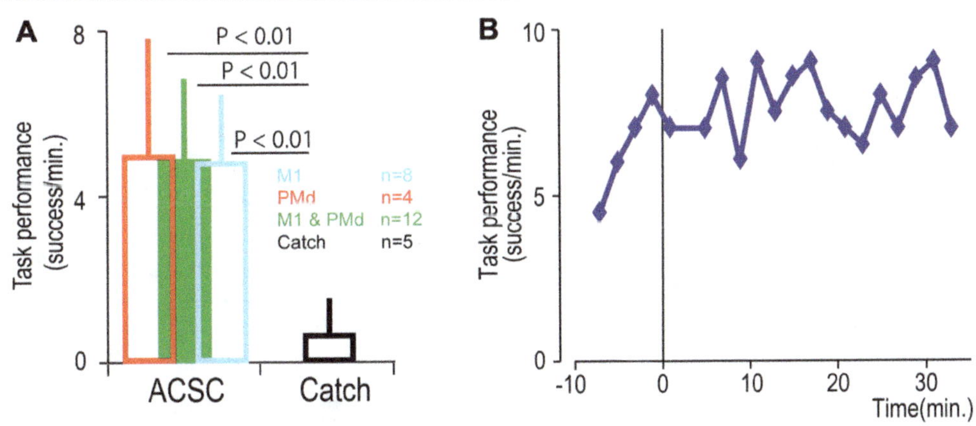

FIGURE 4 | Task performance in the artificial corticospinal connection (ACSC). **(A)** Average task performance with the ACSC and during catch trials. Error bars represent standard deviation. **(B)** Time course of task performance. Before time zero the monkey was required to control the cursor with LFP activity. After time zero the task involved ACSC, using the same cortical electrode in digit area of M1.

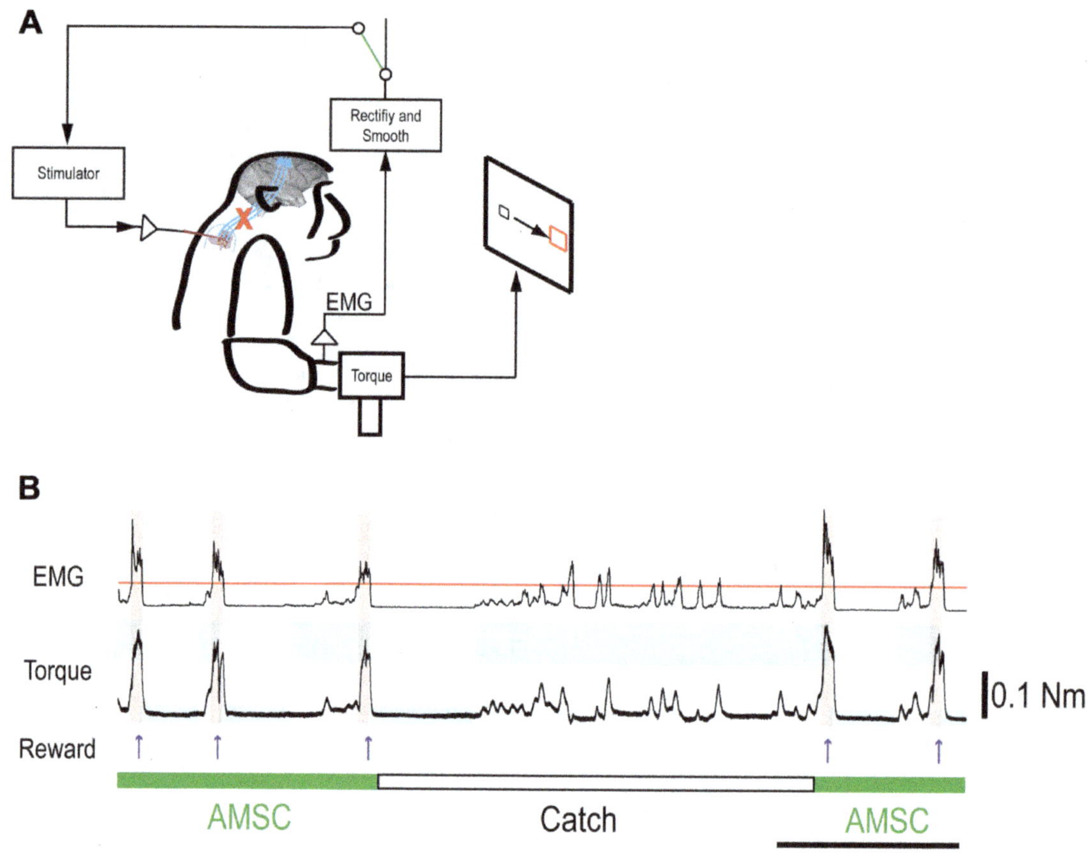

FIGURE 5 | Muscle-controlled spinal cord stimulation. (A) Schematic shows EMG activity gating a train of stimuli to a spinal site below the lesion. **(B)** Five successful trials with AMSC (green) and unsuccessful catch trials (white). During the catch trial, the monkey made several unsuccessful attempts to produce wrist torque, as seen in the EMG and torque. The blue rectangles indicate duration and force range of target. The pink bars indicate duration of electrical stimulation in the spinal site. The red line in top row represents the threshold for gating spinal stimulation. The upper and lower traces are the EMG from ECR and wrist torque generated by the monkey, during stimulation (AMSC, in green) or without stimulation (Catch, in white). Arrows indicate times of successful task completion and reward.

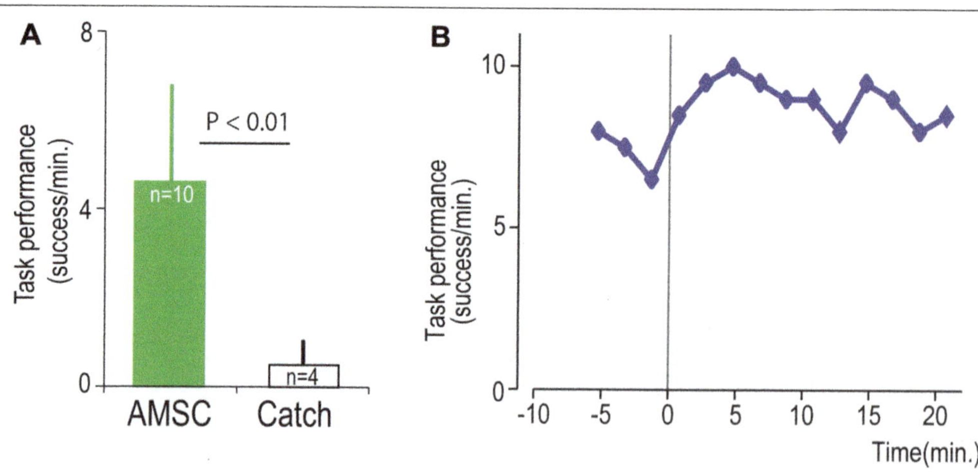

FIGURE 6 | Task performance with the artificial musculospinal connection (AMSC). (A) Average task performance for AMSC and catch trials. Error bars represent standard deviation. **(B)** Time course of task performance in AMSC session. Before time zero the monkey controlled the cursor with EMG activity. After time zero the monkey controlled wrist torque via spinal stimulation triggered from the same muscle with the AMSC.

conditioning task was identical to that with the ACSC and AMSC artificial neural connections. Thus, an arbitrary cortical or muscle signal could be brought under volitional control using biofeedback, to substantially expand the sources of control signals for brain–computer interfaces.

Implementation of the artificial connections with a portable bidirectional neural interface will enable adaptive learning over much longer times and under more varied conditions (Jackson et al., 2006b; Nishimura et al., 2010). The autonomous 'Neurochip' system can discriminate brain or muscle activity and deliver stimulation during free behavior (Zanos et al., 2011). Such autonomous low-power circuits could allow subjects to practice continuously with an artificial connection, without requiring complex decoding algorithms or external devices such as robotic arms. Further development of such direct control of a paretic extremity may lead to implantable devices that could help restore volitional movements to individuals with impaired motor control. Furthermore, recent evidence suggests that continuous activity-dependent stimulation promotes plasticity in motor cortex (Jackson et al., 2006a) and corticospinal connections (Fetz et al., 2010). Thus, activity-dependent stimulation during free behavior may produce both adaptive learning to exploit artificial connections (Nishimura et al., 2010) as well as Hebbian strengthening of spared pathways after neural damage in descending pathway (Fetz et al., 2010). Furthermore, long-term exposure to artificial neural connections could induce reorganization of cortical and spinal circuitry and facilitate functional recovery.

In conclusion, this study demonstrates that artificial neural connections that bridge impaired pathways can ameliorate functional loss. Closed-loop control with intraspinal microstimulation driven by brain or muscle activity could control synergistic muscle activities in upper limb in a monkey with spinal cord injury. The success of our protocol suggests that neurorehabilitative treatment could exploit similar paradigms for restoring volitional control of the extremity for individuals with spinal cord injury or stroke.

CONTRIBUTIONS

Yukio Nishimura and Steve I. Perlmutter conducted the experiments. Yukio Nishimura analyzed the data. Yukio Nishimura, Steve I. Perlmutter, and Eberhard E. Fetz conceived the study and wrote the manuscript.

ACKNOWLEDGMENTS

We thank A. Price, R. Robinson, and J. Skiver-Thompson for technical help, T. Eto for histology and L. Shupe for programming. The work was supported by grants from the National Institutes of Health NS 12542, Christopher & Dana Reeve Foundation, Life Sciences Discovery Fund, and the W. M. Keck Foundation for E. F., the National Institutes of Health NS 40867 for Steve I. Perlmutter and Precursory Research for Embryonic Science and Technology, Japan Science and Technology Agency for Yukio Nishimura.

REFERENCES

Alstermark, B., Pettersson, L. G., Nishimura, Y., Yoshino-Saito, K., Tsuboi, F., Takahashi, M., et al. (2011). Motor command for precision grip in the macaque monkey can be mediated by spinal interneurons. *J. Neurophysiol.* 106, 122–126.

Carmena, J. M., Lebedev, M. A., Crist, R. E., O'Doherty, J. E., Santucci, D. M., Dimitrov, D. F., et al. (2003). Learning to control a brain–machine interface for reaching and grasping by primates. *PLoS Biol.* 1:e42. doi: 10.1371/journal.pbio.0000042

Chao, Z. C., Nagasaka, Y., and Fujii, N. (2010). Long-term asynchronous decoding of arm motion using electrocorticographic signals in monkeys. *Front. Neuroeng.* 3:3. doi: 10.3389/fneng.2010.00003

Chiken, S., Hatanaka, N., and Tokuno, H. (2001). Distribution of median, ulnar and radial motoneurons in the monkey spinal cord: a retrograde triple-labeling study. *Neurosci. Lett.* 307, 143–146.

Choi, K., Hirose, H., Sakurai, Y., Iijima, T., and Koike, Y. (2009). Prediction of arm trajectory from the neural activities of the primary motor cortex with modular connectionist architecture. *Neural Netw.* 22, 1214–1223.

Ethier, C., Oby, E. R., Bauman, M. J., and Miller, L. E. (2012). Restoration of grasp following paralysis through brain-controlled stimulation of muscles. *Nature* 485, 368–371.

Fetz, E. E., and Baker, M. A. (1973). Operantly conditioned patterns on precentral unit activity and correlated responses in adjacent cells and contralateral muscles. *J. Neurophysiol.* 36, 179–204.

Fetz, E. E., and Finocchio, D. V. (1975). Correlations between activity of motor cortex cells and arm muscles during operantly conditioned response patterns. *Exp. Brain Res.* 23, 217–240.

Fetz, E. E., Nishimura, Y., Eaton, R. W., and Perlmutter, S. I. (2010). "Primate corticospinal connections can be strengthened by prolonged spike-triggered stimulation of spinal cord during free behavior," in *Proceeding of 40th Annual Meeting of Society for Neuroscience, 899.2/HHH43,* San Diego, CA.

Flint, R. D., Ethier, C., Oby, E. R., Miller, L. E., and Slutzky, M. W. (2012). Local field potentials allow accurate decoding of muscle activity. *J. Neurophysiol.* 108, 18–24.

Gaunt, R. A., Prochazka, A., Mushahwar, V. K., Guevremont, L., and Ellaway, P. H. (2006). Intraspinalmicrostimulation excites multisegmental sensory afferents at lower stimulus levels than local alpha-motoneuron responses. *J. Neurophysiol.* 96, 2995–3005.

Gustafsson, B., and Jankowska, E. (1976). Direct and indirect activation of nerve cells by electrical pulses applied extracellularly. *J. Physiol.* 258, 33–61.

Jackson, A., Mavoori, J., and Fetz, E. E. (2006a). Long-term motor cortex plasticity induced by an electronic neural implant. *Nature* 444, 56–60.

Jackson, A., Moritz, C. T., Mavoori, J., Lucas, T. H., and Fetz, E. E. (2006b). The Neurochip BCI: towards a neural prosthesis for upper limb function. *IEEE Trans. Neural Syst. Rehabil. Eng.* 14, 187–190.

Jenny, A. B., and Inukai, J. (1983). Principles of motor organization of the monkey cervical spinal cord. *J. Neurosci.* 3, 567–575.

Kennedy, P. R., Bakay, R. A., Moore, M. M., Adams, K., and Goldwaithe, J. (2000). Direct control of a computer from the human central nervous system. *IEEE Trans. Rehabil. Eng.* 8, 198–202.

Koike, Y., Hirose, H., Sakurai, Y., and Iijima, T. (2006). Prediction of arm trajectory from a small number of neuron activities in the primary motor cortex. *Neurosci. Res.* 55, 146–153.

Krüger, J., Caruana, F., Volta, R. D., and Rizzolatti, G. (2010). Seven years of recording from monkey cortex with a chronically implanted multiple microelectrode. *Front. Neuroeng.* 3:6. doi: 10.3389/fneng.2010.00006

Leuthardt, E. C., Schalk, G., Wolpaw, J. R., Ojemann, J. G., and Moran, D. W. (2004). A brain–computer interface using electrocorticographic signals in humans. *J. Neural Eng.* 1, 63–71.

Maier, M. A., Perlmutter, S. I., and Fetz, E. E. (1998). Response patterns and force relations of monkey spinal interneurons during active wrist movement. *J. Neurophysiol.* 80, 2495–2513.

Miller, K. J., Zanos, S., Fetz, E. E., den-Nijs, M., and Ojemann, J. G. (2009). Decoupling the cortical power spectrum reveals real-time representation of individual finger movements in humans. *J. Neurosci.* 29, 3132–3137.

Moritz, C. T., and Fetz, E. E. (2011). Volitional control of single cortical neurons in a brain–machine interface. *J. Neural Eng.* 8, 025017.

Moritz, C. T., Lucas, T. H., Perlmutter, S. I., and Fetz, E. E. (2007). Forelimb movements and muscle responses evoked by microstimulation of cervical spinal cord in sedated monkeys *J. Neurophysiol.* 97, 110–120.

Moritz, C. T., Perlmutter, S. I., and Fetz, E. E. (2008). Direct control of paralysed muscles by cortical neurons. *Nature* 456, 639–642.

Morrow, M. M., and Miller, L. E. (2003). Prediction of muscle activity by populations of sequentially recorded primary motor cortex neurons. *J. Neurophysiol.* 89, 2279–2288.

Mushahwar, V. K., Collins, D. F., and Prochazka, A. (2000). Spinal cord microstimulation generates functional limb movements in chronically implanted cats. *Exp. Neurol.* 163, 422–429.

Mushahwar, V. K., and Horch, K. W. (1998). Selective activation and graded recruitment of functional muscle groups through spinal cord stimulation. *Ann. N. Y. Acad. Sci.* 860, 531–535.

Mushahwar, V. K., and Horch, K. W. (2000). Muscle recruitment through electrical stimulation of the lumbosacral spinal cord. *IEEE Trans. Rehabil. Eng.* 8, 22–29.

Mussa-Ivaldi, F. A., and Bizzi, E. (2000). Motor learning through the combination of primitives. *Philos. Trans. R. Soc. Lond. B. Biol. Sci.* 355, 1755–1769.

Nishimura, Y., Perlmmutter, S. I., and Fetz, E. E. (2010). "Changes in directional tuning of motor cortex cells driving an artificialcorticospinal connection in monkeys," in *Proceeding of 40th Annual Meeting of Society for Neuroscience, 899.1/HHH42*, San Diego, CA.

Pohlmeyer, E. A., Oby, E. R., Perreault, E. J., Solla, S. A., Kilgore, K. L., Kirsch, R. F., et al. (2009). Toward the restoration of hand use to a paralyzed monkey: brain-controlled functional electrical stimulation of forearm muscles. *PLoS ONE* 4:e5924. doi: 10.1371/journal.pone.0005924

Pohlmeyer, E. A., Solla, S. A., Perreault, E. J., and Miller, L. E. (2007). Prediction of upper limb muscle activity from motor cortical discharge during reaching. *J. Neural Eng.* 4, 369–379.

Polikov, V. S., Tresco, P. A., and Reichert, W. M. (2005). Response of brain tissue to chronically implanted neural electrodes. *J. Neurosci. Methods* 148, 1–18.

Popovic, M. R., Popovic, D. B., and Keller, T. (2002). Neuroprostheses for grasping. *Neurol. Res.* 24, 443–452.

Saigal, R., Renzi, C., and Mushahwar, V. K. (2004). Intraspinal microstimulation generates functional movements after spinal-cord injury. *IEEE Trans. Neural Syst. Rehabil. Eng.* 12, 430–440.

Sanchez, J. C., Gunduz, A., Carney, P. R., and Principe, J. C. (2008). Extraction and localization of mesoscopic motor control signals for human ECoG neuroprosthetics. *J. Neurosci. Methods* 167, 63–81.

Santucci, D. M., Kralik, J. D., Lebedev, M. A., and Nicolelis, M. A. L. (2005). Frontal and parietal cortical ensembles predict single-trial muscle activity during reaching movements in primates. *Eur. J. Neurosci.* 22, 1529–1540.

Schalk, G., Kubanek, J., Miller, K. J., Anderson, N. R., Leuthardt, E. C., Ojemann, J. G., et al. (2007). Decoding two-dimensional movement trajectories using electrocorticographic signals in humans. *J. Neural Eng.* 4, 264–275.

Schieber, M. H., and Rivlis, G. (2007). Partial reconstruction of muscle activity from a pruned network of diverse motor cortex neurons. *J. Neurophysiol.* 97, 70–82.

Schmidlin, E., Wannier, T., Bloch, J., and Rouiller, E. M. (2004). Progressive plastic changes in the hand representation of the primary motor cortex parallel incomplete recovery from a unilateral section of the corticospinal tract at cervical level in monkeys. *Brain Res.* 1017, 172–183.

Serruya, M. D., Hatsopoulos, N. G., Paninski, L., Fellows, M. R., and Donoghue, J. P. (2002). Instant neural control of a movement signal. *Nature* 416, 141–142.

Shin, D., Watanabe, H., Kambara, H., Nambu, A., Isa, T., Nishimura, Y., et al. (2012). Prediction of muscle activities from electrocorticograms in primary motor cortex of primates. *PLoS ONE* 7:e47992. doi: 10.1371/journal.pone.0047992

Simeral, J. D., Kim, S. P., Black, M. J., Donoghue, J. P., and Hochberg, L. R. (2011). Neural control of cursor trajectory and click by a human with tetraplegia 1000 days after implant of an intracortical microelectrode array. *J. Neural Eng.* 8, 025027.

Vargas-Irwin, C. E., Shakhnarovich, G., Yadollahpour, P., Mislow, J. M., Black, M. J., and Donoghue, J. P. (2010). Decoding complete reach and grasp actions from local primary motor cortex populations. *J. Neurosci.* 30, 9659–9669.

Wessberg, J., Stambaugh, C. R., Kralik, J. D., Beck, P. D., Laubach, M., Chapin, J. K., et al. (2000). Real-time prediction of hand trajectory by ensembles of cortical neurons in primates. *Nature* 408, 361–365.

Zanos, S., Richardson, G., Shupe, L., Miles, F. A., and Fetz, E. E. (2011). The Neurochip-2: an autonomous head-fixed computer for recording and stimulating in freely behaving monkeys. *IEEE Trans. Neural Syst. Rehabil. Eng.* 19, 427–435.

Zhuang, J., Truccolo, W., Vargas-Irwin, C., and Donoghue, J. P. (2010). Decoding 3-D reach and grasp kinematics from high-frequency local field potentials in primate primary motor cortex. *IEEE Trans. Biomed. Eng.* 57, 1774–1784.

Zimmermann, J. B., Seki, K., and Jackson, A. (2011). Reanimating the arm and hand with intraspinal microstimulation. *J. Neural Eng.* 8, 054001.

12

Closing the loop in primate prefrontal cortex: inter-laminar processing

Ioan Opris[1]*, Joshua L. Fuqua[1], Peter F. Huettl[2], Greg A. Gerhardt[2], Theodore W. Berger[3], Robert E. Hampson[1] and Sam A. Deadwyler[1]*

[1] *Department of Physiology and Pharmacology, Wake Forest University School of Medicine, Winston-Salem, NC, USA*
[2] *Department of Anatomy and Neurobiology, University of Kentucky, Lexington, KY, USA*
[3] *Department of Biomedical Engineering, University of Southern California, Los Angeles, CA, USA*

Edited by:
Steve M. Potter, Georgia Institute of Technology, USA

Reviewed by:
Manuel Casanova, University of Louisville, USA
Randy M. Bruno, Columbia University, USA

****Correspondence:***
Ioan Opris, Department of Physiology and Pharmacology, Wake Forest University School of Medicine, Winston-Salem, NC, USA.
e-mail: ioopris@wfubmc.edu
Sam A. Deadwyler, Department of Physiology and Pharmacology, Wake Forest University School of Medicine, Medical Center Boulevard, Winston-Salem, NC 27157, USA.
e-mail: sdeadwyl@wfubmc.edu

Prefrontal cortical (PFC) activity in the primate brain emerging from minicolumnar microcircuits plays a critical role in cognitive processes dealing with executive control of behavior. However, the specific operations of columnar laminar processing in prefrontal cortex (PFC) are not completely understood. Here we show via implementation of unique microanatomical recording and stimulating arrays, that minicolumns in PFC are involved in the executive control of behavior in rhesus macaque nonhuman primates (NHPs) performing a delayed-match-to-sample (DMS) task. PFC neurons demonstrate functional interactions between pairs of putative pyramidal cells within specified cortical layers via anatomically oriented minicolumns. Results reveal target-specific, spatially tuned firing between inter-laminar (layer 2/3 and layer 5) pairs of neurons participating in the gating of information during the decision making phase of the task with differential correlations between activity in layer 2/3 and layer 5 in the integration of spatial vs. object-specific information for correct task performance. Such inter-laminar processing was exploited by the interfacing of an online model which delivered stimulation to layer 5 locations in a pattern associated with successful performance thereby closing the columnar loop externally in a manner that mimicked normal processing in the same task. These unique technologies demonstrate that PFC neurons encode and process information via minicolumns which provides a closed loop form of "executive function," hence disruption of such inter-laminar processing could form the bases for cognitive dysfunction in primate brain.

Keywords: prefrontal cortex, inter-laminar correlated firing, nonhuman primates, columnar correlates of target selection, columnar correlates of task difficulty, spatial vs. object tuning

INTRODUCTION

The prefrontal cortex (PFC) with its privileged position at the top of sensory-motor processing hierarchy (Alexander et al., 1986; Fuster, 2001) has been traditionally viewed as the seat of higher cognitive functions such as working memory and executive control of behavior (Fuster and Alexander, 1971; Funahashi et al., 1989; Miller, 2000). According to many theories of cognition, cortical mechanisms of executive function coordinate and control "online" cognitive processes underlying memory storage, behavioral selection and motor planning (Posner and Snyder, 1975; Goldman-Rakic, 1996; Shallice and Burgess, 1996; Miyaki et al., 2000; Miller and Cohen, 2001; Baddeley, 2002; Graybiel, 2008). Prefrontal neural activity in the primate brain that emerges from cortical laminar minicolumns is hypothesized to play a critical role in cognitive processes dealing with working memory and executive control of behavior (Goldman-Rakic, 1996; Mountcastle, 1997; Rao et al., 1999; Miller and Cohen, 2001; Baddeley, 2002; Casanova et al., 2007, 2009).

Cortical minicolumns consist of vertically-oriented "aggregates" of cell bodies that represent the basic anatomic and physiologic microcircuitry of the cerebral cortex (Mountcastle, 2003) that consist of pyramidal cells and several types of GABAergic, inhibitory interneurons (i.e., double-bouquet, basket, and chandelier cells) (Casanova et al., 2002a,b, 2007; Sokhadze et al., 2012). Minicolumns in PFC are interconnected to each other through horizontal "long range" projections in layer 2/3 (Kritzer and Goldman-Rakic, 1995), inter-laminar mini-loops (Weiler et al., 2008; Takeuchi et al., 2011) and "reverberatory loops" through projections to the subcortical basal ganglia nuclei and thalamus (Alexander et al., 1986). Such "reverberatory loops" combine incoming signals from thalamus in layer 4 and inputs from cortical horizontal projections in layer 2/3, in order to compare inputs to a threshold criterion triggering an output response under specific conditions.

The ability to make behavioral selections in humans involves attention, target/goal choice, planning and monitoring of actions, and is regarded as a facet of decision making based on sensory evidence, expected costs, and benefits associated with the outcome (Opris and Bruce, 2005; Opris et al., 2005a,b; Heekeren et al., 2008; Pesaran et al., 2008; Resulaj et al., 2009). In order to make optimal selections or decisions, many areas in the primate brain with converging inputs to the supra-granular layers of the PFC are activated (Kritzer and Goldman-Rakic, 1995; Opris et al., 2011; Takeuchi et al., 2011), thus raising the question as to how the PFC processes information required for selection of a particular behavioral response necessary for achieving functional objective. It has been shown that neurons in PFC recorded from rhesus macaque nonhuman primates (NHPs) demonstrate functional interactions between inter-laminar "cell pairs" synaptically connected via cortical minicolumns (Kritzer and Goldman-Rakic, 1995; Mountcastle, 1997; Buffalo et al., 2011; Opris et al., 2011; Takeuchi et al., 2011) and that these cells coordinate activity required to encode spatial location and select the target location or target features.

In the studies presented here this presumed executive function of PFC minicolumns was examined via custom designed conformal multielectrode arrays (MEAs) implemented to record the firing of inter-laminar cell pairs oriented in cortical "microstrips" in NHPs (Opris et al., 2011). The recording pads on the MEAs matched the dimensions of two interconnected cell layers in PFC (layer 2/3 and layer 5) which allowed simultaneous monitoring of columnar oriented cells in each layer in order to characterize the control of arm movements in a cognitive task requiring working memory and image-based target selection (Deadwyler et al., 2007; Hampson et al., 2011). The results reveal target-specific, spatially tuned firing between columnar oriented pairs of inter-laminar PFC neurons, during the decision making and/or motor planning phase of the task (Hampson et al., 2011).

METHODS

All animal procedures were reviewed and approved by the Institutional Animal Care and Use Committee of Wake Forest University, in accordance with U.S. Department of Agriculture, International Association for the Assessment and Accreditation of Laboratory Animal Care, and National Institutes of Health guidelines.

VISUAL DELAYED-MATCH-TO-SAMPLE (DMS) TASK

The NHPs utilized as subjects in this study ($n = 4$) were trained for at least 2 years to perform a well characterized, custom-designed visual delayed-match-to-sample (DMS) task (Hampson et al., 2011; Opris et al., 2011) shown in **Figure 1A**. Animals were seated in a primate chair with a platform in front of a display screen in which position of the arm on the platform was tracked via a UV-fluorescent reflector affixed to the back of the wrist, illuminated via a 15 W UV lamp, and detected by an LCD camera positioned 30 cm above. Hand position and movement was digitized and displayed as a bright yellow cursor on the screen and horizontal positions of illuminated clip-art targets were computed from the video image using a Plexon Cineplex scanner. The DMS task paradigm is shown in **Figure 1A**. Trials were initiated by the animal placing the cursor inside a yellow 3" circle or square randomly illuminated in one of the nine spatial positions on the screen. The presence of either the circle or square constituted the "Start" signal for the trial and indicated "trial type" with respect to the Match reward contingency on the same trial (**Figure 1A**). Placement of the cursor into the Start signal image produced a trial unique clip-art image randomly displayed in one of eight peripheral screen positions on each trial for 2, 0 s, which characterized the "Sample Phase" of the task. Movement of the cursor into the Sample image (Sample Response) blanked the screen and initiated the Delay phase for 10–60 s, randomly selected on each trial. Timeout of the Delay interval initiated the onset of the Match phase of the task (Match phase "onset") in which 2–7 trial unique clip-art images, including the Sample image, were presented on the screen with position selected randomly on each trial. Placing the cursor into either, (1) the Sample image (*Object* trial) or (2) the same location as the prior Sample Response (*Spatial* trial), during the Match phase constituted the correct "Match Response (MR)" which produced a drop of juice as the reward, delivered via a sipper tube located near the animal's mouth, and blanked the screen for 10 s until the next trial. Placement of the cursor into one of the non-match (distracter) images on an *Object* trial, or a different spatial location on the screen during a *Spatial* trial, constituted a MR error that blanked the screen without reward delivery and initiated the 10 s inter-trial interval (ITI). All clip-art images (sample and distracter) were unique for each trial in sessions of 100–150 trials and were chosen from a 10,000 image selection buffer which was updated to replace 20% of the images every month. The four NHPs were trained to overall performance levels of 70–75% correct with respect to the above described DMS task parameters.

SURGERY

Animals were surgically prepared with cylinders for attachment of a microelectrode manipulator over the specified brain regions of interest. During surgery animals were anesthetized with ketamine (10 mg/kg), then intubated and maintained with isoflurane (1–2% in oxygen 6 l/min). Recording cylinders (Crist Instruments, Hagerstown, MD) were placed over 20 mm diameter craniotomies for electrode access to stereotaxic coordinates of the Frontal Cortex (25 mm anterior relative to interaural line and 12 mm lateral to midline/vertex) in the caudal region of the Principal Sulcus (**Figure 2A**), the dorsal limb of Arcuate Sulcus in area 8 and the dorsal part of premotor area 6 (Hampson et al., 2011), areas previously shown by PET imaging to become activated during task performance (Hampson et al., 2009). Two titanium posts were secured to the skull for head restraint with titanium steel screws embedded in bone cement. Following surgery, animals were given 0.025 mg/kg buprenorphine for analgesia and penicillin to prevent infection. Recording cylinders were disinfected thrice weekly with Betadine during recovery and daily during recording. Vascular access ports (Norfolk Medical Products, Skokie, IL) for drug infusions were implanted subcutaneously in the mid-scapular region, the end of the catheter threaded subcutaneously, to a femoral incision, inserted into the femoral vein, and threaded for a distance calculated to terminate in the vena cava and flushed daily with 5 ml heparinized saline needed for IV drug administration.

ELECTROPHYSIOLOGY: RECORDING AND STIMULATION

Electrophysiological procedures and analysis utilized the MAP Spike Sorter by Plexon, Inc. (Dallas, TX) for 64 channels

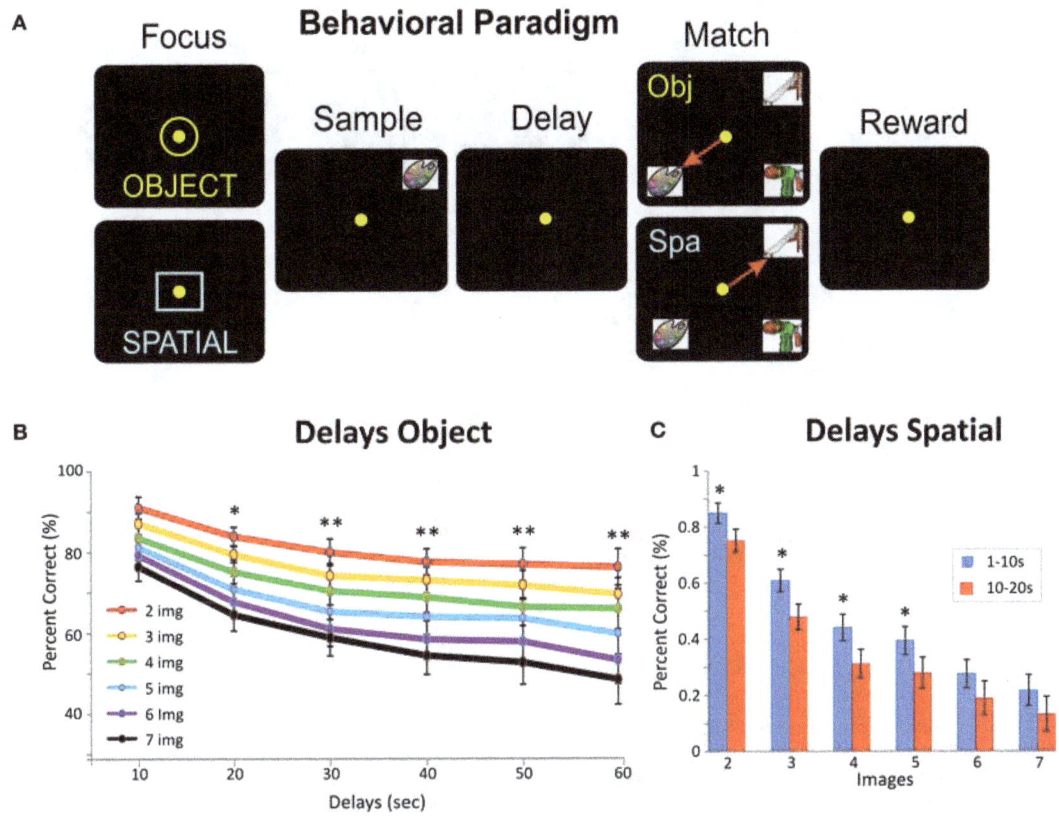

FIGURE 1 | Delayed match to sample task (DMS) in NHPs. (A) Behavioral paradigm shows the DMS task in which two types of trials (*Object* of *Spatial*) were signaled by presentation of one of the two "Focus" signals into which the animal placed the cursor to start the trial. On *Object* trials (yellow ring) reward was delivered for selection of the same clip-art image to be presented in the Sample phase, when it appeared later in the Match phase of the trial, irrespective of position on the screen. On *Spatial* trials (blue square) reward was delivered in the Match phase for selection of the image in the "spatial location on the screen" in which the image was presented in the Sample phase, irrespective of the clip-art image occupying that position in the Match phase. The sequence of events on both types of trials: (1) presentation of "Focus signal" to initiate the trial with cursor placement into the signal, (2) presentation of the 'Sample' clip-art image requiring cursor movement into the image "Sample Response" (3) initiation of a variable "Delay" interval of 1–60 s with the screen blank, (4) upon timeout of the delay interval the Match phase is initiated in which the Sample image is presented on the screen at random locations accompanied by 1–6 other non-match (distracter) images. On *Object* trials placement of the cursor into the (Sample) image for = 0.5 s was the correct Match response (MR) for that trial type. On *Spatial* trials placement of the cursor into the same position in which the image appeared in the Sample phase of the trial was the correct MR. Both correct MRs produced a juice reward via a sipper tube mounted next to the animal's mouth. Placement of the cursor into an inappropriate image or location for = 0.5 s caused the trial to terminate and the screen to blank without reward delivery. The inter-trial interval (ITI) was 10.0 s, and Object and Spatial trials were randomly presented 0.6 and 0.4 percent of trials per session, respectively. **(B)** DMS performance averaged over all animals (mean % correct MRs) for *Object* trials as a function of number of Match phase distracter images (number of images 2–7) and length of delay interval (10–60 s) Asterisks: $^*F_{(1,\ 486)} = 7.98$, $p < 0.01$, $^{**}F_{(1,\ 486)} = 12.24$, $p < 0.001$, ANOVA. **(C)** Behavioral performance averaged over all animals (mean % correct MRs) for *Spatial* trials as a function of length of delay interval (1–20 s) and number of Match phase distracter images (number of images 2–7) Asterisks: $^*F_{(1,\ 486)} = 7.98$, $p < 0.01$, ANOVA.

simultaneous recordings. Customized conformal designed ceramic MEAs were constructed at the University of Kentucky, Center for Microelectrode Technology—CenMet, Lexington, KY, and consisted of etched platinum pads (**Figure 2B**) for recording multiple single neuron activity (Hampson et al., 2004, 2011). Single extracellular action potentials (**Figure 2B**) were isolated and analyzed with respect to activity on specific recording pads (mpedance range 0.5–3.0 MOhms) during different events within DMS trials (**Figure 2C**). The configuration of the MEA (**Figure 2B**) was specially designed to conform to the columnar anatomy of the PFC such that the top four recording pads recorded activity from neurons in the supra-granular layer 2/3 (L2/3) while the lower set of four pads, separated vertically by 1350 μm, simultaneously recorded neuron activity in the infra-granular layer 5 (L5) of the PFC (**Figures 2B** and **C**). Recordings from multiple pads in designated locations on the MEAs were analyzed by a nonlinear model previously perfected for assessing and extracting spatiotemporal multineuron firing patterns in PFC using the same MEAs and to deliver task-contingent electrical stimulation to L5 in the same pattern as recorded during correct trial performance (Hampson et al., 2012). Stimulation consisted of 1.0 ms bipolar pulses (50–70 uA) delivered to L5 recording locations following presentation of the Match phase screen and prior to the completion of the MR (**Figure 7**).

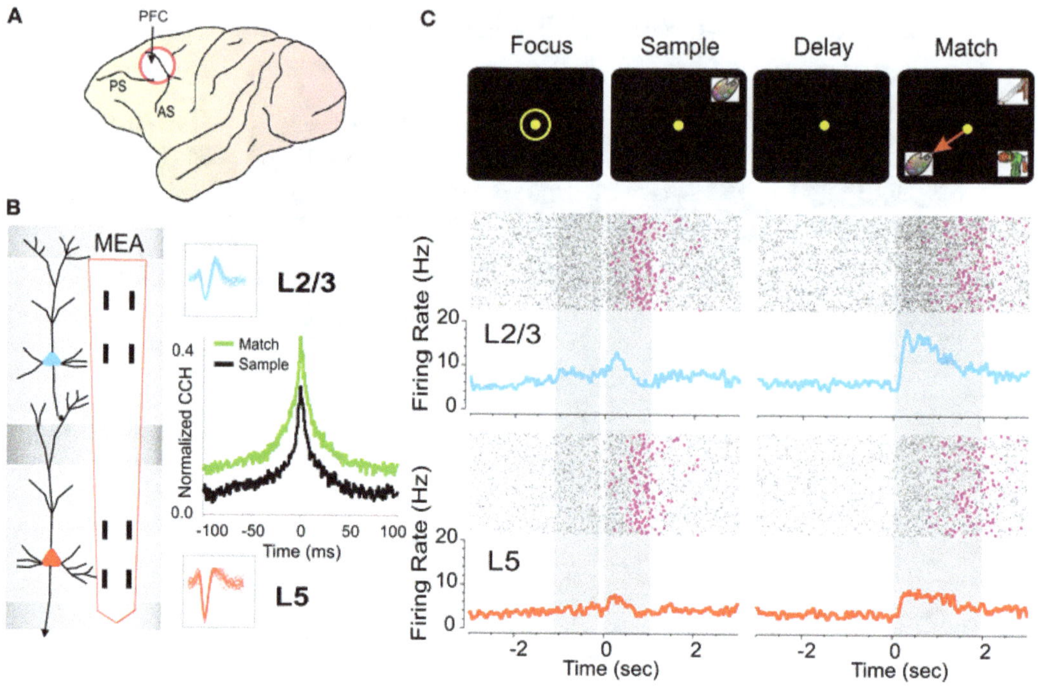

FIGURE 2 | Inter-laminar recording in primate prefrontal cortex during delayed-match-to-sample (DMS) task. (A) Diagram of NHP brain showing PFC recording locations in cortical areas 46, 8, 6 (white circle). **(B)** Recording Array: Diagram of a cortical minicolumn consisting of a "columnar pair" of L2/3 (blue) and L5 (red) PFC cells. Diagram shows conformal multielectrode recording array (MEA) positioned for simultaneous inter-laminar columnar recording from a PFC minicolumn with corresponding L2/3 and L5 cell waveforms (blue and red) corresponding to the task specific neural firing shown in **(C)**. **(C)** Individual trial rasters and average perievent histograms (PEHs) over 50 trials obtained from the inter-laminar "cell pair" recorded simultaneously from L2/3 (blue) and L5 (red) in the minicolumn format shown in **(B)** over ±2.0 s relative to both the Sample and Match phase onset (0.0 s) in a single DMS session. The occurrence of behavioral responses (reaction time plus movement time) in the Match phase on each trial is indicated by pink dots in the rasters. **(B,C)**: Cross-correlation histograms (CCHs) of L2/3 and L5 cell pair activity in **(C)** from the same cell pair in **(B)** for the Sample and Match phases of the task. The larger "green" CCH peak shows increased inter-laminar synchronization during target selection in the Match phase relative to the CCH constructed from the same cell pair during the Sample phase (black) of the task shown in **(C)**.

ELECTROCHEMICAL RECORDING

Ceramic MEAs similar to those utilized above for electrophysiological recording were also prepared for electrochemical recording (Burmeister et al., 2004, 2008; Quintero et al., 2007, 2011; Hascup et al., 2008, 2011; Fuqua et al., 2010). The electrochemistry arrays consisted of four recording sites ($15 \times 333\,\mu M$) in two rows, separated by 500 μm, with a 7 cm polyimide shaft for depth positioning. The electrodes were configured to record from Layer 2/3 with the reference in Layer 1. MEAs were dip coated with Nafion®, a fluoropolymer which excludes the passage of anions, thus ensuring that only cations would reach the platinum recording surface. The dorsal ("sentinel" or reference) recording sites were coated with bovine serum albumin (BSA) plus glutaraldehyde; ventral recording sites were coated with Glutamate oxidase and BSA + glutaraldehyde. The GluOx coating allowed the ventral pads to be sensitive to glutamate release through the enzymatic production of H_2O_2. A +0.7V charging potential was applied to the MEA once per second (using an Ag/AgCl reference electrode) to oxidize the H_2O_2 resulting from detection of glutamate at the electrode. The "relaxation" current from H_2O_2 oxidation was proportional to second-by-second changes in glutamate concentration at the electrode (Quintero et al., 2011).

DATA ANALYSIS

Task performance was determined for each animal ($n = 4$) as percent correct trials within and across sessions and related to simultaneous MEA recordings on individual trials during Match phase image selection MR in the task (Hampson et al., 2011). Cell types were identified as regular firing pyramidal cells in terms of baseline (nonevent) firing rate (Opris et al., 2009) and significant changes ($z > 3.09$, $p < 0.001$) in firing (see below) on single trials in perievent histograms (PEHs) derived for intervals of ±2.0 s relative to the time of Match screen presentation that signaled onset of the Match phase of the task (**Figure 2C**). Task-related neural activity was classified according to locations on the conformal MEA which were positioned specifically in L2/3 and L5 (**Figure 2B**) upon insertion in PFC prior to the start of the DMS session. To account for neuronal responses in terms of columnar microcircuit organization neurons recorded on the MEAs were characterized by (1) simultaneous cell activity on both sets of vertical separated (1350 μm) pads (L2/3 cell upper and L5 cell lower), during electrode positioning (**Figure 2B**), and (2) whether the same cell pair firing was modulated similarly during the Match phase of the DMS task (Hampson et al., 2012). Standard (Z) scores of increased firing rates relative to nonevent baseline values were calculated for individual cells for each DMS task event. Firing rate was analyzed in 250 ms bins for ±2.0 s relative to time of initiation (0.0 s) task events. Only neurons with firing rates significantly elevated from that in pre-event phases (−2.0 to 0.0 s) baseline period were included for analysis. Differences in cross-correlation between neuron spikes of L2/3 and L5 cell pairs on the same vertical sets of MEA pads (**Figure 2B**) were assessed for the same temporal intervals using standardized distributions of correlation coefficients assessed under different conditions related to performance in the Match Phase (**Figures 2–5**). Mean cross-correlation histograms (CCHs) were calculated and compared relative to mean coefficients normalized relative to probability of firing for the same populations of cell pairs under different experimental conditions (**Figures 2B, 3C, 4C,** and **5C**), all of which satisfied the 99% confidence requirement (Opris et al., 2011). CCHs were generated using a shift predictor algorithm built into NeuroExplorer version 4 (http://www.neuroexplorer.com/), which computed chance cross-correlation levels by randomizing the actual spike sequence and calculating cross-correlations five different times for a given pair of neurons, which was then subtracted from the true coefficients for CCHs to adjust for correlated firing due to differences in cell firing rates and frequency of bursting (Opris et al., 2011; Takeuchi et al., 2011). Population (mean) CCHs, normalized as a function of probability, were computed by averaging coefficients across multiple cell pairs and plotting the mean values (±SEM) in 1.0 ms bins (**Figures 2B, 3C, 4C,** and **5C**).

IDENTIFICATION OF CORTICAL LAYERS AND MINICOLUMNS

The conformal MEA (model W3) probe (**Figure 2B**) was designed so that the two sets of recording pads could only record simultaneous activity from neurons separated by ~1350 μm, which given the orientation of insertion into PFC (**Figure 1B**) could only consist of infra-granular layer 5 and supra-granular layer 2/3 cell activity (Hansen and Dragoi, 2011; Opris et al., 2011; Takeuchi et al., 2011). Misplacement of the probe due to a different angular penetration relative to columnar orientation in PFC was detectable by the absence of simultaneous cell recordings on the sets of vertically separated (1350 μm) pads. In addition, the MEA (Hampson et al., 2004; Opris et al., 2011) employed here allowed simultaneous recording of two PFC minicolumns (**Figure 2B**) since, with proper vertical alignment (<5.0°), activity from adjacent minicolumns could be detected, since MEA

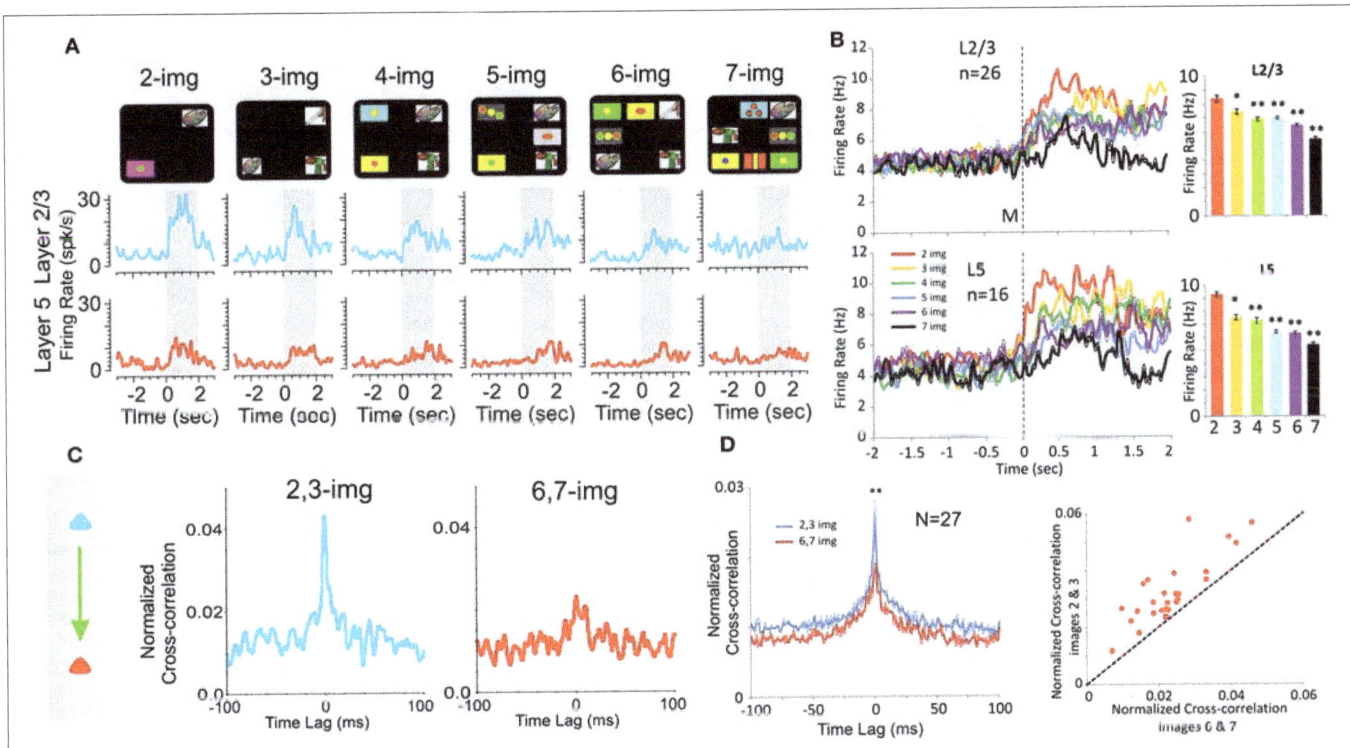

FIGURE 3 | Effect of number of images on PFC columnar firing. (A) Example peri-event histograms comparing neuron firing in PFC layers L2/3 (blue) and L5 (red) as a function of the number of images presented (upper: display screens) in the Match phase on *Object* type trials in the DMS task. **(B)** Population peri-event histograms depicting the activity of prefrontal cells from layers L2/3 ($n = 16$) and L5 ($n = 26$) on all types of trials with different numbers of images (2, 3, 4, 5, 6, and 7) presented during match phase in the DMS task [L2/3: $F_{(6,\ 1039)} = 8.29$, $p < 0.001$; L5: $F_{(6,\ 639)} = 8.64$; $p < 0.001$, ANOVA]. **(C)** Example inter-laminar CCHs for trials with a few (2 and 3 images) vs. many (6 and 7 images) distracter images constructed from the same interlaminar L2/3-L5 cell pair shown in **(A)**. **(D)** Normalized population CCHs for trials with low (2, 3 red) vs. high (6, 7 blue) numbers of images in the Match phase consisting of the average correlation coefficients across individual CCHs from 27 different inter-laminar cell pairs. Scatter plot showing differential distributions of individual CCH peak correlation coefficients on trials with low vs. high numbers of images for the same cell pairs ($n = 27$) comprising the population CCH. $^{**}p < 0.001$, $^{*}p < 0.01$, ANOVA.

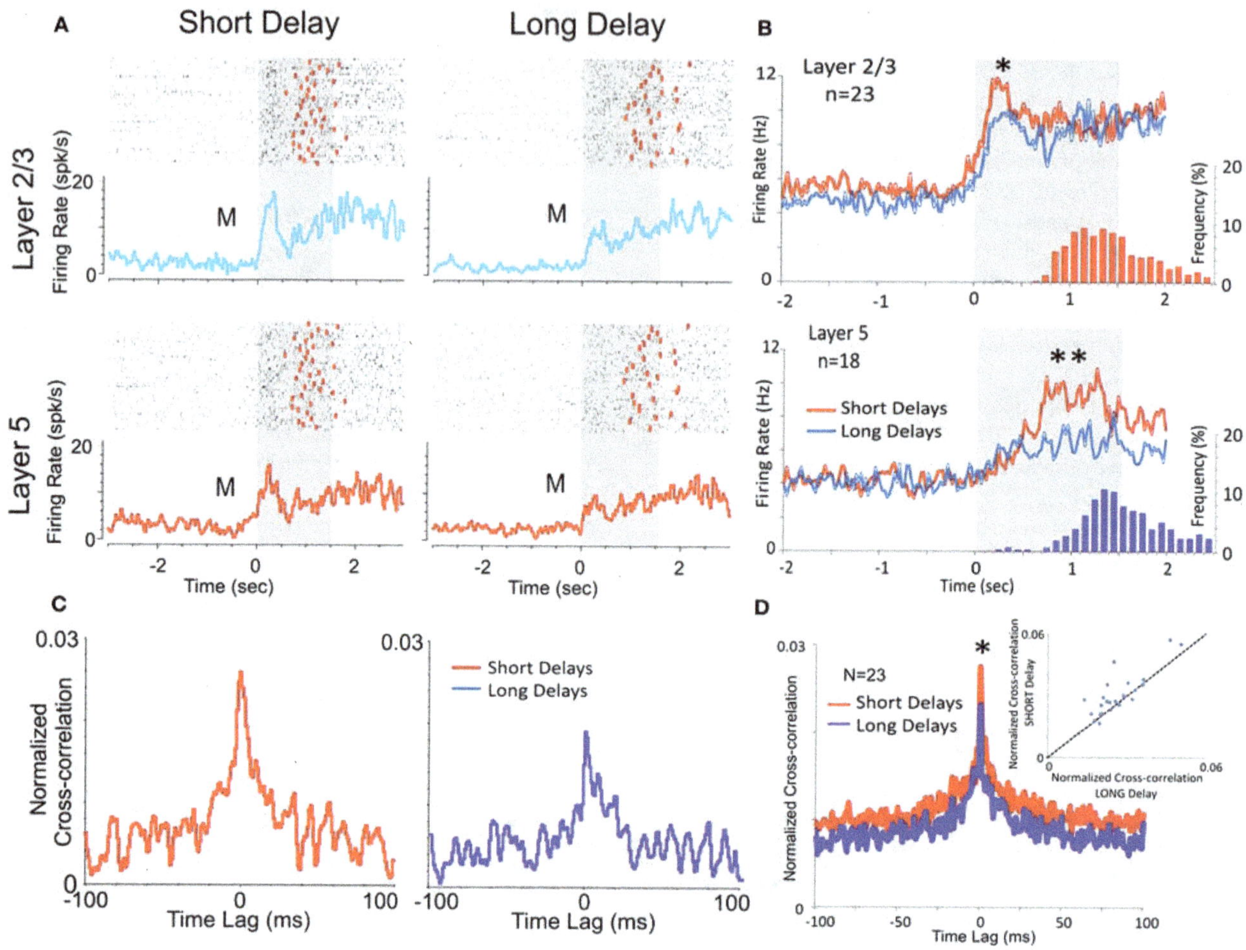

FIGURE 4 | Effect of DMS delay duration on PFC neuronal activity and columnar firing. (A) Raster and peri-event histograms comparing firing of PFC L2/3 and L5 cells in the Match phase as a function of short (≤20 s) vs. long (>40 s) delays in the DMS task. **(B)** Population peri-event histograms depicting the activity of L2/3 and L5 cells during short (≤20 s) vs. long (>40 s) delays ($n = 23$ cells in L2/3, $p < 0.01$ ANOVA and $n = 18$ cells in L5; $p < 0.001$ ANOVA). Histograms show distribution of Match response latencies for short (red) vs. long (blue) delays. **(C)** Example inter-laminar CCHs for L2/3 and L5 cell pairs shown in **(B)** on trials with short vs. long delays. **(D)** Population of inter-laminar CCHs and scatter plot for short vs. long delay trials (see **Figure 3D**). $^{**}p < 0.001$, $^{*}p < 0.01$, ANOVA.

pads were separated laterally by 40 μm which exceeds the distances reported (28 μm) from anatomic assessments (Casanova et al., 2009; Hansen and Dragoi, 2011; Mo et al., 2011; Takeuchi et al., 2011).

TUNING PLOTS

For each inter-laminar cell pair (L2/3 and L5), firing on the same trials was plotted with respect to the position of the target selected in the Match phase (**Figure 6B**). Directionality was assigned according to the eight positions on the screen with reference to placement of the cursor in the center providing angles corresponding to the location of the match image around the periphery of the screen, yielding 0° (directly lateral), 45, 90, 135, 180, 225, 270, 315, and 360° movement directions from center of screen (Rao et al., 1999; Felsen et al., 2002). Mean firing rate commencing at Match phase onset until time of occurrence of the MR (i.e., typically 0.5–1.0 s, **Figures 4D** and **5D**) was calculated and represented for each inter-laminar cell pair in polar coordinates as tuning plots of the average firing rate, over all trials in a single session. Directional biases, or "preferences", for cell pairs were defined as response locations with the highest mean firing rates relative to all the other positions responded to during the session (**Figure 6B**). A *tuning index* plot (Meyer et al., 2011) was employed for comparing the distribution of biases for the same cells on *Object* vs. *Spatial* trials (**Figure 6E**).

RESULTS

The four subjects NHPs trained to perform the DMS task (Hampson et al., 2011) were required to select the same video image presented on-screen in the prior Sample phase from a set of 2–7 images in the subsequent Match Phase after an intervening Delay of 10–60 s (**Figure 1A**). The NHPs made hand tracking movements of a cursor on the screen in the Match phase to obtain a juice reward for selection of the correct (Sample) image

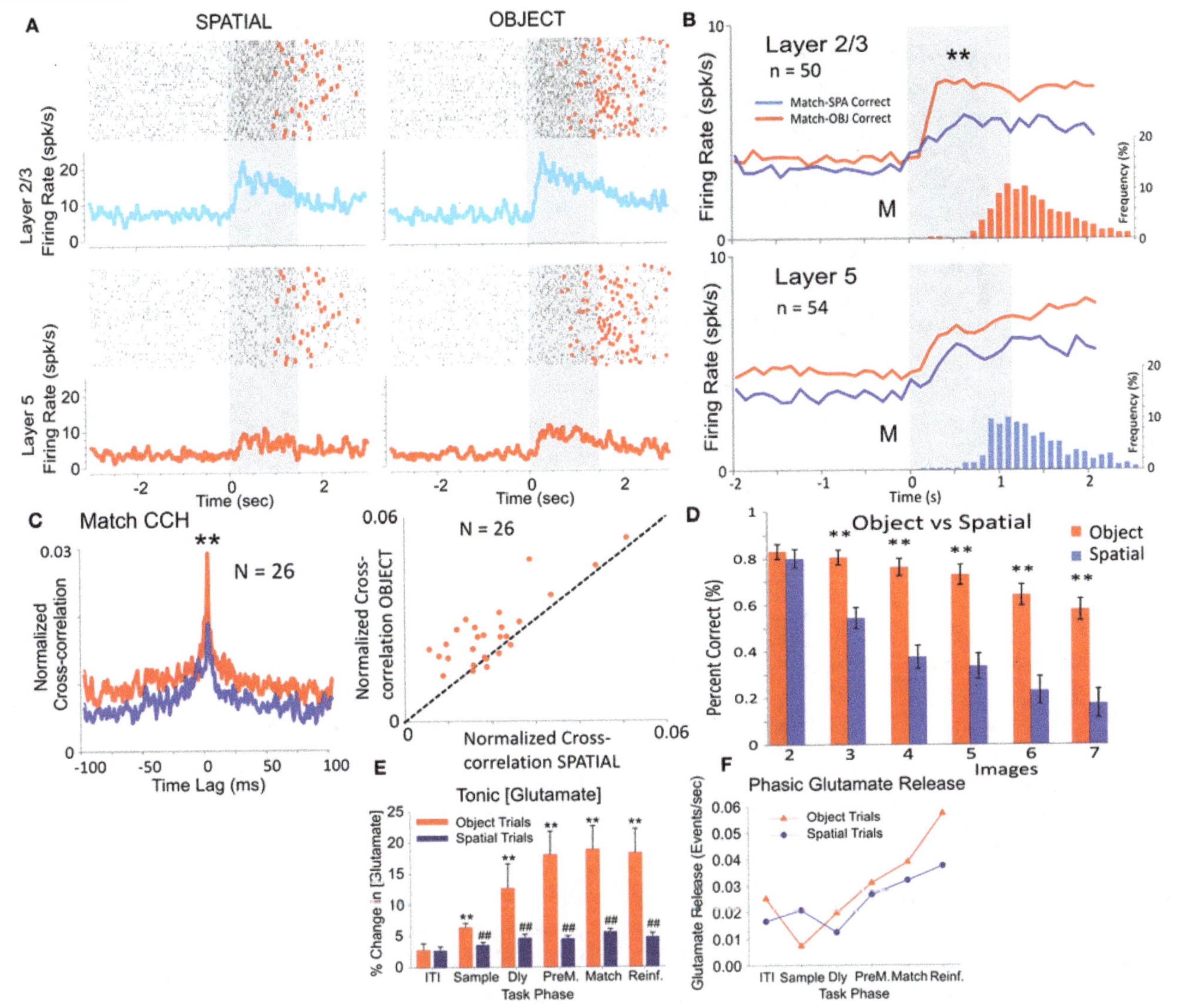

FIGURE 5 | Comparison of PFC inter-laminar firing on *Object* vs. *Spatial* trials. (A) Rasters and Peri-event histograms showing firing in the Match phase of a PFC L2/3-L5 cell pair recorded during *Spatial* vs. *Object* type trials. **(B)** Population peri-event histograms depicting the activity of PFC L2/3 ($n = 50$) and L5 ($n = 54$) cells on *Spatial* (blue) vs. *Object* (red) trials presented during match phase in the DMS task [$F_{(1,\ 1039)} = 12.89$, $p < 0.001$, ANOVA]. Histograms show distribution of match response latencies for *Spatial* (blue) vs. *Object* (red) trials. **(C).** Average inter-laminar cross-correlation for the same cell pairs ($n = 26$) recorded on *Object* vs. *Spatial* trials. Scatter plot of shows differential distribution of peak CCH values for *Object* vs. *Spatial* trials for the same cell pairs. **(D)** Behavioral performance as a function of the number of images (2–7) on *Object* vs. *Spatial* trials. **(E)** Electrochemical recording of tonic glutamate neurotransmitter concentrations in PFC Layer 2/3. Mean (±S.E.M.) glutamate concentration ([Glutamate]) measured as a percentage increase over baseline (average $8.69 \pm 0.77\ \mu$M) glutamate concentration. Horizontal axis indicates phase of DMS task: intertrial interval (ITI), Sample phase, Delay phase (Dly), end of delay phase 5 s prior to Match (PreM), Match phase and reinforcement (Reinf.). Asterisks: $^*p < 0.01$, $^{**}p < 0.001$, *Object* vs. *Spatial* trials; $^{\#}p < 0.01$, $^{\#\#}p < 0.001$ DMS task phases vs. ITI. **(F)** Frequency of phasic glutamate release events measured as transient increase (<2.0 s duration) of at least 5% in [Glutamate] for the same trials shown **(E)**. Frequency normalized to number of events per second per DMS trial (Fuqua et al., 2010).

in different positions which varied on each trial with respect to image-type and screen position. The key variables in the task therefore were: (1) number of distracter images (2–7) presented randomly in different screen positions in the Match phase on each trial, (2) the duration of the intervenning delay interval (1.0–60.0 s) and (3) the random placement of the Sample (target) image in 1 of 7 spatial positions on the screen in the Match phase (after the delay interval). Previous research with the same DMS task has indicated the necessity of attention, short-term memory and response latency, together with influence of type of choice, as factors that affect cognitive workload in the same task (Porrino et al., 2005; Deadwyler et al., 2007). Recent analyses of PFC activity showed that animals execute a "decision process" in the Match phase of the task (**Figure 1A**) involving target selection (Hampson et al., 2011) and that this involved inter-laminar synchrony in cell activity (Hampson et al., 2012). In the study

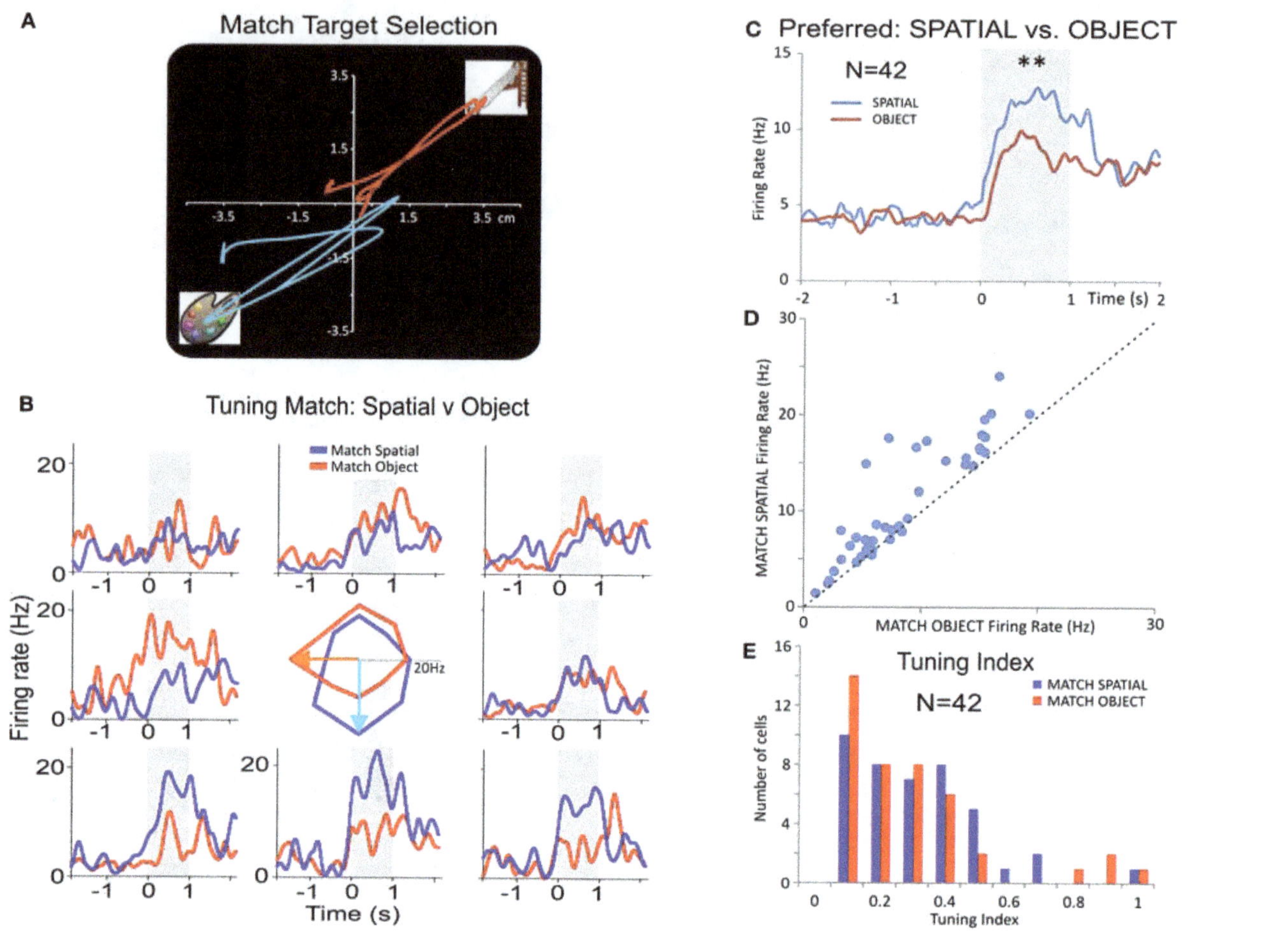

FIGURE 6 | Inter-laminar PFC spatial tuning during DMS task performance. (A) Illustration of two arm movement tracks from a single animal for two opposite target locations on the screen during the Match phase of the DMS task. **(B)** Tuning Plot Multigram PEHs (multigram) and spatial tuning plot (diagram in center) for a PFC L2/3 cell on *Spatial* (blue) and *Object* (red) trials. The tuning plot in the middle displays Match phase mean firing rates (shaded areas in PEHs) along radial axes corresponding to movement of the cursor into each of the eight screen image positions from the screen center summed over all trials in a single session. The spatial (i.e. screen position) "bias" indicated by the highest firing rate for target selection, for the *Object* trial tuning vectors was in the "medial left" position (i.e.,180°), while the bias for *Spatial* trial tuning vectors was in the "down" (i.e., 270°) position. **(C)** Average firing rate for *Spatial* biases (preferred target locations) and Object biases summed across different ($n = 42$) inter-laminar (L2/3 and L5) cells. **(D)** Scatter plot comparing preferred (i.e., highest) firing rate directions for the same cells in **(C)** on *Spatial* vs. *Object* trials, indicating a more biased directional firing on *Spatial* trials. **(E)** Histogram comparing the distribution of preferred firing for the same cells as a function of a tuning index (TI) derived as TI = (PF−NF)/(PF+NF), on *Spatial* (blue) and *Object* (red) trials, where PF represents preferred location/direction firing rate and NF stands for non-preferred direction firing rate. The plot in **(E)** shows that there was a trend for lower TIs, less bias for one position, on *Spatial* vs. *Object* trials by showing more cells with lower TI values. $^{**}p < 0.001$, ANOVA.

presented here PFC columnar inter-laminar pair-wise cell firing from four NHPs (60 cell pairs: 21 in animal K, 16 in B, 12 in E and 11 in G) was characterized for all of the above mentioned task-related parameters shown previously (Porrino et al., 2005; Deadwyler et al., 2007) to control cognitive processing in this DMS task.

MULTIELECTRODE ARRAY RECORDINGS FROM CORTICAL LAYERS AND MINICOLUMNS

Prior reports of neural relationships to executive function and decision making in a sensorimotor hierarchy (Miller and Cohen, 2001; Opris and Bruce, 2005; Heekeren et al., 2008; Pesaran et al., 2008; Opris et al., 2012) referred to recordings made in dorsolateral PFC as shown in **Figures 2A** and **B**, which were also reported to depend on the interaction between neurons in different layers in the same area (Goldman-Rakic, 1996; Opris et al., 2011; Takeuchi et al., 2011). In this study, inter-laminar connectivity was sensed by previously described conformal-designed MEAs (Hampson et al., 2012) positioned to simultaneously record neurons located in PFC layer 2/3 and layer 5 in adjacent "minicolumns" during performance of the DMS task (**Figures 2B** and **C**). The MEA contained two linear sets of four recording pads separated vertically by 1350 μm to conform to the distance between PFC cortical cell layer 2/3 (L2/3) and layer 5 (L5) when inserted perpendicular to the parallel lamellae (see "Methods"). The two sets of dual vertical pads in each upper and lower position on the MEA were separated horizontally by 40 μm in order to exceed the reported 28 μm width of single cortical minicolumns (Casanova et al., 2007; Opris et al., 2011). This allowed simultaneous recording from two adjacent L2/3 and L5 columnar "cell pairs" constituting neural activity from two separate minicolumns on a single MEA probe. This pad configuration insured that only cells in L2/3 and L5 were recorded, since the appearance of cells simultaneously on both sets of vertical pads required 0° angular placement relative to both cell layers (Takeuchi et al., 2011) as shown in **Figure 2B**. In this study spatiotemporal analyses of 180 prefrontal cortical (PFC) pyramidal cells recorded in four NHPs revealed a large number ($n = 60$) of confirmed L2/3 and L5 cell pairs in this region of PFC (**Figure 2A**) that displayed inter-laminar interactions during the Match phase of the DMS task.

INTER-LAMINAR PROCESSING IN PFC DURING DMS TASK

The relevance of minicolumnar activity to decision making has been investigated in several types of cognitive processing tasks (Goldman-Rakic, 1996; Opris and Bruce, 2005; Heekeren et al., 2008; Pesaran et al., 2008; Resulaj et al., 2009; Opris et al., 2011, 2012). An example of this inter-laminar interaction during the target-selection in the Match phase of the DMS task (**Figure 1A**) is shown in **Figure 2C** in raster/PEHs constructed over ±2.0 s for the Sample and Match phases of the trial for a cell pair recorded in the PFC with the MEA (**Figure 2B**). The cell pair was recorded on appropriate sets of pads as shown in the illustration of the two cells in L2/3 and L5 next to the MEA (**Figure 2B**). Neurons in both layers showed significant increases in mean firing during Sample (L2/3: $Z = 7.30$, $p < 0.001$; L5: $Z = 4.16$, $p < 0.001$) and Match (L2/3: $Z = 12.86, p < 0.001$; L5: $Z = 6.20$, $p < 0.001$) screen presentations (post events: 0.0–2.0 s) and during subsequent movements associated with target selection in this task (Hampson et al., 2011). A consistent finding employing this recording configuration was that within neuron pairs significantly higher mean firing rate in the 0.0 + 2.0 s interval were observed for L2/3 cells after Match phase onset [$F_{(1, 153)} = 20.93$, $p < 0.001$] as demonstrated in the upper and lower raster/PEHs in **Figure 2C**. More precise functional connections between individual cells within each minicolumn was determined by cross (CCHs; Opris et al., 2011; Takeuchi et al., 2011; Hong et al., 2012) constructed for the same minicolumn cell pairs. This is shown for the firing displayed in the PEHs in **Figure 2C** and although there was significantly correlated firing (Match: $Z = 12.23$, $p < 0.001$; Sample: $Z = 10.12, p < 0.001$) the differences in peak correlation shown in the CCHs [$F_{(1, 401)} = 9.41, p < 0.001$] indicate that the cell pair firing was more synchronized in the Match than in the Sample phase of the task.

EFFECTS OF TASK DIFFICULTY ON INTER-LAMINAR PROCESSING

Number of match phase images

As shown in prior reports (Porrino et al., 2005; Deadwyler et al., 2007; Hampson et al., 2011) a major cognitive factor influencing target selection in the Match phase of this task was the number of distracter images (number of images) presented with the Sample image on a given trial (**Figure 1A**). **Figure 3A** shows an example of a graded decrease in cell pair firing in both L2/3 and L5 as a function of the number of images presented in the Match phase. In agreement with prior results (Hampson et al., 2011), overall mean firing rates of L2/3 ($n = 26$) and L5 ($n = 16$) neurons (**Figure 3B**) were systematically decreased as a function of the number of images in the Match phase (L2/3: $F_{(6, 1039)} = 8.29$, $p < 0.001$; L5: $F_{(6, 639)} = 8.64$; $p < 0.001$, ANOVA). However, more importantly this decrease was also expressed in terms of correlated firing between L2/3-L5 cell pairs as shown in **Figures 3C** and **D** ($n = 27$) in which Match phase CCHs on trials with few (2 and 3) images showed significantly higher correlations than on trials with more (6 and 7) images [$F_{(1, 53)} = 7.21$; $p < 0.01$, ANOVA]. This finding of decreased inter-laminar correlated firing is consistent with the fact that increasing the number of distracter images decreases task performance (**Figures 1B** and **C**) due to an increase the in cognitive workload of the task (Hampson et al., 2011; Kelley and Lavie, 2011).

Duration of delay

Another factor increasing cognitive workload in the DMS task is memory of the Sample target image across the delay interval (**Figure 1A**) and has been shown to be a factor influencing Match target selection (Deadwyler et al., 2007). Consistent with this relationship as shown in **Figure 4B** was the fact that average firing rates for L2/3 and L5 cell pairs was significantly lower on "long" (>40 s) vs. "short" (=20 s) delay trials [L2/3: $F_{(1, 919)} = 6.67$, $p < 0.01$, $n = 23$; L5: $F_{(1, 719)} = 10.92$; $p < 0.001$, $n = 18$, ANOVA]. **Figure 4C** shows that Match phase (0.0–2.0 s) CCHs for both L2/3 and L5 cells were significantly lower on "short" vs. "long" delay trials [short delay: $F_{(1, 1639)} = 10.87, p < 0.001$; long delay: $F_{(1, 1639)} = 6.71, p < 0.01$] as were the average CCHs for all L2/3 vs. L5 cell pairs (**Figure 4B**) under both conditions [$F_{(1, 45)} = 7.27; p < 0.01$, ANOVA]. The decrease in interlaminar correlation as a function of short vs. long delays is shown more explicitly in the scatterplot in **Figure 4D** where short delay trials produced higher correlation coefficients than long delay trials for the same cell pairs.

EFFECT OF 'TRIAL TYPE' (*OBJECT* vs. *SPATIAL*) ON INTER-LAMINAR PROCESSING

PFC minicolumns are a functional neuronal "module" (Buxhoeveden and Casanova, 2002; Casanova et al., 2003) with basic associative abilities to integrate horizontal and vertical anatomic "components" of the cortex (Mountcastle, 1997; Lund et al., 2003; Tanaka, 2003; Opris et al., 2011). The visual signals carrying *Spatial* information ascend from visual cortex on the dorsal stream to be integrated in PFC minicolumns with signals from the ventral stream that label the clip art image visual features such as color, shape, brightness used on *Object* trials. To compare firing in PFC layers L2/3 and L5 on *Spatial* vs. *Object* trials we examined image selection ability of cortical minicolumns during the Match phase of DMS task in the same cells during both types of trial in the same session. **Figures 5A** and **B** show differences in L2/3 and L5 cells with respect to mean (±SEM) firing rate changes during the Match phase interval of *Spatial* and *Object* trials trials within the same DMS sessions.

Mean firing rates during the Match phase (0.0–2.0 s) were significantly higher for L2/3 vs. L5 cells for both types of trials [$F_{(1, 1039)} = 12.89$, $p < 0.001$, ANOVA], however, **Figure 5B** shows that rates were significantly lower on *Spatial* vs. *Object* trials for L2/3 cells [$F_{(1, 499)} = 10.96$, $p < 0.001$, $n = 50$], but not for L5 [$F_{(1, 539)} = 1.12$, ns, $n = 54$; ANOVA]. **Figure 5C** shows that these differences in firing rates were also associated with significant decreases in mean CCHs for the same L2/3-L5 cell pairs on *Object* vs. *Spatial* trials [$F_{(1, 51)} = 12.20, p < 0.001$] which as indicated in the "Methods" section, were not due to alterations in firing rate *per se* (Hong et al., 2012). These results are consistent with the differences in degree of difficulty between *Object* vs. *Spatial* trials with respect to task performance, as shown in **Figure 5D**.

The contribution of different cellular networks for differential columnar processing on *Object* vs. *Spatial* trials was examined by employing electrochemical recording of glutamate levels in PFC Layer 2/3. Glutamate neurotransmission have been implicated in learning and memory (Dudkin et al., 2003; Riedel et al., 2003), therefore we hypothesized that changes in levels of released glutamate would correlate with differential cognitive processing (Stephens et al., 2010) of DMS trials. Glutamate-sensitive electrochemical recording MEAs were tested in three sessions for each of the four NHPs. The average basal glutamate concentration across animals and sessions was $8.69 \pm 0.77\ \mu M$. **Figure 5E** shows the percent change in *tonic* glutamate concentration (Glutamate) from baseline sorted by individual phases (events) in the DMS task averaged separately across animals for *Object* vs. *Spatial* trials. While both *Object* and *Spatial* trials exhibited significantly increased glutamate concentrations [$F_{(5, 789)} = 11.42, p < 0.001$] in the Delay and Match phases of the task compared to baseline and ITI levels (Fuqua et al., 2010), glutamate levels were significantly elevated on *Object* relative to *Spatial* trials [$F_{(2, 789)} = 32.17, p < 0.001$]. **Figure 5F** depicts the frequency of *phasic* (i.e., transient) glutamate increases putatively related to neurotransmitter release events (Stephens et al., 2010). Although the frequency of glutamate release detected in the vicinity of the electrode was similar, it was still greater for *Object* vs. *Spatial* trials (**Figure 5E**) suggesting that the difference in overall tonic concentration represented activity of a network of glutamate synapses throughout PFC.

Spatial tuning

Another comparison of *Object* vs. *Spatial* trial processing was provided by examining "tuning plots" (Rao et al., 1999; Felsen et al., 2002) of PFC L2/3 and L5 cell pairs constructed for each target location on the screen during Match target selection (**Figure 6A**). **Figure 6B** shows an example of L2/3 cell firing on both *Spatial* (blue) and *Object* (red) trials. This type of comparison clearly dissociates the L2/3 cell biases/preferences on *Spatial*; tuning vector points to lower target location, 270°) vs. *Object* trials (**Figure 6A**; tuning vector points to left target location; 180°). **Figure 6C** shows average PEHs of preferred firing rates on *Spatial* (blue) vs. *Object* (red) trials for 42 neurons which showed significant increases [$F_{(1, 1679)} = 19.63$; $p < 0.001$, ANOVA] on *Spatial* vs. *Object* trials. Finally, a scatter plot of mean firing rates (**Figure 6D**) at biased target locations of the same cells ($n = 42$) as in **Figure 6C** shows a significant difference in preferred firing on *Spatial* vs. *Object* trials ($P < 0.001$; paired T-test). A "tuning index" defined as: $TI = (PF - NF)/(PF + NF)$, where PF represents mean firing rate in the preferred/biased location and NF the non-preferred (lowest) firing location, was calculated to compare firing in the Match phase on *Object* vs. *Spatial* trials. **Figure 6E** shows the comparison of tuning index for Match target selection on *Spatial* vs. *Object* trials, that have comparable magnitudes in selection abilities on different, prior trial-specific instructions via the focus signal (**Figure 1A**), which is consistent with the multifunctional roles of these same cells in executive control. The results shown in **Figures 6D** and **E** indicate dominance of preferred location firing on *Spatial* vs. *Object* trials which was likely the result of the influence of the prior trial type instruction in the Focus phase of the task.

CLOSING THE LOOP WITH INTERLAMINAR REGULATED STIMULATION

The unique properties of conformal MEAs also provide the basis for applying a system specific model to control firing of cells via application of electrical stimulation to the same loci in which columnar firing has been detected and analyzed with respect to DMS task performance (Hampson et al., 2012). This same model was implemented here to test whether it could facilitate performance on trials that show a distinctive difference in performance as a function of the prior instructions as to type of response to make in the Match phase (i.e., *Object* vs. *Spatial* trials). **Figure 7A** shows the integration of a multi-input multi-output (MIMO) nonlinear math model to assess the patterns of firing in L2/3 and L5 cells recorded in the columnar manner with the MEA shown with adjacent vertical pads (Hampson et al., 2012; Opris et al., 2012). **Figure 7B** reflects the type of input and output firing patterns recorded and analyzed by the MIMO model and also illustrates how the output pattern of L5 cell firing is duplicated via a multichannel stimulator that is capable of delivering predetermined patterns of pulses to the same L5 pads to mimic firing on correct trials. The advantage of the MIMO model is that the online recording provides the means to detect when the inappropriate L2/3 firing pattern occurs which triggers the delivery of the appropriate L5 stimulation pattern providing the means to override errors and enhance performance (Hampson et al., 2012). The results of stimulation delivery are shown in **Figures 7C** and **D**, in which the effects on performance are compared to trials in which stimulation was not delivered, irrespective of trial type. **Figure 7C** shows the change in latency to respond on stimulation trials with respect to the time of onset of the Match phase, while **Figure 7D** shows the increase in correct performance on trials as a function of the number of distracter images in the Match phase. Finally in agreement with all prior demonstrations and correlations of columnar specificity with respect to the influence of trial type on DMS performance, **Figure 7E** shows that *Spatial* trials that received MIMO stimulation showed improved performance relative to *Object* trials (with the same number of distracter images and delays 1–20 s). These results indicate that MIMO derived stimulation facilitated cognitive processing required to retrieve the "rule" for successful Match phase selection of the appropriate Sample item as shown in **Figure 6**.

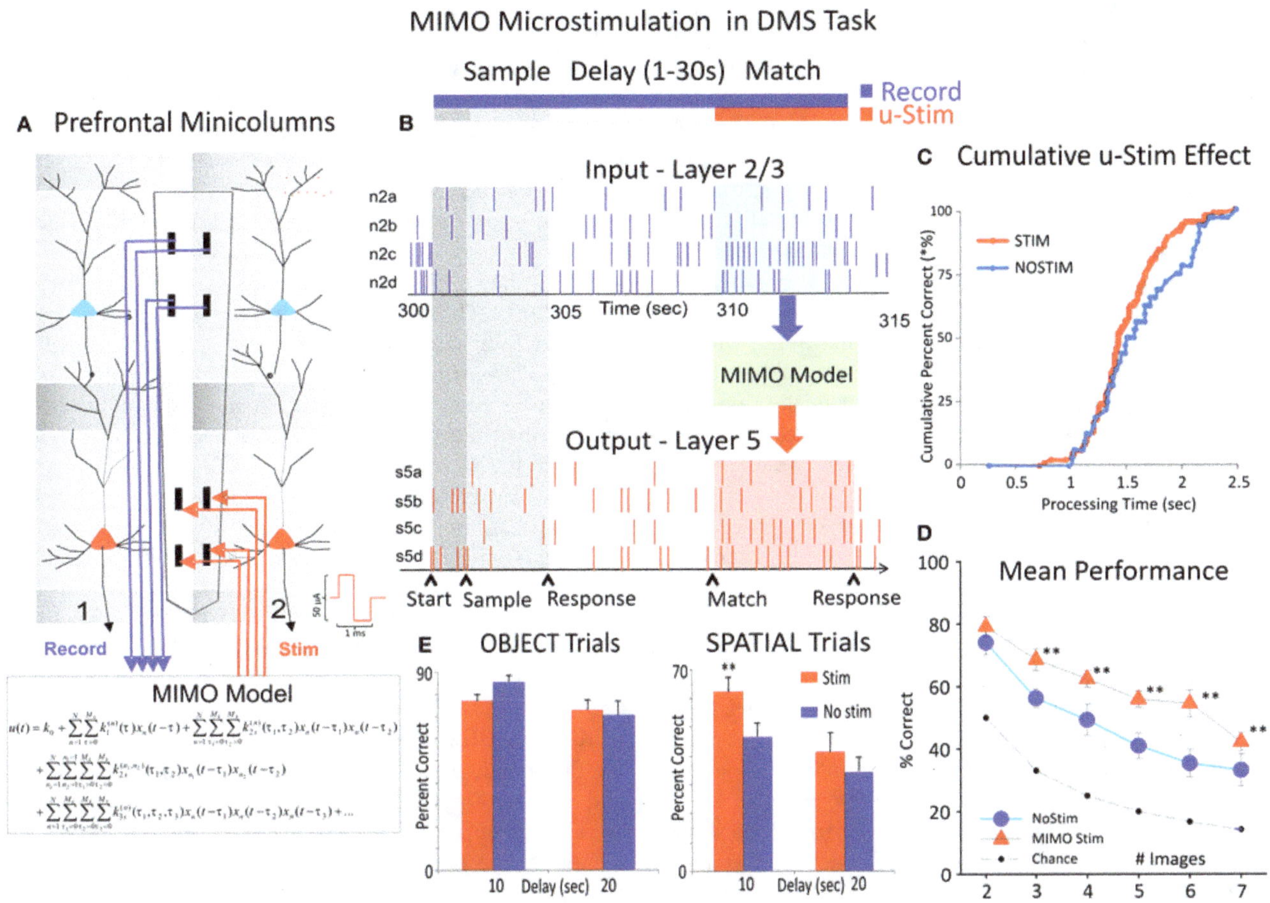

FIGURE 7 | Closing interlaminar loops in PFC with MIMO model generated stimulation. (A) Diagram of the interfacing of MIMO model with conformal MEAs shown in **Figure 2** between L2/3 and L5 during task performance. Electrical stimulation delivered to MEA pads in L5 via patterns of pulses (biphasic) recorded and derived from the same L5 locations on successful trials by the MIMO model. **(B)** Firing of L2/3 and L5 located columnar neurons as shown in **Figure 2** recorded on line and fed to MIMO model shown in **(A)**. Shaded areas indicate time of Match Response execution during DMS trial, and the illustrated firing in L5 which is the same pattern as the delivered stimulation on trials with inappropriate L2/3 firing. **(C)** Changes in cummulative response latencies (processing time) from Match phase onset ("0") during trials with stimulation delivered in the manner shown in **(A)** and **(B)**, **(D)**. Increase in performance across trials with increasing difficulty as a function of the number of Match phase distracter images on trials that received MIMO stimulation in the manner shown in **(A,E)**. Differential effects of MIMO stimulation on *Spatial* vs. *Object* trials showing more enhancement on *Spatial* trials ranging in delays of 1–20 s. $^{**}p < 0.001$, ANOVA.

DISCUSSION

INTER-LAMNAR PROCESSING IN PREFRONTAL CORTEX vs. CLOSING THE LOOP

The findings reported here (**Figures 2**, **3**, and **4**) are consistent with the idea that neurons in the supra- and infra-granular layers form efficient mini-columnar circuits during Match phase target selection required for effective performance of this DMS task (Swadlow et al., 2002; Pesaran et al., 2008; Resulaj et al., 2009; Buffalo et al., 2011; Opris et al., 2011; Takeuchi et al., 2011). The implementation of the unique MEA (**Figure 2B**) provided the basis for the detailed assessment of inter-laminar correlated firing (Opris et al., 2011) that was validated in multiple recordings of L2/3 and L5 cell pairs that yielded similar relations following differential changes in performance-dependent task parameters across animals and sessions (**Figures 3D**, **4D**, and **5D**). The increase in L2/3 and L5 correlations specific to the decision for target selection in the Match phase of the task (**Figures 2**, **3**, and **4**) suggests that a key variable in controlling task performance was activation of L5 neurons via specific minicolumnar input from paired neurons in layers 2 and 3 which have been shown to participate in the integration of "long-range" sensory inputs from the parietal dorsal visual stream (Opris and Bruce, 2005; Heekeren et al., 2008; Pesaran et al., 2008; Resulaj et al., 2009). Such integration was definitely reduced by trial difficulty as indicated by the reduction in firing synchrony between L2/3 and L5 cell pairs relative to trials with less cognitive demand (**Figures 1B**, **3C,D**, and **4C,D**). Prior investigations have shown that the firing of adjacent minicolumns is not correlated with respect to L2/3 and L5 activation during the Match phase of the task (Hampson et al., 2012; Opris et al., 2012). This again supports the notion that specific columnar processing was the basis for effective task performance and that such processing with respect to correlated firing between columns was independent, potentially reflecting processing of different forms of task specific information (Miyaki et al., 2000; Miller and Cohen, 2001; Opris et al., 2011).

Another feature demonstrating the columnar nature of this type of multineuron processing was the fact that classified L2/3–L5 cell pairs also showed the same Match phase spatial tuning biases (Felsen et al., 2002) during the session (**Figure 6**), which indicates the possible presence of previously identified PFC minicolumnar selection biases (Rao et al., 1999; Resulaj et al., 2009; Opris et al., 2011) in the cell pairs reported here (**Figures 3**, **4**, and **5**). This columnar processing trend, with the same tunning bias of L2/3 and L5 cells, reported in 81% of the cell pairs in *Spatial* trials was also present in the same percentage during *Object* trials, although the direction of tuning biases in the same minicolumn varied between these two trial contingencies.

Figures 5B and **C** show a very important distinction with respect to PFC inter-laminar processing which illucidates markedly why animals were less efficient in performing *Spatial* vs. *Object* types of trials with the same delays (**Figure 5D**) in the same behavioral sessions. The reduction in L2/3-L5 cell pair correlation on *Spatial* trials shown in **Figure 5C**, reflects a difference related to a state controlled by "prior" trial specific instruction (**Figure 1A** Focus signal) and suggests a lack of contextual encoding sufficient to maintain the same level of interlaminar communication. This is supported also by the demonstration of the independent influence of trial delay shown in **Figure 4** which clearly had a greater influence on *Spatial* vs. *Object* trials. In addition, the electrochemical measurement of glutamate concentration in Layer 2/3 (**Figures 5E–F**) suggests that different networks, circuits, or even possibly, interlaminar columns of PFC neurons, differentially support the processing of *Spatial* vs. *Object* trials. Thus, Inter-laminar processing likely underlies the putative "executive function" of this brain region. These unique neural recordings demonstrate that relations between prefrontal neurons that encode and process information between cortical layers via minicolumns are likely relevant factors involved in executive dysfunction in which interlaminar disruption could be the basis for the cognitive impairment as shown recently (Hampson et al., 2011, 2012; Opris et al., 2012). This was verified by the fact that delivery of the appropriate firing pattern with MIMO model derived electrical stimulation in the same L5 neural firing pattern as during successful execution of the MR in the task, improved performance when more distracter images were present (**Figure 7D**). However the fact that MIMO stimulation also facilitated performance by avoiding a different type of error with respect to retaining and implementing the "rule" for the type of trial (*Object* or *Spatial*) being executed (**Figure 7E**), suggests that closing PFC columnar loops activates a process that normally functions to enhance cognitive decision making in NHPs performing tasks that require retention of the contexts in which target selections are made.

ACKNOWLEDGMENTS

We thank Joshua Long, Joseph Noto, Brian Parish, Mack Miller, and Shahina Kozhisseri for their assistance on this project. This work was supported by National Institutes of Health Grants DA06634, DA023573, DA026487 and by Defense Advanced Research Projects Agency (DARPA) contract N66601-09-C-2080 to Sam A. Deadwyler.

REFERENCES

Alexander, G. E., DeLong, M. E., and Strick, P. L. (1986). Parallel organization of functionally segregated circuits linking basal ganglia and cortex. *Ann. Rev. Neurosci.* 9, 357–381.

Baddeley, A. (2002). "Fractionating the central executive," in *Principles of Frontal Lobe Function,* eds D. T. Stuss and R. T. Knight (New York, NY: Oxford University Press), 246–260.

Buffalo, E. A., Fries, P., Landmanc, R., Buschman, T. J., and Desimone, R. (2011). Laminar differences in gamma and alpha coherence in the ventral stream. *Proc. Natl. Acad. Sci. U.S.A.* 108, 11262–11267.

Burmeister, J. J., Coates, T. D., and Gerhardt, G. A. (2004). Multisite microelectrode arrays for measurements of multiple neurochemicals. *Conf. Proc. IEEE Eng. Med. Biol. Soc.* 7, 5348–5351.

Burmeister, J. J., Pomerleau, F., Huettl, P., Gash, C. R., Werner, C. E., Bruno, J. P., et al. (2008). Ceramic-based multisite microelectrode arrays for simultaneous measures of choline and acetylcholine in CNS. *Biosens. Bioelectron.* 23, 1382–1389.

Buxhoeveden, D. P., and Casanova, M. F. (2002). The minicolumn hypothesis in neuroscience. *Brain* 125, 935–951.

Casanova, M. F., Buxhoeveden, D. P., Cohen, M., Switala, A. E., and Roy, E. L. (2002a). Minicolumnar pathology in dyslexia. *Ann. Neurol.* 52, 108–110.

Casanova, M. F., Buxhoeveden, D. P., and Brown, C. (2002b). Clinical and macroscopic correlates of minicolumnar pathology in autism. *J. Child Neurol.* 17, 692–695.

Casanova, M. F., Buxhoeveden, D., and Gomez, J. (2003). Disruption in the inhibitory architecture of the cell minicolumn: implications for autism. *Neuroscientist* 9, 496–507.

Casanova, M. F., Switala, A. E., Trippe, J., and Fitzgerald, M. (2007). Comparative minicolumnar morphometry of three distinguished scientists. *Autism* 11, 557–569.

Casanova, M. F., El-Baz, A., Vanbogaert, E., Narahari, P., and Trippe, J. (2009). Minicolumnar width: comparison between supragranular and infragranular layers. *J. Neurosci. Methods* 184, 19–24.

Deadwyler, S. A., Porrino, L., Siegel, J. M., and Hampson, R. E. (2007). Systemic and nasal delivery of orexin-A (Hypocretin-1) reduces the effects of sleep deprivation on cognitive performance in nonhuman primates. *J. Neurosci.* 27, 14239–14247.

Dudkin, K. N., Chueva, I. V., Arinbasarov, M. U., and Bobkova, N. V. (2003). Organization of working memory processes in monkeys: the effects of a dopamine receptor agonist. *Neurosci. Behav. Physiol.* 33, 387–398.

Felsen, G., Shen, Y. S., Yao, H., Spor, G., Li, C., and Dan, Y. (2002). Dynamic modification of cortical orientation tuning mediated by recurrent connections. *Neuron* 36, 945–954.

Funahashi, S., Bruce, C. J., and Goldman-Rakic, P. S. (1989). Mnemonic coding of visual space in the monkey's dorsolateral prefrontal cortex. *J. Neurophysiol.* 61, 331–349.

Fuqua, J. L., Quintero, J. E., Long, J. L., Noto, J. V., Hampson, R. E., Gerhardt, G. A., et al. (2010). *Electrical Stimulation of Glutamate Release in the Hippocampus. 2010 Neuroscience Meeting Planner.* Program No. 610.8. (Washington, DC: Society for Neuroscience).

Fuster, J. M. (2001). The prefrontal cortex–an update: time is of the essence. *Neuron* 30, 319–333.

Fuster, J. M., and Alexander, G. E. (1971). Neuron activity related to short-term memory. *Science* 173, 652–654.

Goldman-Rakic, P. S. (1996). The prefrontal landscape: implications of functional architecture for understanding human mentation and the central executive. *Philos. Trans. R. Soc. Lond. B Biol. Sci.* 351, 1445–1453.

Graybiel, A. M. (2008). Habits, rituals, and the evaluative brain. *Annu. Rev. Neurosci.* 31, 359–387.

Hampson, R. E., Coates, T. D. Jr., Gerhardt, G. A., and Deadwyler, S.

A. (2004). "Ceramic-based microelectrode neuronal recordings in the rat and monkey," in *Proceedings of the Annual International Conference of the IEEE Engineering in Medicine and Biology Society (EMBS),* (Lexington, KY), 25, 3700–3703.

Hampson, R. E., España, R. A., Rogers, G. A., Porrino, L. J., and Deadwyler, S. A. (2009). Mechanisms underlying cognitive enhancement and reversal of cognitive deficits in nonhuman primates by the ampakine CX717. *Psychopharmacology (Berl.)* 202, 355–369.

Hampson, R. E., Gerhardt, G. A., Marmarelis, V., Song, D., Opris, I., Santos, L. M., et al. (2012). Facilitation and restoration of cognitive function in primate prefrontal cortex by a neuroprosthesis that utilizes minicolumn-specific neural firing. *J. Neural Eng.* 9, 056012.

Hampson, R. E., Porrino, L. J., Opris, I., Stanford, T., and Deadwyler, S. A. (2011). Effects of cocaine rewards on neural representations of cognitive demand in nonhuman primates. *Psychopharmacology (Berl.)* 213, 105–118.

Hansen, B., and Dragoi, V. (2011). Adaptation-induced synchronization in laminar cortical circuits. *Proc. Natl. Acad. Sci. U.S.A.* 108, 10720–10725.

Hascup, K. N., Hascup, E. R., Pomerleau, F., Huettl, P., and Gerhardt, G. A. (2008). Second-by-second measures of L-glutamate in the prefrontal cortex and striatum of freely moving mice. *J. Pharmacol. Exp. Ther.* 324, 725–731.

Hascup, K. N., Hascup, E. R., Stephens, M. L., Glaser, P. E., Yoshitake, T., Mathe, A. A., et al. (2011). Resting glutamate levels and rapid glutamate transients in the prefrontal cortex of the Flinders Sensitive Line rat: a genetic rodent model of depression. *Neuropsychopharmacology* 36, 1769–1777.

Heekeren, H. R., Marrett, S., and Ungerleider, L. G. (2008). The neural systems that mediate human perceptual decision making. *Nat. Rev. Neurosci.* 9, 467–479.

Hong, S., Ratté, S., Prescott, S. A., and De Schutter, E. (2012). Single neuron firing properties impact correlation-based population coding. *J. Neurosci.* 32, 1413–1428.

Kelley, T. A., and Lavie, N. (2011). Working memory load modulates distractor competition in primary visual cortex. *Cereb. Cortex* 21, 659–665.

Kritzer, M. F., and Goldman-Rakic, P. S. (1995). Intrinsic circuit organization of the major layers and sublayers of the dorsolateral prefrontal cortex in the rhesus monkey. *J. Comp. Neurol.* 359, 131–143.

Lund, J. S., Angelucci, A., and Bressloff, P. C. (2003). Anatomical substrates for functional columns in macaque monkey primary visual cortex. *Cereb. Cortex* 13, 15–24.

Meyer, T., Qi, X. L., Stanford, T. R., and Constantinidis, C. (2011). Stimulus selectivity in dorsal and ventral prefrontal cortex after training in working memory tasks. *J. Neurosci.* 31, 6266–6276.

Miller, E. K. (2000). The prefrontal cortex and cognitive control. *Nat. Rev. Neurosci.* 1, 59–65.

Miller, E. K., and Cohen, J. D. (2001). An integrative theory of prefrontal cortex function. *Annu. Rev. Neurosci.* 24, 167–202.

Miyaki, A., Friedman, N., Emerson, M., Witzki, A., Howerter, A., and Wagner, T. (2000). The unity and diversity of executive functions and their contributions to complex frontal lobe tasks: a latenet variable analysis. *Cogn. Psychol.* 41, 49–100.

Mo, J., Schroeder, C. E., and Ding, M. (2011). Attentional modulation of alpha oscillations in macaque inferotemporal cortex. *J. Neurosci.* 31, 878–882.

Mountcastle, V. B. (1997). The columnar organization of the neocortex. *Brain* 120(Pt 4), 701–722.

Mountcastle, V. B. (2003). Introduction. Computation in cortical columns. *Cereb. Cortex* 13, 2–4.

Opris, I., Barborica, A., and Ferrera, V. P. (2005a). Microstimulation of dorsolateral prefrontal cortex biases saccade target selection. *J. Cogn. Neurosci.* 17, 893–904.

Opris, I., Barborica, A., and Ferrera, V. P. (2005b). Effects of electrical microstimulation in monkey frontal eye field on saccades to remembered targets. *Vis. Res.* 45, 3414–3429.

Opris, I., and Bruce, C. J. (2005). Neural circuitry of judgment and decision mechanisms. *Brain Res. Rev.* 48, 509–526.

Opris, I., Hampson, R. E., and Deadwyler, S. A. (2009). The encoding of cocaine vs. natural rewards in the striatum of nonhuman primates: categories with different activations. *Neuroscience* 163, 40–54.

Opris, I., Hampson, R. E., Gerhardt, G. A., Berger, T. W., and Deadwyler, S. A. (2012). Columnar processing in primate prefrontal cortex: evidence for executive control microcircuits. *J. Cogn. Neurosci.* 24, 2334–2347.

Opris, I., Hampson, R. E., Stanford, T. R., Gerhardt, G. A., and Deadwyler, S. A. (2011). Neural activity in frontal cortical cell layers: evidence for columnar sensorimotor processing. *J. Cogn. Neurosci.* 23, 1507–1521.

Pesaran, B., Nelson, M. J., and Andersen, R. A. (2008). Free choice activates a decision circuit between frontal and parietal cortex. *Nature* 453, 406–409.

Porrino, L. J., Daunais, J. B., Rogers, G. A., Hampson, R. E., and Deadwyler, S. A. (2005). Facilitation of task performance and removal of the effects of sleep deprivation by an ampakine (CX717) in nonhuman primates. *PLoS Biol.* 3:e299. doi: 10.1371/journal.pbio.0030299

Posner, M., and Snyder, C. (1975). "Attention and cognitive control," in *Information Processing and Cognition: The Loyola Symposium,* ed R. Solso (Hillsdale, NJ: L. Erlbaum Assoc.), 55–85.

Rao, S. G., Williams, G. V., and Goldman-Rakic, P. S. (1999). Isodirectional tuning of adjacent interneurons and pyramidal cells during working memory: evidence for microcolumnar organization in PFC. *J. Neurophysiol.* 81, 1903–1916.

Resulaj, A., Kiani, R., Wolpert, D. M., and Shadlen, M. N. (2009). Changes of mind in decision-making. *Nature* 461, 263–266.

Quintero, J. E., Day, B. K., Zhang, Z., Grondin, R., Stephens, M. L., Huettl, P., et al. (2007). Amperometric measures of age-related changes in glutamate regulation in the cortex of rhesus monkeys. *Exp. Neurol.* 208, 238–246.

Quintero, J. E., Pomerleau, F., Huettl, P., Johnson, K. W., Offord, J., and Gerhardt, G. A. (2011). Methodology for rapid measures of glutamate release in rat brain slices using ceramic-based microelectrode arrays: basic characterization and drug pharmacology. *Brain Res.* 1401, 1–9.

Riedel, G., Platt, B., and Micheau, J. (2003). Glutamate receptor function in learning and memory. *Behav. Brain Res.* 140, 1–47.

Shallice, T., and Burgess, P. (1996). The domain of supervisory processes and temporal organization of behaviour. *Philos. Trans. R. Soc. Lond. B Biol. Sci.* 351, 1405–1411.

Sokhadze, E. M., Baruth, J. M., Sears, L., Sokhadze, G. E., El-Baz, A. S., and Casanova, M. F. (2012). Prefrontal neuromodulation using rTMS improves error monitoring and correction function in autism. *Appl. Psychophysiol. Biofeedback* 37, 91–102.

Stephens, M. L., Pomerleau, F., Huettl, P., Gerhardt, G. A., and Zhang, Z. (2010). Real-time glutamate measurements in the putamen of awake rhesus monkeys using an enzyme-based human microelectrode array prototype. *J. Neurosci. Methods* 185, 264–272.

Swadlow, H. A., Gusev, A. G., and Bezdudnaya, T. (2002). Activation of a cortical column by a thalamocortical impulse. *J. Neurosci.* 22, 7766–7773.

Takeuchi, D., Hirabayashi, T., Tamura, K., and Miyashita, Y. (2011). Reversal of interlaminar signal between sensory and memory processing in monkey temporal cortex. *Science* 331, 1443–1447.

Tanaka, K. (2003). Columns for complex visual object features in the inferotemporal cortex: clustering of cells with similar but slightly different stimulus selectivities. *Cereb. Cortex* 13, 90–99.

Weiler, N., Wood, L., Yu, J., Solla, S. A., and Shepherd, G. M. (2008). Top-down laminar organization of the excitatory network in motor cortex. *Nat. Neurosci.* 11, 360–366

13

Closed-loop response properties of a visual interneuron involved in fly optomotor control

Naveed Ejaz[1,2]*, Holger G. Krapp[2] and Reiko J. Tanaka[2]

[1] *Institute of Cognitive Neuroscience, University College London, London, UK*
[2] *Department of Bioengineering, Imperial College London, London, UK*

Edited by:
Ahmed El Hady, Max Planck Institute for Dynamics and Self Organization, Germany

Reviewed by:
Michael Nitabach, Yale University School of Medicine, USA
Dierk F. Reiff, Albert-Ludwigs-Universität Freiburg, Germany

Correspondence:
Naveed Ejaz, Institute of Cognitive Neuroscience, University College London, Alexandra House, 17 Queen Square, London WC1N 3AR, UK.
e-mail: n.ejaz@ucl.ac.uk

Due to methodological limitations neural function is mostly studied under open-loop conditions. Normally, however, nervous systems operate in closed-loop where sensory input is processed to generate behavioral outputs, which again change the sensory input. Here, we investigate the closed-loop responses of an identified visual interneuron, the blowfly H1-cell, that is part of a neural circuit involved in optomotor flight and gaze control. Those behaviors may be triggered by attitude changes during flight in turbulent air. The fly analyses the resulting retinal image shifts and performs compensatory body and head rotations to regain its default attitude. We developed a fly robot interface to study H1-cell responses in a 1 degree-of-freedom image stabilization task. Image shifts, induced by externally forced rotations, modulate the cell's spike rate that controls counter rotations of a mobile robot to minimize relative motion between the robot and its visual surroundings. A feedback controller closed the loop between neural activity and the rotation of the robot. Under these conditions we found the following H1-cell response properties: (i) the peak spike rate decreases when the mean image velocity is increased, (ii) the relationship between spike rate and image velocity depends on the standard deviation of the image velocities suggesting adaptive scaling of the cell's signaling range, and (iii) the cell's gain decreases linearly with increasing image accelerations. Our results reveal a remarkable qualitative similarity between the response dynamics of the H1-cell under closed-loop conditions with those obtained in previous open-loop experiments. Finally, we show that the adaptive scaling of the H1-cell's responses, while maximizing information on image velocity, decreases the cell's sensitivity to image accelerations. Understanding such trade-offs in biological vision systems may advance the design of smart vision sensors for autonomous robots.

Keywords: brain machine interface, optomotor control, closed-loop system, blowfly, electrophysiology, optic flow, motion vision

INTRODUCTION

In recent years an increasing interest has emerged to apply biological principles of signal processing and control design to autonomous robotics. An enormous body of behavioral and physiological data accumulated over several decades on how the nervous system, mostly of insects, uses sensory signals for motor control (e.g., review: Taylor and Krapp, 2007) led to a significant growth in biomimetic robotics (Floreano et al., 2009; Srinivasan, 2011; Srinivasan et al., 2012). The major drive for this development comes from two directions: engineers are keen to exploit biology for the design of new robust as well as adaptive sensor and control systems, while neurobiologists are interested in robotics as a tool to validate their experimentally derived functional principles (Webb, 2008; Barth et al., 2012)

A prominent example of the joint venture between neurobiologists and engineers is the application of functional principles of insect vision to guidance, navigation, and control in aerial robotics (Srinivasan et al., 2012). Discoveries on how flies and bees process visual motion information to estimate their self-motion and control their flight has sparked a number of projects where the underlying principles were implemented in autonomous small scale air vehicles (Hyslop and Humbert, 2010; Hyslop et al., 2010). Although most control systems, both in biology and engineering operate under closed-loop conditions, many implementations so far were based on experimental data obtained under open-loop conditions.

Invertebrate animal models are ideally suited for studying the response properties of neural control circuits generating movements under both open- and closed-loop conditions. Specifically, flies display a broad repertoire of visually guided behaviors including gaze and flight stabilization reflexes which can readily be quantified at both the behavioral and the electrophysiological level. Visuo-motor stabilization behaviors or optomotor reflexes have been extensively studied at the behavioral level under both open- and closed-loop conditions (Gotz, 1964, 1968; review: Heisenberg and Wolf, 1993). Correspondingly, a great deal is now known about the open-loop response properties of a population of visual interneurons in flies, the lobula plate tangential cells (LPTCs; review: Krapp and Wicklein, 2008), which contribute to the control of optomotor reflexes (review: Hausen, 1993). However, with only a single exception (Warzecha and Egelhaaf, 1996), studies on LPTC response properties were all carried out under open-loop conditions. The specific involvement of the LPTCs in fly visual stabilization behavior naturally poses the question as to whether or not response dynamics observed under closed-loop conditions are comparable with those measured in open-loop.

Here, we compare the open- and closed-loop response properties of an identified visual interneuron, the H1-cell, which is part of a neural circuit that provides optomotor reflexes in the fly (Haag and Borst, 2001). Specifically, we compare the effect of dynamically changed image velocities and accelerations on the instantaneous spike rate of the cell under open- and closed-loop conditions. We report that the response properties are qualitatively similar under both conditions and discuss the implication of our results in the context of fly optomotor reflexes with respect to potential applications to bio-inspired control design.

MATERIALS AND METHODS

FLY-ROBOT INTERFACE

The closed-loop fly-robot interface (FRI; **Figure 1A**) uses the H1-cell of an immobilized fly, placed in front of two cathode ray tube (CRT) displays, as a sensor that provides an estimate of the horizontal angular velocity of a visual pattern (spatial wavelength $\lambda_{sp} = 11°$, contrast $\approx 100\%$). The spike rate of the H1-cell resulting from pattern motion on the CRT displays was used by closed-loop feedback controllers to regulate the angular velocity of the robot (**Figure 1B**). The robot was positioned on a turntable placed inside a cylindrical arena lined with a vertically oriented grating pattern. The dynamic properties of the robot (Arexx Engineering, ASURO Robot Kit) and the turntable represented the real-world actuator components of the FRI. Relative motion between the robot and the visual pattern forced by movement of the turntable mimicked self-motion of the animal resulting in horizontal pattern shifts. High-speed cameras mounted on the robot captured the visual image shifts at 200 fps and presented it on the visual CRT displays.

ELECTROPHYSIOLOGY RECORDINGS

Experiments were carried out on 2–3 day old female blowflies, *Calliphora vicina*. Each animal was immobilized and its symmetrical deep pseudo-pupil (Franceschini, 1975) was used to align the head with respect to the CRT displays. Two small holes were cut in the right and left part of the animal's rear head capsule for placement of the recording and ground electrodes, respectively.

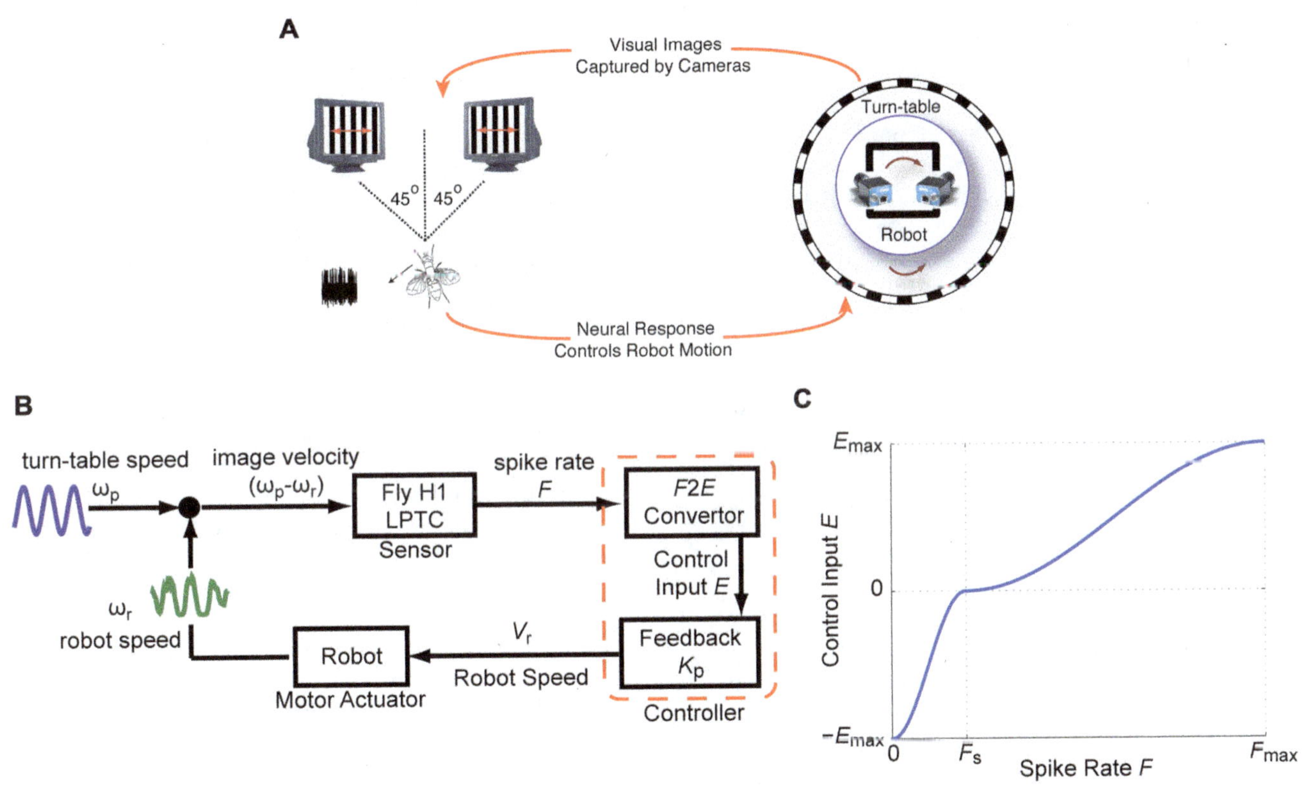

FIGURE 1 | The fly-robot interface (FRI) (A) A fly was placed in front of a visual display consisting of two high-speed CRT displays. Input to the two monitors were provided by two high-speed video cameras mounted on a mobile robot. The robot was positioned on a turntable placed inside a cylindrical arena lined with vertically oriented grating pattern. Robot and turntable movements were limited to rotations around the vertical axis. Visual motion as a result of the rotation of the turntable was captured by the cameras. Electrophysiology recordings from the H1-cell were used to control the rotation of the robot. **(B)** Block diagram of the closed-loop FRI. Relative motion between the turn-table and the robot, ω_p-ω_r, caused spiking in the H1-cell. The responses of the H1-cell (instantaneous spike rate F), were used by a controller to compensate for externally generated turntable movements, by driving the robot in the opposite direction. **(C)** The *F2E* convertor maps F onto the control input E. The piece-wise sigmoid functions, based on which E was used to update the robot speed V_r. (modified from Ejaz et al., 2012).

Tungsten electrodes were used to record the extracellular spike rate of the left H1-cell's telodendritic output arborisation (Krapp et al., 2001) in the right lobula plate. An amplitude threshold was used to digitize the spike times at a resolution of 0.1 ms. The digitized spikes were convolved with a causal half-Gaussian kernel ($\sigma_{fr} = 0.05$ ms) to obtain an estimate of the instantaneous spike rate, F. The instantaneous spike rate, F, is considered to reflect the visual motion ($\omega_p - \omega_r$) under closed-loop conditions and was used as an input for the two closed-loop controllers described in the section below. A video protocol of the fly preparation can be found in Ejaz et al. (2011a).

CLOSED-LOOP CONTROLLERS

For the controller, a non-linear transformation (*F2E* converter) and a feedback gain (K_p) were applied to the instantaneous spike rate, F, in order to obtain an 8-bit value (V_r), which was used to modulate the robot's angular velocity (ω_r; **Figure 1B**). F depends on pattern motion determined by the difference between the turntable and the robot angular velocities. The *F2E* converter converts F into the control input E, based on piece-wise sigmoid functions for $0 \leq F \leq F_S$ and for $F_S \leq F \leq F_{max}$ where F_s and F_{max} represent the spontaneous and maximum spike rates, respectively (**Figure 1C**). $\pm E_{max}$ represents the upper and lower 8-bit values, over which the robot speed is modulated. Using this controller, the robot speed is updated by:

$$V_r(t+1) = K_p \cdot E + V_r(t). \tag{1}$$

Prior to the closed-loop experiments, both F_s (mean ± SE: 19.67 ± 2.3) and F_{max} (mean ± SE: 78 ± 4.27) were determined in open-loop conditions for each fly, using three trails of 5 s stimulation without and with image motion in the preferred direction (PD) of the H1-cell, respectively.

As shown below in more detail, we used two different controllers to close the loop between the visual motion ($\omega_p - \omega_r$) observed by the fly and the instantaneous spiking rate, F, of its H1-cell. The first one is a static gain controller, which consisted of a fixed feedback gain K_p and an *F2E* converter with constant F_{max} (Ejaz et al., 2011a,b). This controller belongs to the class of linear feedback controllers in which the control effort is proportional to the error being controlled for. In our case, the updated robot speed is proportional to the visual motion error (Eq. 1) under closed-loop conditions. Note, that an equivalent proportional controller was previously used by Warzecha and Egelhaaf (1996), to generate a feedback signal based on the differential activity of two H1-cells under closed-loop conditions. In the second controller, the condition of a fixed feedback gain was relaxed in order to obtain an adaptive gain controller. In order to achieve an adaptive feedback gain, every 50 ms, the maximum spike rate, F_{max} is updated over a historical time window of length ΔT_{ws}. Continuously updating F_{max} scaled the sigmoid mapping between F and E during motion in the PD ($F_s \leq F \leq F_{max}$; **Figure 1C**) of the H1-cell, where the updated value for the robot speed was calculated with $K_p = 1$ in Eq. 1. This scaling method provided the basis for the adaptive feedback gain, and was motivated by a neural coding strategy proposed by Laughlin (1994).

Once a value for the updated robot speed is estimated using either controller, it is transmitted to the robot via Bluetooth. As a result, the robot speeds up or down in order to correct for the visual motion error.

CLOSED-LOOP EXPERIMENTS

We carried out two closed-loop experiments using the setup described above.

Constant input with static gain controller

In order to determine the input/output relationship for the H1-cell, we applied a constant angular velocity for 12.5 s set to

$$\omega_p = \begin{cases} 0°/s & \text{for} \quad 0 \leq t < 2.5\,s, \\ 144°/s & \text{for} \quad 2.5\,s \leq t \leq 15\,s, \end{cases} \tag{2}$$

and used the static gain controller to close the loop.

We measured the cell's spike rates (F) and the image velocities ($\omega_p - \omega_r$) for five flies with four different values of K_p, in a total of 111 trials (12 trials for $K_p = 0.01$, 24 trials for $K_p = 0.1$, 15 trials for $K_p = 0.5$, and 60 trials for $K_p = 1.0$) and discretized them at a rate of 100 Hz.

Figure 2A shows the spike rate of the H1 cell plotted against the image velocity. A sigmoid function was fitted (least square fit) to the data shown in the plot:

$$F = \frac{A}{1 + e^{-\beta(\omega_p - \omega_r)}}, \tag{3}$$

where A is the upper asymptote which captures the peak spike rate and β is the growth parameter which determines the slope of the function. We use the fitting parameters A and β to evaluate the effect of different image velocities on the input–output relationship of the H1 cell. Larger values of A correspond to larger peak spike rates the cell generates for a given image velocities over the trial. The value of β specifies the slope of the function. Smaller values of β correspond to shallower and steeper slopes of the function converting image velocity into spike rate.

Sinusoidal input with adaptive gain controller

In order to determine the frequency response of the H1-cell, we applied sinusoidal angular velocities $\omega_p = 72[\sin(2\Pi f_i t) + 1]$ to the closed-loop system, where the input frequency f_i covered a range of $0.03 \leq f_i \leq 1.0$ Hz, and updated the adaptive gain controller based on estimation time windows, $\Delta T_{ws} = [0.05,\ 0.10,\ 0.15]$ ($N = 5$ flies), to close the loop. In previous work, we showed that the adaptive gain controller has a higher cut-off frequency as compared to the static gain controller with the corresponding frequency response gains for the two controllers being approximately equal (Ejaz et al., 2012). The adaptive gain controller was therefore chosen primarily because it allowed us to obtain H1-cell responses over a wider range of frequencies as compared to the static gain controller.

At each input frequency, f_i, the amplitude (power spectral densities) and phase for the H1 input ($\omega_p - \omega_r$), G_i and P_i, and those for the H1 output (spike rate F), G_o and P_o, were calculated using a periodogram. Sequences were pre-multiplied with a Hamming window equal to the length of the sequence. The obtained gain $\left(\frac{G_o}{G_i}\right)$ and phase ($P_o - P_i$) are shown in **Figures 4C,D**, respectively.

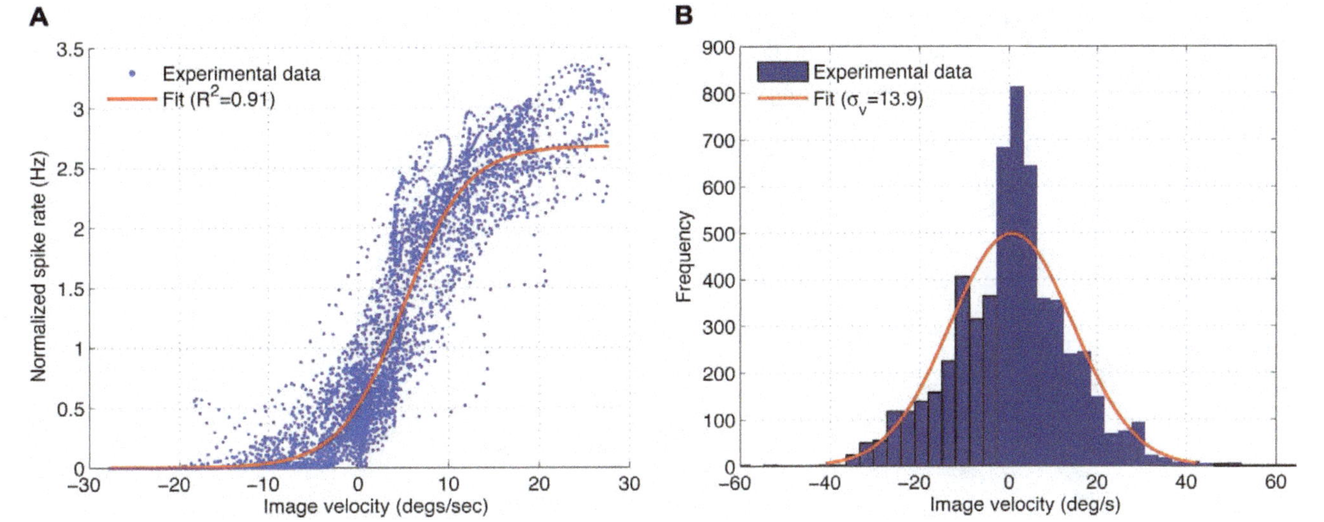

FIGURE 2 | (A) Experimental measurement showing the input–output relationship for the H1-cell under closed-loop conditions (blue) and its least-squares sigmoid fit ($A = 2.68$, $\beta = 0.29$) (red), obtained from the fly robot response with the static gain controller ($K_p = 0.1$) and sinusoidal input ($f_i = 0.03$ Hz). For further explanation see text. **(B)** Distribution of the image velocities observed in closed-loop is approximately Gaussian.

RESULTS

We performed two experiments (described in Materials and Methods) in order to determine whether the responses of the H1-cell were different under open- and closed-loop conditions.

EFFECTS OF THE MOMENTS OF THE IMAGE VELOCITY DISTRIBUTION ON THE H1-CELL INPUT–OUTPUT RELATIONSHIP UNDER OPEN- AND CLOSED-LOOP CONDITIONS

The input–output relationship of the H1 cell, i.e., the relationship between the image velocity (input) and the spike rate (output) was obtained for different gains, K_p, of the static gain controller using a constant angular velocity (**Figure 2A**). Here, the spike rate was normalized by its mean over each trial. The obtained input–output relationship for the H1-cell can be approximated by a sigmoid function, as was suggested by Brenner et al. (2000) for the open-loop experiments, although the variability of the H1-cell response turned out to be much larger under our closed-loop conditions. The highly variable responses are possibly due to the non-stationarity of the image velocity distributions during closed-loop experiments. The image velocities previously used under open-loop conditions by Brenner et al. (2000) and Fairhall et al. (2001) were generated from a normal distribution with zero mean and fixed standard deviation for the duration of each trial, over which the spike rate was measured. In our closed-loop experiments, however, the image velocities observed by the fly depended on the performance of the FRI in minimizing the retinal slip speeds ($\omega_p - \omega_r$). During the course of a closed-loop trial, the performance of the FRI typically varied between perfect image stabilization and short periods of high image velocities. Therefore, while the overall image velocities observed by the fly during a trial are normally distributed (**Figure 2B**), the standard deviation of the image velocities, when calculated over a shorter time interval, are constantly changing during a trial resulting in a highly variable input–output relationship of the H1-cell (**Figure 2A**).

To characterize the H1-cell response under closed-loop conditions, we initially measured the first (mean μ_v) and second (standard deviation σ_v) moments of the input, i.e., the image velocity observed by the fly (**Figure 3A**). Increasing the feedback gain K_p monotonically increases both μ_v and σ_v. The increase in σ_v can be explained by control oscillations particularly pronounced for high feedback gains (Ejaz et al., 2011a). Such control oscillations are not specific to the FRI, but have also been observed as yaw torque fluctuations during closed-loop optomotor tasks in *Drosophila* (Mayer, 1989; Wolf and Heisenberg, 1990; Warzecha and Egelhaaf, 1996). The increase in μ_v can be explained by the fact that we use a single H1-cell for closed-loop control. Ideally, a fly would attempt to maintain optomotor equilibrium by balancing clockwise and counter-clockwise rotations so that the observed image motion is minimized. The two H1-cells would contribute sensitivity to motion in opposing directions based on which the optomotor equilibrium is maintained. However, when a single H1-cell is used for closed-loop control, the optomotor equilibrium is un-balanced which in turn leads to an increased value of μ_v. An un-balanced optomotor equilibrium does not, however, seem to have drastic behavioral consequences for the fly. In a behavioral study, Kern and Egelhaaf (2000) occluded one eye in *Lucilia* and measured the turning responses in both freely flying and walking flies inside a visual arena. The authors concluded that it was hard to tell from the turning responses that the fly had been limited to the use of monocular vision and that while the flies exhibited a slight turning preference toward the stimulated eye (i.e., increased μ_v), no such asymmetry could be observed in individual responses. As a result, while increasing μ_v decreases the overall performance of image stabilization under closed-loop, it does not affect the conclusions that can be drawn regarding the response properties of the H1-cell.

After characterizing the input to the H1-cell by its standard deviation and mean, we investigated the effect of σ_v on the cell's

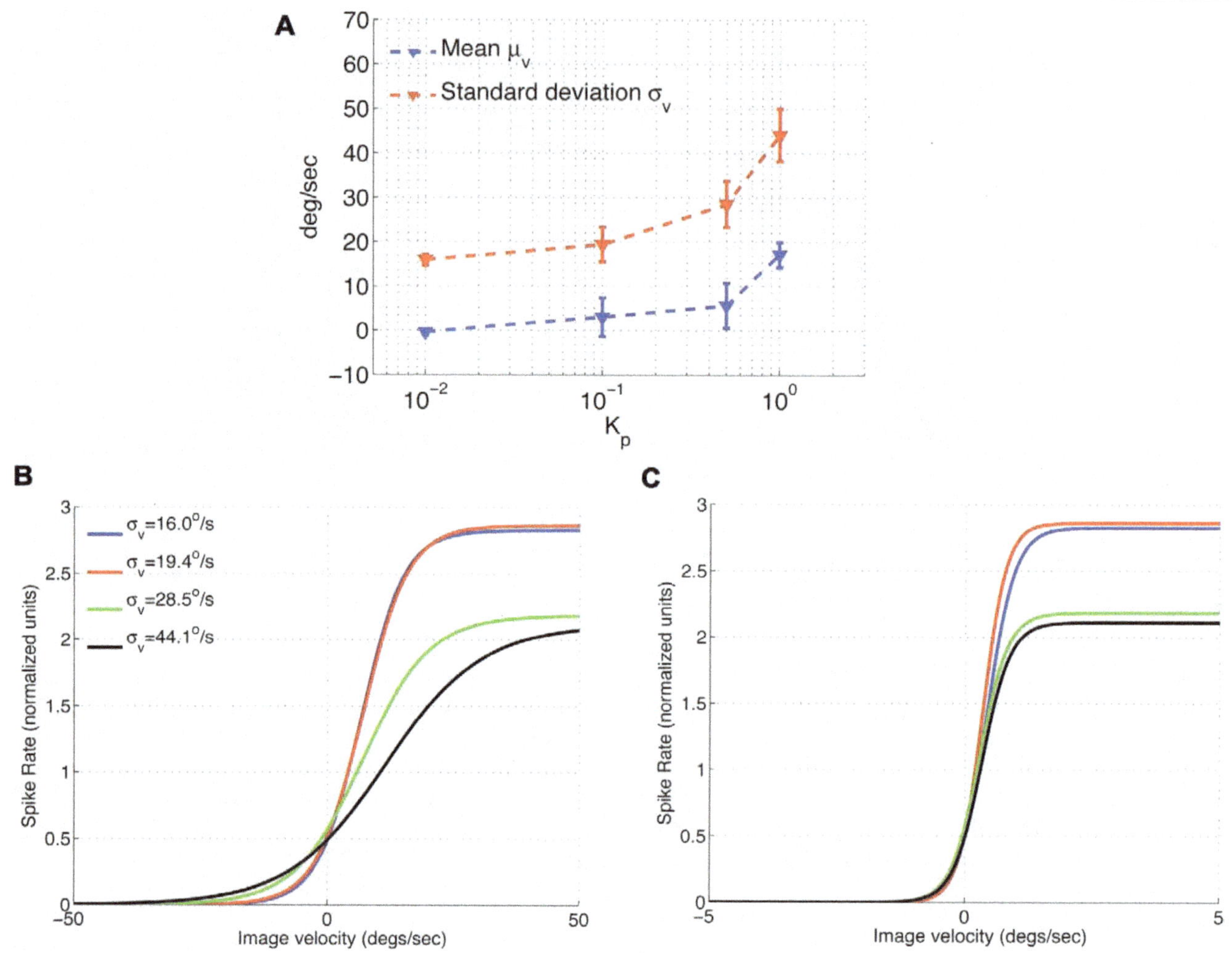

FIGURE 3 | Effect of the image velocity mean and standard deviation on the adaptive scaling properties of the H1-cell response function (A) Mean and standard deviation of the H1 input (slip speed). (B) The fitted H1-cell response functions adapts to accommodate the increased standard deviation of the image velocities **(C)** Normalizing the image velocities in **(B)** by their corresponding standard deviations results in response functions with similar slopes (around $\sigma_V = 0$ deg/s). The respective peak spike rates (normalized), however, remain unchanged.

response properties. Its input–output relationship has previously been shown in open-loop measurements to adapt to the standard deviation, σ_V, of the input image velocity distribution (Brenner et al., 2000; Fairhall et al., 2001). Large values of σ_V cause the input–output function to expand along the *x*-axis (image velocity) leading to a shallower slope, i.e., smaller value for β, for the response function. In comparison, small values of σ_V cause compression along the velocity axis resulting in a steeper slope for the response function and consequently a higher value for β. Our experiments show that the response function also scales in proportion to the standard deviation of the image velocity under closed-loop conditions (**Figures 3B,C**). As reported by Brenner et al. (2000) for open-loop condition, normalizing the input–output relationship by the standard deviation removes differences in cell's adaptation properties under closed-loop condition as well (**Figure 3C**).

Note however, that this normalization does not change the peak spike rate, *A*, in our closed-loop experiments (**Figure 3C**), suggesting that the peak spike rate of the H1-cell may be controlled by another moment of the image velocity distribution, possibly its mean. Further open-loop experiments on the H1-cell have shown that increasing either the mean (Reisenman et al., 2003) or the standard deviation (Borst et al., 2005) of the image velocity results in a decrease of its peak spike rate. In our closed-loop experiments, an approximate 2-fold increase in the standard deviation (from $\sigma_V = 16.0$ deg/s to $\sigma_V = 28.5$ deg/s) results in a spike rate deduction of approximately 18% (**Figure 3C**). Such a decrease is larger than it would be predicted for an increased standard deviation under open-loop conditions (Borst et al., 2005). This suggests that the peak spike rate of the H1-cell under closed-loop conditions depends on both the mean and the standard deviation of the image velocity.

The effects of the moments of the input distribution on the spike rate of the H1-cell for the open- and closed-loop conditions are highly similar in that (i) the H1-cell response is adjusted to the standard deviation of the image velocity and (ii) the H1-cell decreases its peak spike rate when mean and standard deviation of the image velocity distribution are increased.

EFFECTS OF INCREASING IMAGE ACCELERATIONS ON THE GAIN OF THE H1-CELL RESPONSE UNDER OPEN- AND CLOSED-LOOP CONDITIONS

In the second experiments, we induced sinusoidal angular velocity perturbations into the closed-loop system, while varying the length of the spike rate estimation time window ΔT_{ws} for the adaptive gain controller. For each trial, the resulting closed-loop image velocities (**Figure 4A**) and H1-cell spike rates were recorded to investigate the cell's frequency response.

The gain of the H1-cell decreased linearly with increasing input frequencies, with a gradient of approximately 8–9 dB/dec (**Figure 4B**). The linear decrease in gain with frequency did not, by and large, depend on the time window ΔT_{ws} for the adaptive controller. The corresponding phase (**Figure 4C**) of the H1-cell decreased from approximately 35° at a frequency of $f_i = 0.03$ Hz to around 0° for $f_i > 0.03$ Hz.

We are tempted to argue here that, under closed-loop conditions, the frequency-dependent decrease of the H1-cell response gain (**Figure 4C**) is related to the increase in image acceleration. For the sinusoidal image velocity perturbations we used in the second experiment, the increase in the input frequency, f_i, leads to an increase in the image acceleration. Therefore, the gain plot of the H1-cell (**Figure 4B**) represents the relationship between the cell's spike rate and the image accelerations under closed-loop conditions and suggests that the response gain of the cell decreases for increasing image acceleration. Such an approximately linear decrease in response gain of the cell with increasing accelerations was also observed under open-loop conditions (Borst et al., 2005).

The effects of increasing the frequency on the moments of the image velocity distribution are shown in **Figures 4D,E**. As the frequency increased, σ_V increased from around 28° to 46°/s (**Figure 4D**) and the peak spike rate decreased (**Figure 4E**). Actually, the decrease in the peak spike rate is largely the result of the increase in σ_V, as the corresponding mean (μ_V) of the image velocities is very close to 0°/s for the frequency range we examined (**Figure 4D**). It should be noted that increasing σ_V is equivalent to increasing the image velocity amplitudes and therefore produces higher image accelerations, which in turn decreases the response gain of the cell.

DISCUSSION

THE FRI AS A CLOSED-LOOP EXPERIMENTAL SYSTEM

The use of a robotic controller to understand animal behavior provides real-world physical interactions typically missing from modeling studies where a low-pass filter is used to describe the dynamics of the fly flight motor system. As argued by Webb (2006), this lack of physical interaction would mean that complex motion dynamics such as slipping due to friction cannot be accounted for in the computer model. Indeed, recent work by Dickson et al. (2010) showed that both body-inertia and -damping play a significant role in the dynamics of saccadic yaw turns in *Drosophila* flight. While the configuration of the fly in such a closed-loop experimental setup is far removed from conditions during natural flight, the stimulus velocity distributions observed by the fly in the FRI are within range of those used in previous measurements of the H1 cell under open-loop conditions (Warzecha and Egelhaaf, 1996; Brenner et al., 2000; Borst, 2003; Borst et al., 2005).

While H1-cell responses have been studied extensively under open-loop conditions (e.g., Maddess and Laughlin, 1985; Brenner et al., 2000; Borst, 2003; Reisenman et al., 2003), this paper presents the first study of the cell's response properties for a variety of image velocity profiles under closed-loop conditions. Our FRI was used to generate dynamic visual stimuli, i.e., sinusoidal and constant image velocity perturbations to drive the responses of the H1-cell.

In a pioneering study, Warzecha and Egelhaaf (1996) obtained electrophysiology recordings from both the ipsi- and the contralateral H1 LPTC's while the fly compensated for externally imposed visual motion under closed-loop conditions. In that study, however, comparatively small and constant image velocities (18) were used and thus there was little or no modulation of the image accelerations presented to the H1-cells. As a result Warzecha and Egelhaaf (1996) characterized the cell's closed-loop responses only for a rather narrow velocity profile, compared to the dynamic visual stimuli generated by our FRI. While they found the responses of the cell to decrease as the image velocity increased which is in agreement with our findings – they did not observe the dependence of the H1-cell responses on image accelerations we report here.

A limitation of our experiments was that only the activity of one H1-cell had been considered for closed-loop control. During walking and free-flight, a fly receives information about its yaw rotation from both the ipsi- and the contra-lateral H1-cells. Using only the activity of a single cell for visual stabilization reduced the fly's sensitivity to yaw rotations. Given that the peak spike rate of the H1-cell has been found to decrease strongly with an increase of the mean image velocity, in both open- (Reisenman et al., 2003) and closed-loop (**Figure 3B**) measurements, one key function of two H1-cells could be to keep the fly in optomotor equilibrium by trying to minimize the mean image velocity. Such a strategy of minimizing the mean image velocity would remove any restrictions on the peak spike rate of the cell. This in turn would be advantageous as the fly would remain sensitive to differences in image velocities as opposed to absolute values, which appears to be a general feature of biological sensing (Taylor and Krapp, 2007).

Our results with the FRI show that the open- and closed-loop responses are qualitatively similar, in the sense that the H1-cell maximizes the information transmitted about the image velocity distribution by adapting its input–output relationship (Brenner et al., 2000; **Figures 3B,C**). We found in addition that higher image acceleration, as a result of increased standard deviation of the image velocity distribution, decreases the gain of the H1-cell. It is important to note that this dependence is not the result of the dynamic properties of the robot or the turntable. This is because the decrease in the H1-cell response gain is too large (8–9 dB), even for small changes in acceleration (between 0.03 and 0.3 Hz), to be explained by the frequency response of either the robot or the turntable (Ejaz et al., 2011b, 2012).

In the following we will discuss our findings in more detail with an emphasis on coding of visual motion information optomotor control and the translation of closed-loop results into biomimetic applications.

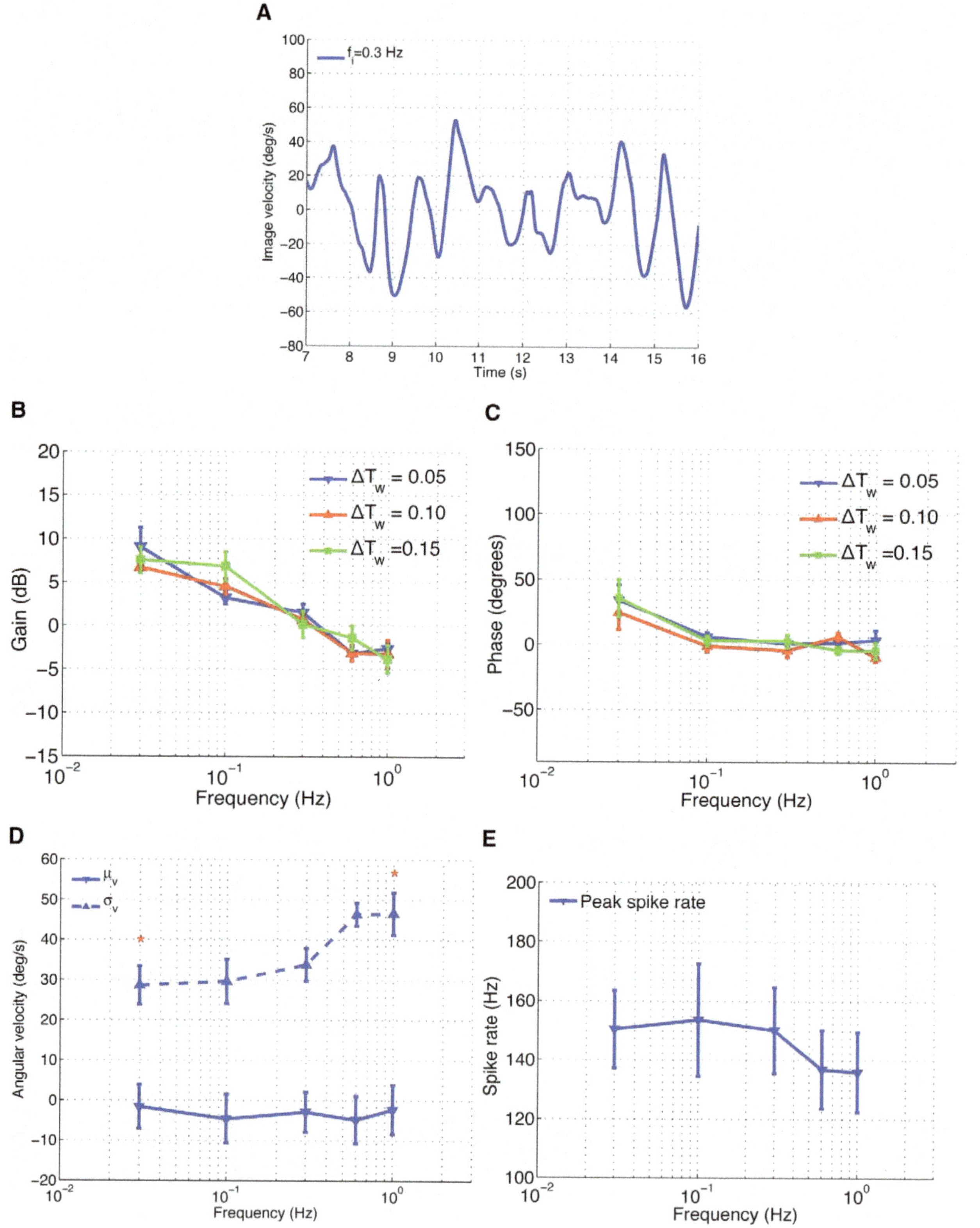

FIGURE 4 | H1-cell frequency response. (A) An example time course data of image velocity observed by the fly for an input frequency $f_i = 0.3$ Hz. The gain **(B)** and phase **(C)** plots over different input frequencies. **(D)** The mean (μ_V) and standard deviation (σ_V) of the image velocities. *Values of σ_V for $f_i = 0.3$ Hz and $f_i = 1.0$ Hz are significantly different (calculated using Wilcoxon rank-sum method with $\alpha = 0.001$). **(E)** Peak spike rate (*) for different input frequencies.

THE DECREASE IN THE RESPONSE GAIN FOR INCREASING IMAGE ACCELERATION IS A DIRECT CONSEQUENCE OF THE ADAPTIVE SCALING PROPERTY OF H1

A key finding of our closed-loop experiments we report here, is that the decrease in sensitivity to image accelerations is a direct result of the H1-cell's adaptive scaling property. To the extent of our knowledge, this relationship has not been explicitly highlighted previously in open-loop measurements and is discussed below.

Figure 5 shows how the H1 cell decreases its sensitivity to acceleration by scaling its response range to fit that of a wider image velocity distribution. Increasing the standard deviation of the image velocities results in a decrease in the gradient, β, of the cells input–output function (**Figures 5A,B**). This decrease in β directly results in a linear decrease in the peak acceleration sensitivity of the cell (**Figures 5C,D**). Furthermore, this decrease in sensitivity to acceleration is linear. The adaptive re-scaling of the H1-cell responses which maximizes information transfer, apparently comes at the expense of a reduced sensitivity to image acceleration. It is tempting to speculate that the trade-off between maximizing information transmission related to the input image velocity and the reduced sensitivity to acceleration might reflect a more general strategy preferred during the evolution of sensory systems. While in the visual system a decreased sensitivity to acceleration might be partly compensated for by signals from other sensory modalities (e.g., the halteres), a decrease in information transmission would be detrimental for the neural representation of visual motion. Given that neurons are required to process information under very strict energy constraints (Laughlin et al., 1998; Laughlin, 2001), inefficiencies in neural coding might come at a high evolutionary cost. In addition, inefficient coding at the sensory system level will most certainly propagate downstream to produce inadequate motor outputs. Altogether, a loss of acceleration sensitivity as a result of adaptive re-scaling might be a comparatively small cost to pay.

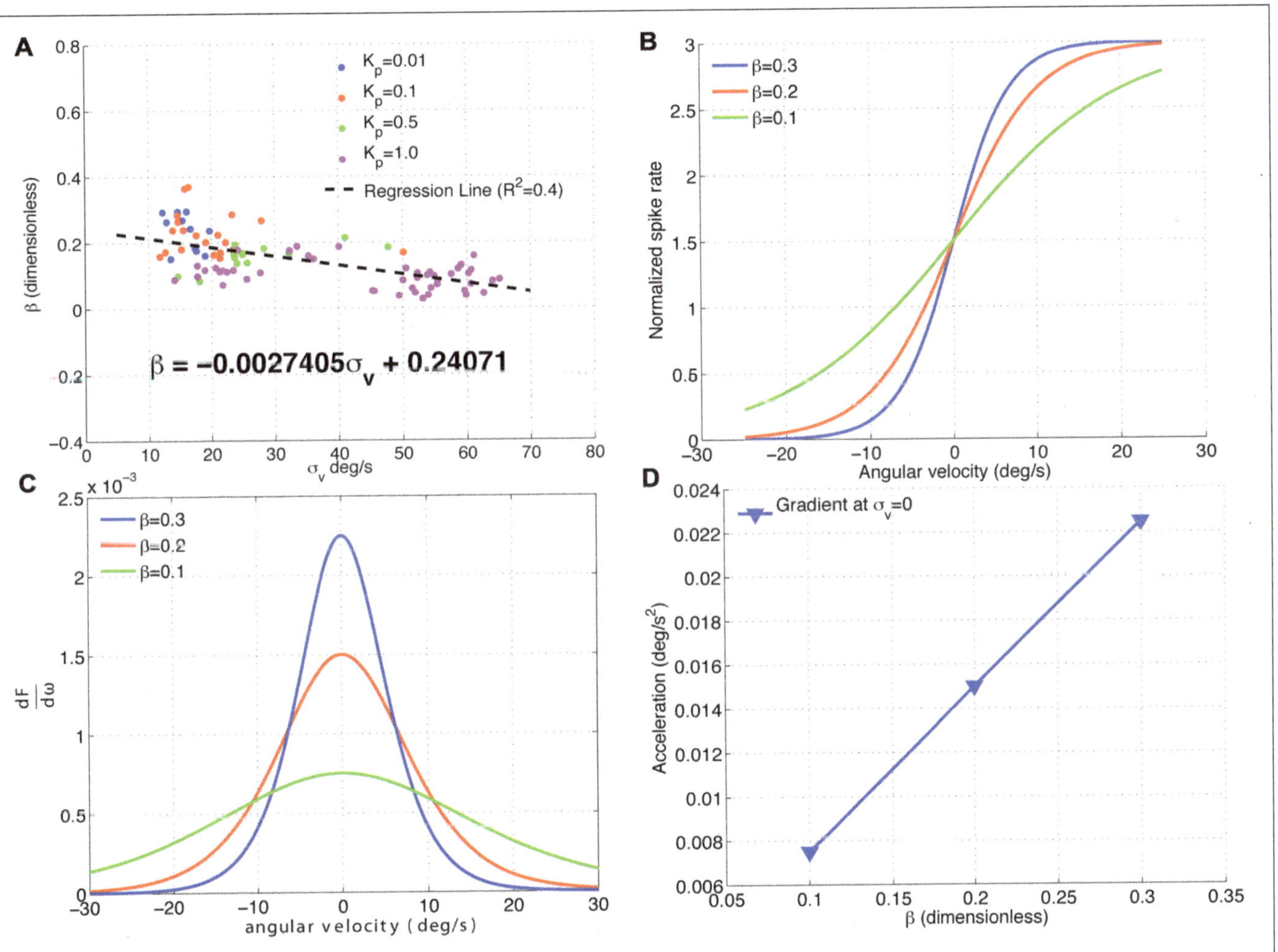

FIGURE 5 | Effect of σ_V on the acceleration sensitivity of the H1-cell. **(A)** The fitted values of β for the proportional controller with gain K_p are plotted against the standard deviation of the velocity distribution, σ_V. Increasing σ_V linearly decreases β as per the relationship specified by the regression line. **(B)** The input–output functions for three different values of β (normalized by the peak spike rate, *F*) show that **(C)** decreasing beta linearly decreases the gradient at the point $\sigma_V = 0$ deg/s **(D)** and this decrease is linear. This reduction in gradient of the H1-cell input–output function represents a decrease in sensitivity to changes in the image velocity i.e., a decrease in sensitivity to image acceleration. The results show that increasing σ_V directly decreases the sensitivity of the H1-cell to image accelerations.

The dependence of the H1-cell frequency response on image acceleration is also found to be qualitatively similar for open- and closed-loop studies. In earlier work, Brenner et al. (2000) showed that the altering the image velocity or acceleration resulted in a modulation of the responses of the H1 cell under open-loop conditions. In subsequent studies open-loop studies, the gain of the H1 cell was proposed to depend on acceleration and other higher-order time derivatives of image velocity (Borst, 2003; Borst et al., 2005). Specifically, the responses of the H1 cell decreased as a result of increasing image accelerations, which is also what we report under closed-loop conditions (**Figure 5**).

Our results also show that the acceleration sensitivity of the H1-cell is highest while there is little or no pattern motion ($\sigma_V = 0^\circ/s$, **Figure 6C**). This is clearly advantageous for the fly, as it enables the H1-cell to respond more quickly to image motion that rapidly changes from null direction to PD, as Lewen et al. (2001) proposed earlier.

While maintaining a high sensitivity to acceleration, i.e., high value of β, might make sense intuitively, it comes with potential risks. An input–output response function with a high value of β means that very small changes in angular velocity result in large changes of spike rate. β therefore partly determines the forward gain in the motion vision pathway of the system. The potential risk, however, is that with a high forward gain in combination with inherent noise in the system may easily drive the responses of downstream neural circuits into saturation. Additionally, if the feedback gain (on top of the forward gain of the H1 cell) is too high and control delays are too long, then the feedback control

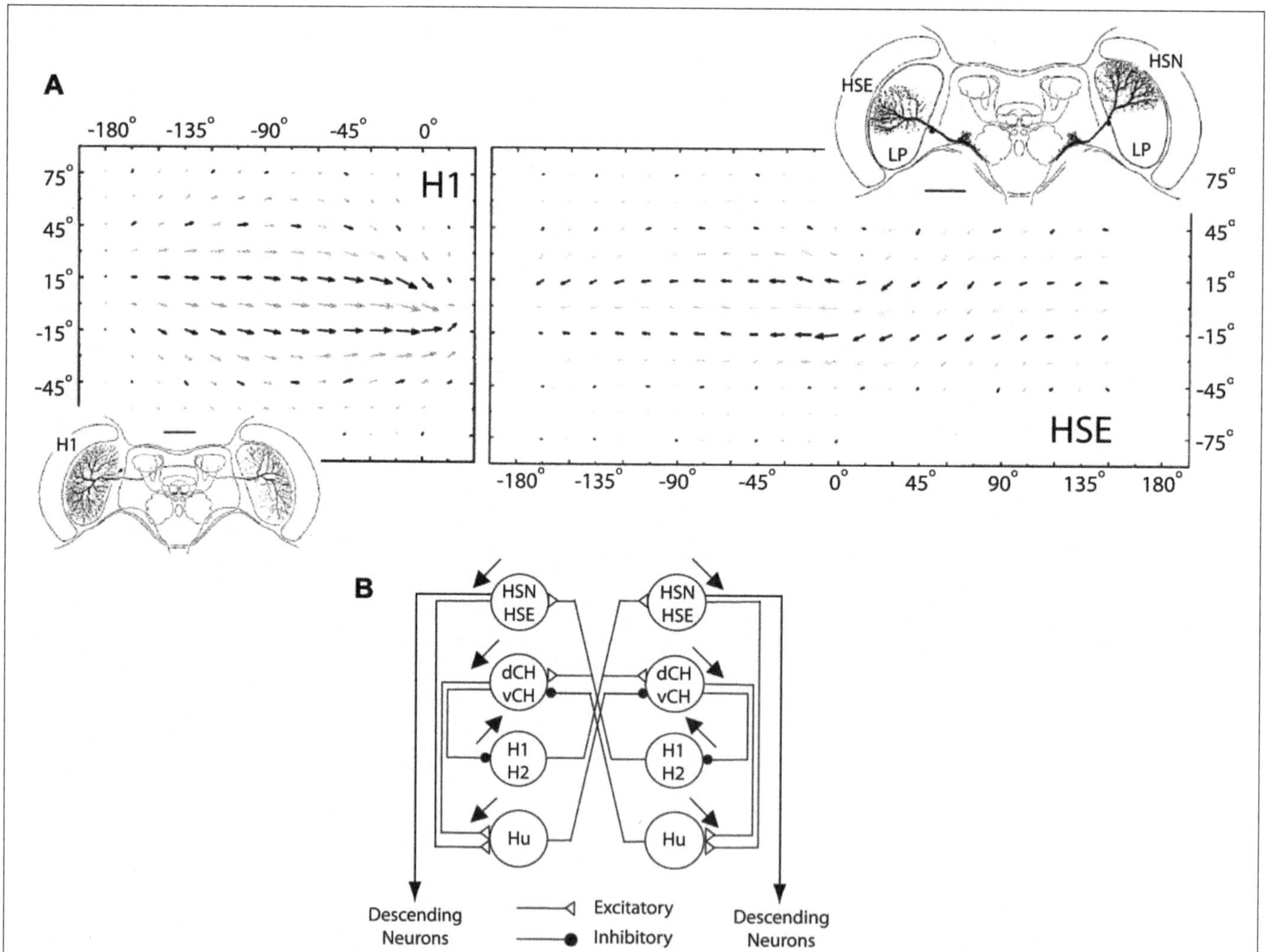

FIGURE 6 | H1 and HSE receptive fields and horizontal network connections. (A) Top row shows monocular and binocular receptive fields of the H1 and the HSE LPTCs, respectively. The insets show the dendritic arborization patterns of both cells in the left lobula plate as well as the HSN LPTC in the right lobula plate. The dendritic input arbourizations and the telo-dendritic output arborizations of the H1 cell are connected via a thin axon that transmits visual motion information from the left to the right lobula plate using action potentials. The HSE and the HSN cells arborize in the equatorial and the north sections of the lobula plate, respectively (modified from Krapp et al., 2001). **(B)** The connectivity in the network of LPTCs sensitive to horizontal motion. Excitatory and inhibitory interactions are depicted with open triangles and filled circles, respectively. The HSE and HSN cells receive excitatory input from the contralateral H1 and H2 cells and project onto descending neurons which in turn supply the neck and flight motor systems of the fly (modified from Krapp et al., 2001).

system is in danger of becoming instable. In this context, decreasing sensitivity to acceleration by having a lower response gain for increasing frequencies is possibly advantageous from a control theoretic point of view and this argument is discussed in the following section.

SIMILARITY IN H1-CELL RESPONSES UNDER OPEN- AND CLOSED-LOOP CONDITIONS AND ITS IMPLICATIONS FOR OPTOMOTOR CONTROL

As a hetero-lateral neuron, the H1 cell helps disambiguate between rotation- and translation-induced optic flow as it is completely inhibited during forward translation but excited during yaw rotations. The cell also provides excitatory input to the HSE and HSN cells (**Figure 6**), two major output neurons of the visual system that respond to visual motion with a graded modulation of their membrane potential (Hausen, 1976, 1982). By connecting to the contralateral HSE and HSN cells, it makes the response of these output cells more specific to yaw rotation. Therefore, the response properties and connectivity of the H1 cell make it an important neuron in the optomotor pathway of the fly.

It is by no means trivial that the response of the H1-cell to the moments of the image velocity distribution (mean, standard deviation, acceleration), are highly similar under open- and closed-loop conditions. This similarity may reflect the way in which the sensory-motor control loops are organized in the fly.

One particular model of the sensory-motor control loop in the fly proposed by Warzecha and Egelhaaf (1996) and Borst et al. (2005) does not require sensory feedback to explain the non-linear response properties of the H1-cell. In this model, the non-linear properties of the H1-cell and the LPTCs in general, can be predicted solely based on the properties of the Reichardt (1987) elementary movement detector (EMD). Warzecha and Egelhaaf (1996) suggested that the reduced gain of the H1-cell at higher image velocities is the result of intrinsic response properties of EMDs. Similarly, Borst et al. (2005) showed that an EMD model could explain the dependence of the H1-cell responses to the standard deviation and the autocorrelation time constant of the image velocities. In both cases, no feedback signals were required to explain the non-linear response properties of the H1-cell, which were suggested to be based on the computational structure of the EMD model. This particular model of control architecture is closely linked to that proposed by Wehner (1987) who argued that architecture and response properties of invertebrate sensory systems reflect a detailed model of the physical world. If the model is true, no feedback signals are necessary and H1-cell responses under closed-loop are simply the result of EMD properties, readily observable under open-loop conditions.

An alternate control architecture involves forward models, in which a copy of a motor command (efference copy) is used to subtract those components of the sensory feedback that are due to the animal's own action (Chan et al., 1998; Wolpert and Ghahramani, 2000; reviews: Webb, 2004; Krapp and Wicklein, 2008). Forward models or efference copies have been proposed to explain the mechanism by which flies adjust their gain parameters when faced with unexpected visual feedback during an optomotor task inside a flight simulator (Kirschfeld, 1989). One possible explanation for the similarity of the H1-cell responses under open and closed-loop conditions could be that in fully restrained animals an efference copy from the motor system may not be sent to the LPTCs. Our FRI did not allow us to assess the potential impact of an efference copy signal. Even though the fly was under closed-loop conditions, it was immobilized for the purpose of obtaining electrophysiology recordings which makes it unlikely that the animal would have generated motor commands similar to those under free flight conditions. At this point, we can only speculate on which control architecture, i.e., with or without feedback control at the level of the LPTCs, best explains the similarity in H1-cell responses as measured under open- and closed-loop conditions.

Finally, in the context of optomotor control, the frequency response of the H1-cell (**Figures 4C** and **5D**) imposes certain limitations on fly's ability to compensate for externally imposed yaw rotations. For the visual system to contribute to the stabilization of visual motion, the reduction of gain and cut-off frequency of the horizontal cells in the lobula plate must be higher than those of the flight muscles which produce compensatory torque. The response delay in the motion vision pathway ($\approx$30 ms) for the fly is long compared to other sensory systems like the ocelli ($\approx$15 ms) and the halteres ($\approx$10 ms) (Taylor and Krapp, 2007). It would therefore make sense for the cell's response not to have a high gain at high frequencies that would potentially result in instabilities of the control system as initially proposed by Warzecha and Egelhaaf (1996). A low gain at high frequencies would be in agreement with the proposed primary function of LPTCs to mainly compensate for slow drifts (Collett et al., 1993). In comparison, the halteres and the ocelli, with their short response delays, would be better suited to control yaw rotations in the higher dynamic range. The importance of keeping delays to a minimum within the optomotor control loop, and in biological control loops, in general (Dickson et al., 2010), is also evidenced by our finding that the response phase of the H1-cell stays close to zero over the tested frequency range.

The surprising qualitative similarity between closed- and open-loop data suggest that it is reasonable, in instance first approximation, to base any implementations of fly inspired (optomotor) control design on experimental open-loop data. This could potentially expedite the translation of biological design principles in technical applications as methodologically more challenging closed-loop experiments may not always be required to conclusively characterize the dynamics of neuronal responses. It should be noted, however, that the present study focused only on a 1 DoF visual stabilization task. Neuronal closed- and open-loop activity supporting multisensory control of higher dimensional tasks may as well show very different response dynamics – in particular if observed in freely or semi-freely moving animals.

ACKNOWLEDGMENTS

We would like to thank K.D. Longden and K.D. Peterson for helping with the electrophysiology experiments; K.D. Longden, M. Wicklein, and D.A. Schwyn for helpful discussions on the work in this manuscript. Research was supported by the Higher Education Commission Pakistan Fellowship to Naveed Ejaz, US Airforce Research Labs [grant FA 8655-09-1-3022] grant to Holger G. Krapp, and an EPSRC Career Acceleration Fellowship to Reiko J. Tanaka.

REFERENCES

Barth, F., Humphrey, J. A., and Srinivasan, M. V. (2012). *Frontiers in Sensing: From Biology to Engineering*. Heidelberg: Springer.

Borst, A. (2003). Noise, not stimulus entropy, determines neural information rate. *J. Comput. Neurosci.* 14, 23–31.

Borst, A., Flanagin, V. L., and Sompolinsky, H. (2005). Adaptation without parameter change: dynamic gain control in motion detection. *Proc. Natl. Acad. Sci. U.S.A.* 102, 6172–6176.

Brenner, N., Bialek, W., and van Steveninck, R. D. R. (2000). Adaptation rescaling maximizes information transmission. *Neuron* 26, 695–702.

Chan, W. P., Prete, F., and Dickinson, M. H. (1998). Visual input to the efferent control system of a fly's "gyroscope". *Science* 280, 289–292.

Collett, T., Nalbach, H., and Wagner, H. (1993). "Visual stabilization in arthropods," in *Visual Motion and its Role in the Stabilization of Gaze*, eds F. A. Miles and J. Wallman (Amsterdam: Elsevier), 239–263.

Dickson, W. B., Polidoro, P., Tanner, M. M., and Dickinson, M. H. (2010). A linear systems analysis of the yaw dynamics of a dynamically scaled insect model. *J. Exp. Biol.* 213, 3047–3061.

Ejaz, N., Peterson, K. D., and Krapp, H. G. (2011a). An experimental platform to study the closed-loop performance of brain-machine interfaces. *J. Vis. Exp.* 10, 3791.

Ejaz, N., Tanaka, R. J., and Krapp, H. G. (2011b). "Closed-loop performance of a proportional controller for visual stabilization using a fly-robot interface," in *IEEE International Conference on Robotics and Biomimetics (ROBIO)*, December 7–11, 2011, Karon Beach, 1509–1515.

Ejaz, N., Tanaka, R. J., and Krapp, H. G. (2012). "Static versus adaptive gain control strategy for visuo-motor stabilization," in *Living Machine 2012: The International Conference on Biomimetic and Biohybrid Systems*, Vol. 7375, eds T. J. Prescott, N. F. Lepora, A. Mura, and P. F. M. J. Verschure (Berlin: Springer), 107–119.

Fairhall, A. L., Lewen, G. D., Bialek, W., and Ruyter van Steveninck, R. R. D. (2001). Efficiency and ambiguity in an adaptive neural code. *Nature* 412, 787–792.

Floreano, D., Zufferey, J. C., Srinivasan, M. V., Ellington, C. (eds). (2009). *Flying Insects and Robots*. Berlin: Springer-Verlag.

Franceschini, N. (1975). "Sampling of the visual environment by the compound eye of the fly: fundamentals and applications," in *Photoreceptor Optics*, eds A. W. Snyder and R. Menzel (Berlin: Springer), 98–125.

Gotz, K. G. (1964). Optomotorische untersuchung des visuellen systems einiger augenmutanten der fruchtfliege *Drosophila*. *Kybernetik* 77–92.

Gotz, K. G. (1968). Flight control in *Drosophila* by visual perception of motion. *Kybernetik* 4,199–208.

Haag, J., and Borst, A. (2001). Recurrent network interactions underlying flow-field selectivity of visual interneurons. *J. Neurosci.* 21, 5685–5692.

Hausen, K. (1976). Functional characterisation and anatomical identification of motion sensitive neurones in the lobula plate of the blowfly *Calliphora erythrocephala*. *Z Naturforsch* 31, 629–633.

Hausen, K. (1982). Motion sensitive interneurons in the optomotor system of the fly. II. The horizontal cells: receptive field organization and response characteristics. *Biol. Cybern.* 46, 67–79.

Hausen, K. (1993). "Decoding of retinal image flow in insects," in *Reviews of Oculomotor Research: Visual motion and its role in the stabilisation of gaze*, eds F. A. Miles and J. Wallman (Amsterdam: Elsevier), 203–235.

Heisenberg, M., and Wolf, R. (1993). "The sensory-motor link in motion dependent flight control of flies" in *Visual Motion and its Role in the Stabilization of Gaze* eds F. A. Miles and J. Wallman (Amsterdam: Elsevier), 265–283.

Hyslop, A., Krapp, H. G., and Humbert, J. S. (2010). A control theoretic interpretation of directional motion preferences in optic flow processing interneurons. *Biol. Cybern.* 103, 353–364.

Hyslop, A. M., and Humbert, J. S. (2010). Autonomous navigation in 3-D urban environments using wide field integration of optic flow. *J. Guid. Control Dyn.* 33, 147–159.

Kern, R., and Egelhaaf, M. (2000). Optomotor course control in flies with largely asymmetric visual input. *J. Comp. Physiol.* 186, 45–55.

Kirschfeld, K. (1989). Automatic gain control in movement detection of the fly: implica- tions for optomotor responses. *Naturwis* 76, 378–380.

Krapp, H. G., Hengstenberg, R., and Egelhaaf, M. (2001). Binocular contributions to optic flow processing in the fly visual system. *J. Neurophysiol.* 85, 724–734.

Krapp, H. G., and Wicklein, M. (2008). "Central processing of visual information in insects," in *The Senses: A Comprehensive Reference*, eds R. Masland and T. D. Albright (San Diego: Academic Press), 131–204.

Laughlin, S. B. (1994). Matching coding, circuits, cells, and molecules to signals – general principles of retinal design in the fly's eye. *Prog. Retin. Eye Res.* 13, 165–196.

Laughlin, S. B. (2001). Energy as a constraint on the coding and processing of sensory information. *Curr. Opin. Neurobiol.* 11, 475–480.

Laughlin, S. B., van Steveninck, R. D. R., and Anderson, J. C. (1998). The metabolic cost of neural information. *Nat. Neurosci.* 1, 36–41.

Lewen, G. D., Bialek, W., and Ruyter van Stevenick, R. R. D. (2001). Neural coding of naturalistic motion stimuli. *Network* 12, 317–329.

Maddess, T., and Laughlin, S. B. (1985). Adaptation of the motion-sensitive neuron H1 is generated locally and governed by contrast frequency. *Proc. R. Soc. Lond. B Biol. Sci.* 225, 251–275.

Mayer, M. (1989). *Raumliche und zeitliche integration von bewegungsinformatiiomn visuellenf lugsystemv on Drosophila melanogaster. modellentwicklunagu f der grundlagev on verhaltens-versuchen.* Doctoral dissertation, Universität Würzburg, Würzburg.

Reichardt, W. (1987). Evaluation of optical motion information by movement detectors. *J. Comp. Physiol.* 161, 533–547.

Reisenman, C., Haag, J., and Borst, A. (2003). Adaptation of response transients in fly motion vision I: Experiments. *Vis. Res.* 43, 1291–1307.

Srinivasan, M. V. (2011). Honeybees as a model for the study of visually guided flight, navigation, and biologically inspired robotics. *Physiol. Rev.* 91, 413–460.

Srinivasan, M. V., Moore, R. J. D., Thurrowgood, S., Soccol, D., and Bland, D. (2012). "From biology to engineering: insect vision and applications to robotics," in *Frontiers in Sensing: From Biology to Engineering*, eds F. G. Barth, J. A. C. Humphrey, and M. V. Srinivasan (Berlin: Springer-Verlag), 19–39.

Taylor, G. K., and Krapp, H. G. (2007). Sensory systems and flight stability: what do insects measure and why? *Adv. Insect Physiol.* 34, 231–316.

Warzecha, A. K., and Egelhaaf, M. (1996). Intrinsic properties of biological motion detectors prevent the optomotor control system from getting unstable. *Philos. Trans. R. Soc. Lond. B Biol. Sci.* 351, 1579–1591.

Webb, B. (2004). Neural mechanisms for prediction: do insects have forward models. *Trends Neurosci.* 5, 278–282.

Webb, B. (2006). Validating biorobotic models. *J. Neural Eng.* 3, 25–35.

Webb, B. (2008). Automatic gain control in movement detection. *Adv. Study Behav.* 38, 1–58

Wehner, R. (1987). Matched filters: neural models of the external world. *J. Comp. Phys. A* 161, 511–531.

Wolf, R., and Heisenberg, M. (1990). Visual control of straight flight in Drosophila melanogaster. *J. Comp. Physiol. A* 167, 269–283.

Wolpert, D. M., and Ghahramani, Z. (2000). Computational principles of movement neuroscience. *Nat. Neurosci.* 3, 1212–1217.

14

Learning and exploration in action-perception loops

Daniel Y. Little*[1] *and Friedrich T. Sommer*[2]

[1] *Department of Molecular and Cell Biology, Redwood Center for Theoretical Neuroscience, University of California, Berkeley, CA, USA*
[2] *Redwood Center for Theoretical Neuroscience, Helen Wills Neuroscience Institute, University of California, Berkeley, CA, USA*

Edited by:
Ahmed El Hady, Max Planck Institute for Dynamics and Self Organization, Germany

Reviewed by:
Richard Hahnloser, ETH University Zurich, Switzerland
Rava Azeredo Da Silveira, Ecole Normale Supérieure, France

****Correspondence:***
Friedrich T. Sommer, Redwood Center for Theoretical Neuroscience, Helen Wills Neuroscience Institute, University of California, 575A Evans Hall, MC #3198, Berkeley, CA 94720-3198, USA.
e-mail: fsommer@berkeley.edu

Discovering the structure underlying observed data is a recurring problem in machine learning with important applications in neuroscience. It is also a primary function of the brain. When data can be actively collected in the context of a closed action-perception loop, behavior becomes a critical determinant of learning efficiency. Psychologists studying exploration and curiosity in humans and animals have long argued that learning itself is a *primary* motivator of behavior. However, the theoretical basis of learning-driven behavior is not well understood. Previous computational studies of behavior have largely focused on the control problem of maximizing acquisition of rewards and have treated learning the structure of data as a *secondary* objective. Here, we study exploration in the absence of external reward feedback. Instead, we take the quality of an agent's learned internal model to be the primary objective. In a simple probabilistic framework, we derive a Bayesian estimate for the amount of information about the environment an agent can expect to receive by taking an action, a measure we term the predicted information gain (PIG). We develop exploration strategies that approximately maximize PIG. One strategy based on value-iteration consistently learns faster than previously developed reward-free exploration strategies across a diverse range of environments. Psychologists believe the evolutionary advantage of learning-driven exploration lies in the generalized utility of an accurate internal model. Consistent with this hypothesis, we demonstrate that agents which learn more efficiently during exploration are later better able to accomplish a range of goal-directed tasks. We will conclude by discussing how our work elucidates the explorative behaviors of animals and humans, its relationship to other computational models of behavior, and its potential application to experimental design, such as in closed-loop neurophysiology studies.

Keywords: knowledge acquisition, information theory, control theory, machine learning, behavioral psychology, computational neuroscience

1. INTRODUCTION

Computational models of exploratory behavior have largely focused on the role of exploration in the acquisition of external rewards (Thrun, 1992; Kaelbling et al., 1996; Sutton and Barto, 1998; Kawato and Samejima, 2007). In contrast, a consensus has emerged in behavioral psychology that learning represents the primary drive underlying explorative behaviors (Archer and Birke, 1983; Loewenstein, 1994; Silvia, 2005; Pisula, 2009). The computational principles underlying learning-driven exploration, however, have received much less attention. To address this gap, we introduce here a mathematical framework for studying how behavior affects learning and develop a novel model of learning-driven exploration.

Machine learning techniques for extracting the structure underlying sensory signals have often focused on passive learning systems that can not directly affect the sensory input. Exploration, in contrast, requires actively pursuing useful information and can only occur in the context of a closed action-perception loop. Learning in closed action-perception loops differs from passive learning both in terms of "what" is being learned as well as "how" it is learned (Gordon et al., 2011). In particular, in closed action-perception loops:

1. Sensorimotor contingencies must be learned.
2. Actions must be coordinated to direct the acquisition of data.

Sensorimotor contingencies refer to the causal role actions play on the sensory inputs we receive, such as the way visual inputs change as we shift our gaze or move our head. They must be taken into account to properly attribute changes in sensory signals to their causes. This tight interaction between actions and sensation is reflected in the neuroanatomy where sensory-motor integration has been reported at all levels of the brain (Guillery, 2005; Guillery and Sherman, 2011). We often take our implicit understanding of sensorimotor contingencies for granted, but in fact they must be learned during the course of development (the exception being contingencies for which we are hard-wired by evolution). This is eloquently expressed in the explorative behaviors of young infants (e.g., grasping and manipulating objects during proprioceptive exploration and then bringing them into visual view during intermodal exploration) (Rochat, 1989; O'Regan and Noë, 2001; Noë, 2004).

Not only are actions part of "what" we learn during exploration, they are also part of "how" we learn. To discover what is inside an unfamiliar box, a curious child must open it. To learn about the world, scientists perform experiments. Directing the acquisition of data is particularly important for embodied agents whose actuators and sensors are physically confined. Since the most informative data may not always be accessible to a physical sensor, embodiment may constrain an exploring agent and require that it coordinates its actions to retrieve useful data.

In the model we propose here, an agent moving between discrete states in a world has to learn how its actions influence its state transitions. The underlying transition dynamics is governed by a Controllable Markov Chain (CMC). Within this simple framework, various utility functions for guiding exploratory behaviors will be studied, as well as several methods for coordinating actions over time. The different exploratory strategies are compared in their rate of learning and how well they enable agents to perform goal-directed tasks.

2. METHODS

2.1. MATHEMATICAL FRAMEWORK FOR EMBODIED ACTIVE LEARNING

CMCs are a simple extension of Markov chains that incorporate a control variable for switching between different transition distributions in each state, e.g., (Gimbert, 2007). Formally, a CMC is a 3-tuple $(\mathscr{S}, \mathscr{A}, \Theta)$ where:

- $\mathscr{S}$ is a finite set of *states* (here representing, the possible locations of an agent in its world) $N = |\mathscr{S}|$.
- $\mathscr{A}$ is a finite set of control values, or *actions*, an agent can choose from $M = |\mathscr{A}|$.
- Θ is a 3-dimensional *CMC kernel* describing the transition probabilities between states for each action (for example, the probability an agent moves from an *originating state* s to a *resultant state* s' when it chooses action a):

$$p(s'|a, s; \Theta) = \Theta_{ass'}$$
$$\Theta_{as\cdot} \in \Delta_{N-1} \quad (1)$$

Here, Δ_{N-1} denotes the standard $(N-1)$-simplex and is used to constrain Θ to describing legitimate probability distributions:

$$\Delta_{N-1} := \{(x_0, x_1, \ldots, x_{N-1}) \in \mathbb{R}^N | \sum_{i=0}^{N-1} x_i = 1 \text{ and } x_i \geq 0 \; \forall i\}$$

CMCs provides a simple mathematical framework for modeling exploration in embodied action-perception loops. At each time step, an exploring agent is allowed to select any action $a \in \mathscr{A}$. This action, along with the agent's current state, then determines which transition distribution its next state is drawn from. For this study, we will make the simplifying assumption that the states can be directly observed by the agent, i.e., the system is not hidden. Since we are interested in the role behavior plays in learning about the world, we consider the exploration task of the agent to be the formation of an accurate estimate, or *internal model* $\widehat{\Theta}$, of the true CMC kernel that describes its *world* Θ.

This framework captures the two important roles actions play in embodied learning. First, transitions depend on actions, and actions are thus a constituent part of "what" is being learned. Second, an agent's immediate ability to interact with and observe the world is limited by its current state. This restriction models the *embodiment* of the agent, and actions are "how" an agent can overcome this constraint on accessing information. Our primary question will be how action policies can optimize the speed and efficiency of learning in embodied action-perception loops as modeled by CMCs.

2.2. INFORMATION-THEORETIC ASSESSMENT OF LEARNING

Following Pfaffelhuber (1972), we define *missing information* $\mathrm{I_M}$ as a measure of the inaccuracy of an agent's internal model. To compute $\mathrm{I_M}$, we first calculate the Kullback–Leibler (KL) divergence of the internal model from the world for each transition distribution:

$$\mathrm{D_{KL}}(\Theta_{as\cdot} \| \widehat{\Theta}_{as\cdot}) := \sum_{s'=1}^{N} \Theta_{ass'} \log_2 \left(\frac{\Theta_{ass'}}{\widehat{\Theta}_{ass'}}\right) \quad (2)$$

The KL-divergence is an information-theoretic measure of the difference between two distributions. Specifically, Equation (2) gives the expected number of bits that would be lost if observations (following the true distribution) were communicated using an encoding scheme optimized for the estimated distribution (Cover and Thomas, 1991). It is large when the two distributions differ greatly and zero when they are identical. Next, missing information is defined as the unweighted sum of the KL-divergences:

$$\mathrm{I_M}(\Theta \| \widehat{\Theta}) := \sum_{s \in \mathscr{S}, a \in \mathscr{A}} \mathrm{D_{KL}}(\Theta_{as\cdot} \| \widehat{\Theta}_{as\cdot}) \quad (3)$$

We will use missing information to assess learning under different explorative strategies. Steeper decreases in missing information over time represent faster learning and thus more efficient exploration. The definition of missing information and those of several other relevant terms that will be introduced later in this manuscript have been compiled into **Table 1** for easy reference.

2.3. BAYESIAN INFERENCE LEARNING

As an agent acts in its world, it observes the state transitions and can use these observations to update its internal model $\widehat{\Theta}$. Taking a Bayesian approach, we assume the agent models its world Θ as a random variable $\boldsymbol{\Theta}$ with an initial *prior distribution* f over the space of possible CMC structures, $\mathscr{W} = \Delta_{N-1}^{NM}$. There is no standard nomenclature for tensor random variables and we will therefore use a bold upright theta $\boldsymbol{\Theta}$ to denote the random variable and a regular upright theta Θ to denote an arbitrary realization of this random variable. Thus, $f(\Theta)$ describes the exploring agent's initial belief that Θ accurately describes its world, i.e., that $\boldsymbol{\Theta} = \Theta$. By Bayes' theorem, an agent can calculate a posterior belief on the structure of its world from its prior and any data it has collected, $\vec{\mathrm{d}}$:

$$f(\Theta|\vec{\mathrm{d}}) = \frac{p(\vec{\mathrm{d}}|\Theta)f(\Theta)}{p(\vec{\mathrm{d}})} \quad (4)$$

Bayes' theorem decomposes the posterior distribution of the CMC kernel into the likelihood function of the data, $p(\vec{\mathrm{d}}|\Theta)$, and the prior, $f(\Theta)$. The normalization factor is calculated by

Table 1 | Table of measures.

Name used here, abbreviation (Equation)	Name used in (References)	Mathematical expression
Missing information, I_M (3)	Missing information (Pfaffelhuber, 1972)	$\sum_{s,a} D_{KL}(\Theta_{as\cdot} \| \widehat{\Theta}_{as\cdot})$
Information gain, I_G (6)		$I_M(\Theta \| \widehat{\Theta}) - I_M(\Theta \| \widehat{\Theta}^{a,s \to s^*})$
Predicted information gain, PIG (7)	Information gain (Nelson, 2005)	$\sum_{s^*} \widehat{\Theta}_{ass^*} D_{KL}(\widehat{\Theta}^{a,s \to s^*}_{as\cdot} \| \widehat{\Theta}_{as\cdot})$
Posterior expected information gain, PEIG (17)	KL-divergence (Storck et al., 1995)	$D_{KL}(\widehat{\Theta}^{\text{current}}_{as\cdot} \| \widehat{\Theta}^{\text{past}}_{as\cdot})$
Predicted mode change, PMC (11)	Probability gain (Nelson, 2005)	$\sum_{s^*} \widehat{\Theta}_{ass^*} \left[\max_{s'} \widehat{\Theta}^{a,s \to s^*}_{ass'} - \max_{s'} \widehat{\Theta}_{ass'}\right]$
Predicted L_1 change, PLC (12)	Impact (Nelson, 2005)	$\sum_{s^*} \widehat{\Theta}_{ass^*} \left[\frac{1}{N} \sum_{s'} \left|\widehat{\Theta}^{a,s \to s^*}_{ass'} - \widehat{\Theta}_{ass'}\right|\right]$

integrating the numerator over $\mathscr{W}$:

$$p(\vec{d}) = \int_{\mathscr{W}} p(\vec{d}|\Theta) f(\Theta) d\Theta$$

We now formulate a Bayesian estimate by directly calculating the posterior belief in transitioning to state s' from state s under action a:

$$\begin{aligned} \widehat{\Theta}_{ass'} &:= p(s'|a, s, \vec{d}) = \int_{\mathscr{W}} p(s', \Theta|a, s, \vec{d}) d\Theta \\ &= \int_{\mathscr{W}} p(s'|a, s; \Theta) f(\Theta|\vec{d}) d\Theta \\ &= \int_{\mathscr{W}} \Theta_{ass'} f(\Theta|\vec{d}) d\Theta = \mathrm{E}_{\boldsymbol{\Theta}|\vec{d}}[\Theta_{ass'}] \end{aligned} \tag{5}$$

For discrete priors the above integrals would be replaced with summations. Equation (5) demonstrates that the Bayesian estimate is simply the expectation of the random variable given the data. While other estimates are possible for inferring world structure, such as Maximum Likelihood, the Bayesian estimate is often employed to avoid over-fitting (Manning et al., 2008). Moreover, as the following theorem demonstrates, the Bayesian estimate is optimal under our minimum missing information objective function.

Theorem 1. *Consider a CMC random variable* $\boldsymbol{\Theta}$ *modeling the ground truth environment* Θ *and drawn from a prior distribution* f. *Given a history of observations* $\vec{d}$, *the expected missing information between* $\boldsymbol{\Theta}$ *and an agent's internal model* Φ *is minimized by the Bayesian estimate* $\Phi = \widehat{\Theta}$. *That is:*

$$\widehat{\Theta} := \mathrm{E}_{\boldsymbol{\Theta}|\vec{d}}[\boldsymbol{\Theta}] = \arg\min_{\Phi} \mathrm{E}_{\boldsymbol{\Theta}|\vec{d}}\left[\mathrm{I}_M(\boldsymbol{\Theta} \| \Phi)\right]$$

Proof. See Appendix A1

The exact analytical form for the Bayesian estimate will depend on the prior distribution. We emphasize that the utility of the Bayesian estimate rests on the accuracy of its prior. In the discussion, we will address issues deriving from uncertain or inaccurate prior beliefs, but for now will provide the agents with priors that match the generative process by which we create new worlds for the agents to explore.

2.4. THREE TEST ENVIRONMENTS FOR STUDYING EXPLORATION

In the course of exploration, the data an agent accumulates will depend on both its behavioral strategy as well as the structure of its world. We reasoned that studying diverse environments, i.e., CMCs that differ greatly in structure, would allow us to investigate how world structure effects the relative performance of different exploratory strategies and to identify action policies that produce efficient learning under broad conditions. We thus constructed and considered three classes of CMCs that differ greatly in structure: Dense Worlds, Mazes, and 1-2-3 Worlds. Dense Worlds are randomly generated from a uniform distribution over all CMCs with $N = 10$ states and $M = 4$ actions (see **Figure A1** in Appendix). They therefore represent very unstructured worlds. Mazes, in contrast, are highly structured and model moving between rooms of a 6-by-6 maze (see **Figure 1**). The state space in mazes consist of the $N = 36$ rooms. The $M = 4$ actions correspond to the noisy translations in the four cardinal directions. To make the task of learning in mazes harder, 30 transporters are randomly distributed amongst the walls which lead to a randomly chosen absorbing state (concentric rings in **Figure 1**). While perhaps not typically abundant in mazes, absorbing states, such as at the bottom of a gravity well, are common in real world dynamics. Finally, 1-2-3 Worlds differ greatly from both Dense Worlds and Mazes in that their transitions are drawn from a discrete distribution rather than a continuous one (see **Figure A2** in Appendix). Since our work is heavily rooted in the Bayesian approach, the consideration of worlds with a different priors was an important addition to understanding the dependency of an exploration strategy on these priors. 1-2-3 Worlds consist of $N = 10$ states and $M = 3$ actions. In a given state, action $a = 1$ moves the agent deterministically to a single target state, $a = 2$ moves the agent with probability 0.5 to one of two target states, and $a = 3$ moves the agent with probability 0.333 to one of three potential target states. The Appendix contains detailed information on the generative distributions used to create examples from each class of environments and also provides the analytical form for the Bayesian estimate in each world (see Appendix A2).

3. RESULTS

3.1. ASSESSING THE INFORMATION-THEORETIC VALUE OF PLANNED ACTIONS

The central question to be addressed in this manuscript is how behavior affects the learning process in embodied action-perception loops. The fast reduction of missing information

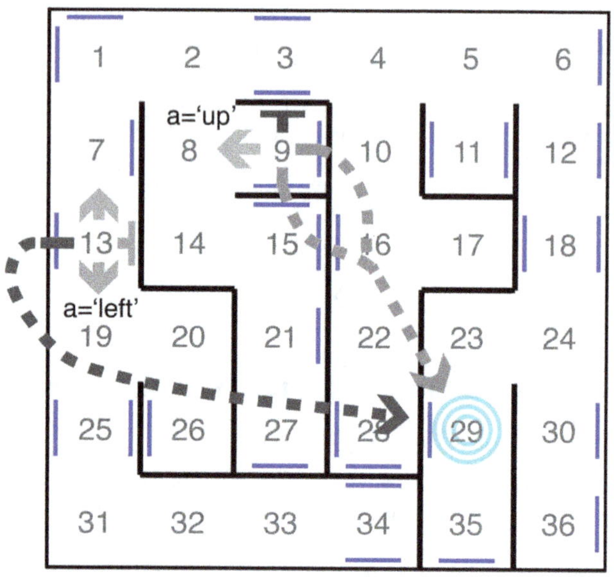

FIGURE 1 | Example maze. The 36 states correspond to rooms in a maze. The four actions correspond to noisy translations in the cardinal directions. Two transition distributions are depicted, each by a set of four arrows emanating from their originating states. Flat-headed arrows represent translations into walls, resulting in staying in the same room. Dashed arrows represent translation into a portal (blue lines) leading to the absorbing state (blue target). The shading of an arrow indicates the probability of the transition (darker color represents higher probability).

is taken to be the agent's objective during learning-driven exploration (Equation 3). As discussed in section 2.3, the Bayesian estimate minimizes the expected missing information and thus solves the inference problem. The control problem of choosing actions to learn quickly nevertheless remains to be solved. We now show that Bayesian inference can also be used to predict how much missing information will be removed by an action. We call the decrease in missing information between two internal models the *information gain* (I_G). Letting $\widehat{\Theta}$ be a current model derived from data $\vec{d}$ and $\widehat{\Theta}^{a,s\to s^*}$ be an updated model after observing a transition from s to s^* under action a, the information gain for this observation is:

$$I_G(a, s, s^*) := I_M(\Theta \| \widehat{\Theta}) - I_M(\Theta \| \widehat{\Theta}^{a,s\to s^*}) = \sum_{s'} \Theta_{ass'} \log_2 \frac{\widehat{\Theta}^{a,s\to s^*}_{ass'}}{\widehat{\Theta}_{ass'}} \quad (6)$$

An exploring agent cannot compute I_G directly because it depends on the true CMC kernel Θ. It also cannot know the outcome s^* of an action until it has taken it. We therefore again take the Bayesian approach introduced in section 2.3 and consider the agent to treat Θ and s^* as random variables. Then, by calculating the expected value of I_G, we show in Theorem 2 that an agent can compute an estimate of information gain from its prior belief on Θ and the data it has collected. We term this estimate the *predicted information gain* (PIG).

Theorem 2. *If an agent is in state s and has previously collected data $\vec{d}$, then the expected information gain for taking action a is given by:*

$$\mathrm{PIG}(a, s) := E_{s^*,\Theta|\vec{d}}[I_G(a, s, s^*)] = \sum_{s^*} \widehat{\Theta}_{ass^*} D_{KL}(\widehat{\Theta}^{a,s\to s^*}_{as\cdot} \| \widehat{\Theta}_{as\cdot}) \quad (7)$$

Proof. See Appendix A3

PIG has an intuitive interpretation. In a sense the agent imagines the possible outcomes s^* of taking action a in state s. It then determines how each of these results would hypothetically change its internal model $\widehat{\Theta}^{a,s\to s^*}$. It compares these new hypothetical models to its current model by computing the KL-divergence between them. The larger this difference the more information the agent would likely gain if it indeed transitioned to state s^*. Finally, it averages these hypothetical gains according to the likelihood of observing s^* under its current model.

For each class of environments, **Figure 2** compares the average PIG with the average realized information gain as successive observation are used to update a Bayesian estimate. In accordance with Theorem 2, in all three environments PIG accurately predicts the average information gain. Thus, theoretically and empirically, PIG represents an accurate estimate of the improvement an agent can expect in its internal model if it takes a planned action in a particular state.

Interestingly, the expression on the RHS of Equation (7) has been previously studied in the field of Psychology where it was introduced *ad hoc* to describe human behavior during hypothesis testing (Klayman and Ha, 1987; Oaksford and Chater, 1994; Nelson, 2005). To our knowledge, its equality to the predicted gain in information (Theorem 2) is novel. In a later section, we will compare PIG to other measures proposed in the field of Psychology.

3.2. CONTROL LEARNERS: UNEMBODIED AND RANDOM ACTION

Before introducing and assessing the performance of different explorative strategies, we first develop positive and negative controls. A naive strategy would be to select actions uniformly randomly. Such random policies are often employed to encourage exploration in reinforcement learning models. We will use a *random action* strategy as a negative control exhibiting the baseline learning rate of an undirected explorer.

An *unembodied* agent that achieves an upper bound on expected performance serves as a positive control. Unlike an embodied agent, the unembodied control is allowed, at every time step, to relocate itself to any state it wishes. For such an agent, optimization of learning decomposes into an independent sampling problem (Pfaffelhuber, 1972). Since the PIG for each transition distribution decreases monotonically over successive observations (**Figure 2**), learning by an unembodied agent can be optimized by always sampling from the state and action pair with the highest PIG. Thus, learning can be optimized in a greedy fashion:

$$(a, s)_{\mathrm{Unemb.}} := \arg\max_{(a,s)} \mathrm{PIG}(a, s) \quad (8)$$

Comparing the learning performances of the random action and unembodied control (red and black curves, respectively in **Figure 3**) we find a notable difference among the three classes of environments. The performance margin between these two controls is significant in Mazes and 1-2-3 Worlds ($p < 0.001$), but not in Dense Worlds ($p > 0.01$). Despite using a naive strategy, the random actor is essentially reaching maximum performance in Dense Worlds, suggesting that exploration of this environment is fairly easy. In contrast, in Mazes and 1-2-3 Worlds, a directed exploration strategy may be necessary to reach learning speeds closer to the unembodied upper bound.

3.3. EXPLORATION STRATEGIES BASED ON PIG

PIG represents a utility function that can be used to guide exploration. Since greedy maximization of PIG is optimal for the unembodied agent, one might expect a similar strategy to be promising for an embodied agent. Unlike the unembodied control, however, the embodied agent [PIG(greedy)] would only be able to select its action, not its state:

$$a_{\mathrm{PIG(greedy)}} := \arg\max_{a} \mathrm{PIG}(a, s) \tag{9}$$

The performance comparison between PIG(greedy) (Equation 9) and the positive control (Equation 8) is of particular interest because they differ only in that one is embodied while the other is not. As shown in **Figure 4** the performance difference is largest in Maze worlds, moderate though significant in 1-2-3 Worlds and smallest in Dense Worlds ($p < 0.001$ for Mazes and 1-2-3 Worlds, $p > 0.001$ for Dense Worlds). To quantify the embodiment constraint faced in a world, we define an *embodiment index* as the relative difference between the areas under the learning curves for PIG(greedy) and the unembodied control. The average embodiment indices for Dense Worlds, Mazes, and 1-2-3 Worlds are 0.02, 2.59, and 1.27, respectively.

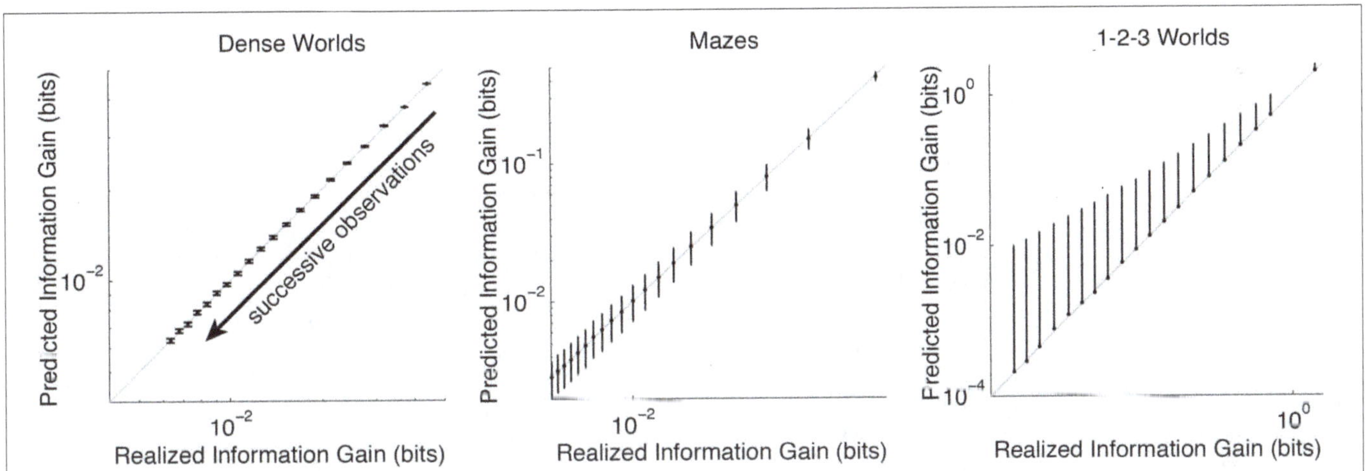

FIGURE 2 | Accuracy of predicted information gain. The average predicted information gain is plotted against the average realized information gain. Averages are taken over 200 CMCs, $N \times M$ transition distributions, and 50 trials. Error bars depict standard deviations (only plotted above the mean for 1-2-3 Worlds). The arrow indicates the direction of increasing numbers of observations (top-right = none, bottom-left = 19). The unity lines are drawn in gray.

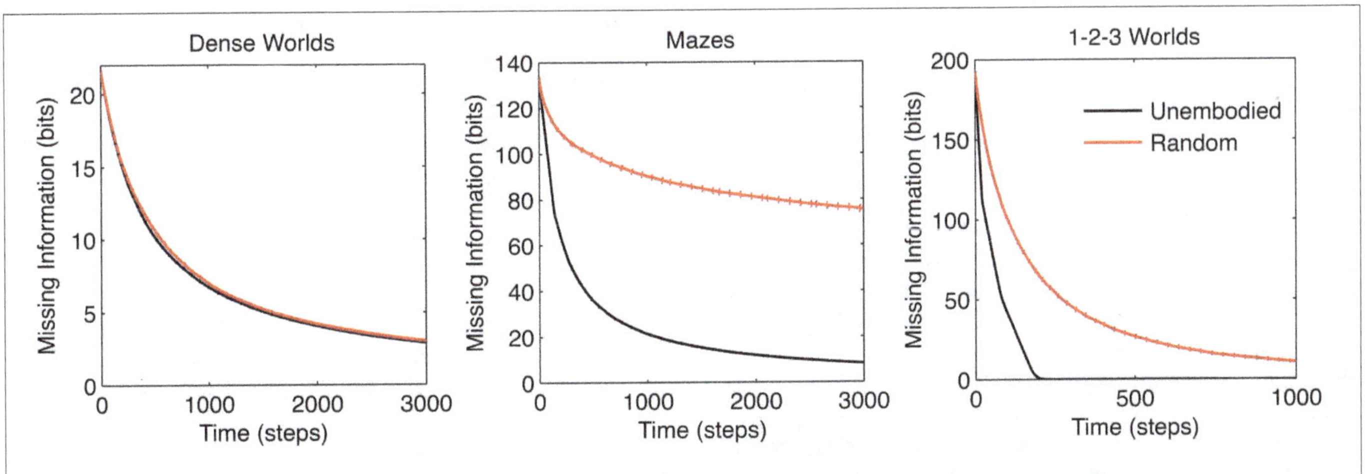

FIGURE 3 | Learning curves for control strategies. The average missing information is plotted over exploration time for the unembodied positive control and random action baseline control. Standard errors are plotted as dotted lines above and below learning curves ($n = 200$).

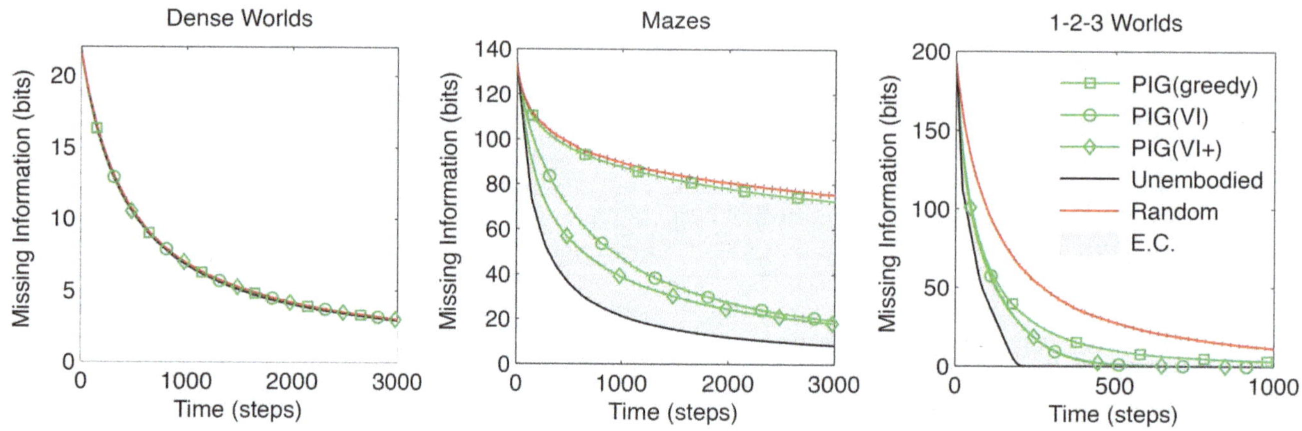

FIGURE 4 | Coordinating exploration using predicted information gain. The average missing information is plotted over exploration time for greedy and value-iterated (VI) maximization of PIG. The standard control strategies and the VI+ positive control are also depicted. Standard errors are plotted as dotted lines above and below learning curves ($n = 200$). EC, embodiment constraint.

We also find that, whereas PIG(greedy) yielded no improvement over random action in Dense Worlds and Mazes ($p > 0.001$), it significantly improved learning in 1-2-3 Worlds ($p < 0.001$), suggesting that this utility function was most beneficial in 1-2-3 Worlds.

Greedy maximization of PIG only accounts for the immediately available information gains and fails to account for the effect an action can have on future utility. In particular, when the potential for information gain is concentrated at remote states in the environment, it may be necessary to coordinate actions over time. Forward estimation of total future PIG is intractable. We therefore employ a back-propagation approach previously developed in the field of economics called *value-iteration* (VI) (Bellman, 1957). The estimation starts at a distant time point (initialized as $\tau = 0$) in the future with initial values equal to the PIG for each state-action pair:

$$Q_0(a, s) := \text{PIG}(a, s)$$

Then propagating backwards in time, we maintain a running total of estimated future value:

$$Q_{\tau-1}(a, s) := \text{PIG}(a, s) + \gamma \sum_{s' \in \mathcal{S}} \widehat{\Theta}_{ass'} \cdot V_\tau(s') \qquad (10)$$

$$\text{where } V_\tau(s) := \max_a Q_\tau(a, s)$$

Here, γ is a discount factor, set to 0.95. Such discount factors are commonly employed in value-iteration algorithms to favor more immediate gains over gains further in the future (Bellman, 1957). As discussed later, discounting may also help, in part, to account for the decreasing return on information from successive observations (see **Figure 2**).

Ideally, the true transition dynamics Θ would be used in Equation (10), but since the agent must learn these dynamics, it employs its internal model $\widehat{\Theta}$ instead. Applying the VI algorithm to PIG, we construct a behavioral policy PIG(VI) that coordinates actions over several time steps toward the approximate maximization of expected information gain:

$$a_{\text{PIG(VI)}} := \arg\max_a Q_{-10}(a, s);$$

As shown in **Figure 4**, the use of VI to coordinate actions yielded the greatest gains in Mazes, with moderate gains also seen in 1-2-3 Worlds. Along with the embodiment indices introduced above, these results support the hypothesis that worlds with high embodiment constraints require agents to coordinate their actions over several time steps to achieve efficient exploration.

Bellman showed that VI accurately estimates future gains when the true transition dynamics Θ is known and when the utility function is stationary (Bellman, 1957). Neither of these are true in our case, and PIG(VI) is therefore only an approximation of future gains. Nevertheless, as we will show, its utility is validated by its superior performance when compared to other previously introduced exploration strategies.

While a learning agent cannot use the true dynamics for VI, we can ascertain how much this impairs its exploration by considering a second positive-control PIG(VI+) which is given the true dynamics for coordinating its actions. That is, this control uses Θ instead of $\widehat{\Theta}$ in Equation (10) above. The performance of PIG(VI+) only differs from PIG(VI) in Mazes, and this difference is relatively small compared to the gains made over the random or greedy behaviors (**Figure 4**). Altogether these results suggest that PIG(VI) may be an effective strategy employable by embodied agents for coordinating explorative actions toward learning.

3.4. STRUCTURAL FEATURES OF THE THREE WORLDS

In the course of exploration, the data an agent accumulates will depend on both its behavioral strategy as well as the dynamical structure of its world. To elucidate this interaction, we next consider how structural differences in the three classes of environments correlate with an agents ability to explore. In particular, we consider three structural features of the worlds: their tendency to draw agents into a biased distribution over states, the amount of control a single action provides an agent over its future states, and the average distance between any two states.

3.4.1. State bias

To assess how strongly a world biases the state distribution of its agents we quantify the unevenness of the equilibrium distribution under a random action policy. The equilibrium distribution Ψ quantifies the likelihood that an agent will be in a particular state at a distant time-point in the future. To quantify the bias of this distribution, we define a *structure index* (SI) as the relative difference between its entropy $H(\Psi)$ and the entropy of the uniform distribution $H(U)$:

$$SI(\Psi) := \frac{H(U) - H(\Psi)}{H(U)}$$

where:

$$H(s) := -\sum_{s \in \mathcal{S}} p(s) \log_2(p(s))$$

In **Figure 5A**, the structure indices for 200 worlds in each class of environment are plotted against the embodiment index (defined in section 3.3). As depicted, the embodiment index correlates strongly with the structure index suggesting that state bias represents a significant challenge embodied agents face during exploration.

3.4.2. Controllability

To measure the capacity for an agent to control its state trajectory we computed a control index as the mutual information between a random action a_0 and an agent's state t time steps in the future s_t averaged uniformly over possible starting states s_0:

$$CI(t) = \sum_{s_0 \in \mathcal{S}} \frac{1}{N} \text{MI}[A_0, S_t | s_0]$$

$$= \sum_{s_0 \in \mathcal{S}} \frac{1}{N} \left(\sum_{a_0 \in \mathcal{A},\, s_t \in \mathcal{S}} p(a_0, s_t | s_0) \log_2 \left(\frac{p(s_t | a_0, s_0)}{p(s_t | s_0)} \right) \right)$$

As shown in **Figure 5B**, an action in a Maze or 1-2-3 Worlds has significantly more impact on future states than an action in Dense Worlds. Controllability is required for effective coordination of actions, such as under PIG(VI). In Mazes, where actions can significantly affect states far into the future, agents yielded the largest gains from coordinated actions. 1-2-3 Worlds also revealed high controllability, but only over the more immediate future. Interestingly, 1-2-3 Worlds also showed moderate gains from coordinating actions.

3.4.3. Mean path length

To assess the size of each CMC, we calculated the average minimum expected path length between every two states. To do this, we first determined the action policy that would minimize the expected path length to any target state. We then calculated the expected number of time-steps it would take an agent to navigate to that target state while employing this optimal policy. The average value of this expected path length taken across start and

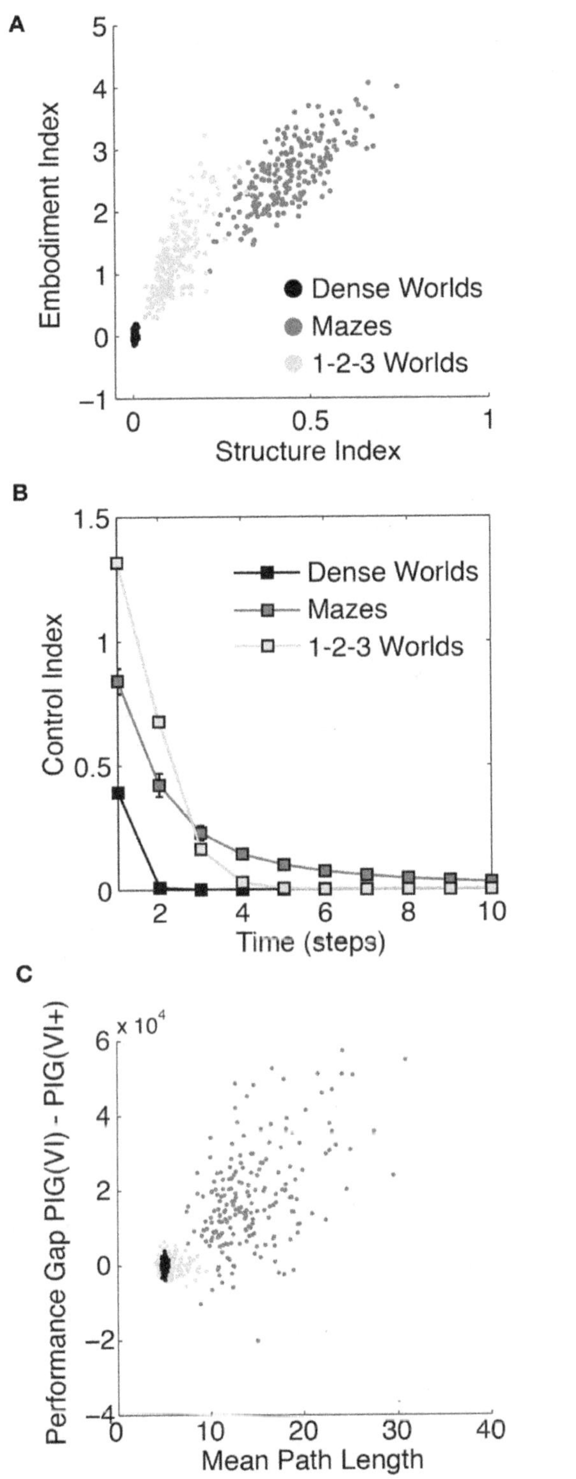

FIGURE 5 | Quantifying the structure of the worlds. (A) The embodiment index, defined in section 3.3, is plotted against the structure index for each of 200 Dense Worlds, Mazes, and 1-2-3 Worlds. **(B)** For the same CMCs, the average controllability is plotted as a function of the number of time steps the state lies in the future. The error bars depict standard deviations. **(C)** Again for the same CMCs, the learning performance gap in between PIG(VI) and PIG(VI+) is plotted against the mean path length between any two states.

target states was used as a measure of the extent of the CMC (see Appendix A4 for details). We had previously found that the three classes of CMCs differed in the relative performance between the PIG(VI) explorer and the PIG(VI+) control. Since these two strategies differ only in that the former uses the agent's internal model to coordinate its actions while the latter is allowed to use the true world dynamics, we wondered if the performance gap between the two (the area between their two learning curves) could be related to the path length to a potential source of information. Indeed, comparing this performance gap to the mean path length for each world, we found a strong correlation, as shown in **Figure 5C**. This suggests that coordination of actions may be more dependent on internal model accuracy for spatially extended worlds. Finally, it is interesting to note that the Mean Path Length is typically larger in mazes than 10 time steps, the planning horizon used in Value Iteration. Ten was chosen simply as a round number and it may be surprising that it works as well as it does in such spatially extended worlds. We believe two factors may contribute to this. First, it is likely that states of high informational value will be close together. Coordinating actions toward a nearby state of high value will therefore likely bring the agent closer to other states of potentially higher value. Second, and we suspect more importantly, since the mean path length is an average, a VI planner can direct its action toward a high information state under the possibility that it might reach that state within 10 time steps even if the expected path length to that location is significantly longer.

3.5. COMPARISON TO PREVIOUS EXPLORATIVE STRATEGIES

Models of exploration have been previously developed in the field of reinforcement learning (RL). Usually, these models focus on the role of exploration in reward acquisition rather than its direct role in learning world structure. Still, several of the principles developed in the RL field can be implemented in our framework. In this section, we compare these various methods to PIG(VI) under our learning objective. Since no rewards are available, we consider only RL strategies that can be implemented without rewards. Random action is perhaps the most common exploration strategy in RL. As we have already seen, random action is only efficient for exploring Dense Worlds. The following directed exploration strategies have also been developed in the RL literature (learning curves are plotted in **Figure 6**):

Least Taken Action (LTA): Under LTA, an agent will always choose the action that it has performed least often in the current state (Sato et al., 1988; Barto and Singh, 1990; Si et al., 2007). Like random action, LTA yields uniform sampling of actions in each state. Across worlds, LTA fails to significantly improve on the learning rates seen under random action ($p > 0.001$ for all three environments).

Counter-Based Exploration (CB): Whereas LTA actively samples actions uniformly, CB attempts to induce a uniform sampling across states. To do this, it maintains a count of the occurrences of each state, and chooses its action to minimize the expected count of the resultant state (Thrun, 1992). CB performs even worse than random action in Dense Worlds and 1-2-3 Worlds ($p < 0.001$). It does outperform random actions in Mazes but falls far short of the performance seen by PIG(VI) ($p < 0.001$).

Q-learning on Surprise [PEIG(Q)]: Storck et al. (1995) developed Surprise as a measure to quantify past changes in an agent's internal model which they used to guide exploration under a Q-learning algorithm (Sutton and Barto, 1998). Interestingly, it can be shown that Surprise as employed by Storck et al. is equivalent to the posterior expected information gain (PEIG), a posterior analog to our PIG utility function (see Appendix A5 and **Table 1**). Q-learning is a model-free approach to maximizing long-term gains of a utility function (Sutton and Barto, 1998). Implementing this strategy, we found that like CB, PEIG(Q) generally performed worse than random action.

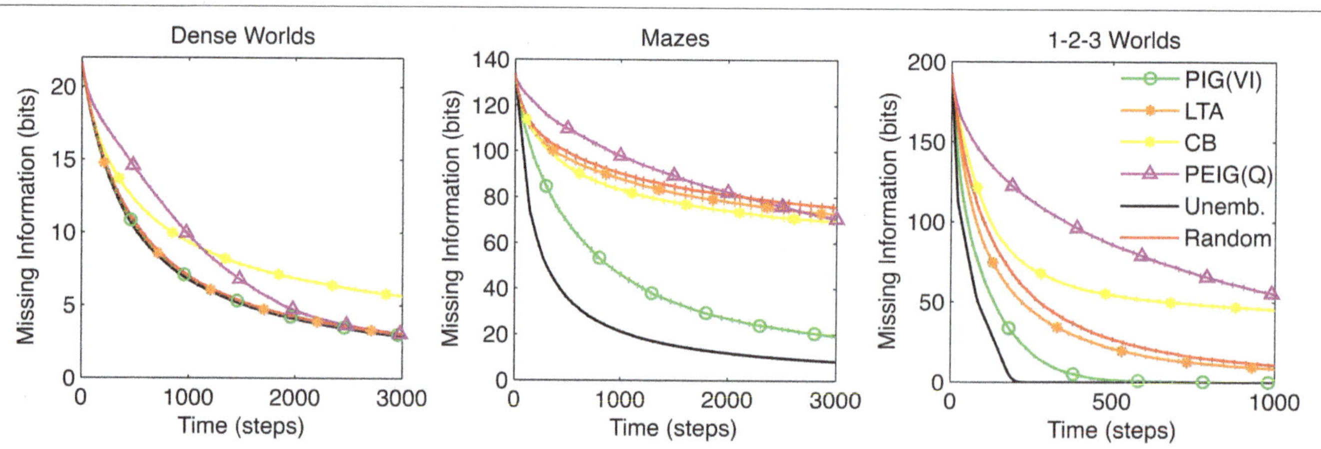

FIGURE 6 | Comparison to previous exploration strategies. The average missing information is plotted over time for PIG(VI) agents along with three exploration strategies from the literature: least taken action (LTA) (Sato et al., 1988; Barto and Singh, 1990; Si et al., 2007), counter-based (CB) (Thrun, 1992), and Q-Learning on posterior expected information gain [PEIG(Q)] (Storck et al., 1995). The standard control strategies are also shown. Standard errors are plotted as dotted lines above and below learning curves ($n = 200$).

The results in **Figure 6** show that PIG(VI) outperforms the previous explorative strategies at learning in structured worlds. We note that all of these strategies were originally developed to encourage exploration for the sake of improving reward acquisition, and their poor performance at our learning objective does not conflict with their previously demonstrated utility under the reinforcement learning framework.

3.6. COMPARISON TO UTILITY FUNCTIONS FROM PSYCHOLOGY

Independent findings in Psychology have suggested that the maximization of PIG can be used to predict human behavior during hypothesis testing (Oaksford and Chater, 1994). Inspired by these results, we investigated two other measures also developed in this context. Like PIG, both are measures of the difference between the current and hypothetical future internal models:

Predicted mode change (PMC) predicts the height difference between the modes of the current and future internal models (Baron, 2005; Nelson, 2005):

$$\mathrm{PMC}(a,s) = \sum_{s^*} \widehat{\Theta}_{ass^*}\left[\max_{s'} \widehat{\Theta}^{a,\,s\to s^*}_{ass'} - \max_{s'} \widehat{\Theta}_{ass'}\right] \quad (11)$$

Predicted L1 change (PLC) predicts the average L1 distance between the current and future internal models (Klayman and Ha, 1987):

$$\mathrm{PLC}(a,s) = \sum_{s^*} \widehat{\Theta}_{ass^*}\left[\frac{1}{N}\sum_{s'}\left|\widehat{\Theta}^{a,\,s\to s^*}_{ass'} - \widehat{\Theta}_{ass'}\right|\right] \quad (12)$$

We tested agents that approximately maximize PMC or PLC using VI. As **Figure 7** reveals, PIG(VI) proved again to be the best performer overall. In particular, PIG(VI) significantly outperforms PMC(VI) in all three environments, and PLC(VI) in 1-2-3 Worlds ($p < 0.001$). Nevertheless, PMC and PLC achieved significant improvements over the baseline control in Mazes and 1-2-3 Worlds, highlighting the benefit of coordinated actions across different utility functions. Interestingly, when performance was measured by an L1 distance instead of missing information, PIG(VI) still outperformed PMC(VI) and PLC(VI) in 1-2-3 Worlds (data not shown).

3.7. GENERALIZED UTILITY OF EXPLORATION

In considering the causes underlying a behavior such as exploration, psychologists often distinguish between the proximate (or behavioral) causes and the ultimate (or evolutionary) causes (Mayr, 1961; Pisula, 2009). Proximate causes are those factors that act directly on the individual in the control of behavior, while ultimate causes are those factors that contribute to the survival value of a behavior upon which natural selection can act. Thus far we have focused on efficient learning as the major objective because it has been identified by psychologists as the primary proximate cause of exploration (Archer and Birke, 1983; Loewenstein, 1994). We now, however, return to the question of the ultimate cause of exploration, which must lie in improved survival or reproductive fitness. The evolutionary advantage of learning-driven exploration is thought to lie in the general usefulness of possessing an accurate internal model of the world (Kaplan and Kaplan, 1983; Renner, 1988, 1990; Pisula, 2003, 2008). Unlike many models of reward-driven exploration, which focus on learning to optimize reward acquisition in a single context, an accurate internal model derived from learning-driven exploration may hold general utility applicable across a wide range of contexts. To compare the general utility of internal models gained through the various exploration methods, we assessed the ability of our agents to apply their internal models toward solving an array of goal-directed tasks. We note that these studies were performed without any changes to the exploration strategies employed by the agent. In essence, we interrupt an agent's exploration at several benchmark time points. We then ask the agent how it would solve, given its internal model, a particular task before allowing it to continue on in its exploration. The agent does not actually perform the task. It is simply asked to solve the task using it internal model. The solution that it provides is then compared by us to the optimal

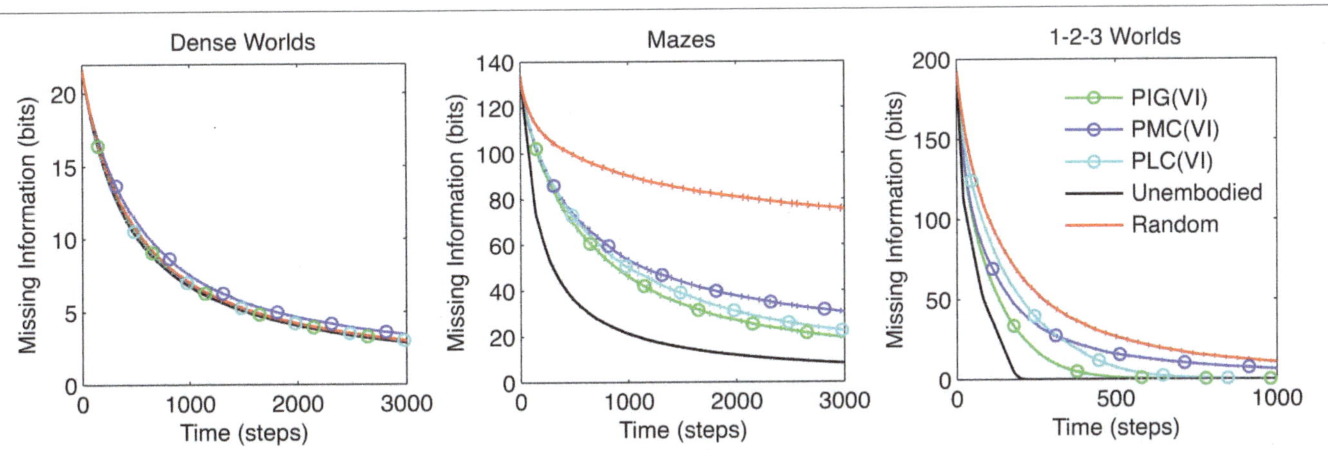

FIGURE 7 | Comparison between utility functions. The average missing information is plotted over time for agents that employ VI to maximize long-term gains in the three objective function, PIG, PMC, or PLC. The standard control strategies are also shown ($n = 200$).

solution. We considered two types of tasks, navigation and reward acquisition:

Navigation: Given a starting state, the agent has to quickly navigate to a target state.

Reward Acquisition: Given a starting state, the agent has to gather as much reward as possible over 100 time steps. Reward values are drawn from a normal distribution and randomly assigned to every state in the CMC. The agent is given the reward value of each state.

After various lengths of exploration, the agent's internal model is assessed for general utility. For each task, we derive the behavioral policy that optimizes performance under the internal model. As a positive control, we also derive an objective optimal policy that maximizes performance given the true CMC kernel. The difference in realized performance between the agent's policy and the control is used as a measure of navigational or reward loss. For detailed methods, please see Appendix A6.

Figure 8 depicts the average rank in the navigational and reward tasks for the different explorative strategies. In all environments, for both navigation and reward acquisition, PIG(VI) always grouped with the top performers ($p > 0.001$), excepting positive controls. PIG(VI) was the only strategy to do so. Thus, the explorative strategy that optimized learning under the missing information objective function also prepared the agent for accomplishing arbitrary goal-directed tasks.

Our test for generalized utility differs from the standard reinforcement learning paradigm in that it tests an agent across multiple tasks. The agent therefore cannot simply learn habitual sensorimotor responses specific to a single task. Though most reinforcement learning studies consider only a stationary, unchanging reward structure, we wanted to compare PIG(VI) to reward-driven explorers. BOSS is a state-of-the-art model-based reinforcement learning algorithm (Asmuth et al., 2009). To implement reward-driven exploration we trained a BOSS reinforcement-learner to navigate to internally chosen target-states. After reaching its target, the BOSS agent would randomly select a new target, updating its model reward structure accordingly. We then assessed the internal model formed by a BOSS explorer under the same navigational and reward acquisition tasks. As can be seen in **Figure 8**, BOSS (black cross) was not as good as PIG(VI) at either class of objectives despite being trained specifically on the navigation task.

4. DISCUSSION

In this manuscript we introduced a parsimonious mathematical framework for studying learning-driven exploration by embodied agents based on information theory, Bayesian inference, and CMCs. We compared agents that utilized different exploration strategies toward optimizing learning. To understand how learning performance depends on the structure of the world, three classes of environments were considered that challenge the learning agent in different ways. We found that fast learning could be achieved in all environments by an exploration strategy that coordinated actions toward long-term maximization of PIG.

4.1. CAVEATS

The optimality of the Bayesian estimate (Theorem 1) and the estimation of information gain (Theorem 2) both require an accurate prior over the transition kernels. For biological agents, such priors could have been learned from earlier exploration of related environments, or may represent hardwired beliefs optimized by evolutionary pressures. Alternatively, an agent could attempt to simultaneously learn a prior while exploring its environment.

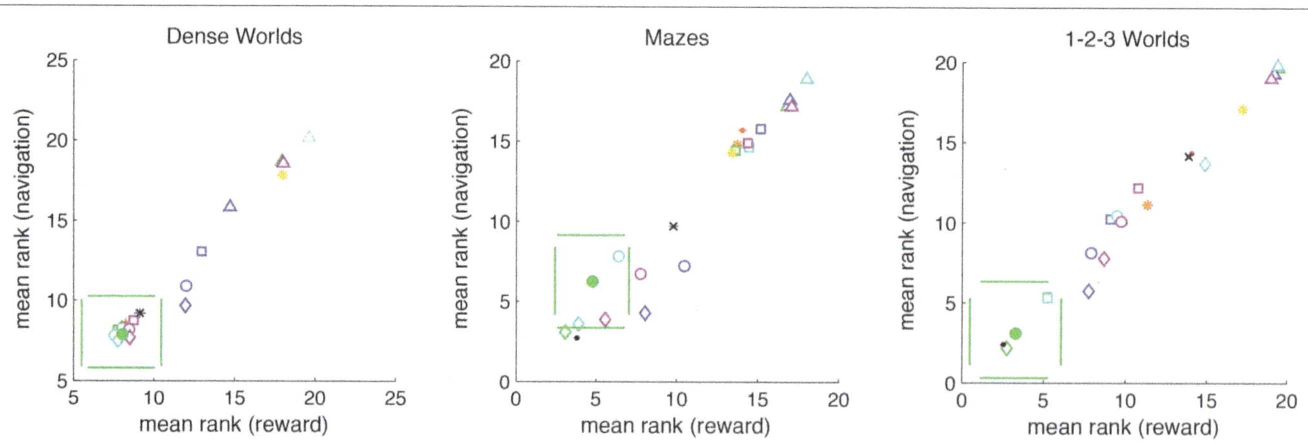

FIGURE 8 | Demonstration of generalized utility. For each world ($n = 200$), explorative strategies are ranked for average performance on the navigational tasks (averaged across N start states and N target states) and the reward tasks (averaged across N start states and 10 randomly generated reward distributions). The average ranks are plotted with standard deviations. PIG(VI) is depicted as a filled green circle. Strategies lying outside the pair of horizontal green lines differ significantly from PIG(VI) in navigational performance. Strategies lying outside the pair of vertical green lines differ significantly from PIG(VI) in reward performance ($p < 0.0001$). The different utility functions and heuristics are distinguished by color: PIG(green), PEIG (magenta), PMC (dark-blue), PLC (cyan), LTA (orange), and CB (yellow). The different coordination methods are distinguished by symbol: Greedy (squares), VI (circles), VI+ (diamonds), Heuristic Strategies (asterisks). The two standard controls are depicted as points as follows: Unembodied (black), Random (red). The BOSS reinforcement learner is depicted by a black cross.

Indeed a simple maximum-likelihood estimation of the concentration parameter for Dense Worlds and Mazes is sufficient for an agent to achieve efficient exploration (data not shown). Nevertheless, biological agents may not always have access to an accurate prior for an environment. For such cases, future work is required to understand exploration under false priors and how they could yield sub-optimal but perhaps biologically realistic exploratory behaviors.

Another potential limitation of our approach occurs from the fact that the VI algorithm is only optimal if the utility function is stationary (i.e., unchanging) (Bellman, 1957). Any utility function, including PIG, that attempts to capture learning progress will necessarily change over time. This caveat may be partially alleviated by the fact that PIG changes only for the sampled distributions. Furthermore, PIG decreases in a monotonic fashion (see **Figure 2**) which can potentially be captured by the discount factor of VI. Interesting future work may lie in accounting for the effect of such monotonic decreases in estimates of future information gains either through direct estimation or through better approximation by a different choice of discounting mechanism. The problem of accounting for diminishing returns on utility has been previously approached in the field of optimal foraging theory. Modeling the foraging behaviors of animals, optimal foraging theory considers an animals decision of when it should leave its present feeding area, or patch, in which it has been consuming the available food and expend energy to seek out a new, undiminished patch (MacArthur and Pianka, 1966). Charnov's Marginal Value Theorem, a pivotal finding in the field, suggests that the decision to transition should be made once the expected utility of the current patch decreases to the average expected utility across all patches accounting for transition costs (Charnov, 1976). Extending this work to our information-theoretic approach in CMCs may provide the necessary insights to address the challenge of diminishing returns on information gain.

Finally, the VI algorithm scales linearly with the size of the state space, and the calculation of PIG can scale linearly with the square of the size of the state space. This means that for larger and larger CMCs, these approaches will become more computationally expensive to perform. For large worlds, clever methods for approximating these approaches or for sparsifying their representation may be necessary. An explicit model of memory may also be necessary to fully capture the limitation on computational complexity biological organisms face. A wealth of literature from Reinforcement Learning and related fields may offer insights in approaching these challenge which we reserve for future work.

4.2. RELATED WORK IN REINFORCEMENT LEARNING

CMCs are closely related to Markov Decision Processes (MDPs) commonly studied in Reinforcement Learning. MDPs differ from CMCs in that they explicitly include a stationary reward function associated with each transition (Sutton and Barto, 1998; Gimbert, 2007). RL research of exploration usually focusses on its role in balancing exploitative behaviors during reward maximization. Several approaches for inducing exploratory behavior in RL agents have been developed. One very common approach is the use of heuristic strategies such as random action, least taken action, and counter-based algorithms. While such strategies may be useful in gathering unchanging external rewards, our results show that they are inefficient for learning the dynamics of structured worlds.

Other RL approaches involve reward-driven exploration. In the absence of external rewards, exploration could still be induced under reward-driven strategies by having the agent work through a series of internally chosen reward problems. This is essentially how the described BOSS agent operates. It was nevertheless insufficient to reach the performance accomplished by PIG(VI).

In addition, several RL studies have investigated intrinsically motivated learning. For example, Singh et al. (2010) have demonstrated that RL guided by saliency, an intrinsic motivation derived from changes in stimulus intensity, can promote the learning of reusable skills. As described in section 3.5, Storck et al. introduced the combination of Q-learning and PEIG as an intrinsic motivator of learning (Storck et al., 1995). In their study, PEIG(Q) outperformed random action only over long time scales. At shorter time scales, random action performed better. Interestingly, we found exactly the same trend, initially slow learning with eventual catching-up, when we applied PEIG(Q) to exploration in our test environments (**Figure 6**).

4.3. BETWEEN LEARNING-DRIVEN AND REWARD-DRIVEN EXPLORATION

While curiosity, as an intrinsic value for learning, is believed to be the primary drive of explorative behaviors, other factors, including external rewards, may play a role either in motivating exploration directly or in shaping the development of curiosity (Archer and Birke, 1983; Loewenstein, 1994; Silvia, 2005; Pisula, 2009). In this manuscript, we wished to focus on a pure learning-based exploration strategy and therefore chose to take an unweighted sum of missing information as a parsimonious objective function (Equation 3). Two points, however, should be noted in considering the relationship of this work to previous work in the literature. First, our objective function considers only the learning of the transition dynamics governing a CMC as this fully describes such a world. When we incorporate additional features into our framework, such as rewards in MDPs, those features too could be learned and assessed under our missing information objective function. Toward this goal, interesting insights may come from comparing our work with the multi-armed bandits literature. Multi-armed bandits are a special class of single state MDPs (Gittins, 1979). By considering only a single state, multi-armed bandits remove the embodiment constraint of multi-state CMCs and MDPs. Thus, CMCs and multi-armed bandits represent complimentary special cases of MDPs. That is, a CMC is an MDP without reward structure, while a multi-armed bandit is an MDP without transition kernels. Recent research has attempted to decouple the exploration and exploitation components of optimal control in multi-armed bandits (Abbeel and Ng, 2005; Bubeck et al., 2009). These studies aim at minimizing, through exploration, a construct termed regret, the expected reward forgone by a recommended strategy. Regret is similar to the navigational and reward acquisition loss values we calculated for ranking our explorers under goal-directed tasks. Importantly, while our work considered a wide array of goal-directed tasks, these multi-armed bandit approaches typically consider only learning a single fixed reward structure. Understanding these difference will be important if one wishes to shift attention from the unbiased information-theoretic view we take to a directed task-dependent view. Identifying a means, perhaps through information theory, of quantifying uncertainty in which strategy will optimize a task, will be an important extension bridging these two approaches. The idea of directed information brings us to our second consideration in relating our work to previous literature. Psychologists have found that curiosity, or interest, can vary greatly both between and within individuals (Silvia, 2001, 2006). While one should be careful to not conflate the valuation of an extrinsic reward with the emotion of interest, it is possible such valuations could act to influence the development of interests. By transitioning away from our non-selective measure of missing information toward a weighted objective function that values certain information over others, we may begin to bridge the learning-driven and reward-driven approaches to exploration. One interesting proposal, put forth by Vergassola et al. suggests that information regarding a reward often falls off with distance as an organism moves away from the source of the reward (Vergassola et al., 2007). Accordingly, a greedy local maximization of information regarding the reward may simultaneously bring the individual closer to the desired reward. The resultant "infotaxis" strategy is closely related to our PIG(greedy) strategy but is applied only to a single question of where a particular reward is located.

4.4. RELATED WORK IN PSYCHOLOGY

In the Psychology literature, PIG, as well as PMC and PLC, were directly introduced as measures of the expected difference between a current and future belief (Baron, 2005; Klayman and Ha, 1987; Oaksford and Chater, 1994; Nelson, 2005). Here, we showed that PIG equals the expected change in missing information (Theorem 2). Analogous theorems do not hold for PMC or PLC. For example, PLC is not equivalent to the expected change in L1 distance with respect to the true world. This might explain why PIG(VI) outperformed PLC(VI) even under an L1 measure of learning.

We applied PIG, PMC, and PLC to the problem of learning a full model of the world. In contrast, the mentioned psychology studies focussed specifically on hypothesis testing and did not consider sequences of actions or embodied action-perception loops. These studies revealed that human behavior during hypothesis testing can be modeled as maximizing PIG, suggesting that PIG may have biological significance (Oaksford and Chater, 1994; Nelson, 2005). However, those results could not distinguish between the different utility functions (PIG, PMC, and PLC) (Nelson, 2005). Our finding that 1-2-3 Worlds give rise to large differences between the three utility functions may help identify new behavioral tasks for disambiguating the role of these measures in human behavior.

To model bottom–up visual saliency and predict gaze attention, Itti and Baldi recently developed an information-theoretic measure closely related to PEIG (Itti and Baldi, 2006, 2009; Baldi and Itti, 2010). In this model, a Bayesian learner maintains a probabilistic belief structure over the low-level features of a video. Attention is believed to be attracted to locations in the visual scene that exhibit high Surprise. Several potential extensions of this work are suggested by our results. First, it may be useful to model the active nature of data acquisition during visual scene analysis. In Itti and Baldi's model, all features are updated for all location of the visual scene regardless of current gaze location or gaze trajectory. Differences in acuity between the fovea and periphery, however, suggest that gaze location will have a significant effect on which low-level features can be transmitted by the retina (Wässle and Boycott, 1991). Second, our comparison between PIG and PEIG (**Figure 6**) suggests that predicting future changes may be more efficient than focusing attention only on those locations where change has occurred in the past. A model that anticipates Surprise, as PIG anticipates information gain, may be better able to explain some aspects of human attention. For example, if a moving object disappears behind an obstruction, viewers may anticipate the reemergence of the object and attend that location. Incorporating these insights into new models of visual saliency and attention could be an interesting course of future research.

4.5. INFORMATION-THEORETIC MODELS OF BEHAVIOR

Recently information-theoretic concepts have become more popular in computational models of behavior. These approaches can be grouped under three guiding principles. The first principle uses information theory to quantify the complexity of a behavioral policy, with high complexity considered undesirable. Tishby and Polani for example, considered RL maximization of rewards under such complexity constraints (Tishby and Polani, 2011).

The second principle is to maximize a measure called *predictive information* which quantifies the amount of information a known (or past) variable contains regarding an unknown (or future) variable (Tishby et al., 1999; Ay et al., 2008; Still, 2009). Predictive information has also been referred to as *excess entropy* (Crutchfield and Feldman, 2003) and should not be confused with PIG. When the controls of a simulated robot were adjusted such that the predictive information between successive sensory inputs was maximized, Ay et al. found that the robot began to exhibit complex and interesting explorative behaviors (Ay et al., 2008). This objective selects for behaviors that cause the sensory inputs to change often but to remain predictable from previous inputs, and we therefore describe the resulting exploration as stimulation-driven. Such exploration generally benefits from a good internal model but on its own, does not drive fast learning. It is therefore more suitable later in exploration, after a learning-driven strategy, such as PIG(VI), has had a chance to form an accurate model. PIG, in contrast, is most useful in the early stages when the internal model is still deficient. These complimentary properties of predictive information and PIG lead us to hypothesize that a simple additive combination of the two objectives may naturally lead to a smooth transitioning from learning-driven exploration to stimulation-driven exploration, a transition that may indeed be present in human behavior (see section 4.6).

Epsilon machines introduced by Crutchfield and Young (1989) and the information bottleneck approach introduced by Tishby et al. (1999) combine these first two principles of maximizing predictive information and constraining complexity. In particular maximizing the information between a compressed internal variable and the future state progression subject to a constraint on the complexity of generating the internal variable from sensory inputs. Recently, Still extended the information bottleneck method to incorporate actions (Still, 2009).

Finally, the third information-theoretic principle of behavior is to minimize of free-energy, an information-theoretic bound on surprise. Friston put forth this Free-Energy (FE) hypothesis as a unified variational principle for governing both the inference of an internal model and the control of actions (Friston, 2009). Under this principle, agents should act to minimize the number of states they visit. This stands in stark contrast to both learning-driven and stimulation-driven exploration. A learning-driven explorer will seek out novel states where missing information is high, while a stimulation-driven explorer actively seek to maintain high variation in its sensory inputs. Still, reduced state entropy may be valuable in dangerous environments where few states permit survival. The balance between cautionary and exploratory behaviors would be an interesting topic for future research.

4.6. TOWARD A GENERAL THEORY OF EXPLORATION

With the work of Berlyne (1966), psychologists began to dissect the different motivations that drive exploration. A distinction between play (or diversive exploration) and investigation (or specific exploration) grew out of two competing theories of exploration. As reviewed by Hutt (1970), "curiosity"-theory proposed that exploration is a consummatory response to curiosity-inducing stimuli (Berlyne, 1950; Montgomery, 1953). In contrast, "boredom"-theory held that exploration was an instrumental response for stimulus change (Myers and Miller, 1954; Glanzer, 1958). Hutt suggested that the two theories may be capturing distinct behavioral modes, with "curiosity"-theory underlying investigatory exploration and "boredom"-theory underlying play. In children, exploration often occurs in two stages, inspection to understand what is perceived, followed by play to maintain changing stimulation (Hutt and Bhavnani, 1972). These distinctions nicely correspond to the differences between our approach and the predictive information approach of Ay et al. (2008) and Still (2009). In particular, we hypothesize that our approach corresponds to curiosity-driven investigation, while predictive information a la Ay et al. and Still may correspond with play. Furthermore, the proposed method of additively combining these two principles (section 4.4), may naturally capture the transition between investigation and play seen in children.

For curiosity-driven exploration, there are many varied theories (Loewenstein, 1994). Early theories viewed curiosity as a drive to maintain a specific level of arousal. These were followed by theories interpreting curiosity as a response to intermediate levels of incongruence between expectations and perceptions, and later by theories interpreting curiosity as a motivation to master one's environment. Loewenstein developed an Information Gap Theory and suggested that curiosity is an aversive reaction to missing information (Loewenstein, 1994). More recently, Silvia proposed that curiosity comprises two traits, complexity and comprehensibility (Silvia, 2005). For Silvia complexity is broadly defined, and includes novelty, ambiguity, obscurity, mystery, etc. Comprehensibility appraises whether something can be understood. It is interesting how well these two traits match information-theoretic concepts, complexity being captured by entropy, and comprehensibility by information gain (Pfaffelhuber, 1972). Indeed, PIG might be able to explain the dual aspects of curiosity-driven exploration proposed by Silvia. PIG is bounded by entropy and thus high values require high complexity. At the same time, PIG equals the expected decrease in missing information and thus may be equivalent to expected comprehensibility.

All told, our results add to a bigger picture of exploration in which the theories for its different aspects fit together like pieces of a puzzle. This invites future work for integrating these pieces into a more comprehensive theory of exploration and ultimately of autonomous behavior.

4.7. APPLICATION TOWARD EXPERIMENTAL DESIGN

In many ways, scientific research itself epitomizes learning-driven exploration. Like our modeled agents, researchers design experiments to maximize their expected gain in information. Recently, there has been growing interest in automated experimental design. While not every experimental paradigm will fit neatly into our CMC framework, our explorative principles may have direct application to closed-loop neurophysiology. Suppose, for example, we are interested in how ongoing activity within a population of neurons affects their receptive fields. To study this, we would want to measure the neurons' responses to different stimuli and determine how those responses are affected by the activity of the neurons just prior to stimulus presentation. Specific sequences of *priming* stimuli may be necessary to drive the neurons into a particular activation state of ongoing activity in which their responses to a *probe* stimulus could be measured. It may be difficult for a researcher to determine before hand which sequences of stimuli are interesting, but PIG(VI) might offer an automated way of choosing appropriate stimuli on the fly. The ongoing activity of a population of neurons can be treated as the states of the system, and the choice of stimuli as the actions. A closed-loop electrophysiology system controlled by PIG(VI) could investigate not only how the neurons responded to presented stimuli but also how to use the stimuli to prime the neurons into interesting states of ongoing activity for probing.

ACKNOWLEDGMENTS

This work was supported by the Redwood Center for Theoretical and Computational Neuroscience Graduate Student Endowment to Daniel Y. Little and NSF Grant (IIS-0713657) to Friedrich T. Sommer. The authors wish to thank Tom Griffiths, Reza Moazzezi, and the Redwood Center for Theoretical Neuroscience for useful discussions.

REFERENCES

Abbeel, P., and Ng, A. (2005). "Exploration and apprenticeship learning in reinforcement learning," in *Proceedings of the 22nd International Conference on Machine Learning* (New York, NY: ACM), 1–8.

Archer, J., and Birke, L. (1983). *Exploration in Animals and Humans.* Berkshire: Van Nostrand Reinhold (UK) Co Ltd.

Asmuth, J., Li, L., Littman, M., Nouri, A., and Wingate, D. (2009). "A Bayesian sampling approach to exploration in reinforcement learning," in *Proceedings of the Twenty-Fifth Conference on Uncertainty in Artificial Intelligence* (Montreal, QC: AUAI Press), 19–26.

Ay, N., Bertschinger, N., Der, R., Güttler, F., and Olbrich, E. (2008). Predictive information and explorative behavior of autonomous robots. *Eur. Phys. J. B* 63, 329–339.

Baldi, P. F., and Itti, L. (2010). Of bits and wows: a Bayesian theory of surprise with applications to attention. *Neural Netw.* 23, 649–666.

Baron, J. (2005). *Rationality and Intelligence.* New York, NY: Cambridge University Press.

Barto, A., and Singh, S. (1990). "On the computational economics of reinforcement learning," in *Connectionist Models: Proceedings of the 1990 Summer School. Morgan Kaufmann* (San Diego, CA: Citeseer).

Bellman, R. E. (1957). *Dynamic Programming.* Princeton, NJ: Princeton University Press.

Berlyne, D. (1950). Novelty and curiosity as determinants of exploratory behaviour1. *Br. J. Psychol.* 41, 68–80.

Berlyne, D. (1966). Curiosity and exploration. *Science* 153, 25.

Bubeck, S., Munos, R., and Stoltz, G. (2009). "Pure exploration in multi-armed bandits problems," in *Algorithmic Learning Theory*, eds R. Gavaldà, G. Lugosi, T. Zeugmann, and S. Zilles (Porto: Springer), 23–37.

Charnov, E. (1976). Optimal foraging, the marginal value theorem. *Theor. Popul. Biol.* 9, 129–136.

Cover, T., and Thomas, J. (1991). *Elements of Information Theory.* Vol. 6. New York, NY: Wiley Online Library.

Crutchfield, J., and Feldman, D. (2003). Regularities unseen, randomness observed: levels of entropy convergence. *Chaos* 13, 25. (Woodbury, NY).

Crutchfield, J. P., and Young, K. (1989). Inferring statistical complexity. *Phys. Rev. Lett.* 63, 105–108.

Friston, K. (2009). The free-energy principle: a rough guide to the brain? *Trends Cogn. Sci.* 13, 293–301.

Gimbert, H. (2007). "Pure stationary optimal strategies in markov decision processes," in *STACS 2007, Vol. 4393,* eds W. Thomas and P. Weil (Aachen: Springer), 200–211.

Gittins, J. (1979). Bandit processes and dynamic allocation indices. *J. R. Stat. Soc. B* 41, 148–177.

Glanzer, M. (1958). Curiosity, exploratory drive, and stimulus satiation. *Psychol. Bull.* 55, 302.

Gordon, G., Kaplan, D., Lankow, B., Little, D., Sherwin, J., Suter, B., et al. (2011). Toward an integrated approach to perception and action: conference report and future directions. *Front. Syst. Neurosci.* 5:20. doi: 10.3389/fnsys.2011.00020

Guillery, R. W. (2005). Anatomical pathways that link perception and action. *Prog. Brain Res.* 149, 235–256.

Guillery, R. W., and Sherman, S. M. (2011). Branched thalamic afferents: what are the messages that they relay to the cortex? *Brain Res. Rev.* 66, 205–219.

Hutt, C. (1970). Specific and diversive exploration1. *Adv. Child Dev. Behav.* 5, 119.

Hutt, C., and Bhavnani, R. (1972). Predictions from play. *Nature* 237, 171–172.

Itti, L., and Baldi, P. (2006). Bayesian surprise attracts human attention. *Adv. Neural Inf. Process. Syst.* 18, 547.

Itti, L., and Baldi, P. F. (2009). Bayesian surprise attracts human attention. *Vis. Res.* 49, 1295–1306.

Kaelbling, L., Littman, M., and Moore, A. (1996). Reinforcement learning: a survey. Arxiv preprint: cs/9605103.

Kaplan, R., and Kaplan, S. (1983). *Cognition and Environment: Functioning of an Uncertain World.* Ann Arbor, MI: Ulrichs Books.

Kawato, M., and Samejima, K. (2007). Efficient reinforcement learning: computational theories, neuroscience and robotics. *Curr. Opin. Neurobiol.* 17, 205–212.

Klayman, J., and Ha, Y. (1987). Confirmation, disconfirmation, and information in hypothesis testing. *Psychol. Rev.* 94, 211.

Loewenstein, G. (1994). The psychology of curiosity: a review and reinterpretation. *Psychol. Bull.* 116, 75.

MacArthur, R., and Pianka, E. (1966). On optimal use of a patchy environment. *Am. Nat.* 100, 603–609.

MacKay, D., and Peto, L. (1995). A hierarchical dirichlet language model. *Nat. Lang. Eng.* 1, 1–19.

Manning, C. D., Raghavan, P., and Schütze, H. (2008). *Introduction to Information Retrieval, Vol. 1.* Cambridge: Cambridge University Press.

Mayr, E. (1961). Cause and effect in biology. *Science* 134, 1501.

Montgomery, K. (1953). Exploratory behavior as a function of "similarity" of stimulus situation. *J. Comp. Physiol. Psychol.* 46, 129.

Myers, A., and Miller, N. (1954). Failure to find a learned drive based on hunger; evidence for learning motivated by "exploration." *J. Comp. Physiol. Psychol.* 47, 428.

Nelson, J. (2005). Finding useful questions: on bayesian diagnosticity, probability, impact, and information gain. *Psychol. Rev.* 112, 979.

Noë, A. (2004). *Action in Perception.* Cambridge, MA: MIT Press.

Oaksford, M., and Chater, N. (1994). A rational analysis of the selection task as optimal data selection. *Psychol. Rev.* 101, 608.

O'Regan, J., and Noë, A. (2001). A sensorimotor account of vision and visual consciousness. *Behav. Brain Sci.* 24, 939–972.

Pfaffelhuber, E. (1972). Learning and information theory. *Int. J. Neurosci.* 3, 83–88.

Pisula, W. (2003). Costs and benefits of curiosity: the adaptive value of exploratory behavior. *Polish Psychol. Bull.* 34, 183–186.

Pisula, W. (2008). Play and exploration in animals – a comparative analysis. *Polish Psychol. Bull.* 39, 104–107.

Pisula, W. (2009). *Curiosity and Information Seeking in Animal and Human Behavior.* Boca Raton, FL: Brown Walker Press.

Renner, M. (1990). Neglected aspects of exploratory and investigatory behavior. *Psychobiology* 18, 16–22.

Renner, M. J. (1988). Learning during exploration: the role of behavioral topography during exploration in determining subsequent adaptive behavior. *Int. J. Comp. Psychol.* 2, 43–56.

Rochat, P. (1989). Object manipulation and exploration in 2-to 5-month-old infants. *Dev. Psychol.* 25, 871.

Sato, M., Abe, K., and Takeda, H. (1988). Learning control of finite markov chains with an explicit trade-off between estimation and control. *IEEE Trans. Syst. Man Cybern.* 18, 677–684.

Si, B., Herrmann, J. M., and Pawelzik, K. (2007). "Gain-based exploration: from multi-armed bandits to partially observable environments," in *Proceedings of the Third International Conference on Natural Computation, Vol. 1* (Washington, DC: IEEE Computer Society), 177–182.

Silvia, P. (2001). Interest and interests: the psychology of constructive capriciousness. *Rev. Gen. Psychol.* 5, 270.

Silvia, P. (2005). What is interesting? Exploring the appraisal structure of interest. *Emotion* 5, 89.

Silvia, P. (2006). *Exploring the Psychology of Interest.* Oxford: Oxford University Press.

Singh, S., Lewis, R., Barto, A., and Sorg, J. (2010). Intrinsically motivated reinforcement learning: an evolutionary perspective. *IEEE Trans. Auton. Ment. Dev.* 2, 70–82.

Still, S. (2009). Information-theoretic approach to interactive learning. *EPL* 85, 28005.

Storck, J., Hochreiter, S., and Schmidhuber, J. (1995). "Reinforcement driven information acquisition in non-deterministic environments," in *ICANN'95* eds F.-S. Françoise and G. Patrick (Paris: Citeseer), 159–164.

Sutton, R., and Barto, A. (1998). *Reinforcement Learning.* Vol. 9. Cambridge, MA: MIT Press.

Thrun, S. (1992). *Efficient Exploration in Reinforcement Learning.* Technical report, School of Computer Science, Carnegie-Mellon University.

Tishby, N., Pereira, F., and Bialek, W. (1999). "The information bottleneck method," in *Proceedings of the 37th Allerton Conference on Communication,*

Control and Computation (Monticello, IL).

Tishby, N., and Polani, D. (2011). "Models, Architectures, and Hardward, Chapter 19," in *Perception-Action Cycle,* eds V. Cutsuridis, A. Hussain, and J. G. Taylor (New York, NY: Springer), 601–636.

Vergassola, M., Villermaux, E., and Shraiman, B. (2007). 'infotaxis' as a strategy for searching without gradients. *Nature* 445, 406–409.

Wässle, H., and Boycott, B. (1991). Functional architecture of the mammalian retina. *Physiol. Rev.* 71, 447.

APPENDIX A

A1 PROOF OF THEOREM 1

Claim. *Consider a CMC random variable* $\boldsymbol{\Theta}$ *modeling the ground truth environment* Θ *and drawn from a prior distribution* f. *Given a history of observations* $\vec{d}$, *the expected missing information between* $\boldsymbol{\Theta}$ *and an agent's internal model* Φ *is minimized by the Bayesian estimate* $\Phi = \widehat{\Theta}$. *That is:*

$$\widehat{\Theta} := \mathrm{E}_{\boldsymbol{\Theta}|\vec{d}}[\boldsymbol{\Theta}] = \arg\min_{\Phi} \mathrm{E}_{\boldsymbol{\Theta}|\vec{d}}\left[\mathrm{I_M}(\boldsymbol{\Theta}\|\,\Phi)\right]$$

Proof. Minimizing missing information is equivalent to independently minimizing the KL-divergence of each transition kernel.

$$\begin{aligned}
&\arg\min_{\Phi_{as\cdot}} \mathrm{E}_{\boldsymbol{\Theta}|\vec{d}}\left[\mathrm{D_{KL}}\left(\boldsymbol{\Theta}_{as\cdot}\|\,\Phi_{as\cdot}\right)\right] \\
&= \arg\min_{\Phi_{as\cdot}} \mathrm{E}_{\boldsymbol{\Theta}|\vec{d}}\left[\sum_{s'} \boldsymbol{\Theta}_{ass'} \log_2\left(\frac{\Theta_{ass'}}{\Phi_{ass'}}\right)\right] \\
&= \arg\min_{\Phi_{as\cdot}} \mathrm{E}_{\boldsymbol{\Theta}|\vec{d}}\left[\sum_{s'} \boldsymbol{\Theta}_{ass'} \log_2 \boldsymbol{\Theta}_{ass'} - \boldsymbol{\Theta}_{ass'} \log_2 \Phi_{ass'}\right] \\
&= \arg\min_{\Phi_{as\cdot}} \; -\mathrm{E}_{\boldsymbol{\Theta}|\vec{d}}\left[\sum_{s'} \boldsymbol{\Theta}_{ass'} \log_2 \Phi_{ass'}\right] \\
&= \arg\min_{\Phi_{as\cdot}} \; -\sum_{s'} \mathrm{E}_{\boldsymbol{\Theta}|\vec{d}}\left[\boldsymbol{\Theta}_{ass'}\right] \log_2 \Phi_{ass'} \\
&= \arg\min_{\Phi_{as\cdot}} \mathrm{H}\left[\mathrm{E}_{\boldsymbol{\Theta}|\vec{d}}\left[\boldsymbol{\Theta}_{as\cdot}\right];\, \Phi_{as\cdot}\right]
\end{aligned}$$

Here H denotes cross-entropy (Cover and Thomas, 1991). Finally, by Gibb's inequality (Cover and Thomas, 1991):

$$\arg\min_{\Phi_{as\cdot}} \mathrm{H}\left[E_{\boldsymbol{\Theta}|\vec{d}}\left[\boldsymbol{\Theta}_{as\cdot}\right];\, \Phi_{as\cdot}\right] = \mathrm{E}_{\boldsymbol{\Theta}|\vec{d}}\left[\boldsymbol{\Theta}_{as\cdot}\right] = \widehat{\Theta}_{as\cdot}$$

A2 GENERATIVE DISTRIBUTIONS AND BAYESIAN ESTIMATES FOR THE 3 CLASSES OF ENVIRONMENTS

(1) *Dense Worlds* correspond to complete directed probability graphs with $N = 10$ states and $M = 4$ actions. An example is depicted in **Figure A1**. Each transition distribution is independently drawn from a Dirichlet distribution over the standard $(N-1)$-simplex:

$$f(\Theta_{as\cdot}) = \mathrm{Dir}(\boldsymbol{\alpha}) = \frac{1}{Z(\boldsymbol{\alpha})} \cdot \prod_{s'} \Theta_{ass'}{}^{\alpha_{s'}-1}$$

The normalizing constant Z brings the area under the distribution to 1:

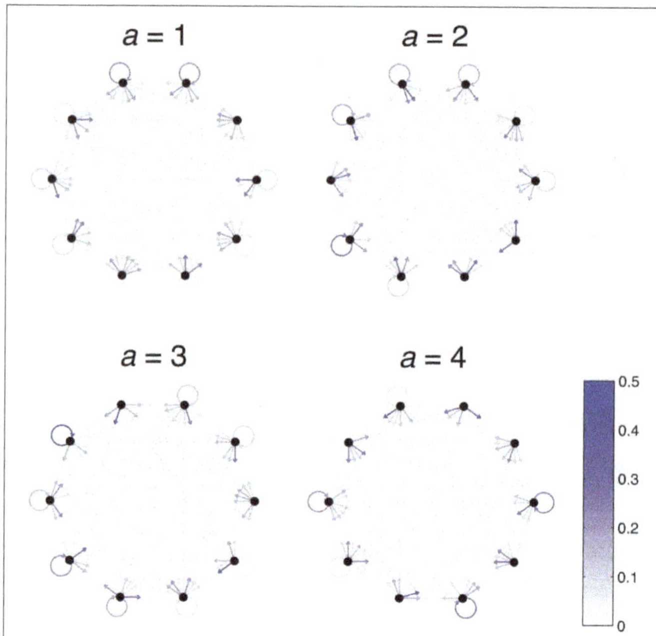

FIGURE A1 | Example Dense World. Dense Worlds consist of 4 actions (separately depicted) and 10 states (depicted as nodes of the graphs). The transition probabilities associated with taking a particular action are depicted as arrows pointing from the current state to each of the possible resultant states. Arrow color depicts the likelihood of each transition.

$$Z(\boldsymbol{\alpha}) := \int_{\Delta_{N-1}} \prod_{s'} \Theta_{ass'}{}^{\alpha_{s'}-1} d\Theta_{as\cdot} = \frac{\prod_{s'} \Gamma(\alpha_{s'})}{\Gamma(\sum_{s'} \alpha_{s'})}$$

$$\text{where } \Gamma(x) := \int_0^\infty t^{x-1} e^{-t} dt$$

The mean of a Dirichlet distribution takes on a simple form:

$$\int_{\Delta_{N-1}} \Theta_{as\cdot} \frac{\prod_{s'} \Theta_{ass'}{}^{\alpha_{s'}-1}}{Z(\boldsymbol{\alpha})} d\Theta_{as\cdot} = \frac{\boldsymbol{\alpha}}{\sum_{s'} \alpha'_s}$$

We will assume a symmetric prior setting $\boldsymbol{\alpha}_{s'}$ equal to α for all s'. The vector form of the Dirichlet distribution will nevertheless still be useful in deriving the Bayesian estimate. The parameter α determines how much probability weight is centered at the midpoint of the simplex and is known as the *concentration factor*. For Dense Worlds, we use a concentration parameter $\alpha = 1$ which results in a uniform distribution over the simplex.

To derive an analytic form for the Bayesian estimate of Dense Worlds, we define the matrix $\boldsymbol{F}$ such that $\boldsymbol{F}_{ass'}$ is a count of the number of times $a, s \rightarrow s'$ has occurred in the data. Since each layer $\widehat{\Theta}_{as\cdot}$ of the CMC kernel is independently distributed, its posterior distribution can be computed as follows:

$$f(\Theta|\boldsymbol{F}) = \frac{\prod_{s'} \Theta_{ass'}^{F_{ass'}} \cdot \prod_{s'} \Theta_{ass'}{}^{\alpha-1}/Z(\alpha)}{p(\boldsymbol{F})}$$

$$= \frac{\prod_{s'} \Theta_{ass'}^{F_{ass'}+\alpha-1}}{Z(\alpha)p(\boldsymbol{F})} = \mathrm{Dir}(\boldsymbol{F}+\alpha)$$

Thus, the posterior distribution is also Dirichlet and the Bayesian estimate $\widehat{\Theta}$ is simply the mean of the distribution:

$$\widehat{\Theta}_{ass'} = \frac{F_{ass'} + \alpha}{\sum_{s^*} F_{ass^*} + \alpha} = \frac{F_{ass'} + 1}{\sum_{s^*} F_{ass^*} + 1} \quad (13)$$

In this form, we find that the Bayesian estimate for Dense Worlds is simply the relative frequencies of the observed data with the addition of fictitious counts of size α to each bin. The incorporation of this fictitious observation is referred to as Laplace smoothing and is often performed to avoid over-fitting (Manning et al., 2008). The derivation of Laplace smoothing from Bayesian inference over a Dirichlet prior is a well known result (MacKay and Peto, 1995).

(2) *Mazes* consist of $N = 36$ states corresponding to rooms in a randomly generated 6 by 6 maze and $M = 4$ actions corresponding to noisy translations, each biased toward one of the four cardinal directions. An example is depicted in **Figure 1**. Walking into a wall causes the agent to remain in its current location. Thirty transporters are randomly distributed amongst the walls which lead to a randomly chosen absorbing state (concentric rings in **Figure 1**). States that are not one step away from the originating state (either directly, through a portal, or against a wall) are assumed to have zero probability of resulting from any action. Transition probabilities for states that are one step away are drawn from a Dirichlet distribution with concentration parameter $\alpha = 0.25$, and the highest probability is assigned to the state corresponding to the preferred direction of the action. The small concentration parameter distributes more probability weight in the corners of the simplex resulting in less entropic transitions.
Letting N_s denote the number of states one-step away from state s, the Bayesian estimate for maze transitions is given by:

$$\widehat{\Theta}_{a,s,s'} = \frac{F_{ass'} + \alpha}{N_s \cdot \alpha + \sum_{s^*} F_{ass^*}} \quad (14)$$

As with Dense Worlds, the Bayesian estimate (Equation 14) for mazes is a Laplace smoothed histogram.

(3) *1-2-3 Worlds* consists of $N = 20$ states and $M = 3$ actions. In a given state, action $a = 1$ moves the agent deterministically to a single target state, $a = 2$ brings the agent with probability 0.5 to one of two possible target states, and $a = 3$ brings the agent with probability 0.333 to one of three potential target states. The target states are randomly and independently selected for each transition distribution. An absorbing state is form by universally increasing the likelihood that state 1 is chosen as a target. Explicitly, letting Ω_a be the set of all admissible transition distributions for action a:

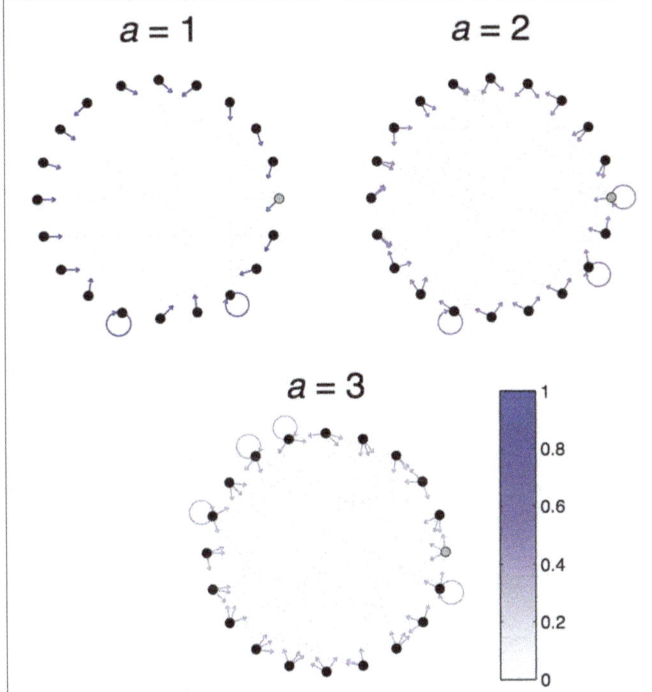

FIGURE A2 | Example 1-2-3 World. 1-2-3 Worlds consist of 3 actions (separately depicted) and 20 states (depicted as nodes of the graphs). The transition probabilities associated with taking a particular action are depicted as arrows pointing from the current state to each of the possible resultant states. Arrow color depicts the likelihood of each transition. The absorbing state is depicted in gray.

$$\Omega_a := \left\{ \Theta \in \mathbb{R}^N | \sum_{s'} \Theta_{s'} = 1 \text{ and } \Theta_{s'} \in \left\{0, \frac{1}{a}\right\} \forall s' \right\}$$

the transition distributions are drawn from the following distribution:

$$p(\Theta_{as\cdot}) = \begin{cases} 0 & \text{if } \Theta_{as\cdot} \notin \Omega_a \\ \dfrac{1-0.75^a}{\binom{N-1}{a-1}} & \text{else if } \Theta_{as1} = \frac{1}{a} \\ \dfrac{1-(1-0.75^a)}{\binom{N-1}{a}} & \text{otherwise} \end{cases} \quad (15)$$

Bayesian inference in 1-2-3 Worlds differs greatly from Mazes and Dense Worlds because of its discrete prior. If $a, s \rightarrow s'$ has been previously observed, then the Bayesian estimate for $\widehat{\Theta}_{ass'}$ is given by:

$$\widehat{\Theta}_{ass'} = \frac{1}{a}$$

If $a, s \rightarrow s'$ has not been observed but $a, s \rightarrow 1$ has, then the Bayesian estimate is given by:

$$\widehat{\Theta}_{ass'} = \frac{1 - \frac{|\mathcal{S}^*|}{a}}{N - T}$$

Here T is the number of target states that have already been observed. Finally, if neither $a, s \rightarrow s'$ nor $a, s \rightarrow 1$ have been observed, then the Bayesian estimate is:

$$\widehat{\Theta}_{ass'} = \begin{cases} \frac{1}{a} \cdot \dfrac{1 - 0.75^a}{1 + \left(\binom{a-1}{T} - 1\right) \cdot 0.75^a} & \text{if } s' = 1 \\ \dfrac{1 - \left(\frac{T}{a} + \widehat{\Theta}_{as1}\right)}{N - T - 1} & \text{otherwise} \end{cases}$$

A3 PROOF OF THEOREM 2

Claim. *If an agent is in state s and has previously collected data $\vec{d}$, then the expected information gain for taking action a is given by:*

$$\begin{aligned} \text{PIG}(a, s) : &= \text{E}_{s^*, \boldsymbol{\Theta}|\vec{d}}[\text{I}_\text{G}(a, s, s^*)] \\ &= \sum_{s^*} \widehat{\Theta}_{ass^*} \text{D}_\text{KL}(\widehat{\Theta}^{a, s \rightarrow s^*}_{as\cdot} \| \widehat{\Theta}_{as\cdot}) \end{aligned} \tag{16}$$

Proof.

$$\begin{aligned} \text{E}_{s^*, \boldsymbol{\Theta}|\vec{d}}[\text{I}_\text{G}(a, s, s^*)] &= \text{E}_{s^*, \boldsymbol{\Theta}|\vec{d}}\left[\sum_{s'} \boldsymbol{\Theta}_{ass'} \log_2 \left(\frac{\widehat{\Theta}^{a, s \rightarrow s^*}_{ass'}}{\widehat{\Theta}_{ass'}}\right)\right] \\ &= \text{E}_{s^*|\vec{d}}\left[\sum_{s'} \text{E}_{\boldsymbol{\Theta}|\vec{d}, s^*}[\boldsymbol{\Theta}_{ass'}] \log_2 \left(\frac{\widehat{\Theta}^{a, s \rightarrow s^*}_{ass'}}{\widehat{\Theta}_{ass'}}\right)\right] \\ &= \text{E}_{s^*|\vec{d}}\left[\sum_{s'} \widehat{\Theta}^{a, s \rightarrow s^*}_{ass'} \log_2 \left(\frac{\widehat{\Theta}^{a, s \rightarrow s^*}_{ass'}}{\widehat{\Theta}_{ass'}}\right)\right] \\ &= \text{E}_{s^*|\vec{d}}\left[\text{D}_\text{KL}(\widehat{\Theta}^{a, s \rightarrow s^*}_{as\cdot} \| \widehat{\Theta}_{as\cdot})\right] \\ &= \sum_{s^*} p(s^*|a, s, \vec{d}) \text{D}_\text{KL}(\widehat{\Theta}^{a, s \rightarrow s^*}_{as\cdot} \| \widehat{\Theta}_{as\cdot}) \text{ by (5)} \\ &= \sum_{s^*} \widehat{\Theta}_{ass^*} \text{D}_\text{KL}(\widehat{\Theta}^{a, s \rightarrow s^*}_{as\cdot} \| \widehat{\Theta}_{as\cdot}) \end{aligned}$$

A4 DERIVATION OF MEAN PATH LENGTH

To optimize navigation to a target state s^*, we consider modified transition probabilities:

$$p_\text{navigation}(s'|a, s) = \begin{cases} \Theta_{ass'} & \text{if } s \neq s^* \\ 1 & \text{if } s = s' = s^* \\ 0 & \text{otherwise} \end{cases}$$

A navigational utility function is then defined as:

$$U_\text{navigation}(s) = \begin{cases} -1 & \text{if } s \neq s^* \\ 0 & \text{otherwise} \end{cases}$$

An optimal policy π is derived through value-iteration as follows:

$$\begin{aligned} Q_0(a, s) &:= U_\text{navigation}(s) \\ Q_{\tau-1}(a, s) &:= U_\text{navigation}(s) + \sum_{s' \in \mathcal{S}} p_\text{navigation}(s'|a, s) \cdot V_\tau(s') \\ \text{where } V_\tau(s) &:= \max_a Q_\tau(a, s) \end{aligned}$$

Value-iteration is continued until V converges, and the optimal policy is then defined as:

$$\pi(s) = \arg\max_a Q_\text{convergence}(a, s)$$

The expected path length to target s^* is then calculated as:

$$\text{E[steps to } s^*] = \sum_s -\frac{1}{N} V_\text{convergence}(s)$$

The mean path length is then taken to be the average of the expected path length over the N possible target states.

A5 DERIVATION OF PEIG

Claim. *Surprise, as employed by Storck et al. (1995), is equal to the posterior expected information gain. That is, if an agent is in state s and has previously collected data $\vec{d}$, then the expected information gain for taking action a and observing resultant state s^* is given by:*

$$\text{Surprise}(a, s, s') : = \text{D}_\text{KL}(\widehat{\Theta}^{\vec{d} \cup s^*}_{as\cdot} \| \widehat{\Theta}^{\vec{d}}_{as\cdot}) = \text{E}_{\boldsymbol{\Theta}|\vec{d} \cup s^*}[\text{I}_\text{G}(a, s, s^*)] \tag{17}$$

Proof.

$$\begin{aligned} \text{E}_{\boldsymbol{\Theta}|\vec{d} \cup s^*}[\text{I}_\text{G}(a, s, s^*)] &= \text{E}_{\boldsymbol{\Theta}|\vec{d} \cup s^*}\left[\sum_{s'} \boldsymbol{\Theta}_{ass'} \log_2 \left(\frac{\widehat{\Theta}^{\vec{d} \cup s^*}_{ass'}}{\widehat{\Theta}^{\vec{d}}_{ass'}}\right)\right] \\ &= \sum_{s'} \text{E}_{\boldsymbol{\Theta}|\vec{d} \cup s^*}[\boldsymbol{\Theta}_{ass'}] \log_2 \left(\frac{\widehat{\Theta}^{\vec{d} \cup s^*}_{ass'}}{\widehat{\Theta}^{\vec{d}}_{ass'}}\right) \\ &= \sum_{s'} \widehat{\Theta}^{\vec{d} \cup s^*}_{ass'} \log_2 \left(\frac{\widehat{\Theta}^{a, s \rightarrow s^*}_{ass'}}{\widehat{\Theta}^{\vec{d}}_{ass'}}\right) \\ &= \text{D}_\text{KL}(\widehat{\Theta}^{\vec{d} \cup s^*}_{as\cdot} \| \widehat{\Theta}^{\vec{d}}_{as\cdot}) \end{aligned}$$

A6 METHODS FOR ASSESSING PERFORMANCE IN GOAL-DIRECTED TASKS

To assess the general utility of an agent's internal model, the agent is first allowed to explore for a fixed number of times steps. After exploring, the agent is asked, for each goal-directed task, to choose a fixed policy that optimizes performance under its learned model:

Navigation: To optimize navigation to a target state s^* under internal model $\widehat{\Theta}$, we took an approach analogous to our method for calculating the mean path length of a world (see Appendix A4). We first consider modified transition probabilities:

$$p_{\text{navigation}}(s'|a, s; \widehat{\Theta}) = \begin{cases} \widehat{\Theta}_{ass'} & \text{if } s \neq s^* \\ 1 & \text{if } s = s' = s^* \\ 0 & \text{otherwise} \end{cases}$$

A navigational utility function is then defined as:

$$U_{\text{navigation}}(s) = \begin{cases} -1 & \text{if } s \neq s^* \\ 0 & \text{otherwise} \end{cases}$$

An optimal policy $\pi_{\widehat{\Theta}}$ is derived through value-iteration as follows:

$$Q_0(a, s) := U_{\text{navigation}}(s)$$

$$Q_{\tau-1}(a, s) := U_{\text{navigation}}(s) + \sum_{s' \in \mathcal{S}} p_{\text{navigation}}(s'|a, s; \widehat{\Theta}) \cdot V_\tau(s')$$

where $V_\tau(s) := \max_a Q_\iota(a, s)$

This process is iterated a number a times, $\tau_{\text{convergence}} > 1000$, sufficient to allow Q to converge to within a small fixed margin. An optimal policy is then defined as:

$$\pi_{\widehat{\Theta}}(s) = \arg\max_a Q_{-\tau_{\text{convergence}}}(a, s)$$

The realized performance of $\pi_{\widehat{\Theta}}$ is assessed as the expected number of time steps, capped at 20, it would take an agent employing $\pi_{\widehat{\Theta}}$ to reach the target state. A true optimal policy is calculated as above except using Θ instead of $\widehat{\Theta}$. For each world and each exploration strategy, navigation is assessed after $t \in$ {25, 50, 75, 100, 150, 200, 250, 300, 350, 400, 450, 500, 600, 700, 800, 900, 1000, 1500, 2000, 2500, and 3000} exploration time steps and compared to the true optimal strategy. Performance difference from true optimal is calculated is averaged over the tested exploration lengths, all starting states, and all target states. The different explorative strategies are then ranked in performance.

Reward Acquisition: Policies in reward acquisition tasks are derived as above for navigational tasks except as follows:

$$p_{\text{reward}}(s'|a, s; \widehat{\Theta}) = \widehat{\Theta}_{ass'}$$

$$U_{\text{reward}}(s) \sim \text{Uniform}([-1, 1])$$

$$\pi_{\widehat{\Theta}}(s) = \arg\max_a Q_{-100}(a, s)$$

Realized performance is assessed as the expected total rewards accumulated by an agent employing $\pi_{\widehat{\Theta}}$ over 100 time steps.

15

Nonlinear dynamical model based control of *in vitro* hippocampal output

Min-Chi Hsiao[1]*, Dong Song[2] and Theodore W. Berger[3]

[1] Department of Biomedical Engineering, University of Southern California, Los Angeles, CA, USA
[2] Department of Biomedical Engineering, Center for Neural Engineering, University of Southern California, Los Angeles, CA, USA
[3] Department of Biomedical Engineering, Program in Neuroscience, and Center for Neural Engineering, University of Southern California, Angeles, CA, USA

Edited by:
Ahmed El Hady, Max Planck Institute for Dynamics and Self Organization, Germany

Reviewed by:
Karim Oweiss, Michigan State University, USA
Thierry R. Nieus, Italian Institute of Technology, Italy

***Correspondence:**
Min-Chi Hsiao, Department of Biomedical Engineering, University of Southern California, 3641 Watts Way, Los Angeles, CA 90089, USA.
e-mail: mhsiao@usc.edu

This paper describes a modeling-control paradigm to control the hippocampal output (CA1 response) for the development of hippocampal prostheses. In order to bypass a damaged hippocampal region (e.g., CA3), downstream hippocampal signal (e.g., CA1 responses) needs to be reinstated based on the upstream hippocampal signal (e.g., dentate gyrus responses) via appropriate stimulations to the downstream (CA1) region. In this approach, we optimize the stimulation signal to CA1 by using a predictive DG-CA1 nonlinear model (i.e., DG-CA1 trajectory model) and an inversion of the CA1 input–output model (i.e., inverse CA1 plant model). The desired CA1 responses are first predicted by the DG-CA1 trajectory model and then used to derive the optimal stimulation intensity through the inverse CA1 plant model. Laguerre-Volterra kernel models for random-interval, graded-input, contemporaneous-graded-output system are formulated and applied to build the DG-CA1 trajectory model and the CA1 plant model. The inverse CA1 plant model to transform desired output to input stimulation is derived from the CA1 plant model. We validate this paradigm with rat hippocampal slice preparations. Results show that the CA1 responses evoked by the optimal stimulations accurately replicate the CA1 responses recorded in the hippocampal slice with intact trisynaptic pathway.

Keywords: neural prosthesis, Volterra kernel, inverse control, trajectory model, hippocampus

INTRODUCTION

A neural prosthesis is a prosthetic device that interfaces with the nervous system to improve or restore impaired neural function (Berger et al., 1994; Schwartz, 2004; Patil and Turner, 2008). The neuroprosthetic technology has been advancing rapidly (Bernotas et al., 1986; Creasey et al., 2004; Mayberg et al., 2005; Hochberg et al., 2006; Allison et al., 2007; Stacey and Litt, 2008). Neural prostheses can be categorized according to the directions of the signal communication between the device and the nervous system (Turner et al., 2005; Song et al., 2007). The first category of neural prostheses attempts to decode neural signals and then to activate an external object. An example would be the neuroprobes decoding motor cortex signals to control a robotic arm (Donoghue, 2002; Nicolelis, 2003; Taylor et al., 2003). The second kind of neural prostheses encodes external sensory stimuli and intends to activate the nervous system. Examples are cochlear implants and artificial retinas (Middlebrooks et al., 2005; Weiland et al., 2005). The third kind of neural prostheses, which forms a bi-directional closed-loop system with the nervous system, receives incoming neural signals from one nervous region and sends its output to activate another nervous system region (Berger et al., 2001, 2011). For the neural prosthesis that involves stimulation to the nervous system, the output system responses could be influenced by the stimulation parameters such as location, intensity, and frequency. Because the signal transformation in the nervous system is nonlinear, it is also important to consider the nonlinearity between stimulation patterns and the output responses. Without considering this nonlinear relationship, large deviations between the device-evoked responses and the desired responses are expected. In practice, such deviations can be mitigated by tuning the stimulation parameters (Lauer et al., 2000; O'Suilleabhain et al., 2003; McIntyre et al., 2004; Tellez-Zenteno et al., 2006; Rupp and Gerner, 2007; Albert et al., 2009; McLachlan et al., 2010). This optimization procedure is typically performed manually and empirically, e.g., assuming a static and linear relation between the stimulation pattern and the desired responses, and then searching for the optimal ratio between the stimulation intensity and the outcome responses via a trial-and-error procedure. To formally solve this important problem, one needs to develop a rigorous stimulation paradigm that takes the (nonlinear dynamical) relationship between stimulation signals and system responses into account (Liu and Oweiss, 2010; Liu et al., 2011).

We are in the process of developing a neural prosthesis to restore the long-term memory formation function of the hippocampus that is lost in Alzheimer's disease, stroke, epilepsy, or other neurological disorders. Our concept of such a prosthetic device is a biomimetic model of the input–output nonlinear dynamics of the hippocampus—a model that captures how hippocampal circuitry re-encodes, or transforms, incoming spatio-temporal patterns of neural activity (i.e., short-term memories) into outgoing spatio-temporal patterns of neural activity (i.e., long-term memories) (Squire, 1992; Berger et al., 2001, 2005; Burgess et al., 2002). We have shown in rodents, both *in vitro* (Chan et al., 2004; Hsiao et al., 2006) and *in vivo* (Song et al., 2007,

2009; Berger et al., 2011, 2012), that a nonlinear hippocampal model is capable of predicting accurately the output signals based on the ongoing input signals in the hippocampus. In this study, we extend this concept by developing a rigorous stimulation paradigm with control theory, and then implementing it rat hippocampal slices.

The intrinsic circuitry of the hippocampus consists of three major subregions: dentate gyrus (DG), CA3, and CA1 as shown in **Figure 1A**. This trisynaptic circuit can be maintained in a transverse slice preparation (Andersen et al., 1969, 2000; Amaral and Witter, 1989). The signal transformations in all three regions are highly nonlinear and dynamical (Berger et al., 1988; Sclabassi

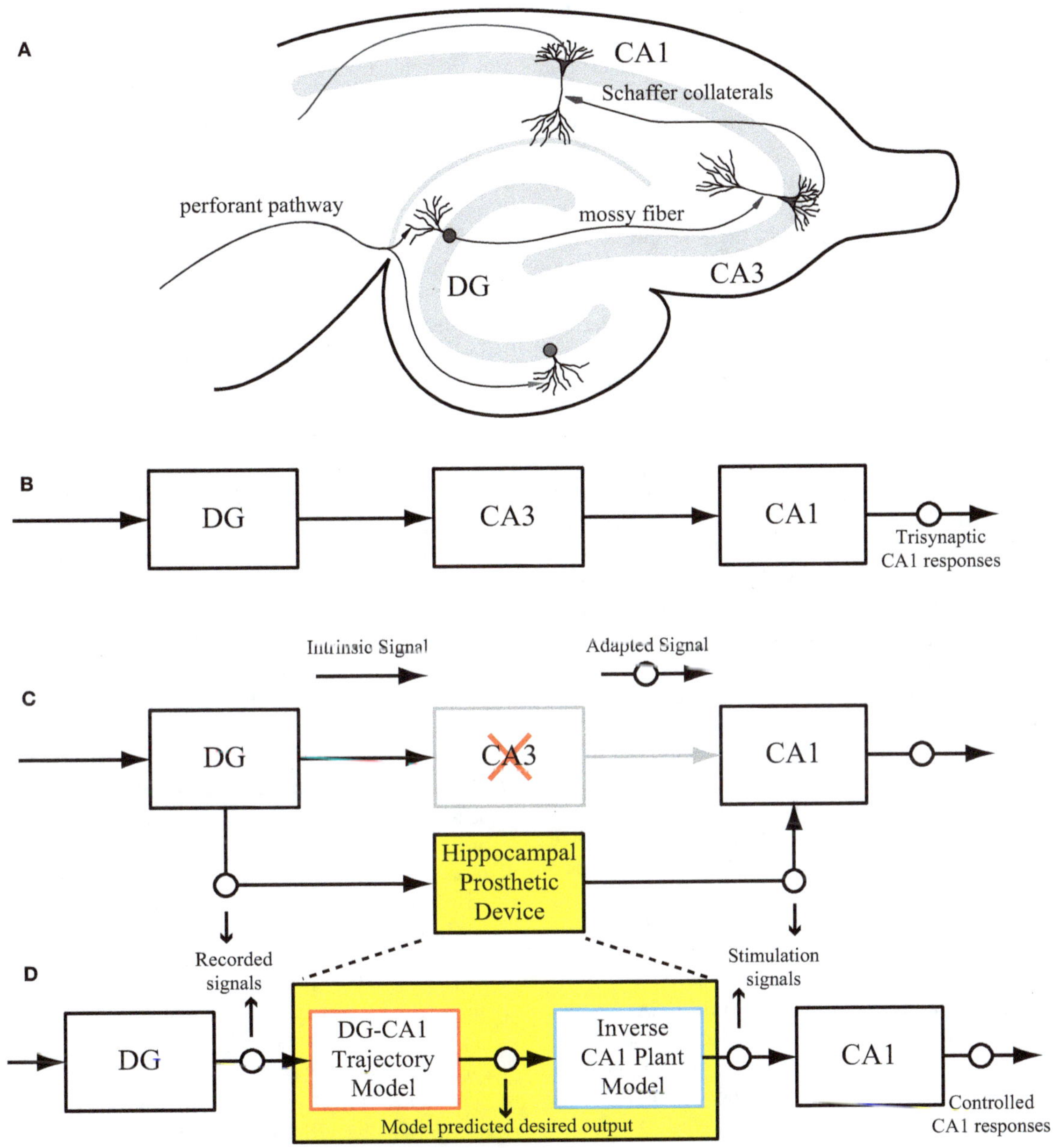

FIGURE 1 | (A) A rat hippocampal slice and its major intrinsic pathways. The input signals from perforant path fibers excite dentate granule cells. Dentate output, in turn, excites CA3 pyramidal cells through mossy fibers. Output from CA3 is transmitted to CA1 pyramidal cells through Schaffer collaterals. This so-called "trisynaptic pathway" is the principal network involved in hippocampal neuronal information processing. **(B)** A block diagram showing the trisynaptic pathway in a hippocampal slice. **(C)** A schematic diagram of a hippocampal prosthesis model functionally replacing the original pathway, where CA3 is damaged, so the signal transmission cannot be completed. This bi-directional prosthetic device receives incoming neural signals from one hippocampal region (DG) and sends its output to stimulate another hippocampal region (CA1). **(D)** The proposed modeling-control paradigm to optimize the stimulation patterns. In this framework, the desired CA1 output is first predicted with the DG signal by the trajectory model, and then converted to the desired stimulation patterns through the inverse model. The desired stimulation patterns then drives the output system (CA1) to the desired output responses.

et al., 1988; Bartesaghi et al., 2006). From an engineering perspective, the hippocampal circuit can be viewed as a cascade of input–output transfer functions between the DG, CA3, and CA1 subregions (**Figure 1B**). In the context of extracellular recording as in this study, the evoked field potentials in each subsystem are measured as input–output signals. For example, the CA3 response (field excitatory postsynaptic potentials amplitude, fEPSP) can be used as the input signal to CA1, and the CA1 response can be considered as the final system output. A schematic diagram of such a hippocampal prosthesis is shown in **Figure 1C**, where CA3 is damaged, thus the signal transmission from DG to CA1 cannot be completed. In the replacement scenario, the prosthesis model processes the DG signals and generates optimal stimulations to elicited desired output response in the CA1 region.

The successful implementation of such a device depends on three sequential components. First, the device must capture incoming neuronal signals reliably from the input region. Second, it must mimic the damaged system precisely through a computational model. Finally, the device should reproduce the desired responses in the output region through electrical stimulation. Thus, through bi-directional communication with the brain, the prosthetic device could essentially bypass the damaged region and substitute the lost function.

This paper describes the procedure of deriving optimal stimulation patterns using an inverse control concept (Houk, 1988; Widrow and Walach, 1996; Camacho and Bordons, 2003; Normann, 2007). The "trajectory model" is a model that predicts the desired output response based on the input patterns. This model can be developed using available knowledge or built directly from experimental input–output data. The stimulation-response properties of the output system is described as the "plant model." The "inverse plant model" describes a system whose transfer function is the inverse transformation of the plant model (Widrow and Bilello, 1993; Widrow and Plett, 1997; Karniel et al., 2001). This inverse transformation can be determined once the input–output transformation of the plant model is fully explored. Once these three models (i.e., trajectory, plant, and inverse plant models) are built, the signals flow like what is shown in **Figure 1D**. Signals recorded from the DG (input) system pass through the trajectory model to predict the desired output. The inverse plant model is then used to derive the desired stimulation amplitudes from desired output. Finally, the CA1 (output) region generates the controlled output responses. Results show that the strategy described in this paper is able to control CA1 output activities (shown in **Figure 1D** as "Controlled CA1 responses") to replicate the CA1 activities recorded from the hippocampal slice with intact trisynaptic pathway (shown in **Figure 1B** as "Trisynaptic CA1 responses").

MATERIALS AND METHODS

The proposed modeling-control paradigm was verified using an *in vitro* rat hippocampal slice preparation. Section "Experimental Procedures" provides an explanation of the methodology used to prepare the hippocampal slices, and the description of our electrophysiology experimental setup. Section "Modeling-Control Paradigm Implementation and Data Collection" describes the estimations and validations of the trajectory model, the plant model and the inverse plant model, and the associated data collection and analysis procedures. The overall experimental protocol is described in section "Modeling-Control Framework Experiment Protocol."

EXPERIMENTAL PROCEDURES

Acute hippocampal slice preparation

Hippocampal slices from 8 to 10-week-old male Sprague-Dawley rats (250–300 gm) were prepared. The animals were first anesthetized with halothane (Halocarbon Laboratory, USA) and then decapitated. Their skulls were rapidly removed and the brain was carefully extracted. Hippocampi were separated from the cortices in an iced sucrose buffer solution (Sucrose 206 mM; KCl 2.8 mM; NaH_2PO_4 1.25 mM; $NaHCO_3$ 26 mM; Glucose 10 mM; $MgSO_4$ 2 mM; Ascorbic Acid 2 mM). Hippocampal slices 400 micrometers thick were sliced transversely from the ventral hippocampi using a vibratome (Leica VT1000S, Germany). The slices were incubated for at least 1 h in 2 mM $MgSO_4$ artificial cerebral spinal fluid (aCSF) at room temperature, to equilibrate. During each electrophysiological recording session, one slice at a time was transferred to the planar multielectrode array. The array attached with a circular plastic chamber and perfused with normal aCSF (NaCl 128 mM; KCl 2.5 mM; NaH_2PO_4 1.25 mM; $NaHCO_3$ 26 mM; Glucose 10 mM; $MgSO_4$ 1 mM; Ascorbic Acid 2 mM; $CaCl_2$ 2 mM) maintained at room temperature (24~26°C). In the recording chamber, each slice was held down by a metallic ring with nylon mesh attached to it. The positioning of the slice was accomplished by manipulating the ring with a small brush. All the solutions were bubbled with 95% O_2 and 5% CO_2 mixed gas. The protocol described above was approved by the Department of Animal Resources and Institutional Animal Care and Use Committee at the University of Southern California.

Electrophysiological recording setup and procedures

Electrophysiology data were collected through an extracellular recording technique using an MEA60 system (Multi Channel Systems, Germany), as seen in **Figure 2**. This system consisted of pre-amplifiers (1200× gain), a data acquisition device (MC_Card), and an 8-channel stimulus generator (STG1008), all operated using software provided by Multi Channel Systems (MC_Rack V3.2.0 and MC_Stimulus V2.0.6). A conformal 60-channel planar multielectrode array was made specifically for this study. The geometry of this conformal array was designed to match the cytoarchitecture of the hippocampus slices (**Figure 2C**) and was platinum based. Details in fabrication and the arrangement of the array can be found in Gholmieh et al. (2006) and Taketani and Baurdy (2006). Collected data were sampled at a frequency of 10 kHz per channel and were recorded using MC_Rack. The MEA60 system was assembled over an inverted microscope (Leica DM-IRB, Germany). In each experiment, the position of the slice on the MEA was captured by a digital image capture system (Diagnostic Instruments, Spot RT Digital Camera, USA) with SPOT (V4.6.4.3) software and Adobe Photoshop (Adobe V7.0, USA).

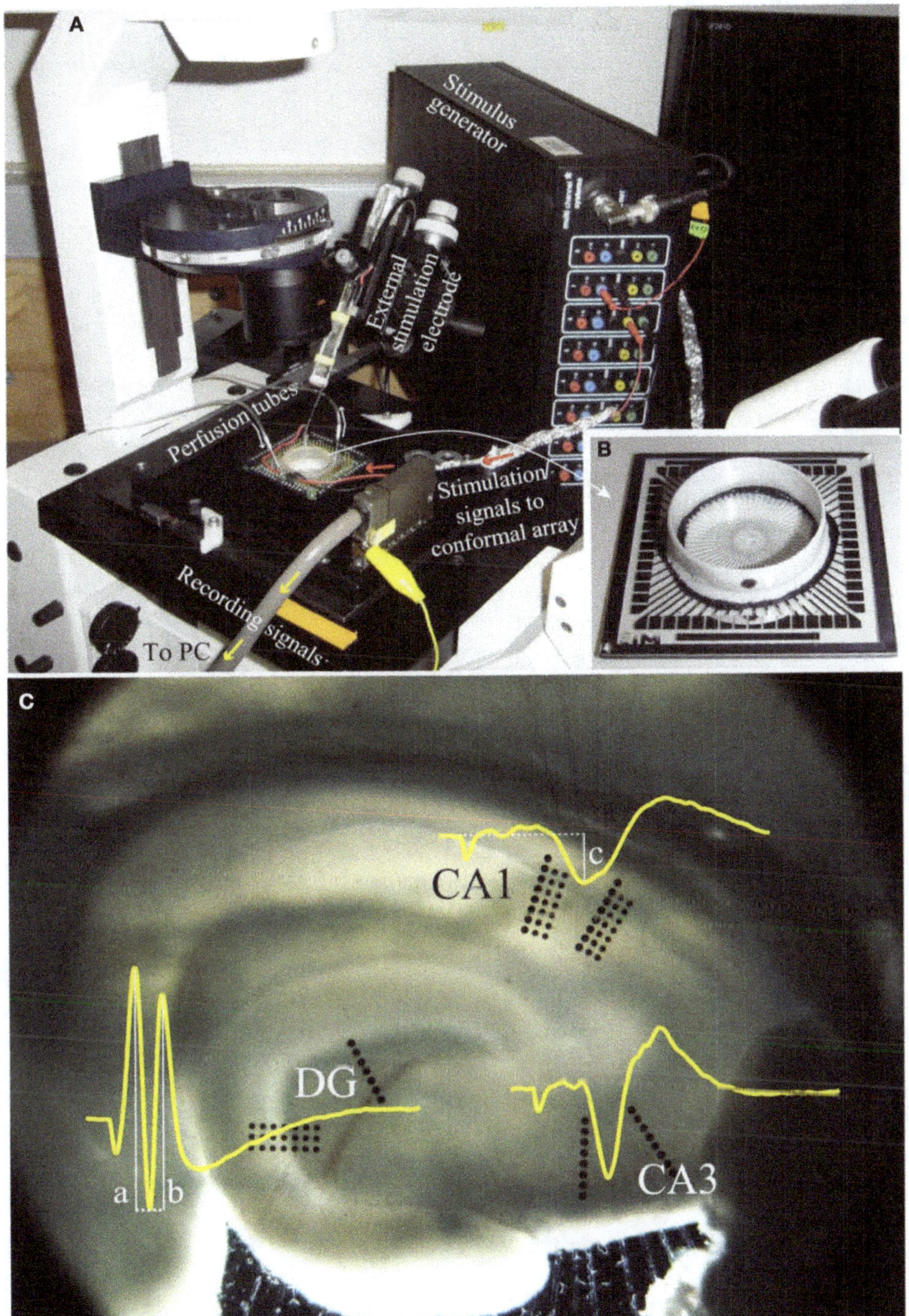

FIGURE 2 | A photo of the electrophysiological recording system. **(A)** The MEA60 system and **(B)** the conformal planar MEA (Gholmieh et al., 2006; Taketani and Baurdy, 2006). **(C)** A photomicrograph of a hippocampal slice on the conformal MEA. The set alignment of this array is according to rat hippocampal cytoarchitecture covering major subregions of DG, CA3, and CA1. The waveforms represent the trisynaptic response of the hippocampal slice recorded in each region. The white lines indicate the amplitude measurement of DG population spike amplitude and CA1 fEPSP amplitude (see section "FARIT-Induced Trisynaptic Data Collection and Analysis").

Stimulation and data collection procedures

In this study, biphasic currents with a 100 μs duration in each phase were applied to all stimulation patterns. Different stimulation trains were programmed in MC_Stimulus and used to study the nonlinear properties of different regions. There was a 5–7 min waiting period between each stimulus train. The evoked neural responses were simultaneously recorded from different regions. The channels were first selected based on the placement of the recording electrodes on the cytoarchitecture of the slices (i.e., DG channels must be in the DG region, CA3 channels must be in the CA3 region, etc). Among those channels, the channels with the largest response (dendritic population spike or EPSP) amplitudes are further selected and analyzed. The main purpose of this procedure is to find the most representative responses for each region, channels with small responses or inappropriate placements are not analyzed because their recordings may reflect a non-cell-body placement or a mixture of activities from multiple regions.

MODELING-CONTROL PARADIGM IMPLEMENTATION AND DATA COLLECTION

DG-CA1 trajectory model implementation

FARIT-induced trisynaptic data collection and analysis. An external bipolar electrode of twisted Nichrome wires was used to elicit the trisynaptic response. Paired-pulse or quadruplet-pulse electrical stimulation was applied to the perforant pathway of each slice using the external electrode to generate electrophysiological responses throughout the trisynaptic pathway (evoked field potentials in DG, CA3, and CA1, as seen in **Figure 2C**). When the full trisynaptic response was observed, we stimulated the slice with a series of fixed-amplitude, random inter-impulse-interval trains (FARITs). Four 300-pulse Poisson distributed FARITs of a fixed current intensity (biphasic, 150–300 μA) were delivered to the perforant path (1200 impulses; range of intervals: 2 ms to 5 s; mean frequency: 2 Hz). Response amplitudes from selected channels in DG and CA1 regions were analyzed to build the DG-CA1 trajectory model. The neuron response measurement in DG was population spike amplitude, the amplitude was calculated by averaging the distance between the negative peak and the first positive peak (measure "a" in **Figure 2C**) and the distance between the negative peak and the second positive peak (measure "b" in **Figure 2C**) (Houk, 1988). To measure responses in the CA1 regions, the field potential amplitude was defined as the negative peak of the waveform (measure "c" in **Figure 2C**).

Trajectory model configuration. A single-input, single-output discrete model was derived from Volterra series as expressed below (Marmarelis and Orme, 1993; Marmarelis, 2004):

$$y(n) = k_0 + \sum_{m=0}^{M} k_1(m)x(n-m) + \sum_{m_1=0}^{M}\sum_{m_2=0}^{M} k_2(m_1, m_2)x(n-m_1)x(n-m_2) + \ldots \tag{1}$$

The zeroth order kernel k_0 is the value of output y when the input is absent. First order kernels k_1 describe the relationship between each single input $x(n-m)$ and output y. Second order kernels k_2 describe the relationship between the output y and each unique pair of input $x(n-m_1), x(n-m_2)$. The term n represents time of occurrence of the present impulse in the input–output sequence and m represents the interval of the impulses prior to the present impulse within the kernel memory window M, $m = 0$ denotes the present input. The input to the system can be expressed as a series of variable-amplitude, random-interval delta functions:

$$x(t_i) = \sum_{i=1}^{I} A_i \delta(t - t_i) \tag{2}$$

where i is the index number of impulses and I is the total number of impulses. The time of occurrence of the ith impulse is t_i. In the DG-CA1 trajectory model experiment, DG population spike amplitude were used as input (A_i) and CA1 fEPSP amplitude were used as output $y(n)$. Because the input amplitude is varied, in order to isolate influence from present input, we considered the zero-lag terms in the original Volterra series (1) independently, as follows:

$$\begin{aligned} y(n) = {} & k_0 + k_1(0)x(n) + \sum_{m=1}^{M} k_1(m)x(n-m) \\ & + k_2(0,0)x(n)x(n) + \sum_{m_1=1}^{M} k_2(m_1, 0)x(n-m_1)x(n) \\ & + \sum_{m_2=1}^{M} k_2(0, m_2)x(n)x(n-m_2) \\ & + \sum_{m_1=1}^{M}\sum_{m_2=1}^{M} k_2(m_1, m_2)x(n-m_1)x(n-m_2) + \ldots \end{aligned}$$

and can be then rearranged as:

$$\begin{aligned} y(n) = {} & k_0 + k_1(0)x(n) + k_2(0,0)x(n)^2 + \sum_{m=1}^{M} k_1(m)x(n-m) \\ & + \sum_{m_1=1}^{M}\sum_{m_2=1}^{M} k_2(m_1, m_2)x(n-m_1)x(n-m_2) \\ & + 2\sum_{m=1}^{M} k_2(m)x(n)x(n-m) + \ldots \end{aligned} \tag{3}$$

The first three terms on right represent the static input–output curve. The last three terms describe the nonlinear dynamical effect of the inputs on the output. In order to reduce the number of open parameters, an estimation of the kernels is facilitated by expanding them on the orthonormal Laguerre basis functions L (Marmarelis, 1993):

$$L_l(m) = \alpha^{(m-l)/2}(1-\alpha)^{1/2}\sum_{k=0}^{l}(-1)^k \binom{m}{k}\binom{l}{k}\alpha^{l-k}(1-\alpha)^k$$

where α is the Laguerre parameter ($0 < \alpha < 1$) and affects the time extent of the basis functions. The convolution of Laguerre basis functions L and inputs x can be represented as

$$v_l(t_i) = \sum_{t_i - \mu < t_j \leq t_i} A_j L_l(t_i - t_j)$$

where A_j is the input spike amplitude in (2), t_i is the time of occurrence of the current impulse in the input–output sequence and t_j is the time of occurrence of the jth impulse prior to the present impulse within the kernel memory window μ. The adapted Laguerre expansion of Volterra kernels with L basis functions can be rewritten as:

$$\begin{aligned} y(t_i) &= c_0 + A_i c_1(0) + A_i^2 c_2(0,0) + \sum_{l=1}^{L} c_1(l) v_l(t_i) \\ &+ \sum_{l_1=1}^{L}\sum_{l_2=1}^{L} c_2(l_1,l_2) v_{l_1}(t_i) v_{l_2}(t_i) \\ &+ 2A_i \sum_{l=1}^{L} c_2(l) v_l(t_i) + \ldots \end{aligned} \quad (4)$$

where $c_0, c_1, c_2, \ldots$ are the kernel expansion coefficients. Since the number of basis functions can be made much smaller than the memory length, the number of open parameters is greatly reduced by this expansion technique. The kernel expansion coefficients ($c_0, c_1, c_2, \ldots$) can be estimated via the least-squares method, and can be used to reconstruct the Volterra kernels (k_i) using Laguerre basis functions (L)

$$k_0 = c_0, \quad k_1 = \sum_{l=1}^{L} c_l L_l, \quad k_2 = \sum_{l_i=1}^{L}\sum_{l_i=1}^{L} c_{l_1,l_2} L_{l_1,l_2}$$

CA1 plant model implementation

RARIT-induced monosynaptic data collection and analysis. After collecting the FARIT data for building DG-CA1 trajectory model, in the same slice, paired-pulse stimulation was applied to the *stratum radiatum* from a pair of stimulation electrodes in the conformal array in order to elicit the monosynaptic CA1 response. The pair of stimulation electrodes was selected according to their location and their ability to evoke typical paired-pulse facilitation. In this set of experiments, the amplitudes of the FARITs were modified to formulate a random-amplitude, random-interval trains (RARITs, Gaussian distributed, mean amplitude: 150 μA, which is the mean CA1 evoked postsynaptic potential amplitude observed in the FARIT-induced trisynaptic dataset). Once the pair of stimulation electrodes were determined, four 300-pulse RARITs were delivered to the slice. A channel from the CA1 region was selected and fEPSP amplitudes were analyzed for suitability in constructing the CA1 plant model.

CA1 plant model configuration. The same Laguerre-Volterra (LV) modeling approach described in section "Trajectory Model Configuration" was applied to build a CA1 plant model. In this set of experiments, the amplitudes of the RARITs (from previous section) were used as measures of the input signal A_i in (2), and the fEPSP amplitudes of CA1 were used as measures of output. Once the input–output transformation of the CA1 system was fully explored, the inverse model can be further derived.

Inverse CA1 plant model implementation

Inverse CA1 plant model configuration. The inverse model was built to transform the output (i.e., desired output of a CA1 region) to the input (i.e., desired input stimulation to a CA1 region). To develop the inverse model based on the LV model, the original Equation (4) was rearranged to:

$$\begin{aligned} &[c_2(0,0)]A_i^2 + \left[c_1(0) + 2\sum_{l=1}^{L} c_2(l) v_l(t_i)\right] A_i \\ &+ \left[c_0 + \sum_{l=1}^{L} c_1(l) v_l(t_i) + \sum_{l_1=1}^{L}\sum_{l_2=1}^{L} c_2(l_1,l_2) v_{l_1}(t_i) \right. \\ &\left. \times v_{l_2}(t_i) - y(t_i)\right] = 0 \end{aligned} \quad (5)$$

In (5), the desired output y and the coefficients $c_0, c_1, c_2, \ldots$ were obtained during process of model estimation. All the convolution terms could also be determined using the coefficients and previous stimulation amplitudes $A_{i-1}, A_{i-2}, \ldots$. Once all the terms are determined, (5) became a quadratic equation with unknown desired input stimulation (A). It can be simplified as:

$$aA^2 + bA + c = 0 \quad (6)$$

where

$$a = c_2(0,0), \quad b = c_1(0) + 2\sum_{l=1}^{L} c_2(l) v_l(t_i),$$

$$c = c_0 + \sum_{l=1}^{L} c_1(l) v_l(t_i) + \sum_{l_1=1}^{L}\sum_{l_2=1}^{L} c_2(l_1,l_2) v_{l_1}(t_i) v_{l_2}(t_i) - y(t_i)$$

such that the transformation of the inverse model (output to input) became an operation of solving A in (6). In this study, the roots of the quadratic equation can all be calculated from

$$A = \frac{-b + \sqrt{b^2 - 4ac}}{2a} \quad (7)$$

The validation of this inverse model implementation is shown in the result (section "Inverse CA1 Plant Model Implementation and Validation Results"). All the calculated stimulation amplitude were used to recompose to the new stimulation trains, called desired-amplitude RITs (DARITs) as described below.

DARIT-induced monosynaptic data collection and analysis. In this set of experiments, the amplitude of the RARITs (as used in section "RARIT-Induced Monosynaptic Data Collection and Analysis") were reformed using the optimal stimulation amplitudes calculated from the inverse CA1 plant model (from previous section "Inverse CA1 Plant Model Configuration"), named DARITs. Four 300-pulse DARITs were delivered to the slice through the same pair of stimulation electrodes as RARIT experiments. A channel from the CA1 region was selected and the fEPSP amplitudes were analyzed.

Model validation

In this study, data were evaluated using the Variance Accounted For (VAF) and the Normalized Mean Square Error (NMSE) as described below:

$$VAF = (1 - \mathrm{var}(Y_i - X_i)/\mathrm{var}(Y_i))$$

$$NMSE = \sum_i (Y_i - X_i)^2 \Big/ \sum_i Y^2$$

where X is the predicted amplitude of the model, Y is the amplitude analyzed from the recorded data, and *var* is the variance of the data. Specific data sets were chosen for comparison and are presented in the result section. To evaluate the prediction power of the models, we have used a cross-validation method, i.e., independent datasets are used for model estimation and model prediction. All model goodness-of-fit reported in this paper are obtained using this method.

MODELING-CONTROL FRAMEWORK EXPERIMENT PROTOCOL

The experiment protocol to verify our modeling-control paradigm for an *in vitro* hippocampal prosthesis involves following steps:

1. Stimulating the perforant path (DG input) with FARITs, and analyzing the trisynaptic responses in DG and CA1; applying DG population spike patterns as input and CA1 fEPSP patterns as output, building a DG-CA1 trajectory model using an LV kernel modeling approach (**Figure 3A**).
2. Stimulating the Schaffer collaterals (CA1 input) with RARITs, and analyzing the monosynaptic responses in CA1; applying RARITs patterns as input and CA1 fEPSP patterns as output, building a CA1 plant model using the LV kernel modeling

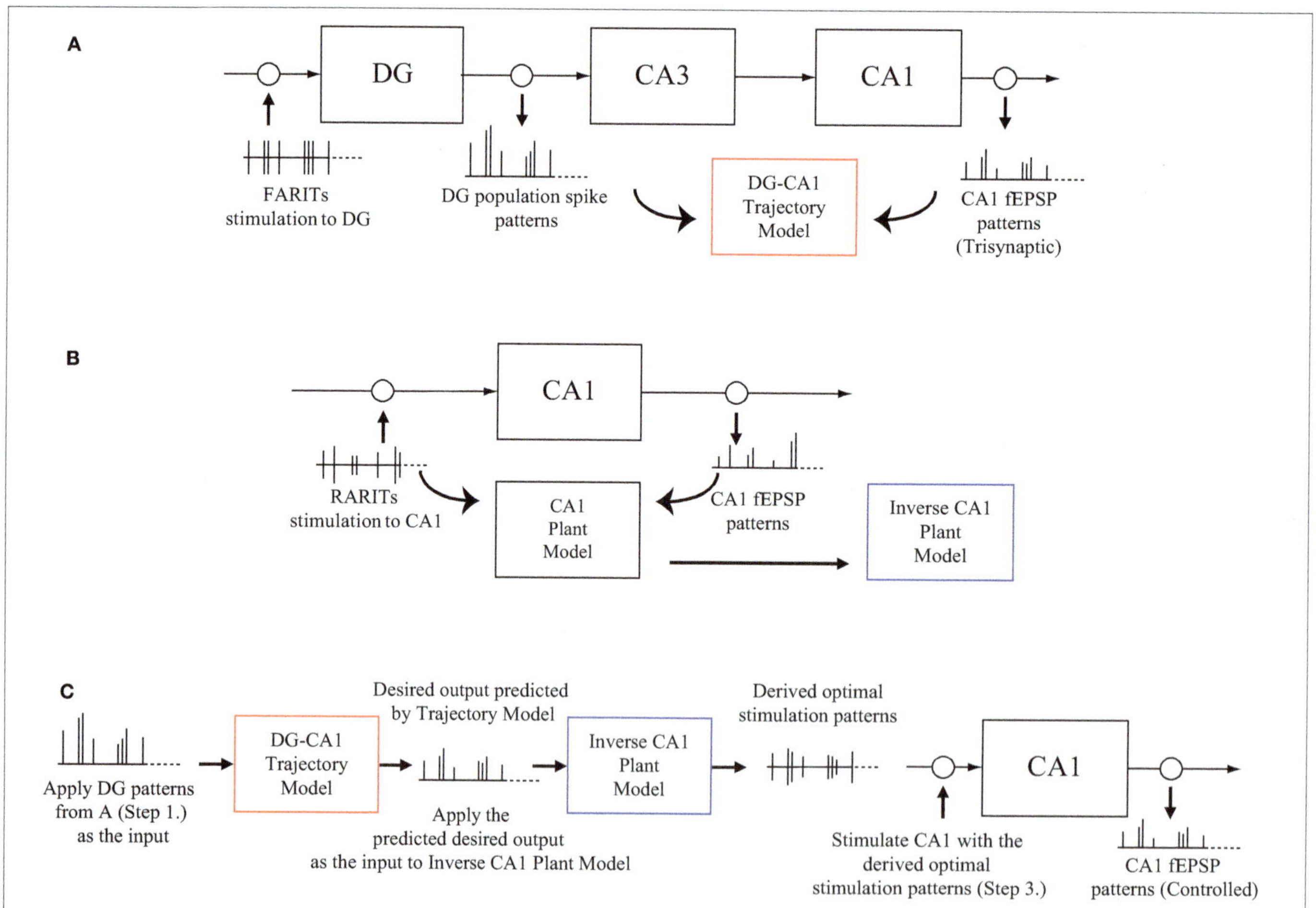

FIGURE 3 | A schematic diagram of the modeling-control experimental protocol. (A) Stimulating the perforant path with FARITs, and analyzing the trisynaptic responses in DG and CA1, to build a DG-CA1 trajectory model. **(B)** Stimulating the Schaffer collaterals with RARITs, and analyzing the monosynaptic responses in CA1, to build a CA1 plant model. The inverse CA1 plant model can then be formulated. **(C)** Applying DG patterns (from **A**) as the input to DG-CA1 trajectory model (built in **A**) to predict desired CA1 output patterns; applying the predicted desired CA1 output as the input to the inverse CA1 plant model (built in **B**) to derive the optimal stimulation patterns; stimulating at the Schaffer collaterals with the derived optimal stimulation patterns, and then analyzing the responses in CA1. CA1 fEPSP amplitudes from **A** and **C** can then be compared.

approach, and then formulating an inverse CA1 plant model (**Figure 3B**).

3. Applying DG patterns as the input to DG-CA1 trajectory model to predict desired CA1 output patterns; applying the predicted desired CA1 output as the input to inverse CA1 plant model, to derive the optimal stimulation patterns; stimulating at the Schaffer collaterals with the derived optimal stimulation patterns, and then analyzing the responses in CA1 (**Figure 3C**).
4. Comparing the CA1 fEPSP amplitudes from Step 1 to those in Step 3.

RESULTS

The diagrams and performance of the DG-CA1 trajectory and CA1 plant model prediction, and the inverse CA1 plant model implementation are presented in this section. The presented protocol was conducted in six experiments. In each experiment, two sets of data were collected from a hippocampal slice. The first dataset was composed of the FARIT-induced trisynaptic data and was used to build the DG-CA1 trajectory model. The second dataset was composed of the RARIT-induced monosynaptic data and was used to build the CA1 plant model. The resulting two built models and their predictions are presented. This section also include the implementation of the inverse CA1 plant model, and lastly, the validation of the modeling-control paradigm used for regulating CA1 nonlinear dynamics.

DG-CA1 TRAJECTORY MODEL AND THE PREDICTION RESULTS

The FARIT-induced hippocampal trisynaptic data were analyzed for use in building the DG-CA1 trajectory model. The amplitudes of evoked DG population spikes were used as measures of the input to the system, and the amplitudes of evoked CA1 fEPSPs were used as measures of output of the system. An LV kernel model was applied to study the nonlinearity of this system. Examples of the first and the second order LV kernels are shown in **Figures 4A,B**, respectively.

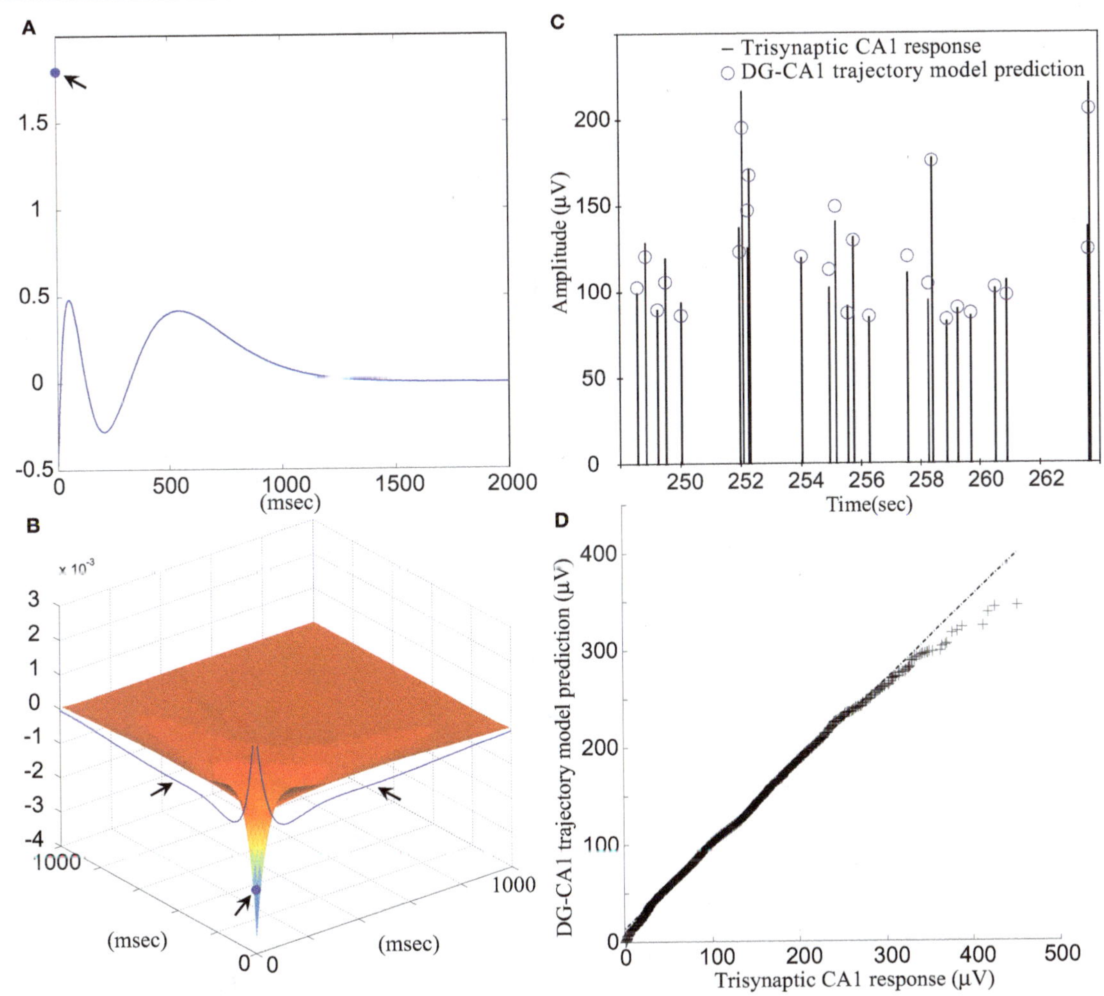

FIGURE 4 | (A) The first order and **(B)** the second order LV kernel of the DG-CA1 trajectory model. The singular points and lines showing on the edge of each figure (indicated by arrows) represent the effect of present input. **(C)** A segment of comparison between a FARIT-induced trisynaptic CA1 response amplitude and the amplitude predicted by the DG-CA1 trajectory model. **(D)** The Q–Q plot of the data distribution between actual trisynaptic CA1 responses recorded from the slice and the outputs predicted by the DG-CA1 trajectory model.

It should be noted that in **Figure 4A**, the singular point represents the $K_1(0)$ term in (3). The different polarity in **Figure 4A** manifests the importance of isolating the zero lag terms. In **Figure 4B**, the singular point represents the $K_2(0,0)$ term in (3), and the two lines indicated by arrows represent the $\sum_{m_1=1}^{M}\sum_{m_2=1}^{M} k_2(m_1, m_2)$ term, while one of the input pairs is the present input ($m = 0$).

Model estimation was completed using population spike amplitudes and the intervals of the input–output sequences. From all datasets, the slice response amplitudes were analyzed and compared with the predicted amplitudes. The mean VAF was 65.97 ± 17.30%. In **Figure 4C**, a segment of FARIT-induced trisynaptic CA1 fEPSP amplitudes is compared to its counterpart predicted from the DG-CA1 trajectory model. The result is further confirmed by an overall comparison between the actual responses and model predicted outputs, as shown in **Figure 4D**. The quantile–quantile (Q–Q) plot demonstrates that the actual trisynaptic CA1 responses recorded from the slice are accurately predicted by the DG-CA1 trajectory model.

CA1 PLANT MODEL AND THE PREDICTION RESULTS

The RARIT-induced CA1 monosynaptic data were analyzed for use in building the CA1 plant model. The random amplitudes of the RARITs were used as measures of input into the system, and the amplitudes of evoked CA1 fEPSPs were used as measures of the output of the system. The LV kernel model was applied to study the nonlinearity of the CA1 system. Examples of the first and the second order LV kernels are shown in **Figures 5A,B**, respectively.

Model estimation was completed using stimulation intensities and intervals of the input–output sequences. The VAF between slice response and model prediction was 85.56 ±

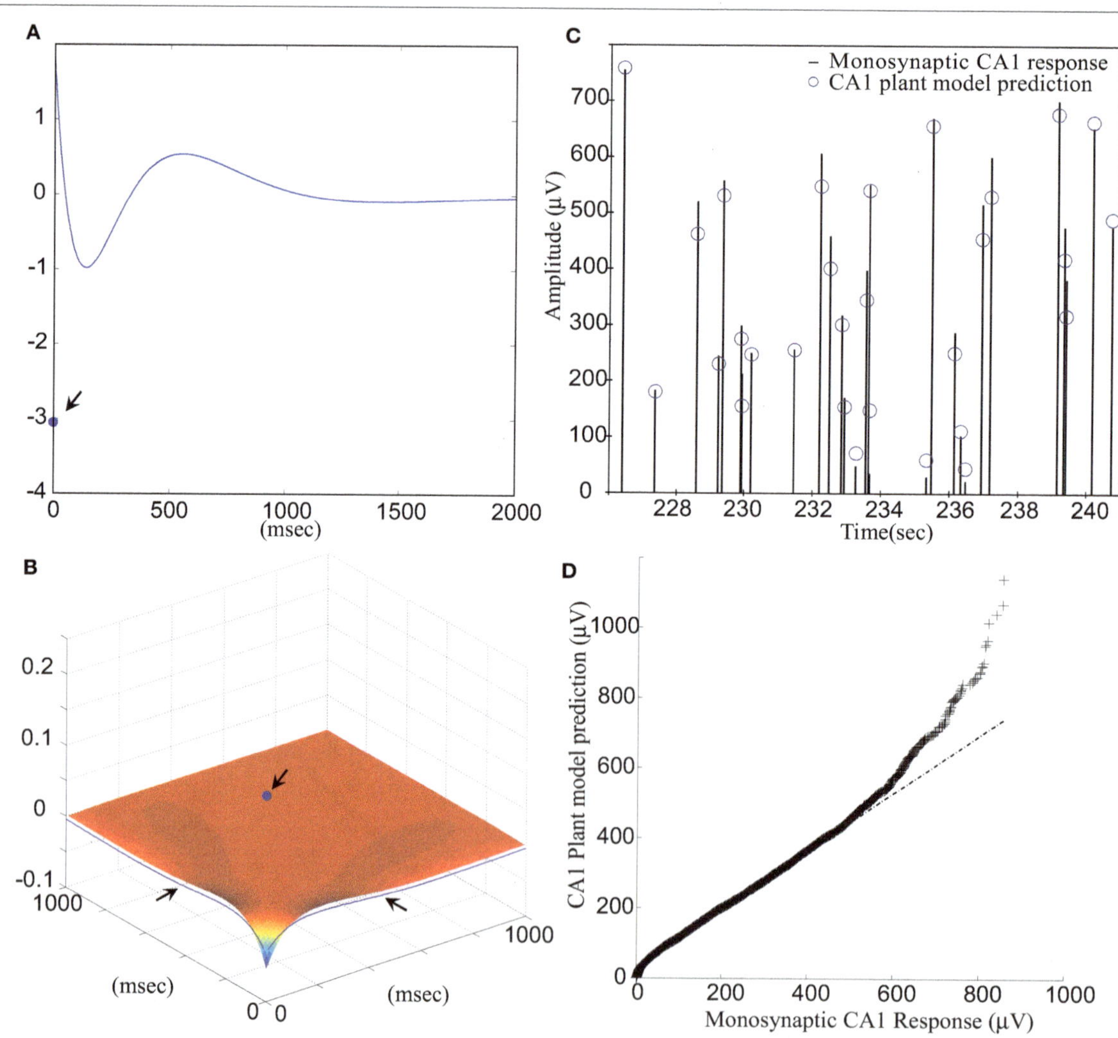

FIGURE 5 | (A) The first order and **(B)** the second order LV kernel of the CA1 plant model. The singular points and lines showing on the edge of each figure (indicated by arrows) represent the effect of present input. **(C)** A segment of comparison between RARIT-induced monosynaptic CA1 response amplitudes and the amplitudes predicted by the CA1 plant model. **(D)** The Q–Q plot of the data distribution between actual monosynaptic CA1 responses recorded from the slice and the outputs predicted by the CA1 plant model.

13.91%, averaged from six datasets. This shows that the CA1 plant model can accurately predict CA1 amplitudes based on stimulation amplitudes. A segment of the RARIT-induced monosynaptic CA1 fEPSP amplitudes is compared to its counterpart predicted by the CA1 plant model, as shown in **Figure 5C**. **Figure 5D** displays the Q–Q plot of the overall monosynaptic CA1 responses and CA1 plant model predicted results.

INVERSE CA1 PLANT MODEL IMPLEMENTATION AND VALIDATION RESULTS

The implementation of the inverse CA1 plant model is accomplished using RARIT-induced monosynaptic data. The purpose for formulating such an inverse model is to transform output predictions into input stimulations. The output predictions were acquired from the CA1 plant model, and applied as the y in (5). The coefficients $c_0, c_1, c_2, \ldots$ were obtained during process of model estimation. Three terms involved the convolution of Laguerre basis functions and input amplitude were unknown, which include

$$\sum_{l=1}^{L} c_2(l)v_l(t_i), \quad \sum_{l=1}^{L} c_1(l)v_l(t_i), \text{ and } \sum_{l_1=1}^{L}\sum_{l_2=1}^{L} c_2(l_1, l_2)v_{l_1}(t_i)v_{l_2}(t_i).$$

Based on our experimental design, no stimulation existed before the stimulation train was sent, so these unknown terms were equal to zero. Thus, the first stimulation amplitude can be calculated by (7). After the first stimulation amplitude was calculated, it was then applied to convolve with the Laguerre basis function and formulate the unknown terms for calculating the next stimulation amplitude. The operations for solving the root were run through all data points in order to process the transformation from output into input. As a result, the inverse model allows us to convert the desired output response amplitudes to input stimulation amplitudes in a dynamic, recursive manner.

The validation of this inverse model was completed by comparing the calculated stimulation amplitudes with the RARIT amplitudes. The scatter plot in **Figure 6** shows that the calculated stimulation amplitudes and the RARIT stimulation amplitudes are identical, showing that: (1) the real roots could all be calculated; and (2) this inverse model implementation can successfully derive optimal stimulations based on desired response amplitudes.

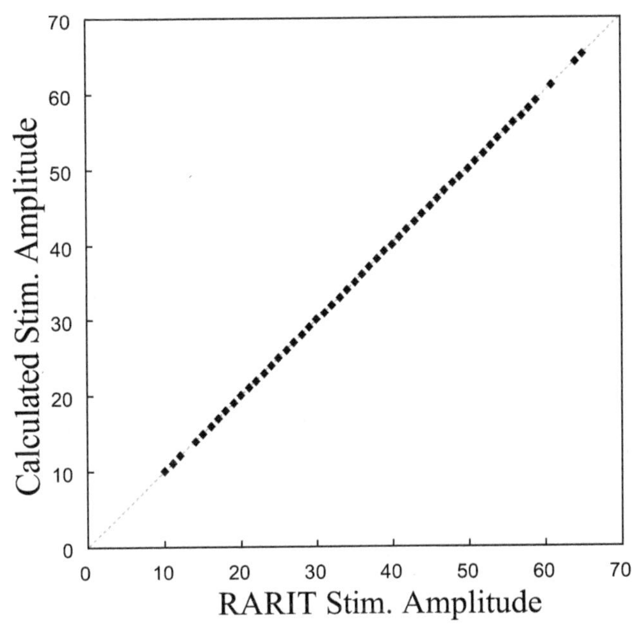

FIGURE 6 | The comparison between stimulation amplitude in RARIT that sent into CA1 and the amplitude calculated from inverse CA1 plant model.

MODELING-CONTROL RESULTS

Following the protocol in this modeling-control framework experiment, CA1 desired output is first predicted through DG-CA1 trajectory model, and then applied into the inverse CA1 plant model to derive the optimal stimulation amplitudes. These amplitudes were used to formulate DARITs and were then sent into the slice, and the monosynaptic CA1 responses were recorded. The proposed modeling-control framework was intended to evoke CA1 to produce activities similar to the original CA1 activities. Thus, DARIT-induced monosynaptic CA1 amplitudes were compared with FARIT-induced trisynaptic CA1 response amplitudes. Two examples are shown in **Figure 7**.

Each panel illustrates results from one experiment: amplitudes of fEPSPs recorded from the CA1 region are shown as a function of 50 impulses chosen from among 2400 impulses of the stimulation trains (1200 administered with FARIT stimulation; 1200 administered with DARIT stimulation). In order to collapse the x axis to comprise more data points, time intervals between impulses are not represented in the figures; only "Input Event" number (sequence of sample impulses) is shown. Data for the FARIT-induced trisynaptic CA1 responses (CA1-trisynaptic) are shown in blue diamonds; data for the DARIT-induced monosynaptic CA1 responses (CA1-Controlled) are shown in red squares. As seen in **Figure 7**, the variation in CA1 fEPSP amplitudes was also captured in our model controlled paradigm. The accuracy was evaluated using NMSE of the amplitude, and the average NMSE was 15.41 ± 8.35%. A Q–Q plot compared through the entire data sets is shown in **Figure 8**.

DISCUSSIONS

One of the essential objectives of a neural prosthetic device is to recreate the desired neural responses. While it is important to develop a reliable hardware model to represent the computational functions of a system, the control between device stimuli and actual responses is equally important. For example, in the application of deep brain stimulation (DBS), many efforts have been made in calibrating the stimulation parameters to achieve the desired effect (Mayberg et al., 2005; Okun et al., 2005). DBS devices depend on a trial-and-error process for finding the optimal stimulation pattern. Patients must repeatedly perform an exercise for a neurologist to adjust the stimulation parameters such as voltage, amplitude, pulse width, frequency, and electrode position (Moro et al., 2002; Volkmann et al., 2002; O'Suilleabhain et al., 2003). Another example is the application of functional electrical stimulation (FES) (Riener, 1999; Duffell et al., 2008;

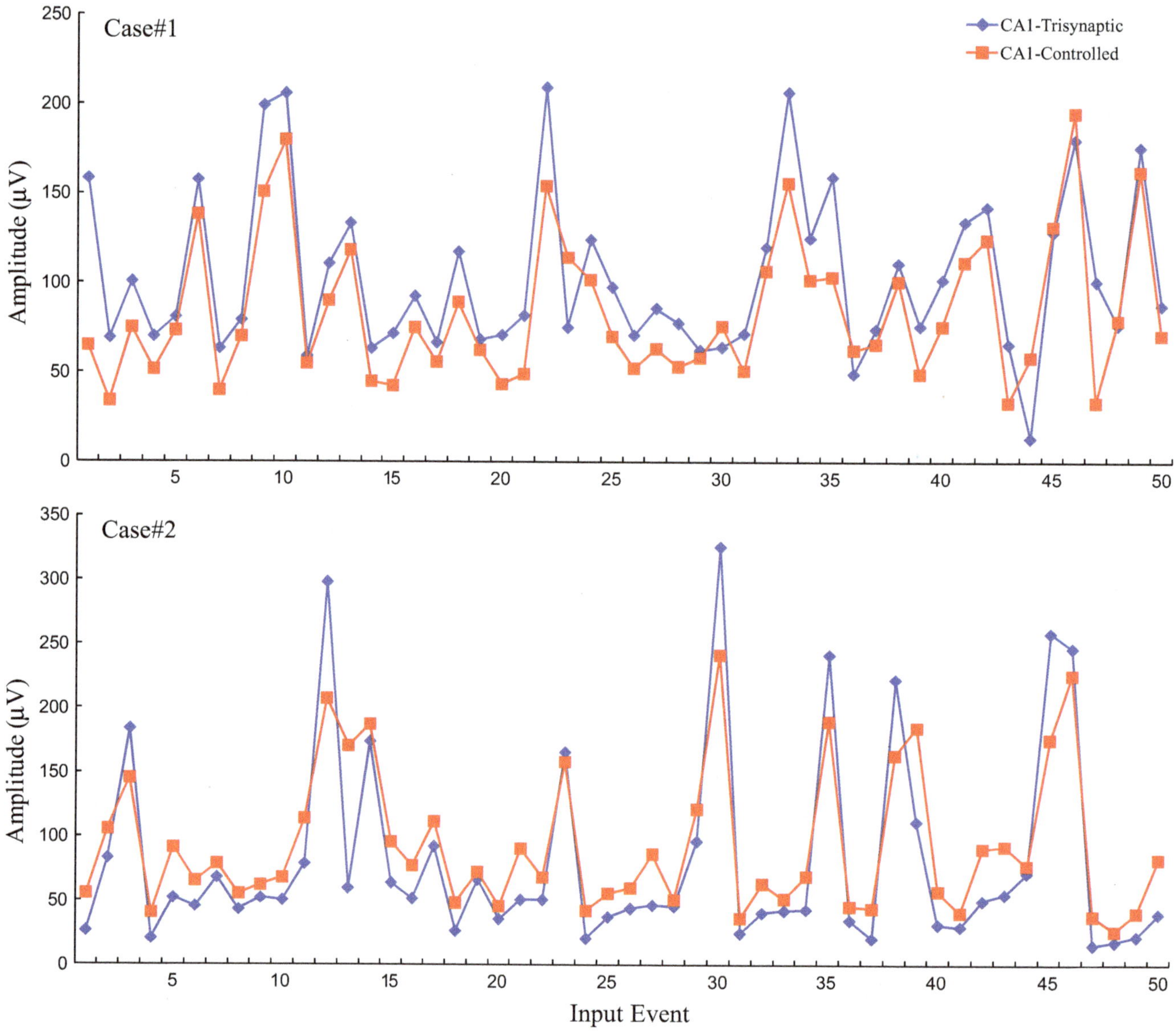

FIGURE 7 | A comparison of CA1 fEPSP amplitudes in response to FARIT-induced trisynaptic response (CA1-trysynaptic in blue diamonds) and DARIT-induced monosynaptic response (CA1-Controlled in red squares). The NMSE from 6 datasets was 15.41 ± 8.35%.

Donovan-Hall et al., 2011). The basic principle of FES is the generation of action potentials in the uninjured lower motor neurons by external electrical stimulation. This device faces problems such as muscle fatigue, spasticity, and limited force in the stimulated muscle. Using control strategies is one way to avoid internal disturbances and improve the time-consuming trial-and-error adjustment (Matjacic et al., 2003; Braz et al., 2009). Current neural prostheses face the same problem—the stimulation signals need to be adjusted manually or empirically based on the output response. In this article, we describe a rigorous approach to generate the stimulation patterns using a modeling-control framework. In the hippocampal slice preparation, with the purpose of restoring the CA1 output responses observed in the intact trisynaptic (DG to CA3 to CA1) circuitry, a nonlinear trajectory model was built to predict the CA1 desired output based on DG input. The predicted CA1 output was then converted to optimal stimulation through an inverse plant model of CA1 (i.e., an inverse transformation of CA1 input–output properties). Thus, the stimulation was essentially derived based on the desired output response, and was used to reactivate the CA1 response. An experimental validation of this modeling-control paradigm using hippocampal slices is provided. One of our preliminary studies was to stimulate CA1 region with non-optimal stimulation parameters, which means the nonlinearity of CA1 input–output relationship was not take into concern. The average NMSE from four experiments was 35.23 ± 18.21%, which is much higher than the modeling-control paradigm results.

In current experimental paradigm, the only open parameters is the stimulation intensity, since the desired output responses are single EPSPs, the stimulations are the standard biphasic pulses, and there is no frequency (multiple impulses will elicit undesired multiple EPSPs). We are aware of the fact that in other applications (e.g., DBS), the phase and frequency are equally important parameters and also could be optimized. Our current modeling-control paradigm can be extended and used as a platform for the optimization of those parameters in the future. We understand that the stimulation site is also critical for this kind of devices, sometimes the misplacement of the electrode lead could cause poor efficacy or adverse effects (Richardson et al., 2009; van den Munckhof et al., 2010). Current clinical DBS surgeries were assisted with preoperative images analysis (MRI or CT), and intra-operatively guided with computerized stereotactic techniques. The lead could also be switched with limited-adjustability to compensate the inappropriate placement issue. By applying the stimulation electrode array in current experimental setup, the optimal stimulation site and its influence to the model can be further evaluated.

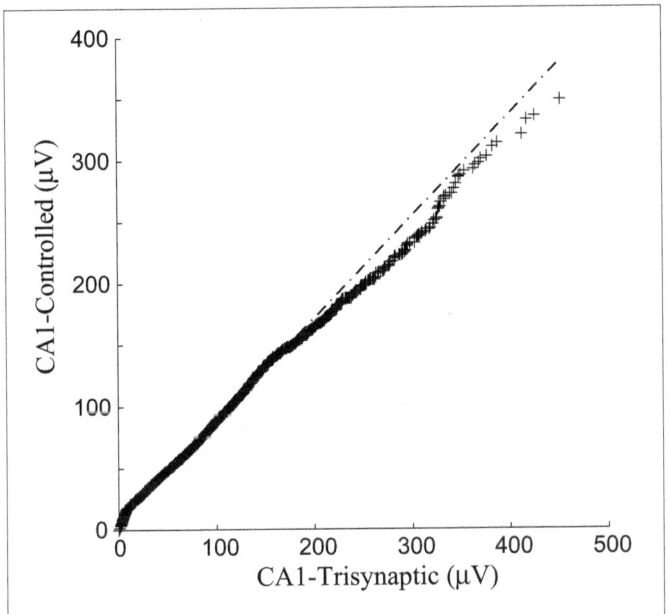

FIGURE 8 | A Q–Q plot demonstration of the data comparison between the trisynaptic CA1 responses and the paradigm controlled CA1 responses.

Our demonstrations also show that implementing a bidirectional neural prosthesis implicitly replaces the damaged system. In this approach, we do not need to explicitly estimate the transformational property of the CA3 region in the trisynaptic circuit. As long as we have the trajectory responses of the output system and once we identify the nonlinear input–output relationship of the output system, we are able to drive it to the desired output through its inverse model. One potential issue here would be "How to know the desired trajectory responses in the intact system?" In our opinion, there are several solutions/mechanisms that can mitigate this problem. First, we may develop a "generic model" from data recorded in normal animals. Previous studies have shown that there are significant amount of common features in the functional input–output properties across different animals, despite the animal-to-animal variations. In the case described in this study, all trajectory models are qualitatively similar in terms of the kernel polarity, kernel duration and kernel shape. Using model derived from other animals is imperfect, but at least provides a good approximation. Second, in behaving animal applications, the "imperfect" outputs generated by the "imperfect model" will be read out by the downstream brain regions. Neural plasticity, which is ubiquitous in the central nervous system, may play a role in adapting the system to the imperfect outputs or model. Third, more sophisticated computational methods such as reinforcement learning can potentially be used to develop self-adaptive or co-adaptive models.

The paradigm introduced in this paper did not include the error feedback. This was based on the assumption that the error observed in the output responses is instantaneous and does not influence the future output. In order to extend the paradigm to a closed-loop feedback system (Bernotas et al., 1986; Houk, 1988; Veltink et al., 1992; Abbas and Riener, 2001; Liu et al., 2011), the output error, that may caused by the interface between electrodes and nervous systems, the variation of the system, or the internal disturbance, need to be considered. The trajectory model

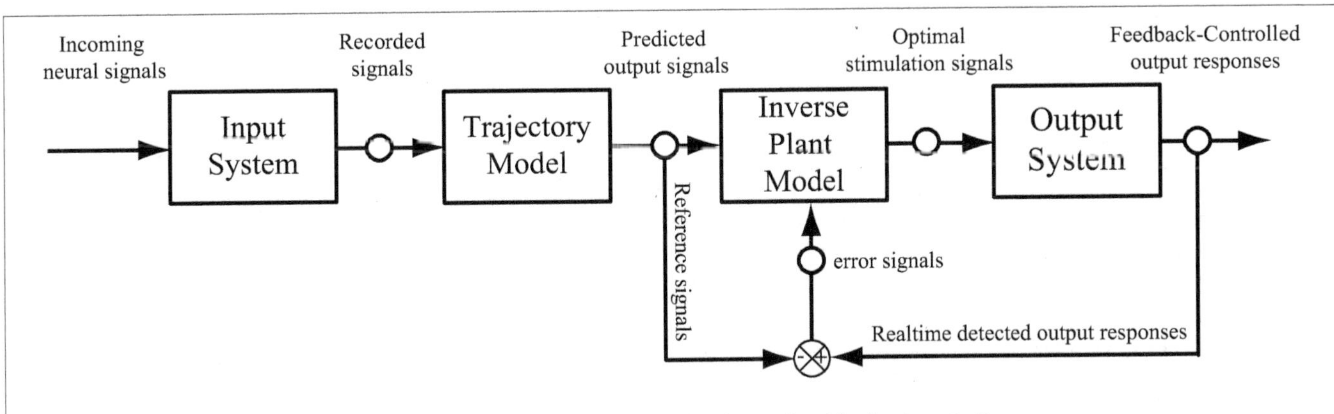

FIGURE 9 | A schematic diagram of a neuroprosthesis implemented with a feedforward and feedback controller.

developed in this study can be used as a reference model, which provide the desired output responses to compare with the actual responses recorded from output system, to calculate the error signal (**Figure 9**). In this case, the feedback error will be used as an external input signal and sent to adjust the properties of the inverse model. The influence of the previous errors on the current output may be taken in to account in a dynamic manner. In such a scheme, the optimal stimulation signals are calculated by the inverse plant model based on both the input and error signals.

ACKNOWLEDGMENTS

This work was supported in part by the NSF (BMES ERC and BITS Program), DARPA (HAND Project), ONR (Adaptive Neural System Program), NIBIB, and the Brain Restoration Foundation.

REFERENCES

Abbas, J. J., and Riener, R. (2001). Using mathematical models and advanced control systems techniques to enhance neuroprosthesis function. *Neuromodulation* 4, 187–195.

Albert, G. C., Cook, C. M., Prato, F. S., and Thomas, A. W. (2009). Deep brain stimulation, vagal nerve stimulation and transcranial stimulation: an overview of stimulation parameters and neurotransmitter release. *Neurosci. Biobehav. Rev.* 33, 1042–1060.

Allison, B. Z., Wolpaw, E. W., and Wolpaw, J. R. (2007). Brain-computer interface systems: progress and prospects. *Expert Rev. Med. Dev.* 4, 463–474.

Amaral, D. G., and Witter, M. P. (1989). The three-dimensional organization of the hippocampal formation: a review of anatomical data. *Neuroscience* 31, 571–591.

Andersen, P., Soleng, A. F., and Raastad, M. (2000). The hippocampal lamella hypothesis revisited. *Brain Res.* 886, 165–171.

Andersen, P., Bliss, T. V., Lomo, T., Olsen, L. I., and Skrede, K. K. (1969). Lamellar organization of hippocampal excitatory pathways. *Acta Physiol. Scand.* 76, 4A–5A.

Bartesaghi, R., Migliore, M., and Gessi, T. (2006). Input-output relations in the entorhinal cortex-dentate-hippocampal system: evidence for a non-linear transfer of signals. *Neuroscience* 142, 247–265.

Berger, T. W., Ahuja, A., Courellis, S. H., Deadwyler, S. A., Erinjippurath, G., Gerhardt, G. A., et al. (2005). Restoring lost cognitive function. *IEEE Eng. Med. Biol. Mag.* 24, 30–44.

Berger, T. W., Baudry, M., Brinton, R. D., Liaw, J.-S., Marmarelis, V. Z., Yoondong Park, A., et al. (2001). Brain-implantable biomimetic electronics as the next era in neural prosthetics. *Proc. IEEE* 89, 993–1012.

Berger, T. W., Chauvet, G., and Sclabassi, R. J. (1994). A biologically based model of functional properties of the Hippocampus. *Neural Netw.* 7, 1031–1064.

Berger, T. W., Eriksson, J. L., Ciarolla, D. A., and Sclabassi, R. J. (1988). Nonlinear systems analysis of the hippocampal perforant path-dentate projection. III. Comparison of random train and paired impulse stimulation. *J. Neurophysiol.* 60, 1095–1109.

Berger, T. W., Hampson, R. E., Song, D., Goonawardena, A., Marmarelis, V. Z., and Deadwyler, S. (2011). A cortical neural prosthesis for restoring and enhancing memory. *J. Neural Eng.* 8, 046017.

Berger, T. W., Song, D., Chan, R. H. M., Marmarelis, V. Z., LaCoss, J., Wills, J.,et al. (2012). A hippocampal cognitive prosthesis: multi-input, multi-output nonlinear modeling and VLSI implementation. *IEEE Trans. Neural Syst. Rehabil. Eng.* 20, 198–211.

Bernotas, L. A., Crago, P. E., and Chizeck, H. J. (1986). A discrete-time model of electrically stimulated muscle. *IEEE Trans. Biomed. Eng.* 33, 829–838.

Braz, G. P., Russold, M., and Davis, G. M. (2009). Functional electrical stimulation control of standing and stepping after spinal cord injury: a review of technical characteristics. *Neuromodulation* 12, 180–190.

Burgess, N., Maguire, E., and O'Keefe, J. (2002). The human hippocampus and spatial and episodic memory. *Neuron* 35, 625–641.

Camacho, E. F., and Bordons, C. (2003). *Model Predictive Control.* London, New York: Springer, xxii, 405.

Chan, C.-H., Srinivasan, V., Hsiao, M.-C., Khanna, S., Wills, J. D., Gholmieh, G., et al. (2004). "Real time hardware neural spike amplitude extraction," in *IEEE International Workshop on Biomedical Circuits and Systems 2004* (Singapore), 437–440.

Creasey, G. H., Ho, C. H., Triolo, R. J., Gater, D. R., DiMarco, A. F., Bogie, K. M., et al. (2004). Clinical applications of electrical stimulation after spinal cord injury. *J. Spinal Cord Med.* 27, 365–375.

Donoghue, J. P. (2002). Connecting cortex to machines: recent advances in brain interfaces. *Nat. Neurosci.* 5(Suppl), 1085–1088.

Donovan-Hall, M. K., Burridge, J., Dibb, B., Ellis-Hill, C., and Rushton, D. (2011). The views of people with spinal cord injury about the use of functional electrical stimulation. *Artif. Organs* 35, 204–211.

Duffell, L. D., Donaldson, N. D. N., Perkins, T. A., Rushton, D. N., Hunt, K. J., Kakebeeke, T. H., et al. (2008). Long-term intensive electrically stimulated cycling by spinal cord-injured people: effect on muscle properties and their relation to power output. *Muscle Nerve* 38, 1304–1311.

Gholmieh, G., Courellis, S., Dimoka, A., Wills, J. D., LaCoss, J., Granacki, J. J., et al. (2004). An algorithm for real-time extraction of population EPSP and population spike amplitudes from hippocampal field potential recordings. *J. Neurosci. Methods* 136, 111–121.

Gholmieh, G., Soussou, W., Han, M., Ahuja, A., Hsiao, M.-C., Song, D., et al. (2006). Custom-designed high-density conformal planar multielectrode arrays for brain slice electrophysiology. *J. Neurosci. Methods* 152, 116–129.

Hochberg, L. R., Serruya, M. D., Friehs, G. M., Mukand, J. A., Saleh, M., Caplan, A. H., et al. (2006). Neuronal ensemble control of prosthetic devices by a human with tetraplegia. *Nature* 442, 164–171.

Houk, J. C. (1988). Control strategies in physiological systems. *FASEB J.* 2, 97–107.

Hsiao, M.-C., Chan, C., Srinivasan, V., Ahuja, A., Erinjippurath, G., and Zanos, T. P. (2006) VLSI implementation of a nonlinear neuronal model: a 'neural prosthesis' to restore hippocampal trisynaptic dynamics. *Conf. Proc. IEEE Eng. Med. Biol. Soc.* 4396–4399.

Karniel, A., Meir, R., and Inbar, G. F. (2001). Best estimated inverse versus inverse of the best estimator. *Neural Netw.* 14, 1153–1159.

Lauer, R. T., Peckham, P. H., Kilgore, K. L., and Heetderks, W. J. (2000). Applications of cortical signals to neuroprosthetic control: a critical review. *IEEE Trans. Rehabil. Eng.* 8, 205–208.

Liu, J., Khalil, H. K., and Oweiss, K. G. (2011). Neural feedback for instantaneous spatiotemporal modulation of afferent pathways in bi-directional brain-machine interfaces. *IEEE Trans. Neural Syst. Rehabil. Eng.* 19, 521–533.

Liu, J., and Oweiss, K. (2010). "Feedback control of the spatiotemporal firing patterns of neural microcircuits," in *49th IEEE Conference on Decision and Control* (Atlanta, GA), 4679–4684.

Marmarelis, V. Z. (1993). Identification of nonlinear biological systems using Laguerre expansions of kernels. *Ann. Biomed. Eng.* 21, 573–589.

Marmarelis, V. Z. (2004). *Nonlinear Dynamic Modeling of Physiological Systems.* Hoboken, NJ: Wiley-Interscience, xvi, 541.

Marmarelis, V. Z., and Orme, M. E. (1993). Modeling of neural systems by use of neuronal modes. *IEEE Trans. Biomed. Eng.* 40, 1149–1158.

Matjacic, Z., Hunt, K., Gollee, H., and Sinkjaer, T. (2003). Control of posture with FES systems. *Med. Eng. Phys.* 25, 51–62.

Mayberg, H. S., Lozano, A. M., Voon, V., McNeely, H. E., Seminowicz, D., Hamani, C., et al. (2005). Deep brain stimulation for treatment-resistant depression. *Neuron* 45, 651–660.

McIntyre, C. C., Savasta, M., Walter, B. L., and Vitek, J. L. (2004). How does deep brain stimulation work? Present understanding and future questions. *J. Clin. Neurophysiol.* 21, 40–50.

McLachlan, R. S., Pigott, S., Tellez-Zenteno, J. F., Wiebe, S., and Parrent, A. (2010). Bilateral hippocampal stimulation for intractable temporal lobe epilepsy: impact on seizures and memory. *Epilepsia* 51, 304–307.

Middlebrooks, J. C., Bierer, J. A., and Snyder, R. L. (2005). Cochlear implants: the view from the brain. *Curr. Opin. Neurobiol.* 15, 488–493.

Moro, E., Esselink, R. J. A., and Xie, J. (2002). The impact on Parkinson's disease of electrical parameter settings in STN stimulation. *Neurology* 59, 706–713.

Nicolelis, M. A. L. (2003). Brain-machine interfaces to restore motor function and probe neural circuits. *Nat. Rev. Neurosci.* 4, 417–422.

Normann, R. A. (2007). Technology insight: future neuroprosthetic therapies for disorders of the nervous system. *Nat. Clin. Pract. Neurol.* 3, 444–452.

Okun, M. S., Tagliati, M., Pourfar, M., Fernandez, H. H., Rodriguez, R. L., Alterman, R. L., et al. (2005). Management of referred deep brain stimulation failures: a retrospective analysis from 2 movement disorders centers. *Arch. Neurol.* 62, 1250–1255.

O'Suilleabhain, P. E., Frawley, W., Giller, C., and Dewey, R. B. (2003). Tremor response to polarity, voltage, pulsewidth and frequency of thalamic stimulation. *Neurology* 60, 786–790.

Patil, P. G., and Turner, D. A. (2008). The development of brain-machine interface neuroprosthetic devices. *Neurotherapeutics* 5, 137–146.

Richardson, R. M., Ostrem, J. L., and Starr, P. (2009). Surgical repositioning of misplaced subthalamic electrodes in Parkinson's disease: location of effective and ineffective leads. *Stereotact. Funct. Neurosurg.* 87, 297–303.

Riener, R. (1999). Model-based development of neuroprosthesis for paraplegic patients. *Philos. Trans. R. Soc. Lond. B Biol. Sci.* 354, 877–894.

Rupp, R., and Gerner, H. J. (2007). Neuroprosthetics of the upper extremity–clinical application in spinal cord injury and challenges for the future. *Acta Neurochir. Suppl.* 97(Pt 1), 419–426.

Schwartz, A. B. (2004). Cortical neural prosthetics. *Annu. Rev. Neurosci.* 27, 487–507.

Sclabassi, R. J., Eriksson, J. L., Port, R. L., Robinson, G. B., and Berger, T. W. (1988). Nonlinear systems analysis of the hippocampal perforant path-dentate projection. I. Theoretical and interpretational considerations. *J. Neurophysiol.* 60, 1066–1076.

Song, D., Chan, R. H. M., Marmarelis, V. Z., Hampson, R. E., Deadwyler, S. A., and Berger, T. W. (2007). Nonlinear dynamic modeling of spike train transformations for hippocampal-cortical prostheses. *IEEE Trans. Biomed. Eng.* 54(6 Pt 1), 1053–1066.

Song, D., Chan, R. H. M., Marmarelis, V. Z., Hampson, R. E., Deadwyler, S. A., and Berger, T. W. (2009). Nonlinear modeling of neural population dynamics for hippocampal prostheses. *Neural Netw.* 22, 1340–1351.

Squire, L. R. (1992). Memory and the hippocampus: a synthesis from findings with rats, monkeys, and humans. *Psychol. Rev.* 99, 195–231.

Stacey, W. C., and Litt, B. (2008). Technology insight: neuroengineering and epilepsy-designing devices for seizure control. *Nat. Clin. Pract. Neurol.* 4, 190–201.

Taketani, M., and Baurdy, M. (2006). *Advances in Network Electrophysiology: Using Multi-Electrode Arrays, 1st Edn.* Michigan: Springer, 127–152.

Taylor, D. M., Tillery, S. I. H., and Schwartz, A. B. (2003). Information conveyed through brain-control: cursor versus robot. *IEEE Trans. Neural Syst. Rehabil. Eng.* 11, 195–199.

Tellez-Zenteno, J. F., McLachlan, R. S., Parrent, A., Kubu, C. S., and Wiebe, S. (2006). Hippocampal electrical stimulation in mesial temporal lobe epilepsy. *Neurology* 66, 1490–1494.

Turner, D. A., Dimitrov, D. F., and Ncolelis, M. A. L. (2005). "Neuroprosthetics and clinical realization of brain-machine interfaces, Chapter 7," in *Modern neurosurgery: Clinical Translation of Neuroscience Advances, 1st Edn.* ed D. A. Turner (Danvers, MA: CRC Press), 117–138.

van den Munckhof, P., Contarino, M. F., Bour, L. J., Speelman, J. D., de Bie, R. M., and Schuurman, P. R. (2010). Postoperative curving and upward displacement of deep brain stimulation electrodes caused by brain shift. *Neurosurgery* 67, 49–53; discussion 53–54.

Veltink, P. H., Chizeck, H. J., Crago, P. E., and El-Bialy, A. (1992). Nonlinear joint angle control for artificially stimulated muscle. *IEEE Trans. Biomed. Eng.* 39, 368–380.

Volkmann, J., Herzog, J., Kopper, F., and Deuschl, G. (2002). Introduction to the programming of deep brain stimulators. *Mov. Disord.* 17(Suppl 3), S181–S187.

Weiland, J. D., Liu, W., and Humayun, M. S. (2005). Retinal prosthesis. *Annu. Rev. Biomed. Eng.* 7, 361–401.

Widrow, B., and Bilello, (1993). "Adaptive inverse control," in *Proceedings of the 1993 IEEE International Symposium on Intelligent Control 1993* (Chicago, IL), 1–6.

Widrow, B., and Plett, G. L. (1997). "Nonlinear adaptive inverse control," in *Proceedings of the 36th IEEE Conference on Decision and Control 1997, Vol. 2* (San Diego, CA), 1032–1037.

Widrow, B., and Walach, E. (1996). *Adaptive Inverse Control.* Upper Saddle River, NJ: Prentice Hall PTR, xvii, 508.

16

Carbon nanotube-based multi electrode arrays for neuronal interfacing: progress and prospects

Lilach Bareket-Keren[1,2] and Yael Hanein[1,2]*

[1] School of Electrical Engineering, Tel-Aviv University, Tel-Aviv, Israel
[2] Tel-Aviv University Center for Nanoscience and Nanotechnology, Tel-Aviv University, Tel-Aviv, Israel

Edited by:
Ahmed El Hady, Max Planck Institute for Dynamics and Self Organization, Germany

Reviewed by:
Graham W. Knott, University of Lausanne, Switzerland
David J. Margolis, University of Zurich, Switzerland

***Correspondence:**
Yael Hanein, School of Electrical Engineering, Tel-Aviv University, 69978 Tel-Aviv, Israel.
e-mail: yaelha@tauex.tau.ac.il

Carbon nanotube (CNT) coatings have been demonstrated over the past several years as a promising material for neuronal interfacing applications. In particular, in the realm of neuronal implants, CNTs have major advantages owing to their unique mechanical and electrical properties. Here we review recent investigations utilizing CNTs in neuro-interfacing applications. Cell adhesion, neuronal engineering and multi electrode recordings with CNTs are described. We also highlight prospective advances in this field, in particular, progress toward flexible, bio-compatible CNT-based technology.

Keywords: carbon nanotubes, multi electrode array, neuronal recording, stimulation

INTRODUCTION

Extensive investigations over the past 50 years revealed the great potential of implanted electrodes for recording and stimulating neuronal signals. Such devices are currently being employed for the treatment of a wide range of conditions such as deafness, Parkinson's disease and chronic pain, to name just a few (Schwartz, 2004; Clark, 2006; Wichmann and DeLong, 2006; McCreery, 2008; Plow et al., 2012). Recent studies also suggested the use of neuro-stimulation in a growing number of additional disabling conditions, such as schizophrenia and Alzheimer's disease (George et al., 2007; Laxton et al., 2010). As high resolution, multi-site recording and stimulation devices are very attractive for neural recording and stimulation applications, the concept of multi electrode array (MEA) has gained increased attention in this field. A MEA device consists of an array of electrically conducting microelectrodes (typically 20–200 μm in diameter), connected to an external circuitry to allow recording or stimulation of neural electrical activity. Extensive effort has indeed demonstrated the potential of MEAs as an effective tool in various neurological applications. In particular, micro-fabrication technologies were employed to form finely shaped metallic [e.g., gold, platinum, and titanium nitride (TiN)] electrodes. The realization of such electrodes is readily achieved using a toolbox borrowed from the micro electro mechanical system (MEMS) field. This toolbox includes fabrication processes as well as materials with improved performances.

The scope of the current review is to explore, within the framework of micro fabricated neuro-electrodes, the employment of carbon nanotubes (CNTs) as a novel material with unique properties for neuro-applications. To this end, the CNT properties will be reviewed as well as their processing and fabrication into devices. The general field of micro fabricated neuro-electrodes will be introduced briefly and is beyond the scope of this review. We refer the reader for further reading on micro fabricated neuro-electrodes to HajjHassan et al. (2008), on the biocompatibility of CNTs to Warheit et al. (2004), Bottini et al. (2006), Carrero-Sanchez et al. (2006), and Firme and Bandaru (2010), and on the use of CNTs in biology to Bekyarova et al. (2005), Tarakanov et al. (2010), and Bottini et al. (2011).

We begin by reviewing the fundamental chemical, physical and electrical properties of CNTs (Thostenson et al., 2001; Harris, 2009; Lan et al., 2011). We then examine studies in which the neuron-CNT interface was explored. Next, the use of CNTs for neuronal patterning is discussed followed by a review of the electrical interfacing between CNTs and neurons and the study of CNT MEAs for neuronal applications. Finally, we discuss the progress toward flexible, bio-compatible CNT technology.

BEYOND CONVENTIONAL MICRO-FABRICATION

Despite a rapid recent development, contemporary MEAs for neuronal applications are still typified by relatively low signal to noise ratio (SNR), low spatial resolution (leading to poor site specificity) and limited biocompatibility. Clearly, further development is needed to make better electrodes suited for seamless integration between electronic devices and neuronal systems. The limited performances of these MEA systems stem primarily from the challenging interface between the biological systems and the artificial, electronic systems. The design of an interface between a living tissue and an electronic device must consider the dramatic structural and chemical differences between these two systems: Living tissues are soft, whereas electronic devices are usually rigid. Tissue conducts charges by ionic transport, whereas electronic devices conduct electrons and holes. Therefore, neural electrodes should accommodate differences in mechanical properties, bioactivity, and mechanisms of charge transport. Proper electrode-neuron interface is critical in ensuring both the viability of the cells and the effectiveness of the electrical interface.

A fundamental limiting feature of many contemporary MEAs is large electrode dimensions. Smaller electrodes would allow better spatial resolution and specific cell recording or stimulation. Also, reduction in electrode size (and therefore the dimensions of the entire device) is related to decreased tissue injury and immune response (Szarowski et al., 2003; Biran et al., 2005; Polikov et al., 2005; McConnell et al., 2009). While manufacturing small electrodes is technologically possible; the reduction in electrode size, needed for improving both stimulation and recording, is challenging. Small electrodes fail to provide sufficient charge injection owing to their high interface impedance. Low reversible charge storage capacity (CSC) means that the electrode cannot inject enough current to the tissue at small enough overpotential to avoid irreversible electrochemical reactions (i.e., electrolysis) and the ensuing damage to the electrode and the tissue (Cogan, 2008). Thus, to reduce electrode size without sacrificing the electrode ability to transfer charge, electrodes with high specific area are desired. High impedance also contributes to increased overall noise levels in recorded signals, thus reducing the recording sensitivity. An additional concern is the polarity of the electrode. For better biocompatibility, polar electrodes are desired (Merrill et al., 2005). These issues are further discussed later in the text.

Coupling neural cells intimately to the electrodes is also important otherwise the efficacy of both recording and stimulation are compromised. Recording is compromised by background noise of nearby neurons. Also, the conductance of the solution effects both recording and stimulation (Grattarola and Martinoia, 1993). The most common means to promote neural adhesion is through the use of cell adhesion proteins (Sorribas et al., 2001; Heller et al., 2005). Synthetic positively charged polymers, such as polylysine (Crompton et al., 2007) and poly(ethyleneimine) (PEI) (Ruardij et al., 2000) are commonly used to promote neural cell attachment (He and Bellamkonda, 2005; Khan and Newaz, 2010). The temperature sensitive Poly(N-isopropylacrylamide) (PNIPAm) was used to improve the binding between a retinal implant and the retina (Tunc et al., 2007). Conducting polymers (CPs), such as poly(ethylenedioxythiophene) (PEDOT), and polypyrrole (PPy) were used as neural growth substrate and electrode coating and are of particular interest due to their combined electronic and ionic conductivity (George et al., 2005; Abidian and Martin, 2008; Asplund et al., 2009; Abidian et al., 2010). The main disadvantage of CPs is their low stability under continued stimulation and exposure to ultra-violate (UV) radiation or heat. Applied voltage results with the insertion or removal of counter ions, so the CPs undergo swelling, shrinkage or breaking that gradually degrades their conductance (Yamato et al., 1995; Marciniak et al., 2004). Additionally, synthetic and CPs are often fabricated using complex or toxic polymerization schemes that are not well suited for cell interfacing applications. These residues are often not easily removed (Wan, 2008).

SURFACE ROUGHNESS AND CARBON NANOTUBES IN NEURONAL INTERFACING

Recent studies have shown that surface topography is an important parameter affecting neuronal anchoring and branching (Seidlits et al., 2008; Hoffman-Kim et al., 2010; Roach et al., 2010). In fact, cells preferentially adhere to rough surfaces when exposed to the same chemistry (Fan et al., 2002). Therefore, new electrode materials were investigated to realize electrodes with improved electrical properties, affinity to neuronal cells and biocompatibility utilizing the electrode morphological properties rather than their chemical ones.

An ideal material to meet these requirements is CNTs. CNTs are well suited for neural electrical interfacing applications owing to their large surface area, superior electrical and mechanical properties, as well as their ability to support excellent neuronal cell adhesion (Malarkey and Parpura, 2007; Ben-Jacob and Hanein, 2008; Voge and Stegemann, 2011). Recent studies have indeed confirmed the great potential of CNT surfaces as a biocompatible substrate on which neurons can readily adhere. This affinity was linked to surface properties including roughness, polarity, charge, and chemistry (Hu et al., 2004; Gabay et al., 2005a,b; Malarkey et al., 2009; Sorkin et al., 2009). CNT high surface area can lead to a significant increase in charge injection capacity and decreased interfacial impedance (Gabay et al., 2007; Keefer et al., 2008).

Investigations so far focused on several main themes: The effect of chemically modified CNTs on the viability of neuronal cells, process outgrowth and branching (Mattson et al., 2000; Hu et al., 2004; Matsumoto et al., 2007), electrical interfacing with neurons (Gheith et al., 2006; Wang et al., 2006; Gabay et al., 2007; Shein et al., 2009), and the development of neural implants (Webster et al., 2004; Nunes et al., 2012). CNTs are now widely investigated as an interfacing material for neuronal applications (Malarkey and Parpura, 2007; Ben-Jacob and Hanein, 2008; Pancrazio, 2008; Lee and Parpura, 2009; Voge and Stegemann, 2011). As highlighted above, both surface-chemistry and surface-topography are critically important parameters determining the formation of effective electrodes. Many schemes have been developed addressing these challenges using CNT coatings (pristine and chemically modified) offering exciting opportunities as will be further explored below.

CARBON NANOTUBES

We begin our review with a brief overview of the physical properties of CNTs. CNTs are hollow cylinders formed in the shape of a rolled graphite sheet. Single walled CNTs (SWCNTs) are the simplest of these objects with a diameter ranging between 0.4 and 2.5 nm and lengths of up to a few millimeters. Multi walled carbon nanotubes (MWCNTs) are composed of a set of coaxially organized SWCNTs and are 2–100 nm in diameter while their length can vary from one to several hundred micrometers (Harris, 2009). The arrangement of the carbon atoms in the graphene sheet can be of different chirality: armchair, chiral, or zigzag. The chirality, as well as the tube diameter and the number of graphene walls, determine the CNT conductivity. Generally, SWCNTs can be metallic or semiconducting with MWCNTs featuring metallic behavior (Charlier et al., 2007). CNTs are also mechanically stable with very high tensile strengths and chemical inertness (Ciraci et al., 2004; Hayashi et al., 2007). CNTs are commonly synthesized from a catalyst by a variety of methods including: chemical vapor deposition (CVD), electric arc discharge and laser ablation (Thostenson et al., 2001; Seah et al., 2011). Their physical properties make CNTs a durable nanomaterial for biological applications, especially where a long lasting material is desired (e.g., scaffolds for support of cellular growth). Although the surface of CNTs is fundamentally inert, it can be readily functionalized with different polymers or bioactive molecules, such as peptides and proteins to improve their biocompatibility and bioactivity (Bekyarova et al., 2005; Yang et al., 2007; Lu et al., 2009; Bottini et al., 2011).

CARBON NANOTUBES AND NEURONS

The first investigations into the use of CNTs in neuro-interfacing applications focused on characterizing neuronal adhesion and proliferation on CNT coated surfaces. Mattson and co-workers were the first to discuss the use of CNTs as a substrate for neuronal growth (Mattson et al., 2000). The researchers grew embryonic rat hippocampal neurons on cover slips covered with PEI and MWCNTs. They found that pristine MWCNT substrates allowed neuronal attachment but did not support neurite branching as elaborate as that of cells cultured on PEI-coated coverslips. However, when MWCNTs were non-covalently functionalized (by physiosorption) with 4-hydroxynonenal (4-HNE), a molecule that promotes neurite outgrowth, large increases in the number of neurites per cell and in the overall neurite lengths were observed. This study demonstrated that MWCNTs can serve as a permissive substrate for neuronal cell adhesion and growth and that modifying MWCNTs with a biologically relevant molecule can be used to modulate neuronal growth and neurite outgrowth (Mattson et al., 2000).

The pioneering work of Mattson and co-workers was followed by a succession of studies aiming to further elucidate the observed effects. Hu et al. studied the effect of charge. Longer neurites and more elaborate branching were observed on positively charged CNT substrates (Hu et al., 2004). The charge of a MWCNT substrate was modified by functionalization with carboxyl groups, poly-m-aminobenzene sulfonic (PABS) acid or ethylenediamine (EN) to create negatively, zwitterionic or positively charged nanotubes, respectively. The number of neurites was counted depending on the nature of the nanotubes and their functionalization. Xie and co-workers determined that MWCNT mats functionalized with carboxyl groups are a permissive substrate for rat dorsal root ganglion (DRG) neurons growth, as confirmed by scanning electron microscopy (SEM) imaging. The researchers further suggested that the functional groups act as anchoring seeds enhancing neural cells and neurite adhesion (Xie et al., 2006).

Covalent modifications of CNTs with neurotrophins, protein growth factors that promote the survival and differentiation of neurons, were studied by Matsumoto et al. (2007). MWCNTs were functionalized with nerve growth factor (NGF) and brain-derived neurotrophic factor (BDNF). Embryonic chick DRG neurite outgrowth on modified MWCNTs was similar to that seen with soluble NGF and BDNF in culturing media, indicating that the covalently attached factors were still bioactive. Pristine MWCNTs were also shown to support the growth of neurons (Gabay et al., 2005a,b; Galvan-Garcia et al., 2007). This effect is nicely illustrated in **Figure 1** which shows the strong affinity between dissociated locust neurons and pristine CNT islands

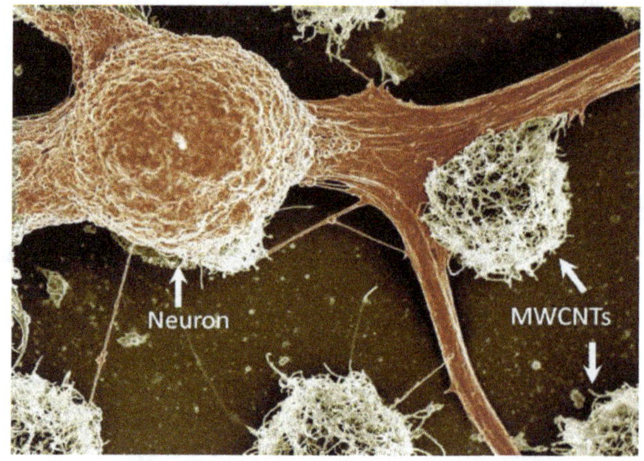

FIGURE 1 | A false-colored SEM image of fixed locust frontal ganglion neuronal cells cultured on carbon nanotube islands. The carbon nanotube islands were grown using the chemical vapor deposition method directly on a quartz support. For further details see Sorkin et al. (2009). Width of field of view is 77 μm.

after several days of incubation. Galvan-Garcia and co-workers reported that MWCNTs in the form of sheets or yarns supported long-term growth of a variety of cell types ranging from skin fibroblasts and Schwann cells, to postnatal cortical and cerebellar neurons. When highly purified, these CNT sheets allowed neurons to extend processes in a similar number and length to those grown on planar polyornithine substrates (a permissive support). Thus, these results suggest that the interaction between neurons and CNTs may be affected by the purity of the CNTs, as well as by the three-dimensional organization of the CNT substrate.

Although initial investigations focused on MWCNTs, SWCNTs were also studied as neuronal substrates. Hu and co-workers synthesized a PEI functionalized SWCNT graft copolymer (SWCNT-PEI) (Hu et al., 2005). Covalent functionalization was used to turn SWCNTs to be soluble in aqueous media. Next, rat hippocampal neurons were cultured on coverslips coated with SWCNT-PEI and the results were compared with those of pristine MWCNT or PEI substrates. Fluorescent microscopy was used to examine neuronal viability, as indicated by their ability to accumulate the vital stain, calcein. It was found that SWCNT functionalization diluted the effect of the PEI's positive charge, resulting in neurite outgrowth and branching with intermediate extent to that of as-prepared CNT films or PEI alone. These results were consistent with the initial findings of Mattson and colleagues using fixed cells. Modified MWCNTs were found to be inferior to PEI as a culturing substrate (Hu et al., 2005). Gheith and co-workers demonstrated that free-standing SWCNT-polymer films prepared by the layer-by-layer (LBL) technique are compatible with neuronal cell culturing. The films were prepared by layering SWCNT with a negatively charged polyacrylic acid polymer. The SWCNTs were coated with amphiphilic poly (*N*-cetyl-4-vinylpyridinium bromide-*co*-*N*-ethyl-4-vinylpyridinium bromide-*co*-4-vinylpyridine). The presence of positively charged groups on the surface of this polymer promoted cell adhesion. Cell cultures of the neuronal model cell line NG108 effectively grew and proliferated on these substrates. Moreover, the number of neurites spun from individual cells exceeded those developed on traditional cell growth substrates (Gheith et al., 2005). However, not all CNT functionalization lead to the design of substrates that enhance neural cell growth. Liopo and co-workers showed that 4-tertbutylphenyl or 4-benzoic acid functionalized SWCNTs were less supportive of NG108 cell attachment and growth than pristine nanotubes (Liopo et al., 2006).

Carbon nanofibers (CNFs) are a form of carbon material closely related to MWCNTs and were also tested as a neuronal substrate. CNFs consist of multi-walled graphene structures stacked on top of each other like a stack of ice cream cones (Rodriguez, 1993). Nugen-Vu and co-workers directly grew forest-like vertically aligned CNFs (VACNFs) on a substrate with a lithographically patterned catalyst. After the CNF film was submerged in a liquid and dried, the CNFs irreversibly stuck together to form microbundles. A uniform freestanding film was achieved after coating the CNF with a thin layer of the CP PPy by electrochemical deposition. PC12 cell line grew as monolayers on the CNF films only after further coating with a collagen film. Otherwise cells appeared to float on top of the CNF surface (Nguyen-Vu et al., 2006). In a subsequent study, the neuronal marker NGF was introduced to the VACNF surface to promote the formation of well-differentiated cells with mature neurites. The freestanding VACNFs coated with PPy and NGF were found to bend toward the cell body and adhere to it. Therefore, it was suggested that the soft PPy coating contributes to better mechanical contact with cells due to a reduction in the local mechanical stress (Nguyen-Vu et al., 2007).

CNT CONDUCTIVITY

Since CNTs may vary between being conducting and semi-conducting, their electrical properties were also studied. Malarkey and co-workers varied the conductivity of SWCNT-polyethylene glycol (PEG) graft copolymer coatings by changing the film thickness, while maintaining a constant surface roughness (Malarkey et al., 2009). Rat hippocampal neurons were then seeded. It was shown that thinner, less conducting SWCNT films, resulted in longer neurite processes, while thicker, more conductive films, produced larger cell bodies. Smooth, positively charged PEI substrates resulted in a larger number of growth cones per cell body. This study demonstrated that differences in conductance, roughness, and surface charge can modulate neuronal cell growth and morphology.

CARBON NANOTUBE SURFACE ROUGHNESS

Overall, the origin of the neuron-CNT interaction appears to be strongly affected by surface roughness. It was suggested that the roughness of CNTs contributes to anchoring neural cells (Zhang et al., 2005; Xie et al., 2006; Sorkin et al., 2009). Zhang et al. (2005) fabricated patterned vertical MWCNT surfaces. CNTs were then functionalized with poly-L-lysine (PLL). Cell cultures of the neuronal cell line H19-7 preferentially adhered to the MWCNT patterns. Neuronal growth cones were found to make contact with the nanotube surface, and these strong interactions allowed the neurons to spread along patterns and form interactions with one another. It was established that guided neurite growth was formed preferably on long vertical MWCNTs compared to short ones. This behavior was attributed by the authors to a possible increased adsorption of the PLL molecules onto the long nanotubes. Additional mechanism may be that long nanotubes are flexible and undergo deformation to accommodate the proliferating neurites.

Sorkin and co-workers characterized the arrangement of neurons and glia cells on CNT surfaces (see **Figure 2**). Three-dimensional, small, isolated and pristine CNT islands were fabricated and plated with cells. Two biological model systems were used: cortical neurons from rats, and ganglion cells from locusts. Neurons were found bound and preferentially anchored to the rough surfaces. For both model systems, the morphology of neuronal processes on the small, isolated islands of high density

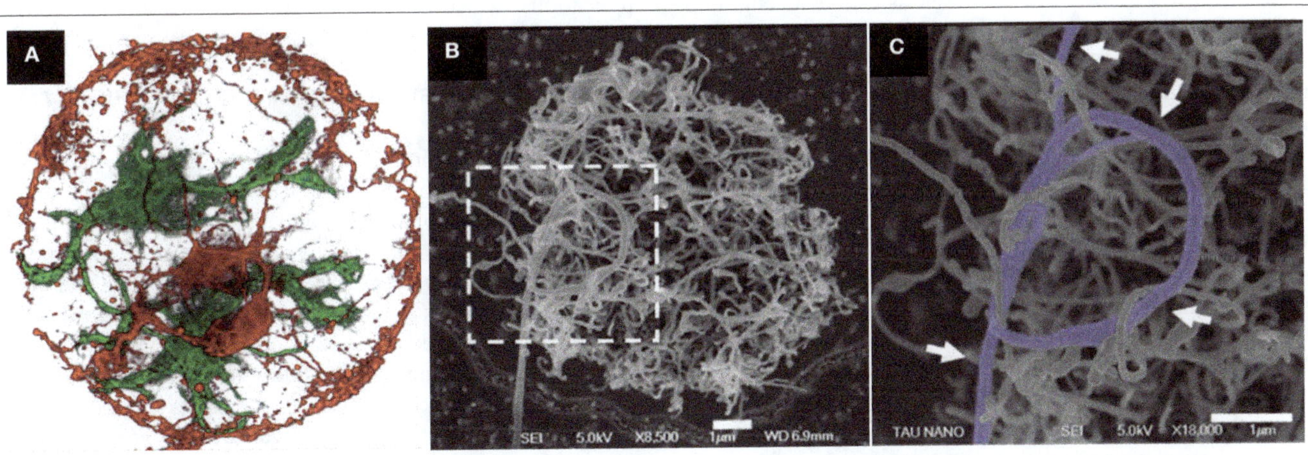

FIGURE 2 | Rat neuronal cultures on CNT islands. (A) Fluorescent confocal image of fixed neurons (red) and glia cells (green) cultured on a carbon nanotube island. Disk diameter is 20 μm. **(B,C)** HRSEM images of a neuronal process forming a loop around several CNTs (designated by arrows). The image in **(C)** corresponds to the area marked by the dashed box in **(B)**. Clearly identifiable process segments were manually highlighted. Processes appear to bind to the carbon nanotube surface in a manner akin to that of tendrils. Adopted from Sorkin et al. (2009).

CNTs was found to be conspicuously curled and entangled. In this study, it was demonstrated that the roughness of the surface must match the diameter of the neuronal processes in order to allow them to bind. It was suggested that entanglement, a mechanical effect, may constitute an additional mechanism by which neurons anchor themselves to rough surfaces (Sorkin et al., 2009).

Table 1 summarizes the main results described above, emphasizing how different CNTs and CNT modifications affect neuronal adhesion. Overall the general picture that emerges from these investigations is that MWCNTs, SWCNTs, and CNFs are permissive substrate for neuronal growth and proliferation. Neuronal interaction with CNTs is affected by CNT surface chemical modification, conductivity, charge, and roughness. Positive charge had a positive effect on neurite branching and length. Altering conductivity resulted with morphological changes in neurite length and cell body size. Surface roughness contributed to anchoring neurons to the surface. Chemical modifications of the CNT surface with 4-HNE, and PEI had a positive effect on neurite branching and growth, whereas modification with 4-tertbutylphenyl and 4-benzoic acid modified substrate diminished neuronal cell growth.

CARBON NANOTUBES FOR NEURONAL PATTERNING

Patterned CNT films, such as those discussed above, provide a unique scheme for creating and studying engineered neuronal networks. Studies using patterned CNTs can provide insight into the collective activity of neural networks. CNT patterns also offer a route for developing three-dimensional scaffolds as a step toward designing circuits for bio-computational purposes and neuro-prosthetics applications. This approach can also be used to build advanced neuro-chips for bio-sensing applications (e.g., drug and toxin detection) where the structure and stability of the networks are important.

Zhang and co-workers cultured neurons on micron-scale patterns with different geometries. These patterns were designed to support an investigation into mechanisms underlying neuronal extension, guidance, and interaction. Straight lines, squares and circular features were used, as well as different lengths of the nanotubes. It was found that neurons preferentially adhered to MWCNT patterns. Growth cones were attached to the nanotube surface, allowing the neurons to spread along patterns and interact with one another (Zhang et al., 2005).

CNT islands were also used extensively by us to engineer neuronal networks into a system with well-defined geometry (see **Figure 3**), so the interplay between geometry and neuronal activity can be systematically investigated (Gabay et al., 2005a,b; Sorkin et al., 2006, 2009; Greenbaum et al., 2009; Shein et al., 2009) (see **Figure 2** for a typical example). In one of the first publications to use MWCNTs for neuronal interfacing applications, Gabay and co-workers imprinted a pattern of iron nanoparticle catalyst on quartz substrates using a poly (dimethylsiloxane) (PDMS) stamp and then grew CNTs from the iron catalyst islands. Rat cortical neurons and glial cells accumulated preferentially on the MWCNT islands and formed interconnected networks, bridging across the non-permissive quartz to form connections between adjacent islands. Using the patch clamp technique, cultured neurons were found to be electro-physiologically active with normal resting membrane potentials, demonstrating that the MWCNT did not alter the neuronal integrity (Gabay et al., 2005a,b).

In a successive work, Sorkin and co-workers examined the dynamics of neuronal network organization by placing rat cortical and hippocampal neurons on patterned MWCNT or poly-D-lysine patterned substrates. Cell clusters were found to spontaneously anchor to patterned islands with neurites, connecting nearby islands through a single non-adherent straight bundle composed of axons and dendrites. Square, triangular and circular structures of connectivity were successfully realized. Monitoring the dynamics of the networks in real time revealed that the self-assembly process is mainly driven by the ability of the cells to move while continuously stretching neurite bundles in between. The patterned networks were stable for as long as 11 weeks (Sorkin et al., 2006). In a subsequent study, Sorkin and co-workers cultured rat cortical neurons, as well as locust frontal ganglion neurons on micro-patterned MWCNT islands. Neuronal processes tended to wrap and entangle with the rough MWCNT islands. It appears that the similar dimensions of the CNTs (within the island) and the neurites supports an anchoring mechanism allowing neurons to attach (Sorkin et al., 2009). Greenbaum and co-workers demonstrated the use of specially designed CNT substrates to form small networks of locust frontal ganglion neurons. It was suggested that mechanical tension is created along the cell's processes and pulls the cell's soma; neuronal activity was recorded from single cells (Greenbaum et al., 2009). These effects were further explored (Anava et al., 2009; Hanein et al., 2011) to show that indeed mechanical effects are ubiquitous in these developing networks.

CARBON NANOTUBES FOR ELECTRICAL NEURONAL INTERFACING

As discussed in the "Introduction" section, contemporary electrodes used for neuro-prosthetic applications have relatively high impedance and poor CSC. In order to better appreciate these challenges and to evaluate CNTs potential in neuronal electrode applications, we begin with a brief overview of the electrical processes taking place at the neuron-electrode interface.

EXTRACELLULAR RECORDING AND STIMULATION OF NEURONAL ACTIVITY

Signal transmission in neuronal systems is the result of ionic currents passing through specific ion channels across the cell membrane. Extracellular recording methods monitor the electrical field associated with this dynamic. The time course of the extracellular action potential is typically ~1 ms and the amplitude is in the range of a few tens to a few hundreds of microvolts (Cogan, 2008; Buzsaki et al., 2012). This amplitude is significantly smaller than the corresponding intracellular spike, which is in the tens of millivolt range. Additionally, extra cellular signals diminish rapidly as a function of distance from the cell. A reverse process takes place during stimulation; charges are delivered from the electrode and induce a buildup of membrane potential. Under a strong enough field, voltage sensitive ions in the cell membrane trigger the generation of an action potential (Roth, 1994; Tehovnik, 1996; Basser and Roth, 2000).

Table 1 | Neuronal adhesion on CNT coated surfaces.

	References	CNT surface	CNT modification	*In vitro* bio-testing scheme	Results
MWCNTs	Mattson et al., 2000	MWCNTs coated cover slip	Pristine	Embryonic rat hippocampal cultures	Neuronal growth
			4-HNE		Increased neurites branching and length on modified CNTs
	Hu et al., 2004	MWCNTs coated cover slip	COO PABS EN	Rat hippocampal cultures	Increased neurites branching and length on positively charged CNTs
	Matsumoto et al., 2007	MWCNTs soluble in growth medium	NGF or BDNF	Embryonic chick DRG neurons	CNT attached factors and soluble factors had similar effect on neurite outgrowth
	Gabay et al., 2005a,b	MWCNT islands directly grown on catalyst patterned substrate	Pristine	Rat cortical cultures	Neuronal aggregation on CNT islands and formation of a neurite interconnected network
	Galvan-Garcia et al., 2007	Directionality oriented MWCNT sheets and yarns	Pristine	Rat shwan cells Mice primary cortical and cerebral neurons Mice DRG neurons	Multiple cell types permissiveness Neuronal interaction with CNTs may be affected by CNT purity and 3D structure
	Zhang et al., 2005	Vertical MWCNT arrays directly grown on catalyst patterned substrate	PLL	H19-7 cell line	Preferred guided neurite growth on longer flexible MWCNTs
	Xie et al., 2006	MWCNT mats	COOH	Rat DRG neurons	Longer neurites on modified CNTs Neurites intertwined with CNTs
	Sorkin et al., 2009	MWCNT islands directly grown on catalyst patterned substrate	Pristine	Rat cortical cultures Locust ganglion cells	Neurite morphology on high density CNT islands was curled and entangled
SWCNTs	Hu et al., 2005	SWCNT coated cover slip	Pristine PEI	Rat hippocampal cultures	Increased neurite outgrowth and branching on modified CNTs
	Gheith et al., 2005	SWCNT-PAA coated cover slip (by LBL)	Amphiphilic polymer	NG108 cell line	Neuronal growth
	Liopo et al., 2006	SWCNT coated PET film	4-tertbutylphenyl 4-benzoic acid	NG108 cell line Rat primary peripheral neurons	Decreased neurites branching and length on modified CNTs

(Continued)

Table 1 | Continued

	References	CNT surface	CNT modification	*In vitro* bio-testing scheme	Results
	Malarkey et al., 2009	SWCNT coated cover slips	PEG	Rat hippocampal cultures	Longer neuritis on less conducting films Larger cell bodies on more conductive films
CNFs	Nguyen-Vu et al., 2006	VACNFs directly grown on an catalyst patterned substrate	PPy	PC12 cell line	Soft PPy contributes to better mechanical coupling between cells and CNTs
	Nguyen-Vu et al., 2007		PPy and NGF		

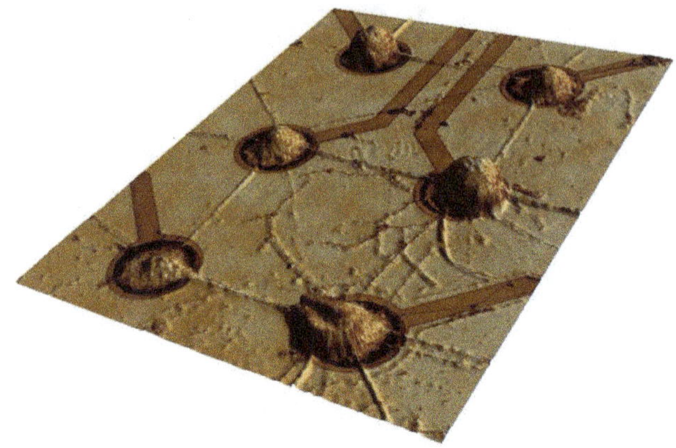

FIGURE 3 | A neuro-glia cortical culture from embryonic rats grown on a carbon nanotube micro electrode array. Clusters of cells self-organized during culture development to position themselves on the electrodes. The distance between electrodes is 200 μm. Image acquired using a 3D confocal microscope (Shein et al., 2009).

Stimulating neurons and recording extracellular signals can be achieved using a conducting electrode placed close to the cell or its processes. The electrode electrochemical properties are fundamental to its performances as a stimulating or recording electrode. Clearly, an effective interface is a prerequisite for both stimulation and recording. While neuronal stimulation and recording are related in nature, these two applications have somewhat different requirements. Foremost, the amount of charge required for stimulation is orders of magnitude higher than what is recorded. Recording may often be impossible with electrodes which are well suited for stimulation. In neuronal recording, the typically small signals make noise considerations very important (Musial et al., 2002). For safe stimulation purpose, however, delivering the appropriate charge to the tissue without causing electrode or tissue damage is the main consideration (McCreery et al., 1988, 1990; Cogan, 2008).

The electrode material and the reactions at the electrode-tissue interface (the reactions mediating the transition from electron flow in the electrode to ion flow in the tissue) are the main parameters determining the safe range for stimulation. The reactions taking place during charge injection can be capacitive or Faradaic (**Figure 4A**). Capacitive reactions involve displacement current and are associated with the charging and discharging of the electrode-electrolyte double layer due to redistribution of charged species in the electrolyte. Faradaic reactions, on the other hand, involve the transfer of electrons across the electrode-electrolyte interface and require that some species, on the surface of the electrode or in solution, are oxidized or reduced. These reactions can lead to irreversible processes that cause electrode or tissue damage. Therefore, while maximizing the current injected through an electrode is important, it has to be achieved ideally by using non-Faradaic electrodes. Capacitive charge delivery is therefore a critical consideration in the design of electrodes both for recording and stimulation.

The capacitive and Faradic reactions at the electrode-electrolyte are modeled by a simple electrical circuit consisting

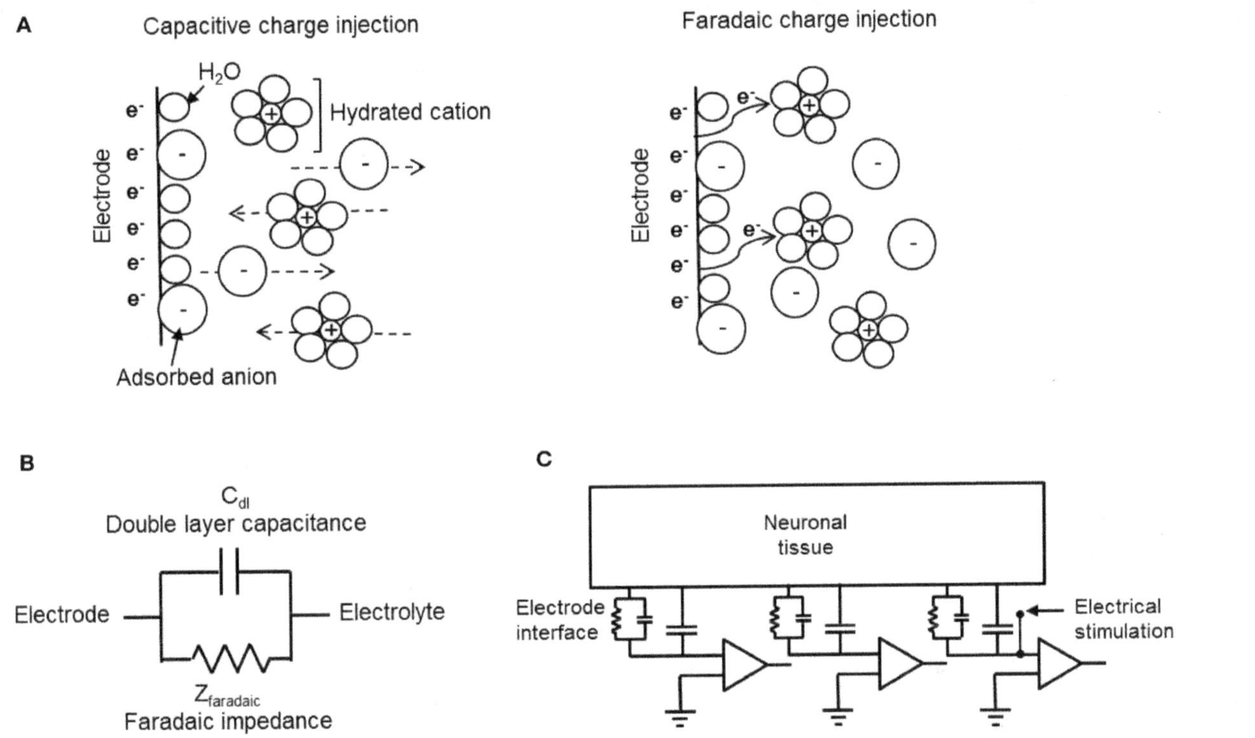

FIGURE 4 | Electrode-electrolyte interface and charge injection. **(A)** Schematic representation of capacitive (left) and Faradaic (right) charge injection mechanisms. While capacitive charge injection includes redistribution of charge in the electrode-electrolyte interface, Faradaic process includes transfer of electrons. **(B)** An electrical circuit model for mechanisms of charge transfer at the electrode-electrolyte interface. **(C)** A circuit model for extracellular recording and stimulation from neuronal tissue using a MEA linked to external amplifiers. The model demonstrates the electrochemical interface resistance and capacitance of the CNT electrode and the solution derived shunt capacitance as well as the point of stimulation.

of two elements, a capacitor and a resistive element in parallel. **Figures 4B,C** illustrate circuit models of electrode-electrolyte interface and extracellular recording and stimulation of neuronal tissue, respectively. The capacitive mechanism, which represents the ability of the electrode to cause charge flow in the electrolyte without electron transfer, is modeled as a simple electrical capacitor called the double layer capacitor (Bard and Falkner, 2000; Merrill et al., 2005). Faradaic processes are modeled as a Faradaic impedance (Bard and Falkner, 2000; Merrill et al., 2005). There are two limiting cases derived from this model: The ideally polarizable electrode, and the ideally non-polarizable electrode (Bard and Falkner, 2000; Merrill et al., 2005). The ideally non-polarizable electrode has a zero Faradaic resistance, therefore current flows readily in Faradaic reactions and there is no change in voltage across the interface upon the passage of current. Thus, the electrode potential remains near equilibrium, even upon current flow. The ideally polarizable electrode has infinite Faradaic impedance element and is modeled by a pure capacitor. In an ideally polarizable electrode, all the current is transferred through capacitive action, thus the electrode potential is easily perturbed away from the equilibrium potential. Real electrode interfaces are modeled by the double layer capacitor in parallel with finite Faradaic impedance, together in series with the solution resistance. A highly polarizable electrode is one that can accommodate a large amount of injected charge on the double layer prior to initiating Faradaic reactions. Thus, for improved biocompatibility, highly polarizable electrodes are desired. An additional important parameter used is the description of neuronal stimulation electrodes is the reversible CSC, also known as the reversible charge injection limit (Robblee and Rose, 1990; Merrill et al., 2005). The CSC of an electrode is the total amount of charge that may be stored reversibly, including storage in the double layer capacitance, pseudocapacitance, or any reversible Faradaic reaction. The material used for the electrode, the size and shape of the electrode, the electrolyte composition, and parameters of the electrical stimulation waveform, all influence the CSC. We refer the reader for a detailed description of the electrochemical electrode-electrolyte interface of recording and stimulation neuronal electrodes (Bard and Falkner, 2000; Merrill et al., 2005; Cogan, 2008).

Overall, increased capacitance results in decreased impedance, and reduction in noise levels, as well as allowing wider voltage windows for safe electrical stimulation. Contemporary Faradaic electrode materials include mainly noble metals such as gold, platinum, titanium, and iridium, as well as alloys of these metals, iridium oxide, stainless steel, and highly doped semiconductors such as silicon. Capacitive electrode materials include TiN, tantalum-tantalum oxide, and the more recently investigated CNTs. The capacitive nature of CNT electrodes is therefore yet another major advantage.

CARBON NANOTUBES FOR RECORDING AND STIMULATION OF NEURONAL ACTIVITY

As we discussed above, CNTs have several fundamental properties which make them ideally suited for neuronal interfacing. They support neuronal proliferation, they are conducting and they form extremely high specific area, capacitive electro-chemical electrodes. Accordingly, many recent studies have employed CNTs as a coating material for neuro-electrodes.

Direct stimulation of isolated neurons in culture using SWCNT coated substrate was demonstrated recently by several groups (Gheith et al., 2006; Liopo et al., 2006; Mazzatenta et al., 2007). Gheith and co-workers incorporated positively charged SWCNTs and poly acrylic acid into LBL multilayers with sufficiently high electrical conductivity to electrically stimulate a model neuronal cells line (NG108). The use of the SWCNT LBL films as culturing substrates did not perturb the key electrophysiological features of the NG108 cells, which confirms previous observations (Gheith et al., 2006). The electrical coupling of NG108 cells, as well as rat primary peripheral neurons to unmodified, as well as 4-tertbutylphenyl or 4-benzoic acid modified SWCNTs deposited onto polyethylene terephthalate (PET) films, were assessed by Liopo et al. (2006). Neurons showed voltage activated currents when electrically stimulated through the conducting SWCNT film. The same issue was subsequently addressed by Mazzatenta and co-workers who used electrophysiological measurements and computational modeling in order to understand the nature of the electrical coupling between neurons and pure SWCNTs (Mazzatenta et al., 2007). The authors cultured rat hippocampal neuronal on glass cover slips coated with pristine SWCNT films. SEM revealed contacts between neuronal membranes and SWCNTs. Electrical recordings using a patch clamp indicated that neurons grown on SWCNT substrates displayed spontaneous electrical activity. Stimulation of cultured neurons was achieved by applying current through the nanotube substrate. Finally, a mathematical model describing the electrical coupling between the SWCNT and the neurons was suggested (Mazzatenta et al., 2007).

Some studies suggested that CNTs boost neuronal electrical activity (Lovat et al., 2005; Cellot et al., 2009). Lovat and co-workers functionalized CNTs with pyrrolidine groups. This functionalization removed impurities and improved the CNT solubility in organic solvents. Glass cover slips were then coated with a drop of the solution. Evaporation of the solvent and heat treatment resulted with defunctionalization, leaving purified MWCNTs on the glass. Neurons grown on MWCNT films showed a six-fold increase in the frequency of the spontaneous postsynaptic currents and spontaneous action potential generation when compared to those grown on untreated glass. The authors proposed that the high conductivity of the CNT substrate might have affected the voltage-dependent membrane processes resulting in the increased activity (Lovat et al., 2005). Cellot and co-workers have suggested that CNTs improve electrical communication between neurons through the formation of tight contacts with the cell membranes. They used thin CNT films formed by solution deposition on glass followed by thermal treatment. Rat hippocampal neurons were seeded onto the films and showed an increase in synaptic firing (Cellot et al., 2009), enhanced formation of synapses as well as changes in synaptic dynamics (Cellot et al., 2011).

Composite CNT coatings enhance recording and stimulation of neurons *in vitro* and *in vivo* by decreasing the impedance and increasing charge transfer. Keefer and co-workers successfully coated electrodes with MWCNTs using different deposition schemes (Keefer et al., 2008). Commercial tungsten and stainless steel sharpened wire electrodes were coated with CNTs, using covalent attachment of the CNT coating, electrodeposition of CNT-gold coating or electrodeposition of CNT combined with CP (PPy). The different CNT coatings resulted with lower impedance and higher charge transfer capacity compared with bare metal electrodes. *In vivo* recording quality of CNT-coated sharp electrodes was tested in the motor cortex of anesthetized rats and in the visual cortex of monkeys. Compared with bare metal electrodes, CNT coated electrodes had reduced noise and improved detection of spontaneous activity (Keefer et al., 2008). Baranauskas and co-workers tested PPy-CNT coated platinum/tungsten microelectrodes. PPy-CNT coating significantly reduced the microelectrode impedance and induced a significant improvement of the SNR, up to four-fold on average. *In vivo* signals were recorded from rat cortex (Baranauskas et al., 2011). Other CPs-CNT composite coatings including PPy-CNT (Lu et al., 2010; Chen et al., 2011a) and PEDOT-CNT (Luo et al., 2011) were tested. These coatings similarly resulted with enhanced electrochemical properties and were found biocompatible. The devices were not used in recording or stimulation. The PPy-CNT coatings highly improve the electrochemical performance of the test electrodes and further investigation into the durability of these coatings under long-term stimulation and recording use would be important to reveal their full potential.

Collectively, the studies reviewed above show that CNTs may provide a superior mean for electrical coupling between devices and neuron. We shall now discuss the use of CNTs electrodes for both electrical recordings and stimulation of neurons in the form of MEAs.

CARBON NANOTUBE MEA FOR NEURONAL RECORDING AND STIMULATION

A major development in the use of CNT in neuro-applications is the design and fabrication of CNT MEAs (Gabay et al., 2007). Such MEAs were made by synthesizing islands of high density CNTs. Both MWCNTs and SWCNTs structures were used. CNTs were either deposited as a coating on top of metal electrodes (Keefer et al., 2008; Gabriel et al., 2009; Fuchsberger et al., 2011) or directly grown from a catalyst patterned substrate (Wang et al., 2006; Gabay et al., 2007; Yu et al., 2007).

MWCNT-gold coated indium-tin oxide MEAs were used to record and stimulate mice cortical cultures by Keefer and co-workers. The CNT coated electrodes were found to be suited for recording and improved the effectiveness of stimulation (Keefer et al., 2008). Pristine CNT coatings were also used. Gabriel et al. coated standard platinum MEAs with SWCNTs which were directly deposited onto electrodes by drop coating and drying. CNT coating resulted with enhanced electrical properties, decreased impedance and increased capacitance. The researchers successfully performed extracellular recordings from ganglion cells of isolated rabbit retinas (Gabriel et al., 2009). Fuchsberger and co-workers proposed the deposition of MWCNT layers onto TiN microelectrode arrays by means of a micro-contact printing technique using PDMS stamps. The coated MEA was applied for the electrochemical detection of dopamine and electrophysiological measurements of rat hippocampal neuronal cultures. MWCNT coated microelectrodes were found to have recording properties superior to those of commercial TiN microelectrodes (Fuchsberger et al., 2011). Drop coating and micro-contact printing methods are quite simple to impalement. However, the film may have weak adhesion to the surface compared with covalent or electrochemical techniques, therefore careful validation of the coating adhesion is important.

CNT MEAs based on top–down fabrication approaches were also reported. Superior electrical properties of CNT microelectrodes were presented by Gabay and co-workers. We fabricated the CNT MEAs by synthesizing high density MWCNT islands on a silicon dioxide substrate. The three-dimensional nature of the CNT electrodes contributes to a very large surface area, and consequently to high electrode specific capacitance (non-Fradaic behavior was validated) and low frequency dependence of the electrode impedance. Spontaneous activity of rat cultured neurons was recorded (Gabay et al., 2005a,b, 2007). Direct electrical interfacing between pristine CNT microelectrodes and rat cultured neurons was also demonstrated by Shein et al. (2009). Each electrode recorded the activity from a cluster of several neurons; this activity was characterized by bursting events (see **Figure 5**). The same CNT MEAs were further used to study the electrical activity of neuronal networks (Shein Idelson et al., 2010) as well as to interface with mice retina (Shoval et al., 2009).

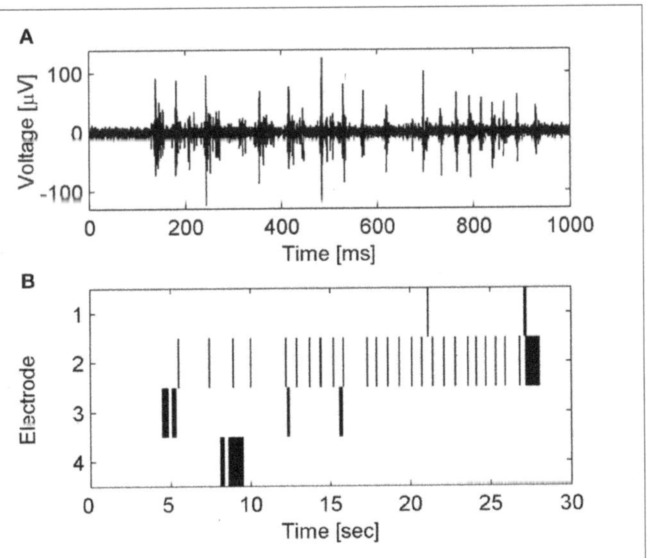

FIGURE 5 | Spontaneous electrical activity of neuronal clusters on CNT MEA. (A) Voltage traces of spontaneous electrical activity recorded from a CNT electrode. **(B)** Raster plot of the spontaneous spiking activity in several CNT electrodes. Activity patterns are characterized by bursting events; short time windows (several hundreds of milliseconds) of rapid collective neuronal firing, which are followed by long intervals (seconds) of sporadic firing. For further details see Shein et al. (2009).

The retina tests revealed that SNR of CNT electrode improved over time suggesting a gradual (over 2 days) improvement in the tissue-electrode coupling. Recent stimulation tests by the same group revealed a similar improvement in the stimulation threshold (Eleftheriou et al., 2012).

Wang and co-workers presented a prototype of vertically aligned MWCNT pillars as microelectrodes on a quartz substrate (Wang et al., 2006). The nanotubes were functionalized with PEG to create a hydrophilic surface. The obtained hydrophilic CNT microelectrodes offer a high charge injection limit without Faradic reactions. *In vitro* electrical stimulation of embryonic rat hippocampal neurons was then achieved and detected by observing intracellular calcium level change using a calcium indicator (Wang et al., 2006). VACNF MEA was fabricated and tested for potential electrophysiological applications by Yu et al. (2007). Extracellular stimulation and recording of both spontaneous and evoked activity in organotypic hippocampal slices was reported. de Asis and co-workers systematically compared PPy-coated VACNF MEA with tungsten wire electrodes, a planar platinum MEA, and an as-grown VACNF MEA for the recording of evoked signals from acute hippocampal slices (de Asis et al., 2009). Recently Su and co-workers synthesized CNTs on a cone-shaped silicon tip by catalytic thermal CVD. Oxygen plasma treatment was used to modify the CNT surface to change the CNT surface characteristics from hydrophobic to hydrophilic in order to improve CNT wettability and electrical properties. Electrochemical characterization of the oxygen plasma-treated three dimensional CNT probes revealed lower impedance and higher capacitance compared with the bare silicon tip. Furthermore, the oxygen treated CNT probes were employed to record signals of a crayfish nerve cord (Su et al., 2010).

The development of CNT MEAs has a few important advantages over silicon probes commonly used in current neuroscience research and clinical applications. Silicon probes typically consist of a silicon support, silicon nitride, and silicon dioxide insulation layer. The electrodes are usually coated with iridium, gold or platinum. The first designs include the Michigan array (Wise et al., 1970; Wise and Angell, 1975) and the Utah array (Campbell et al., 1991). The Michigan probe includes several microelectrode sites patterned on each shank of the structure and the Utah array is a three-dimensional electrode array which consists of multiple sharpened silicon needles. However, a major shortcoming of these devices is the electrode material which is metallic and therefore Faradaic (compared with the capacitive CNT electrodes) and has no affinity to neuronal cells compared with the preferred neuronal adhesion to the rough CNT surfaces.

FLEXIBLE CNT MEA FOR RECORDING AND STIMULATION OF NEURONAL ACTIVITY

Typical MEMS electrodes, despite their many advantages, are rigid and therefore are poorly suited for long-term neural *in vivo* applications. Accordingly, there is an increased interest in the development of flexible MEAs. Specifically, the combination of flexible substrates and CNTs electrodes for neuronal applications has gained attention.

Lin and co-workers were the first to fabricate and implement a flexible CNT-based electrode array for neuronal recording. The

CNT electrode array was grown and patterned on a silicon substrate and was then transferred onto a flexible Parylene-C film. The four-step process included: CNT growth, polymer binding, flexible film transfer, and partial isolation. The resulting vertically aligned CNTs were partially embedded into the polymer film. Recording the electrophysiological response of a crayfish nerve cord was performed with two teflon-coated silver-wires used as a stimulation and a reference electrode. The SNR of the flexible CNT electrode was 257 (Lin et al., 2009).

Direct growth of CNTs on flexible polyimide substrates by catalyst-assisted CVD was also demonstrated (Hsu et al., 2010). The length of the MWCNTs was controlled and increased approximately linearly with the growth time resulting with decreased impedance and increased capacitance. UV-ozone exposure improved the interfacial properties between the CNT electrodes and the electrolyte by increasing the surface wettability (changing it from super hydrophobic to hydrophilic). UV-ozone treatment yielded a 50-fold impedance reduction. Furthermore, flexible CNT electrodes were found to exhibit resistive characteristics, in contrast to the results described above (Nguyen-Vu et al., 2006) which suggested that capacitive conduction dominates. Examination of neuronal cell cultures indicated good biocompatibility. Finally, recordings of evoked action potential from lateral giant neurons in the abdominal ganglia of crayfish were achieved. SNR was about 150, as good as that of a suction pipette and better than gold electrodes (SNR of 122 and 36, respectively). In a subsequent study, a flexible CNT MEA integrated with a chip containing 16 recording amplifiers was presented (Chen et al., 2011b). CNTs were again grown directly on a polyimide flexible substrate. The CNT microelectrode had ten times lower electrode impedance and six times higher capacitance, resulting with better charge injection capacity compared with a gold microelectrode of the same size. Tests with cultured neurons validated the biocompatibility of the device. *In vitro* spontaneous spikes were recorded from a caudal photoreceptor from the tail of the crayfish neuron with SNR of 6.2. The flexible CNT MEA was also applied to record the electrocorticography (ECoG) of a rat motor cortex.

Our group has recently developed a novel all-CNT flexible electrode suited for recording and stimulation of neuronal tissue. Flexible devices were realized by transferring high density MWCNT films onto a flexible PDMS film (Hanein, 2010). A deliberate poor adhesion between the CNT film and the substrate allowed the transfer of the CNTs to the PDMS substrate (**Figure 6A**). This poor adhesion resulted from direct growth of the CNTs on SiO_2. The technology is simple and the resulting stimulating electrodes are nearly purely capacitive. The electrodes exhibit a capacitance of $2\,mF/cm^2$ which is similar to that of TiN and pristine MWCNTs electrodes fabricated on a rigid silicon substrate with 2 and $10\,mF/cm^2$, respectively (Gabay et al., 2007). Recent recording and stimulation tests with chick retina (**Figure 6B**) validate the device suitability for high-efficacy neuronal stimulation applications (David-Pur et al., submitted).

Table 2 summarizes the main findings related to CNT-based neuronal electrical recording and stimulation. The overall picture that emerges from these data is that CNTs were used for neuronal electrical interfacing in three main schemes: CNT coated substrates, CNT coated sharpened wire metal electrodes and CNT MEAs. CNT substrates were used as an *in vitro* growth substrate for neurons and the electrical activity was recorded using intracellular patch clamp technique. Electrical stimulation through these CNT coated surface was also demonstrated. CNT coated sharpened wire electrodes were used for both *in vitro* and *in vivo* neuronal extracellular recording and stimulation. The CNT MEA scheme allows for *in vitro* patterned neuronal growth in conjugation with extracellular recording and stimulation. The final and most recent scheme is the development of flexible CNT MEAs which represents a major step toward implantable neuro-prosthetics applications.

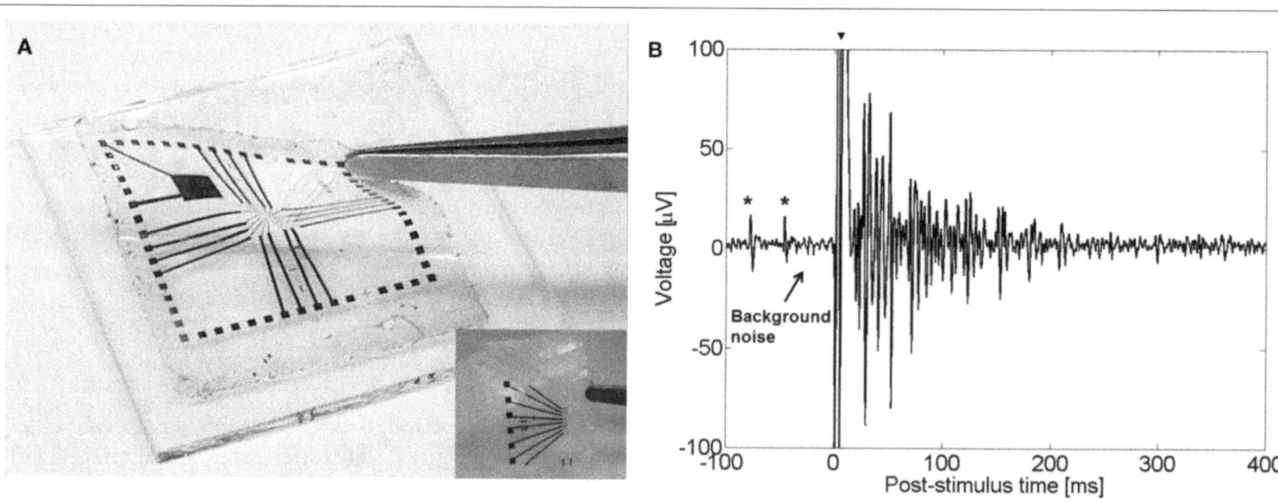

FIGURE 6 | (A) A flexible CNT-based MEA. Inset: flexible CNT-based MEA designed for *in vivo* applications. **(B)** Evoked electrical activity recorded from an embryonic chick retina (day 14) by a CNT electrode (one out of sixteen 50 µm diameter electrodes in the array) using a biphasic anodic first pulse of 20 nC. Retina was flattened on the flexible CNT MEA with retinal ganglion cells layer facing down. The large signal at $t = 0$ (marked with arrow) is an artifact of the stimulation. Spontaneous activity prior to stimulation is marked with asterisks.

Table 2 | Neuronal electrical interfacing CNT technologies.

	References	Electrode/surface description	Bio-testing scheme	Electrical recording	Electrical stimulation
CNT substrates	Lovat et al., 2005	MWCNTs coated cover slip	*In vitro* rat hippocampal cultures	Intracellular patch clamp	Not applied
	Gheith et al. 2006	SWCNTs-PAA coated cover slip	*In vitro* NG108 cell line	Intracellular patch clamp	Intracellular patch clamp
	Liopo et al., 2006	4-tertbutylphenyl or 4-benzoic acid modified SWCNTs coated PET film	*In vitro* NG108 cell line *In vitro* rat peripheral neurons	Intracellular patch clamp	Extracellular
	Mazzatenta et al., 2007	SWCNTs coated cover slip	*In vitro* rat hippocampal cultures	Intracellular patch clamp	Extracellular
	Cellot et al. 2009, 2011	MWCNTs coated cover slip	*In vitro* rat hippocampal cultures	Intracellular patch clamp	Intracellular patch clamp
CNT electrodes	Keefer et al., 2008	PPy-MWCNTs, Au-MWCNTs coated sharpened wire metal electrode	*In vitro* mice frontal cortex cultures *In vivo* rats motor cortex *In vivo* monkeys visual cortex area	Extracellular	Extracellular (*in vitro* tests)
	Baranauskas et al., 2011	PPy-MWCNTs coated sharpened wire metal electrode	*In vivo* rat cortex	Extracellular	Not applied
CNT MEAs	Wang et al., 2006	Vertically aligned MWCNT MEA directly grown on a catalyst patterned substrate and coated with PEGPL for hydrophilic surface	*In vitro* embryonic rat hippocampal neurons	Not applied	Extracellular
	Gabay et al., 2007	MWCNT MEA directly grown on a catalyst patterned substrate	*In vitro* rat cortical cultures	Extracellular	Not applied
	Yu et al., 2007	VACNF MEA directly grown on a catalyst patterned substrate	*In vitro* organotypic rat hippocampal slices	Extracellular	Extracellular
	Keefer et al., 2008	ITO MEA (CNNS) coated with MWCNTs-Au	*In vitro* mice frontal cortex cultures	Extracellular	Extracellular
	de Asis et al., 2009	VACNF MEA directly grown on a catalyst patterned substrate and coated with PPy	*In vitro* rat hippocampal slices	Extracellular	Extracellular
	Gabriel et al., 2009	Pt MEA coated with SWCNTs (drop coating)	*In vitro* isolated rabbit retina	Extracellular	Not applied
	Su et al., 2010	Cone-shaped Si MEA coated with MWCNTs (CVD) after oxygen plasma treatment	*In vitro* crayfish giant neurons	Extracellular	Not applied
	Fuchsberger et al., 2011	TiN MEA coated with MWCNTs (micro-contact printing).	*In vitro* rat postnatal hippocampal cultures	Extracellular	Not applied

(Continued)

Table 2 | Continued

	References	Electrode/surface description	Bio-testing scheme	Electrical recording	Electrical stimulation
Flexible CNT MEAs	Lin et al., 2009	Vertically aligned CNT MEA embedded in Parylene-C film	*In vitro* crayfish nerve cord	Extracellular	Not applied
	Hsu et al., 2010; Chen et al., 2011b	CNT MEA directly grown on a catalyst patterned polyimide after UV-ozone treatment	*In vitro* crayfish giant neurons *In vitro* crayfish caudal photoreceptor *In vitro* EcoG of rat motor cortex	Extracellular	Not applied
	David-Pur et al., submitted	all CNT MEA on PDMS	*In vitro* chick retina	Extracellular	Extracellular

CONCLUSIONS AND PERSPECTIVES

In this review we explored the different properties that make CNT uniquely suited for neuronal interfacing. We have also shown that intensive investigations over the past 10 years have explored CNTs for neuronal interfacing, from surface properties effecting cell adhesion and proliferation to the development of CNT-based MEAs and flexible electrode arrays for *in vivo* applications. This intensive research was motivated by the need to find therapies for neural disorders which require the use of electrical stimulation, as well as by the need to address basic questions in neuroscience. In particular, the study of engineered neuronal circuits can greatly benefit from such CNT-based platforms. Neuronal circuits study aims at rebuilding damaged neuronal tissues. Natural circuits are not prone to manipulations and have highly complex structure and thus are extremely challenging to study. Engineered *in vitro* neuronal networks, however, allow monitoring and systematic investigation and provide unique platform for the study of activity patterns, morphology-activity relationship as well as network damage and repair methods. All These applications can greatly benefit from an efficient neuronal scaffold having the ability to record and stimulate neuronal electrical activity.

The challenging requirements in the field of neural prosthetics, namely, reduction of electrode size while maintaining efficient electrochemical function, as well as reduction of immune response to the implanted device (linked to both size and rigidity of the implanted device), are only poorly fulfilled by commonly used materials. Thus, the development of an efficient neuroprosthetic platform will highly benefit from the realization of CNT electrodes on a flexible substrate.

The emerging applications of CNTs in the field of neuroscience must take into account cytotoxicity considerations. The potential toxicity of CNTs was extensively studied and so far revealed mixed results (Shvedova et al., 2003, 2009, 2010; Dumortier et al., 2006; Firme and Bandaru, 2010; Zhao and Liu, 2012). Better understanding of the interaction between CNTs and the biological environment is required in order to facilitate efficient development of both safe and effective CNT-based neural technologies. Further testing of CNT electrodes corrosion resistance as well as stress durability is required. Another essential step is further study of the nature of neuron-CNT electrical interfacing. Also, comprehensive long-term recording and stimulation studies in animal models followed by clinical trials and approval by administrative authorities such as the US food and drug administration (FDA) must be accomplished to allow routine use of CNT MEAs in neuroscience. The vast literature reviewed here, along with recent studies using CNTs embedded in polymeric support; show that CNTs, if handled properly, are safe as an implantable coating.

Several very promising directions in the study of CNT-based neuro-prosthetic devices currently exist: First is the integration of drug elution coatings. These coatings will allow the reduction of inflammation caused by the insertion of the neuronal implant to the tissue and improve survival of neurons in contact with the device. There is a growing interest in the study of such coatings (Zhong and Bellamkonda, 2005; Wadhwa et al., 2006; He et al., 2007), such studies will also benefit from addressing the development of a coating that will not impair the electrical activity of the device. Second, is the research toward realization of CNT-based flexible MEAs as elaborated in the text above. Some very recent work done in this area by our group and others revealed great potential of such devices. Finally, combining light-sensitive function with the enhanced neuronal interfacing properties of CNTs will be highly beneficial for the development of novel retinal implants.

To conclude, CNT enhanced electrochemical properties, their flexible and simple micro-fabrication preparation procedure, as well as their bio-compatibility and durability, suggest that CNT electrodes are a promising platform for high resolution neuronal applications. The resemblance of CNT surfaces to the nanostructured features of natural neural tissue makes CNTs a suitable platform for tissue engineering and regeneration (Tran et al., 2010; Voge and Stegemann, 2011). Also, the high electrical conductivity of CNTs allows direct electrical interfacing with neurons (Shein-Idelson et al., 2011). Clearly, CNTs have enormous potential in the development of neuronal interfaces and further study will enable the utilization of CNT-based technology to expand the understanding of the nervous system and for the realization of therapeutic approaches.

ACKNOWLEDGMENTS

The authors thank many useful discussions with Moshe David-Pur, Giora Beit-Yaakov, and Dr. Dorit Raz-Prag. They also acknowledge the support of a grant from the Israel Ministry of Science and Technology, the Israel Science Foundation and the European Research Council funding under the European Community's Seventh Framework Programme (FP7/2007–2013)/ERC grant agreement FUNMANIA-306707.

REFERENCES

Abidian, M. R., Corey, J. M., Kipke, D. R., and Martin, D. C. (2010). Conducting-polymer nanotubes improve electrical properties, mechanical adhesion, neural attachment, and neurite outgrowth of neural electrodes. *Small* 6, 421–429.

Abidian, M. R., and Martin, D. C. (2008). Experimental and theoretical characterization of implantable neural microelectrodes modified with conducting polymer nanotubes. *Biomaterials* 29, 1273–1283.

Anava, S., Greenbaum, A., Ben Jacob, E., Hanein, Y., and Ayali, A. (2009). The regulative role of neurite mechanical tension in network development. *Biophys. J.* 96, 1661–1670.

Asplund, M., Thaning, E., Lundberg, J., Sandberg-Nordqvist, A. C., Kostyszyn, B., Inganas, O., et al. (2009). Toxicity evaluation of PEDOT/biomolecular composites intended for neural communication electrodes. *Biomed. Mater.* 4, 1–12.

Baranauskas, G., Maggiolini, E., Castagnola, E., Ansaldo, A., Mazzoni, A., Angotzi, G. N., et al. (2011). Carbon nanotube composite coating of neural microelectrodes preferentially improves the multiunit signal-to-noise ratio. *J. Neural Eng.* 8, 1–12.

Bard, A. J., and Falkner, L. R. (2000). *Electrochemical Methods Fundamentals and Applications.* New York, NY: Wiely.

Basser, P. J., and Roth, B. J. (2000). New currents in electrical stimulation of excitable tissues. *Annu. Rev. Biomed. Eng.* 2, 377–397.

Bekyarova, E., Ni, Y. C., Malarkey, E. B., Montana, V., McWilliams, J. L., Haddon, R. C., et al. (2005). Applications of carbon nanotubes in biotechnology and biomedicine. *J. Biomed. Nanotechnol.* 1, 3–17.

Ben-Jacob, E., and Hanein, Y. (2008). Carbon nanotube micro-electrodes for neuronal interfacing. *J. Mater. Chem.* 18, 5181–5186.

Biran, R., Martin, D. C., and Tresco, P. A. (2005). Neuronal cell loss accompanies the brain tissue response to chronically implanted silicon microelectrode arrays. *Exp. Neurol.* 195, 115–126.

Bottini, M., Bruckner, S., Nika, K., Bottini, N., Bellucci, S., Magrini, A., et al. (2006). Multi-walled carbon nanotubes induce T lymphocyte apoptosis. *Toxicol. Lett.* 160, 121–126.

Bottini, M., Rosato, N., and Bottini, N. (2011). PEG-modified carbon nanotubes in biomedicine: current status and challenges ahead. *Biomacromolecules* 12, 3381–3393.

Buzsaki, G., Anastassiou, C. A., and Koch, C. (2012). The origin of extracellular fields and currents – EEG, ECoG, LFP and spikes. *Nat. Rev. Neurosci.* 13, 407–420.

Campbell, P. K., Jones, K. E., Huber, R. J., Horch, K. W., and Normann, R. A. (1991). A silicon based 3-dimentional neural inerface – manufacturing processes for an intracortical electrode array. *IEEE Trans. Biomed. Eng.* 38, 758–768.

Carrero-Sanchez, J. C., Elias, A. L., Mancilla, R., Arrellin, G., Terrones, H., Laclette, J. P., et al. (2006). Biocompatibility and toxicological studies of carbon nanotubes doped with nitrogen. *Nano Lett.* 6, 1609–1616.

Cellot, G., Cilia, E., Cipollone, S., Rancic, V., Sucapane, A., Giordani, S., et al. (2009). Carbon nanotubes might improve neuronal performance by favouring electrical shortcuts. *Nat. Nanotechnol.* 4, 126–133.

Cellot, G., Toma, F. M., Varley, Z. K., Laishram, J., Villari, A., Quintana, M., et al. (2011). Carbon nanotube scaffolds tune synaptic strength in cultured neural circuits: novel frontiers in nanomaterial-tissue interactions. *J. Neurosci.* 31, 12945–12953.

Charlier, J. C., Blase, X., and Roche, S. (2007). Electronic and transport properties of nanotubes. *Rev. Mod. Phys.* 79, 677–732.

Chen, H. L., Guo, L. H., Ferhan, A. R., and Kim, D. H. (2011a). Multilayered polypyrrole-coated carbon nanotubes to improve functional stability and electrical properties of neural electrodes. *J. Phys. Chem. C* 115, 5492–5499.

Chen, Y. C., Hsu, H. L., Lee, Y. T., Su, H. C., Yen, S. J., Chen, C. H., et al. (2011b). An active, flexible carbon nanotube microelectrode array for recording electrocorticograms. *J. Neural Eng.* 8, 1–7.

Ciraci, S., Dag, S., Yildirim, T., Gulseren, O., and Senger, R. T. (2004). Functionalized carbon nanotubes and device applications. *J. Phys. Condens. Matter* 16, R901–R960.

Clark, G. M. (2006). The multiple-channel cochlear implant: the interface between sound and the central nervous system for hearing, speech, and language in deaf people a per sonal perspective. *Phil. Trans. R. Soc. B* 361, 791–810.

Cogan, S. F. (2008). Neural stimulation and recording electrodes. *Annu. Rev. Biomed. Eng.* 10, 275–309.

Crompton, K. E., Goud, J. D., Bellamkonda, R. V., Gengenbach, T. R., Finkelstein, D. I., Horne, M. K., et al. (2007). Polylysine-functionalised thermoresponsive chitosan hydrogel for neural tissue engineering. *Biomaterials* 28, 441–449.

de Asis, E. D., Nguyen-Vu, T. D. B., Arumugam, P. U., Chen, H., Cassell, A. M., Andrews, R. J., et al. (2009). High efficient electrical stimulation of hippocampal slices with vertically aligned carbon nanofiber microbrush array. *Biomed. Microdevices* 11, 801–808.

Dumortier, H., Lacotte, S., Pastorin, G., Marega, R., Wu, W., Bonifazi, D., et al. (2006). Functionalized carbon nanotubes are non-cytotoxic and preserve the functionality of primary immune cells. *Nano Lett.* 6, 1522–1528.

Eleftheriou, C. G., Zimmermann, J., Kjeldsen, H., David-Pur, M., Hanein, Y., and Sernagor, E. (2012). "Towards the development of carbon nanotube based retinal implant technology: electrophysiological and ultrastructural evidence of coupling at the hybrid interface," in *Proceedings of the 8th International MEA Meeting on Substrate Integrated Microelectrode Arrys* (Reutlingen, Germany).

Fan, Y. W., Cui, F. Z., Hou, S. P., Xu, Q. Y., Chen, L. N., and Lee, I. S. (2002). Culture of neural cells on silicon wafers with nano-scale surface topograph. *J. Neurosci. Methods* 120, 17–23.

Firme, C. P., and Bandaru, P. R. (2010). Toxicity issues in the application of carbon nanotubes to biological systems. *Nanomedicine* 6, 245–256.

Fuchsberger, K., Le Goff, A., Gambazzi, L., Toma, F. M., Goldoni, A., Giugliano, M., et al. (2011). Multiwalled carbon-nanotube-functionalized microelectrode arrays fabricated by microcontact printing: platform for studying chemical and electrical neuronal signaling. *Small* 7, 524–530.

Gabay, T., Ben-David, M., Kalifa, I., Sorkin, R., Abrams, Z. R.,

Ben-Jacob, E., et al. (2007). Electrochemical and biological properties of carbon nanotube based multi-electrode arrays. *Nanotechnology* 18, 1–6.

Gabay, T., Jakobs, E., Ben-Jacob, E., and Hanein, Y. (2005a). Engineered self-organization of neural networks using carbon nanotube clusters. *Physica A* 350, 611–621.

Gabay, T., Kalifa, I., Ezra, L., Jakobs, E., Ben-Jacob, E., and Hanein, Y. (2005b). "Carbon nanotube based neuro-chip for engineering, recording and stimulation of cultured networks," in *The 13th International Conference on Solid-State Sensors, Actuators and Microsystems* (Seoul, Korea), 1226–1229.

Gabriel, G., Gomez, R., Bongard, M., Benito, N., Fernandez, E., and Villa, R. (2009). Easily made single-walled carbon nanotube surface microelectrodes for neuronal applications. *Biosens. Bioelectron.* 24, 1942–1948.

Galvan-Garcia, P., Keefer, E. W., Yang, F., Zhang, M., Fang, S., Zakhidov, A. A., et al. (2007). Robust cell migration and neuronal growth on pristine carbon nanotube sheets and yarns. *J. Biomater. Sci. Polym. Ed.* 18, 1245–1261.

George, M. S., Nahas, Z., Borckardt, J. J., Anderson, B., Foust, M. J., Burns, C., et al. (2007). Brain stimulation for the treatment of psychiatric disorders. *Curr. Opin. Psychiatry* 20, 250–254.

George, P. M., Lyckman, A. W., LaVan, D. A., Hegde, A., Leung, Y., Avasare, R., et al. (2005). Fabrication and biocompatibility of polypyrrole implants suitable for neural prosthetics. *Biomaterials* 26, 3511–3519.

Gheith, M. K., Pappas, T. C., Liopo, A. V., Sinani, V. A., Shim, B. S., Motamedi, M., et al. (2006). Stimulation of neural cells by lateral layer-by-layer films of single-walled currents in conductive carbon nanotubes. *Adv. Mater.* 18, 2975–2979.

Gheith, M. K., Sinani, V. A., Wicksted, J. P., Matts, R. L., and Kotov, N. A. (2005). Single-walled carbon nanotube polyelectrolyte multilayers and freestanding films as a biocompatible platformfor neuroprosthetic implants. *Adv. Mater.* 17, 2663–2670.

Grattarola, M., and Martinoia, S. (1993). Modeling the neuron-microtransducer junction – from extracellular to patch recording. *IEEE Trans. Biomed. Eng.* 40, 35–41.

Greenbaum, A., Anava, S., Ayali, A., Shein, M., David-Pur, M., Ben-Jacob, E., et al. (2009). One-to-one neuron-electrode interfacing. *J. Neurosci. Methods* 182, 219–224.

HajjHassan, M., Chodavarapu, V., and Musallam, S. (2008). NeuroMEMS: neural probe microtechnologies. *Sensors* 8, 6704–6726.

Hanein, Y. (2010). Carbon nanotube integration into MEMS devices. *Phys. Status Solidi B* 247, 2635–2640.

Hanein, Y., Tadmor, O., Anava, S., and Ayali, A. (2011). Neuronal soma migration is determined by neurite tension. *Neuroscience* 172, 572–579.

Harris, P. J. F. (2009). *Carbon Nanotube Science.* New York, NY: Cambridge University Press.

Hayashi, T., Kim, Y. A., Natsuki, T., and Endo, M. (2007). Mechanical properties of carbon nanomaterials. *Chemphyschem* 8, 999–1004.

He, W., and Bellamkonda, R. V. (2005). Nanoscale neuro-integrative coatings for neural implants. *Biomaterials* 26, 2983–2990.

He, W., McConnell, G. C., Schneider, T. M., and Bellamkonda, R. V. (2007). A novel anti-inflammatory surface for neural electrodes. *Adv. Mater.* 19, 3529–3533.

Heller, D. A., Garga, V., Kelleher, K. J., Lee, T. C., Mahbubani, S., Sigworth, L. A., et al. (2005). Patterned networks of mouse hippocampal neurons on peptide-coated gold surfaces. *Biomaterials* 26, 883–889.

Hoffman-Kim, D., Mitchel, J. A., and Bellamkonda, R. V. (2010). "Topography, cell response, and nerve regeneration," in *Annual Review of Biomedical Engineering, Vol 12*, eds M. L. Yarmush, J. S. Duncan, and M. L. Gray (Palo Alto, CA: Annual Reviews), 203–231.

Hsu, H. L., Teng, I. J., Chen, Y. C., Hsu, W. L., Lee, Y. T., Yen, S. J., et al. (2010). Flexible UV-ozone-modified carbon nanotube electrodes for neuronal recording. *Adv. Mater.* 22, 2177–2181.

Hu, H., Ni, Y. C., Mandal, S. K., Montana, V., Zhao, N., Haddon, R. C., et al. (2005). Polyethyleneimine functionalized single-walled carbon nanotubes as a substrate for neuronal growth. *J. Phys. Chem. B* 109, 4285–4289.

Hu, H., Ni, Y. C., Montana, V., Haddon, R. C., and Parpura, V. (2004). Chemically functionalized carbon nanotubes as substrates for neuronal growth. *Nano Lett.* 4, 507–511.

Keefer, E. W., Botterman, B. R., Romero, M. I., Rossi, A. F., and Gross, G. W. (2008). Carbon nanotube coating improves neuronal recordings. *Nat. Nanotechnol.* 3, 434–439.

Khan, S., and Newaz, G. (2010). A comprehensive review of surface modification for neural cell adhesion and patterning. *J. Biomed. Mater. Res. A* 93A, 1209–1224.

Lan, Y. C., Wang, Y., and Ren, Z. F. (2011). Physics and applications of aligned carbon nanotubes. *Adv. Phys.* 60, 553–678.

Laxton, A. W., Tang-Wai, D. F., McAndrews, M. P., Zumsteg, D., Wennberg, R., Keren, R., et al. (2010). A phase I trial of deep brain stimulation of memory circuits in Alzheimer's disease. *Ann. Neurol.* 68, 521–534.

Lee, W., and Parpura, V. (2009). "Carbon nanotubes as substrates/scaffolds for neural cell growth," in *Nanoneuroscience and Nanoneuropharmacology,* ed H. S. Sharma (Amsterdam: Elsevier Science BV), 111–125.

Lin, C. M., Lee, Y. T., Yeh, S. R., and Fang, W. L. (2009). Flexible carbon nanotubes electrode for neural recording. *Biosens. Bioelectron.* 24, 2791–2797.

Liopo, A. V., Stewart, M. P., Hudson, J., Tour, J. M., and Pappas, T. C. (2006). Biocompatibility of native and functionalized single-walled carbon nanotubes for neuronal interface. *J, Nanosci. Nanotechnol.* 6, 1365–1374.

Lovat, V., Pantarotto, D., Lagostena, L., Cacciari, B., Grandolfo, M., Righi, M., et al. (2005). Carbon nanotube substrates boost neuronal electrical signaling. *Nano Lett.* 5, 1107–1110.

Lu, F. S., Gu, L. R., Meziani, M. J., Wang, X., Luo, P. G., Veca, L. M., et al. (2009). Advances in bioapplications of carbon nanotubes. *Adv. Mater.* 21, 139–152.

Lu, Y., Li, T., Zhao, X. Q., Li, M., Cao, Y. L., Yang, H. X., et al. (2010). Electrodeposited polypyrrole/carbon nanotubes composite films electrodes for neural interfaces. *Biomaterials* 31, 5169–5181.

Luo, X. L., Weaver, C. L., Zhou, D. D., Greenberg, R., and Cui, X. Y. T. (2011). Highly stable carbon nanotube doped poly(3,4-ethylenedioxythiophene) for chronic neural stimulation. *Biomaterials* 32, 5551–5557.

Malarkey, E. B., Fisher, K. A., Bekyarova, E., Liu, W., Haddon, R. C., and Parpura, V. (2009). Conductive single-walled carbon nanotube substrates modulate neuronal growth. *Nano Lett.* 9, 264–268.

Malarkey, E. B., and Parpura, V. (2007). Applications of carbon nanotubes in neurobiology. *Neurodegener. Dis.* 4, 292–299.

Marciniak, S., Crispin, X., Uvdal, K., Trzcinski, M., Birgerson, J., Groenendaal, D., et al. (2004). Light induced damage in poly(3, 4-ethylenedioxythiophene) and its derivatives studied by photoelectron spectroscopy. *Synth. Met.* 141, 67–73.

Matsumoto, K., Sato, C., Naka, Y., Kitazawa, A., Whitby, R. L. D., and Shimizu, N. (2007). Neurite outgrowths of neurons with neurotrophin-coated carbon nanotubes. *J. Biosci. Bioeng.* 103, 216–220.

Mattson, M. P., Haddon, R. C., and Rao, A. M. (2000). Molecular functionalization of carbon nanotubes and use as substrates for neuronal growth. *J. Mol. Neurosci.* 14, 175–182.

Mazzatenta, A., Giugliano, M., Campidelli, S., Gambazzi, L., Businaro, L., Markram, H., et al. (2007). Interfacing neurons with carbon nanotubes: electrical signal transfer and synaptic stimulation in cultured brain circuits. *J. Neurosci.* 27, 6931–6936.

McConnell, G. C., Rees, H. D., Levey, A. I., Gutekunst, C. A., Gross, R. E., and Bellamkonda, R. V. (2009). Implanted neural electrodes cause chronic, local inflammation that is correlated with local neurodegeneration. *J. Neural Eng.* 6, 1–12.

McCreery, D. B. (2008). Cochlear nucleus auditory prostheses. *Hear. Res.* 242, 64–73.

McCreery, D. B., Agnew, W. F., Yuen, T. G. H., and Bullara, L. (1990). Charge density and charge per phase as cofactors in neural injury induced by electrical stimulation. *IEEE Trans. Biomed. Eng.* 37, 996–1001.

McCreery, D. B., Agnew, W. F., Yuen, T. G. H., and Bullara, L. A. (1988). Comparison of neural damage induced by electrical stimulation with faradaic and capacitor electrodes. *Ann. Biomed. Eng.* 16, 463–481.

Merrill, D. R., Bikson, M., and Jefferys, J. G. R. (2005). Electrical stimulation of excitable tissue: design of efficacious and safe protocols. *J. Neurosci. Methods* 141, 171–198.

Musial, P. G., Baker, S. N., Gerstein, G. L., King, E. A., and Keating, J. G. (2002). Signal-to-noise ratio improvement in multiple electrode recording. *J. Neurosci. Methods* 115, 29–43.

Nguyen-Vu, T. D. B., Chen, H., Cassell, A. M., Andrews, R., Meyyappan, M., and Li, J. (2006). Vertically aligned carbon nanofiber arrays: an advance toward electrical-neural interfaces. *Small* 2, 89–94.

Nguyen-Vu, T. D. B., Chen, H., Cassell, A. M., Andrews, R. J., Meyyappan, M., and Li, J. (2007). Vertically aligned carbon nanofiber architecture as a multifunctional 3-D neural electrical interface. *IEEE Trans. Biomed. Eng.* 54, 1121–1128.

Nunes, A., Al-Jamal, K., Nakajima, T., Hariz, M., and Kostarelos, K. (2012). Application of carbon nanotubes in neurology: clinical perspectives and toxicological risks. *Arch. Toxicol.* 86, 1009–1020.

Pancrazio, J. J. (2008). Neural interfaces at the nanoscale. *Nanomedicine* 3, 823–830.

Plow, E. B., Pascual-Leone, A., and Machado, A. (2012). Brain stimulation in the treatment of chronic neuropathic and non-cancerous pain. *J. Pain* 13, 411–424.

Polikov, V. S., Tresco, P. A., and Reichert, W. M. (2005). Response of brain tissue to chronically implanted neural electrodes. *J. Neurosci. Methods* 148, 1–18.

Roach, P., Parker, T., Gadegaard, N., and Alexander, M. R. (2010). Surface strategies for control of neuronal cell adhesion: a review. *Surf. Sci. Rep.* 65, 145–173.

Robblee, L. S., and Rose, T. L. (1990). "Electrochemical guidelines for selection of protocols and electrode materials for neural stimulation," in *Neural Prostheses: Fundamental Studies*, eds W. F. Agnew and D. B. McCreery (Englewood Cliffs, NJ: Prentice Hall), 25–66.

Rodriguez, N. M. (1993). A review of catalytically grown carbon nanofibers. *J. Mater. Res.* 8, 3233–3250.

Roth, B. J. (1994). Mechanisms for electrical stimulation of excitable tissue. *Crit. Rev. Biomed. Eng.* 22, 253–305.

Ruardij, T. G., Goedbloed, M. H., and Rutten, W. L. C. (2000). Adhesion and patterning of cortical neurons on polyethylenimine- and fluorocarbon-coated surfaces. *IEEE Trans. Biomed. Eng.* 47, 1593–1599.

Schwartz, A. B. (2004). Cortical neural prosthetics. *Annu. Rev. Neurosci.* 27, 487–507.

Seah, C. M., Chai, S. P., and Mohamed, A. R. (2011). Synthesis of aligned carbon nanotubes. *Carbon* 49, 4613–4635.

Seidlits, S. K., Lee, J. Y., and Schmidt, C. E. (2008). Nanostructured scaffolds for neural applications. *Nanomedicine* 3, 183–199.

Shein Idelson, M., Ben-Jacob, E., and Hanein, Y. (2010). Innate synchronous oscillations in freely-organized small neuronal circuits. *PLoS ONE* 5: e14443. doi: 10.1371/journal.pone.0014443

Shein, M., Greenbaum, A., Gabay, T., Sorkin, R., David-Pur, M., Ben-Jacob, E., et al. (2009). Engineered neuronal circuits shaped and interfaced with carbon nanotube microelectrode arrays. *Biomed. Microdevices* 11, 495–501.

Shein-Idelson, M., Ben-Jacob, E., and Hanein, Y. (2011). Engineered neuronal circuits: a new platform for studying the role of modular topology. *Front. Neuroeng.* 4:10. doi: 10.3389/fneng.2011.00010

Shoval, A., Adams, C., David-Pur, M., Shein, M., Hanein, Y., and Sernagor, E. (2009). Carbon nanotube electrodes for effective interfacing with retinal tissue. *Front. Neuroeng.* 2:4. doi: 10.3389/neuro.16.004.2009

Shvedova, A. A., Castranova, V., Kisin, E. R., Schwegler-Berry, D., Murray, A. R., Gandelsman, et al. (2003). Exposure to carbon nanotube material: assessment of nanotube cytotoxicity using human keratinocyte cells. *J. Toxicol. Environ. Health A* 66, 1909–1926.

Shvedova, A. A., Kagan, V. E., and Fadeel, B. (2010). Close encounters of the small kind: adverse effects of man-made materials interfacing with the nano-cosmos of biological systems. *Annu. Rev. Pharmacol. Toxicol.* 50, 63–88.

Shvedova, A. A., Kisin, E. R., Porter, D., Schulte, P., Kagan, V. E., Fadeel, B., et al. (2009). Mechanisms of pulmonary toxicity and medical applications of carbon nanotubes: two faces of Janus? *Pharmacol. Ther.* 121, 192–204.

Sorkin, R., Gabay, T., Blinder, P., Baranes, D., Ben-Jacob, E., and Hanein, Y. (2006). Compact self-wiring in cultured neural networks. *J. Neural Eng.* 3, 95–101.

Sorkin, R., Greenbaum, A., David-Pur, M., Anava, S., Ayali, A., Ben-Jacob, E., et al. (2009). Process entanglement as a neuronal anchorage mechanism to rough surfaces. *Nanotechnology* 20, 1–8.

Sorribas, H., Braun, D., Leder, L., Sonderegger, P., and Tiefenauer, L. (2001). Adhesion proteins for a tight neuron-electrode contact. *J. Neurosci. Methods* 104, 133–141.

Su, H. C., Lin, C. M., Yen, S. J., Chen, Y. C., Chen, C. H., Yeh, S. R., et al. (2010). A cone-shaped 3D carbon nanotube probe for neural recording. *Biosens. Bioelectron.* 26, 220–227.

Szarowski, D. H., Andersen, M. D., Retterer, S., Spence, A. J., Isaacson, M., Craighead, H. G., et al. (2003). Brain responses to micro-machined silicon devices. *Brain Res.* 983, 23–35.

Tarakanov, A. O., Goncharova, L. B., and Tarakanov, Y. A. (2010). Carbon nanotubes towards medicinal biochips. *WIREs Nanomed. Nanobiotechnol.* 2, 1–10.

Tehovnik, E. J. (1996). Electrical stimulation of neural tissue to evoke behavioral responses. *J. Neurosci. Methods* 65, 1–17.

Thostenson, E. T., Ren, Z. F., and Chou, T. W. (2001). Advances in the science and technology of carbon nanotubes and their composites: a review. *Composites Sci. Technol.* 61, 1899–1912.

Tran, P. A., Zhang, L. J., and Webster, T. J. (2010). Carbon nanofibers and carbon nanotubes in regenerative medicine. *Adv. Drug Del. Rev.* 61, 1097–1114.

Tunc, M., Cheng, X. H., Ratner, B. D., Meng, E., and Humayun, M. (2007). Reversible thermosensitive glue for retinal implants. *Retina* 27, 938–942.

Voge, C. M., and Stegemann, J. P. (2011). Carbon nanotubes in neural interfacing applications. *J. Neural Eng.* 8, 1–10.

Wadhwa, R., Lagenaur, C. F., and Cui, X. T. (2006). Electrochemically controlled release of dexamethasone from conducting polymer polypyrrole coated electrode. *J. Control. Release* 110, 531–541.

Wan, M. X. (2008). A template-free method towards conducting polymer nanostructures. *Adv. Mater.* 20, 2926–2932.

Wang, K., Fishman, H. A., Dai, H. J., and Harris, J. S. (2006). Neural stimulation with a carbon nanotube microelectrode array. *Nano Lett.* 6, 2043–2048.

Warheit, D. B., Laurence, B. R., Reed, K. L., Roach, D. H., Reynolds, G. A. M., and Webb, T. R. (2004). Comparative pulmonary toxicity assessment of single-wall carbon nanotubes in rats. *Toxicol. Sci.* 77, 117–125.

Webster, T. J., Waid, M. C., McKenzie, J. L., Price, R. L., and Ejiofor, J. U. (2004). Nano-biotechnology: carbon nanofibres as improved neural and orthopaedic implants. *Nanotechnology* 15, 48–54.

Wichmann, T., and DeLong, M. R. (2006). Deep brain stimulation for neurologic and neuropsychiatric disorders. *Neuron* 52, 197–204.

Wise, K. D., and Angell, J. B. (1975). Low-capacitance multielectrode probe for use in extracellular neurophysiology. *IEEE Trans. Biomed. Eng.* BM22, 212–219.

Wise, K. D., Angell, J. B., and Starr, A. (1970). An integrated circuit approach to extracellular microelectrodes. *IEEE Trans. Biomed. Eng.* BM17, 238–247.

Xie, J. N., Chen, L. F., Aatre, K. R., Srivatsan, M., and Varadan, V. K. (2006). Somatosensory neurons grown on functionalized carbon nanotube mats. *Smart Mater. Struct.* 15, N85–N88.

Yamato, H., Ohwa, M., and Wernet, W. (1995). Stability of polypyrrole and poly(3, 4-ethylenedioxythiophene) for biosensor application. *J. Electroanal. Chem.* 397, 163–170.

Yang, W. R., Thordarson, P., Gooding, J. J., Ringer, S. P., and Braet, F. (2007). Carbon nanotubes for biological and biomedical applications. *Nanotechnology* 18, 1–12.

Yu, Z., McKnight, T. E., Ericson, M. N., Melechko, A. V., Simpson, M. L., and Morrison, B. (2007). Vertically aligned carbon nanofiber arrays record electrophysiological signals from hippocampal slices. *Nano Lett.* 7, 2188–2195.

Zhang, X., Prasad, S., Niyogi, S., Morgan, A., Ozkan, M., and Ozkan, C. S. (2005). Guided neurite growth on patterned carbon nanotubes. *Sens. Actuators B Chem.* 106, 843–850.

Zhao, X. C., and Liu, R. T. (2012). Recent progress and perspectives on the toxicity of carbon nanotubes at organism, organ, cell, and biomacromolecule levels. *Environ. Int.* 40, 244–255.

Zhong, Y. H., and Bellamkonda, R. V. (2005). Controlled release of anti-inflammatory agent alpha-MSH from neural implants. *J. Control. Release* 106, 309–318.

17

Controlling the oscillation phase through precisely timed closed-loop optogenetic stimulation: a computational study

Annette Witt[1], Agostina Palmigiano[2], Andreas Neef[3], Ahmed El Hady[3], Fred Wolf[3]* and Demian Battaglia[2]*

[1] *Cognitive Neuroscience Department, German Primate Center, Bernstein Center for Computational Neuroscience, Max Planck Institute for Dynamics and Self-Organization, Göttingen, Germany*

[2] *Bernstein Center for Computational Neuroscience, Max Planck Institute for Dynamics and Self-Organization, Göttingen, Germany*

[3] *Max Planck Institute for Dynamics and Self-Organization, Bernstein Center for Computational Neuroscience and Bernstein Focus Neurotechnology, CRC-889 Cellular Basis of Sensory Processing, Göttingen, Germany*

Edited by:
Steve M. Potter, Georgia Institute of Technology, USA

Reviewed by:
Carmen Canavier, LSU Health Sciences Center, USA
Nathan Urban, Carnegie Mellon University, USA
Robert J. Butera, Butera Lab, Georgia Institute of Technology (Georgia Tech), USA

***Correspondence:**
Fred Wolf and Demian Battaglia, Max Planck Institute for Dynamics and Self-Organization, Am Faßberg 17, D-37077 Göttingen, Germany.
e-mail: fred@nld.ds.mpg.de; demian@nld.ds.mpg.de

Dynamic oscillatory coherence is believed to play a central role in flexible communication between brain circuits. To test this communication-through-coherence hypothesis, experimental protocols that allow a reliable control of phase-relations between neuronal populations are needed. In this modeling study, we explore the potential of closed-loop optogenetic stimulation for the control of functional interactions mediated by oscillatory coherence. The theory of non-linear oscillators predicts that the efficacy of local stimulation will depend not only on the stimulation intensity but also on its timing relative to the ongoing oscillation in the target area. Induced phase-shifts are expected to be stronger when the stimulation is applied within specific narrow phase intervals. Conversely, stimulations with the same or even stronger intensity are less effective when timed randomly. Stimulation should thus be properly phased with respect to ongoing oscillations (in order to optimally perturb them) and the timing of the stimulation onset must be determined by a real-time phase analysis of simultaneously recorded local field potentials (LFPs). Here, we introduce an electrophysiologically calibrated model of Channelrhodopsin 2 (ChR2)-induced photocurrents, based on fits holding over two decades of light intensity. Through simulations of a neural population which undergoes coherent gamma oscillations—either spontaneously or as an effect of continuous optogenetic driving—we show that precisely-timed photostimulation pulses can be used to shift the phase of oscillation, even at transduction rates smaller than 25%. We consider then a canonic circuit with two inter-connected neural populations oscillating with gamma frequency in a phase-locked manner. We demonstrate that photostimulation pulses applied locally to a single population can induce, if precisely phased, a lasting reorganization of the phase-locking pattern and hence modify functional interactions between the two populations.

Keywords: oscillations, functional connectivity, modeling, closed-loop systems, optogenetic stimulation, phase response

INTRODUCTION

Neural activity of brain circuits at many scales has often been reported to display oscillatory components at different frequencies (Eckhorn et al., 1988; Gray et al., 1989; Kreiter and Singer, 1996; Tallon-Baudry et al., 1996; Roelfsema et al., 1997; Varela et al., 2001; Brovelli et al., 2004; Samonds and Bonds, 2004; Melloni et al., 2007; Buffalo et al., 2011). In particular, the *communication-through-coherence* hypothesis (Fries, 2005) suggests that oscillatory coherence between different neural circuits could control functional interactions between them with a high degree of flexibility (Womelsdorf et al., 2007). In particular, evidence for a role of enhanced inter-areal oscillatory coherence in attentional modulation is rapidly accumulating (Fries et al., 2001; Gregoriou et al., 2009; Rotermund et al., 2009; Bosman et al., 2012; Gregoriou et al., 2012; Grothe et al., 2012).

The circuit mechanisms underlying the local generation of oscillations, specifically in the gamma range of frequencies (30–100 Hz) have been explored in studies *in vitro* (Whittington et al., 1995; Bartos et al., 2007) and *in silico* (Brunel and Hakim, 1999; Whittington et al., 2000; Brunel and Hansel, 2006; Wang, 2010). All of these contributions have highlighted the crucial role played by the interplay of GABAergic interneurons in creating time-windows in which excitatory and inhibitory neurons can fire in a sparsely synchronized manner, before being counteracted by strong and delayed feedback inhibition. More recently, the functional involvement of local inhibitory networks could be causally verified *in vivo* by targeted selective optogenetic stimulation of Parvalbumine-positive basket cells in a cortical circuit (Cardin et al., 2006; Sohal et al., 2009).

In an analogous way, optogenetic techniques might be used for direct tests of the communication-through-coherence hypothesis and other suggested functional roles of brain oscillations, like their implication in phase coding (Lisman, 2005; Koepsell et al., 2010; Nadasdy, 2010; Kayser et al., 2012). For such applications, however, improved optogenetic stimulation protocols are needed that allow for precise control of the phase relations between different neuronal populations or assemblies, rather than a pure enhancement of oscillatory power.

Theoretical investigations suggest that, due to non-trivial phase response properties (Pikovsky et al., 2001) of oscillating neuronal populations (Akam et al., 2012), stimulation pulses might have a strong influence on local and long-range phase-relations, but only if properly timed with respect to the ongoing oscillatory dynamics (Tiesinga and Sejnowski, 2010; Battaglia et al., 2012). Application of phase-timed stimuli requires a real-time estimate of the phase from continuously recorded local field potential (LFP) data.

Optogenetic stimulation conditional on recorded activity constitutes a closed-loop setup. The advantage of closed-loop stimulation compared to open-loop stimulation is the possibility to program an artificial feedback with defined rules and constraints dependent on the target system's dynamical history. Closed loop electrical stimulation has been successfully used to clamp network activity (Wallach et al., 2011), to control the firing rate of neurons (Miranda-Dominguez et al., 2010), to control bursting activity (Wagenaar et al., 2005), and to train cultured neuronal networks (Marom and Shahaf, 2002). Closing the loop between living neurons and robotics has also been used to realize embodiment—by using representations generated by network activity either to control a robotic arm (Bakkum et al., 2007) or control autonomous systems (Bandyopadhyay, 2005)—or to study neuronal plasticity (Novellino et al., 2007).

In this study, we explore through a modeling approach the feasibility of closed-loop optogenetic control of the phase of a local oscillation and of inter-areal phase synchronization. To this end, we simulated the activity of populations of excitatory and inhibitory conductance-based neurons with random connectivity. To investigate the case where a sparse transduction with Channelrhodopsin 2 (ChR2) is achieved *in vitro* or *in vivo*, small fractions of these neurons were endowed with a newly developed and data-constrained conductance-based model of a light-activated channel. This case is of particular interest, since it has been shown that low transduction rates achieved through either particle mediated gene transfer or via lipid reagents (Takahashi et al., 2012) can increase the spatial specificity of light stimulation (Schoenenberger et al., 2008). Our model, however, applies robustly also to the case of higher ChR2 transduction rates, as the ones that can be achieved using viral transfection (Adamantidis et al., 2007; Aravanis et al., 2007), in utero electroporation (Petreanu et al., 2007) or in T helper type 1 (Thy1) transgenic mice (Wang et al., 2007).

Demonstrating the reliability of our model, we first simulated phase shifting of LFP oscillations with open-loop optogenetic stimulation, quantitatively reproducing and generalizing experimental results *in vitro* (Akam et al., 2012). We moved then to the analysis of a canonical cortical circuit with two interacting areas. Here, we simulated a realistic closed-loop stimulation protocol which was suited to trigger lasting changes of inter-areal phase relations and, correspondingly, to affect communication-through-coherence. Thus, we intend our modeling exploration to foster the implementation of a new generation of closed-loop optogenetic experiments *in vitro* and *in vivo* aiming at inducing distributed reorganization of functional interactions at the system level.

MATERIALS AND METHODS

ChR2 PHOTOCURRENT EXPERIMENTAL CHARACTERIZATION

Human embryonic kidney cells were transfected with a plasmid encoding a ChR2-YFP fusion protein. The pcDNA 3.1-ChR2-YFP construct was kindly provided by Ernst Bamberg, (MPI for Biophysics, Frankfurt, Germany). After two–four days, successfully transfected cells were identified by their YFP fluorescence. In the whole-cell configuration, the membrane voltage was clamped to −60 mV. Channelrhodopsin's conductance was changed by 500 ms long light pulses. The conductance change was monitored as a time and light-intensity dependent current change (**Figure 1B**). In the case of cultured hippocampal neurons, cell were transfected at 7 DIV with AAV1/2-CAG-ChR2-YFP virus. After 1 week, successfully transduced cells could be identified by their YFP fluorescence.

Whole-field illumination was provided by an extended laser beam (488 nm). Light intensity was controlled by neutral density filters (optical density 1 and 2, respectively) and by means of the software provided for the laser. A comparison of the light-induced current waveforms for 90% attenuation by software and a neutral density filter with an optical density of 1.0 showed excellent agreement, indicating that the software produced the intended attenuation. The laser was switched using a built-in mechanical shutter with a response time in the μs range, achieved through the minute spatial extent of the beam.

BIOPHYSICALLY CALIBRATED MODEL OF ChR2 PHOTOCONDUCTANCE

Based on the results of the previously described experiment, we modeled the evoked photocurrents as the product of activation and inactivation functions. The current activation could be described by a single exponential function and the current inactivation by the sum of two exponential functions (see also **Figure 1B**). This light-induced conductance change could be well described by the functional form:

$$F_{ChR2}(t) = A_{\mathrm{act}}\left(1 - e^{-\frac{t-t_{\mathrm{ON}}-d}{\tau_{\mathrm{act}}}}\right) \cdot \left(A_{\mathrm{persist}} + A^{(1)}_{\mathrm{inact}} e^{-\frac{t-t_{\mathrm{ON}}-d}{\tau^{(1)}_{\mathrm{inact}}}} + A^{(2)}_{\mathrm{inact}} e^{-\frac{t-t_{\mathrm{ON}}-d}{\tau^{(2)}_{\mathrm{inact}}}}\right) \quad (1)$$

Here d represents a latency observed between the times t_{ON} of light onset and the actual start of the conductance rise and A_{persist} is set to $A_{\mathrm{persist}} = 1 - A^{(1)}_{\mathrm{inact}} - A^{(2)}_{\mathrm{inact}}$ in order to prevent the inactivation conductance factor from becoming negative. Note that Equation 1 holds true only as long as the light is switched on. After switching off the light, the response returns to baseline with a single exponential time course with time constant τ_{OFF}. When individual current responses were fitted, the latency d, the amplitude A_{act}, the inactivating fractions $A^{(1)}_{\mathrm{inact}}$ and $A^{(2)}_{\mathrm{inact}}$, and

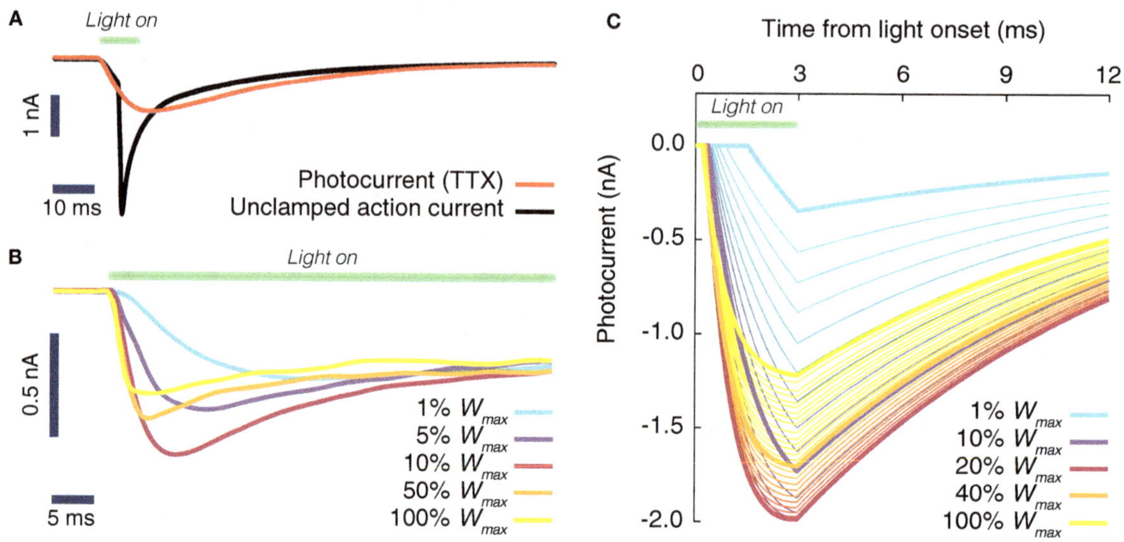

FIGURE 1 | Evoked ChR2 photocurrent: conductance-based model. **(A)** Whole cell voltage clamp recording of a cultured neuron, transduced with Channelrhodopsine 2 (ChR2) and illuminated with LED light (during the time interval shown by a green horizontal bar). Two current intensity recordings have been performed, the first in a physiological solution, i.e., with all channels active (black curve), the second with TTX in the bath, i.e., with blocked Na-channels (red curve). When the Na channels are still active (black curve), even the voltage clamp (−70 mV) at the soma cannot prevent the cell from spiking. **(B)** Activation kinetics of the photo-induced conductance in human embryonic kidney cells (HEK-293) that are transfected with ChR2. For increasing light power density (100% W_{max} corresponds approximately to 130 mW/mm^2) the activation becomes faster. Peak conductance increases from 0 to ~10% of the maximal intensity and decreases for higher light intensities. Note the different scale of evoked currents in neurons and HEK cells. **(C)** Simulated photocurrents generated by the conductance-based model described by Equation (1), for different light intensities (expressed relatively to maximum illumination intensity) and for a rectangular shaped light pulse stimulation with a duration of 3 ms. Model parameters and their dependence on light intensity (see **Table 2**) are obtained from fits to photoconductance recordings analogous to the one shown in panel **(B)**, performed for different light intensities. For short light pulses as used here, the experiments indicate that the largest conductances are obtained for light intensities between 10% and 50% (interpolation of the simulated photocurrent results in an optimal value of 18% of the maximum light intensity).

the activation time constant τ_{act} were found to be dependent on the light-intensity W_{light} when individual current responses were fitted. However, the time constants related to inactivation were almost unchanged for different light intensities. Therefore, for simultaneously fitting current responses evoked by different light intensities (ranging over two orders of magnitude), two global (i.e., light-independent) parameters $\tau^{(1)}_{inact}$ and $\tau^{(2)}_{inact}$ were used. In order to model the dependence on the light intensity of the other parameters (d, τ_{act}, A_{act}, $A^{(1)}_{inact}$, and $A^{(2)}_{inact}$) we fitted the following functions to the recorded data:

$$d = d_A + d_B W_{light} + \frac{d_C}{W_{light}} \tag{2}$$

$$\tau_{act} = \tau^{(0)}_{act} + c_{act} e^{-k_{act} W_{light}} \tag{3}$$

$$A_{act} = a_0 + \frac{a_{min} - 1}{1 + \left(W_{0.5}/W_{light}\right)^2} \tag{4}$$

$$A^{(1)}_{inact} = b_0 + \frac{b_1}{b_2 + \left(W_{light} - W_{inact}\right)^2} \tag{5}$$

$$A^{(2)}_{inact} = c_{inact} e^{-k_{inact} W_{light}} \tag{6}$$

All the parameters of Equations (2–5) are the result of least-squared fits. For Equation (6) k_{inact} has been set manually to assure convergence of the fitting procedure. All fitted parameters of the ChR2 conductance model, together with their standard deviations, are summarized in **Table 1**. Light intensity is measured relatively to the maximum intensity W_{max} that can be achieved in our setup. A precise calibration of the absolute power density at the maximal intensity was not performed. We have estimated it to be approx. $W_{max} = 130\,\text{mW/mm}^2$ for a continuous illumination, which is rather high if compared to 5–6 mW/mm^2 used by Ishizuka et al. (2006) and Ernst et al. (2008) and the maximum (around 20 mW/mm^2) used in Nikolic et al. (2009).

ChR2-TRANSDUCED NEURONAL POPULATIONS MODEL

A local neuronal population was modeled as a random network of $N_E = 4000$ excitatory and $N_I = N_E/4 = 1000$ inhibitory conductance-based model neurons of the Wang-Buzsáki (WB) type (Wang and Buzsáki, 1996). The WB model describes a single compartment neuron endowed with sodium and potassium currents. The membrane potential follows the equation:

$$C\frac{dV}{dt} = -I_L - I_{Na} - I_K + I_{syn} + I_{noise} + \kappa I_{ChR2} \tag{7}$$

where C is the capacitance of the neuron, $I_L = g_L(V - V_L)$ is the leakage current, I_{syn} reflects recurrent interactions with other neurons in the network, I_{noise} models the driving exerted by background noise and I_{ChR2} is the photocurrent-induced by external light stimulation. Sodium and potassium currents are

Table 1 | Parameters of the ChR2 conductance model.

Type of parameter	Parameter	Value ± *SD* l.sq fit (unit)
Latency	d_A	0.27 ± 0.04 (*ms*)
	d_B	-0.05 ± 0.06 (*ms*/[W_{light}])
	d_C	0.0126 ± 0.0006 (*ms* × [W_{light}])
Activation	$\tau_{act}^{(0)}$	0.74 ± 0.20 (*ms*)
	c_{act}	12.0 ± 0.4 (*ms*)
	k_{act}	25 ± 2 (1/[W_{light}])
	a_0	1.00 ± 0.04
	a_{min}	0.4 ± 0.1
	$W_{0.5}$	0.38 ± 0.15 ([W_{light}])
Inactivation (first component)	$\tau_{inact}^{(1)}$	9.06 (*ms*)
	b_0	0.16 ± 0.01
	b_1	0.013 ± 0.004 ([W_{light}]^2)
	b_2	0.027 ± 0.007 ([W_{light}]^2)
	W_{inact}	0.11 ± 0.01 ([W_{light}])
Inactivation (second component)	$\tau_{inact}^{(2)}$	59.6 (*ms*)
	c_{inact}	0.29
	k_{inact}	2.4 (1/[W_{light}])
Deactivation	τ_{off}	10 (ms)
Coupling prefactor	g_{ChR2}	0.007 (μS)

Parameters to simulate time and light-intensity dependent conductance changes mediated by channelrhodopsin 2. Errors are sample standard deviations. Parameters returned from the global fit procedure do not have a measure of uncertainty. See section Materials and methods for the model description.

voltage dependent and given by $I_{Na} = g_{Na} m_\infty^3 h(V - V_{Na})$ and $I_K = g_K n^4 (V - V_K)$. The activation of the sodium current was modeled as instantaneous. We used sodium and potassium current voltage-dependent activation and inactivation functions as given in Wang and Buzsáki (1996).

The synaptic current evoked by a single presynaptic action potential was given by $I_{spike}(t) = -g_\alpha s_{spike}(t)(V - V_\alpha)$, where the reversal potential V_α of the synapse is 0 mV for excitatory AMPA synapses ($\alpha = E$) and -80 mV for inhibitory GABA synapses ($\alpha = I$). The time-course of the postsynaptic conductance was described as a difference of exponentials:

$$s_{spike}(t) \propto \left(e^{-(t + d_{syn} - t_{spike})/\tau_{rise}} - e^{-(t + d_{syn} - t_{spike})\tau_{decay}} \right) \quad (8)$$

for $t > t_{spike}$, 0 otherwise, where t_{spike} is the time of the presynaptic spike, d_{syn} is a combined conduction and synaptic delay, and τ_{rise} and τ_{decay} are respectively the rise- and decay time constants. The normalization constant of $s_{spike}(t)$ was chosen such that its peak value is equal to 1. The peak conductances of all excitatory and inhibitory synapses were set to g_E and g_I, respectively. The total recurrent current $I_{syn}(t)$ was then given by the sum of the contributions $I_{spike}(t)$ from all presynaptic spikes fired before time t.

The background noise input I_{noise} to each neuron was modeled as an additional synaptic current-induced by statistically independent Poisson trains of excitatory spikes with a common firing rate ν_{noise} and a peak conductance g_{noise}.

Excitatory and inhibitory neurons in the populations were transduced by ChR2 with a same probability, given by the transduction rate P_{ChR2}. The photocurrent prefactor κ was set to 1 and 0 respectively for transduced and non-transduced neurons. The induced photocurrent was given by $I_{ChR2}(t) = -g_{ChR2} F_{ChR2} \left[W_{light}(t) \right] (V - V_{ChR2})$. The conductance waveform $F_{ChR2}(t)$ given by Equation (1)—that depends on the applied waveform $W_{light}(t)$ of the optical stimulation—was multiplied by a prefactor g_{ChR2}, such that the peak photocurrent evoked by a pulse with optimal light intensity in the used model neurons (simulated at resting potential) was 2 nA . The reversal potential was $V_{ChR2} \cong 0$.

Excitatory neurons established synapses with other excitatory or inhibitory neurons within the same local circuit with probability P_E, inhibitory neurons with probability P_I. In addition, when considering multiple interconnected local areas, excitatory neurons within a local circuit established long-range connections with excitatory or inhibitory neurons in a remote local area with a probability $P_E^{(lr)}$.

ADOPTED PARAMETERS AND OSCILLATORY SYNCHRONY

The neuronal population model described in the previous section can generate two qualitatively different dynamical regimes, characterized by different degrees of oscillatory coherence. The network resides in one or the other regime depending both on the drive to the network, controlled in this study by varying the background firing rate ν_{noise}, and on the strength of local inhibitory interactions, controlled in this study by varying the probability of inhibitory connection P_I.

The single neuron and network parameters used for all simulations are summarized in **Table 2**. However, we note that qualitatively similar dynamical features, in particular the existence of a smooth transition between a weakly and a strongly synchronous oscillatory regime, would be obtained for a broad range of parameters, with the frequency of the collective oscillation primarily determined by the synaptic time constants, τ_{rise} and τ_{decay}, (Brunel and Wang, 2003). We also find that the transition toward strong synchrony tends to get sharper with increasing network size [not shown, but see as well (Brunel and Hakim, 1999)].

Synchronization of the population activity was quantified through the synchronization index χ (Golomb and Hansel, 2000):

$$\chi = \frac{\sigma_{LFP}^2}{\langle \sigma_{V_i}^2 \rangle} \quad (9)$$

given by the ratio between the variance of the average membrane potential of all excitatory and inhibitory neurons in the local population—here briefly defined conventionally as the "LFP" signal—and the average variance of the membrane potentials

Table 2 | Parameters of the spiking neuronal network model.

Type of parameter	Parameter	Value (unit)
Single neuron	g_L	0.01 (μS)
	V_L	−65 (mV)
	C	100 (pF)
	g_{Na}	3.5 (μS)
	V_{Na}	55 (mV)
	g_k	0.9 (μS)
	V_k	−90 (mV)
	m_∞, h, n	See Wang and Buzsáki (1996)
Population size	N_E	4000
	N_I	1000
Excitatory synapses	τ_{rise}	1 (ms)
	τ_{decay}	3 (ms)
	g_E	0.5 (μS)
Inhibitory synapses	τ_{rise}	1 (ms)
	τ_{decay}	4 (ms)
	g_I	18 (μS)
Synaptic latencies	d_{syn} (local)	1.5 (ms)
	d_{syn} (long-range)	1.0 (ms)
Connection probabilities	P_I	0.3
	P_E	0.12
	$P_E^{(lr)}$	0.06
Background noise	ν_{noise}	3 (kHz)
	g_{noise}	0.5 (μS)

Parameters to simulate the activity of transduced neuronal populations (see section Materials and methods for the model description).

V_i of individual neurons in the population. The synchronization index χ is bounded in the unit range, $\chi = 0$ meaning asynchronous and $\chi = 1$ fully synchronous dynamics.

The dependency of firing rate of excitatory and inhibitory neurons, of the collective oscillation frequency and of the synchrony level χ was studied by systematically varying the parameters ν_{noise} in the range between 2 and 6 kHz and P_I between 0.2 and 0.6 (the reference values, tabulated in **Table 2**, being $\nu_{noise} = 3$ kHz and $P_I = 0.3$). All the quantities were evaluated over simulated time-series lasting 20 s of real time.

ANALYSIS OF PHASE RESPONSE

Although the simulation generates spike trains for all neurons, we focus here on alterations of the ongoing collective activity and, therefore, on the oscillating LFP signal. A single rectangular-shaped light pulse with a given intensity W_{light} and duration T_{light} was applied to the considered network at a specific time of application t_{ON}. For different values of W_{light} and T_{light}, we tested the effects of overall 1500 different light onset times t_{ON}, distributed uniformly over a time interval of approximately 50 oscillation periods. Indeed, averaging over multiple periods was required, because of stochastic fluctuations of the period length. For each stimulation pulse, the activity of the network was further simulated over 60 oscillation cycles following the perturbation.

In every simulation run, the initial conditions, the network topology and the background noise were kept identical, in order to exclusively study the dependence of the induced perturbation on the parameters of the light stimulation and its application time. Pairs of LFP time series were thus generated consisting of a time series after the application of a photostimulation and a time series of the corresponding unperturbed neural dynamics. For every such pair of time series, instantaneous phase values were extracted using a Hilbert transform (Gabor, 1946), an approach extensively used for investigating phase dynamics and synchronization of non-linear oscillators (Pikovsky et al., 2001). The induced phase shift was then measured by averaging the phase difference $\Delta\phi$ between the perturbed and the unperturbed LFPs over the last 50 recorded oscillation cycles. A transient of 10 oscillation cycles immediately following t_{ON} was discarded to ignore transient effects caused by the applied light pulse. The times of perturbation application t_{ON} were translated into phases and binned into 30 equally sized phase bins. The observed phase shifts $\Delta\phi$ were averaged over each bin and plotted as a function of the phase of perturbation application $\phi(t_{ON})$ for different light intensities W_{light} and perturbation pulse duration T_{light}, and also for networks with different transfection rates P_{ChR2}.

The dependency of phase responses on varying values of light intensity, pulse duration and timing of the perturbation were investigated for a specific realization of the network random connectivity. We have repeated our analysis for three different random realizations of connectivity (with the same homogeneous probabilities of connection, P_I and P_E). The corresponding phase responses to light stimuli were qualitatively and quantitatively very similar (not shown). In particular, differences between random network instances were of the same order of magnitude as the error bars shown in **Figure 4**, corresponding to fluctuations of the phase response over time for a same connectivity realization. These similarities are not surprising and match theoretical expectations, since dynamical effects arising from fluctuations due to finite-size connectivity are small for the large network size adopted here (Golomb and Hansel, 2000). Therefore, we can conclude that our results hold in general for random networks with the same (in a probabilistic sense) connectivity features.

ANALYSIS OF PHASE LOCKING CHANGES

If two coupled neuronal populations are simulated with the parameters given in **Table 2**, the oscillations of the two LFPs self-organize in a phase-locked configuration. The temporarily stable relative phase difference, $\Delta\phi$, can have two different values: $\Delta\phi_{locked}$ or $1-\Delta\phi_{locked}$ (phases are measured over the cyclic unit interval $0 \leq \phi \leq 1$). Both phase-locking values correspond to out-of-phase configurations in which either of the two populations leads in phase over the other.

In our simulations, only one of the two local neuronal populations was transduced with ChR2. We applied light stimulation pulses to this transduced population, with a light intensity $W_{light} = 20\%$ (expressed as the percentage of the maximum possible light intensity of our setup W_{max}) and a pulse duration of $T_{light} = 3$ ms. Similar to the protocol used for the phase response analysis of a single population, 1500 different pulse onset times, t_{ON}, were used, which were uniformly distributed over 50 oscillation cycles. Starting from random initial conditions, no perturbation was applied for the first 100 oscillation cycles, to ensure complete convergence to a stable phase-locked attractor. Without loss of generality, we considered the configuration in which the phase of the transduced population leads over that of the not transduced population (i.e., in which the stable inter-circuit phase difference is close to $\Delta\phi_{locked}$ before the perturbation).

Variations of the phase-difference between the two populations were measured in two different time-windows. We first studied the short-term effects of the light stimulation, by averaging the instantaneous Hilbert phase difference over the first 5 oscillation cycles after the perturbation. Binning different onset times according to the corresponding phase of application of the perturbation (as done for the estimation of single population phase response), we quantified the probability $P_{shifting}(\phi)$, that a light pulse induces a relative variation of more than 10% (reduction or increase) of the inter-population phase-difference. For each application phase bin, $P_{shifting}(\phi)$ was compared with the probability of observing similarly large spontaneous fluctuations of $\Delta\phi$ in the unperturbed activity of the same network.

We then studied longer term effects of the light stimulation by averaging the difference of the instantaneous Hilbert phases over the 50 cycles that follow the ten omitted oscillation cycles directly after stimulation. The aim of this long-term analysis was to assess the occurrence of a switching from the phase-locking pattern with phase-difference close to $\Delta\phi_{locked}$ toward the other phase-locking pattern with phase difference close to 1-$\Delta\phi_{locked}$. Once again binning onset times according to the corresponding phase of perturbation application, we quantified the probability $P_{switching}(\phi)$ that the long-term averaged phase difference was within a tolerance interval of $1 - \Delta\phi_{locked} \pm \delta$, with $\delta = 0.05$ (i.e., the transduced population switched steadily from the role of phase leader to phase laggard). For each phase bin, $P_{switching}(\phi)$ was compared to the probability of observing a spontaneous switching of the phase locking (from $\Delta\phi_{locked}$ to 1-$\Delta\phi_{locked}$) over an equivalent time span of 50 cycles, based on time-series of the unperturbed dynamics of the same network.

The probabilities $P_{shifting}(\phi)$ and $P_{switching}(\phi)$ were finally plotted as polar histograms with ten equally-spaced bins for the phase of the onset of the light stimulation $\phi(t_{ON})$, in which the corresponding probabilities of spontaneous shifting or switching were also reported in order to identify phase bins in which the effects induced by the perturbation pulse were significantly low or high (**Figure 5**).

ONLINE PHASE PREDICTION

A closed-loop approach (**Figure 6**) is necessary to estimate a time t_{ON} which corresponds to a future occurrence of a given target phase ϕ_{target}, leading to the largest possible probability of switching of the inter-areal locking (**Figure 5**).

To study the feasibility of such an approach, we modeled its implementation, considering the same bi-areal network used to characterize induced switching between phase-locked states (see previous section and **Figure 5**). Simulated LFPs were recorded from both the stimulation target area and a second coupled area. However, the calculations performed online involved only the LFP time-series $V(t)$ recorded in the target area. The time-series $\tilde{V}(t)$ of the second area were recorded and analyzed offline to determine phase-locking patterns before and after the stimulation.

We approximated the "true" Hilbert phase $\phi_H(t)$ associated to $V(t)$ by a linearly interpolated phase. This approximation could be simply done by interpolating a variable $\phi_L(t)$that was linearly growing in the unit interval $0 \leq \phi_L < 1$ between any two times t_k and t_{k+1} delimiting an oscillation cycle. As shown by **Figure 7B**, the phase variables $\phi_H(t)$ and $\phi_L(t)$ are related by a mildly non-linear map, described as a static non-linearity $\phi_H = f_{LH}(\phi_L)$. However, we systematically ignored this non-linearity in the following by approximating $\phi_H(t)$ directly by $\phi_L(t)$.

The workflow for the prediction of the perturbation onset time t_{ON} is split up into multiple stages (**Figure 6**). First of all, it was necessary, during a *testing stage*, to detect the presence of sufficiently strong local oscillations and to measure their average frequency f_{peak}. It was important to monitor the characteristics of LFP oscillations (band-passed around f_{peak}) in the stimulation target area (*monitoring stage*) and to extract, based on observations of past activity, a model able to approximately predict future phase evolution (*prediction stage*).

Even in the ideal case of an elevated synchrony index χ and sustained oscillations, the duration of oscillation periods T_i fluctuated from cycle-to-cycle around their average $\bar{T}$(cf. **Figure 7A**). Let us suppose that the last oscillation period recorded in the monitoring stage was $T_k = t_k - t_{k-1}$ and that the prediction stage lasts (less than) s oscillation cycles. Neglecting correlations between period lengths of consecutive cycles, the time of beginning of the next cycle after the end of the prediction stage could be estimated via a simple *linear extrapolation*:

$$t^{(0)}_{k+s} = t_k + s\bar{T} \tag{10}$$

However, for our network model, the temporal autocorrelation function of period lengths T_i, $i = 1, \ldots, k$ displayed a fast but not instantaneous decay for increasing lags (measured in oscillation cycles). These weak, positive correlations between consecutive cycle durations could be well captured by a *first order autoregressive process* [AR(1)], $T_i = \bar{T} + a(T_{i-1} - \bar{T}) + \epsilon_i$, with $\bar{T}$ the average oscillation period over the monitoring time-window, a the AR(1) coefficient and $_i$ an i.i.d. Gaussian distributed residual noise term (Brockwell and Davis, 1996). With this AR(1) model, the beginning of the next cycle was estimated as:

$$t^{(1)}_{k+s} = t_k + s\bar{T} + \left(\frac{a^{s+1} - a}{a - 1}\right) \cdot T_k \tag{11}$$

The AR(1) coefficient was derived as:

$$a = \frac{k}{k-1} \frac{\sum_{i=1}^{k-1} (T_i - \bar{T})(T_{i+1} - \bar{T})}{\sum_{i=1}^{k} (T_i - \bar{T})^2} \tag{12}$$

based on the periods T_i, $i = 1, \ldots, k$, measured during the monitoring stage and on their average duration $\bar{T}$.

Spectral analysis of LFPs recorded in the stimulation target area and in a second coupled area was performed during the testing stage. A windowed Fast Fourier Transform (FFT) was applied to demeaned chunks of the LFP signal, to extract a rough estimate of the instantaneous power spectrum. When the power at some frequency f_{peak} in the gamma range exceeded a determined threshold in both recorded areas, the monitoring stage started.

During the monitoring stage, a computationally efficient low-order recursive time domain filter (Percival and Walden, 1993) was applied to clean the oscillating LFP signals. The filtered time-series was computed online as:

$$V_{\text{filtered}}(t) = V(t) + \alpha_1 V_{\text{filtered}}(t-1) + \alpha_2 V_{\text{filtered}}(t-2) \quad (13)$$

Filter coefficients were chosen as $\alpha_2 = -0.99$ and $\alpha_1 = 4\alpha_2 \cos(2\pi(1 - f_{\text{peak}}))/(1 - \alpha_2)$ (assuming a sampling rate of 1 kHz). The pass frequency was then equal to f_{peak} and the main frequency of the activity of recorded areas was maintained. The LFP time-series $V(t)$ and $\tilde{V}(t)$ recorded during the monitoring stage were stored. An analysis of the inter-areal phase-locking pattern before stimulation was then performed offline, while the closed-loop experiment was continuing. A monitoring stage including approximately 20 oscillation cycles was found to be sufficiently long to achieve accurate model estimation.

The limited amount of fast computations to be performed during the prediction stage is summarized as follows:

1. Subtract the mean value from the band-passed LFP time series $V_{\text{filtered}}(t)$ measured during the monitoring window in the stimulation target area.
2. Calculate the timings $t_0, t_1, \ldots, t_k$ at which the LFP $V_{\text{filtered}}(t)$ crosses zero. Their differences $T_i = t_i - t_{i-1}, i = 1, \ldots, k$ are the estimated period lengths of the observed oscillations.
3. Calculate the average period length $\bar{T}$ from the series of T_i.
4. If the AR(1) approach is used, then compute the a coefficient based on equation (12) and compute the perturbation onset time as $t_{\text{ON}}^{(1)} = t_{k+s}^{(1)} + \phi_{\text{target}}\bar{T}$, where $t_{k+s}^{(1)}$ is given by Equation (11).
5. If a simpler linear extrapolation is used, compute the perturbation onset time directly as $t_{\text{ON}}^{(0)} = t_{k+s}^{(0)} + \phi_{\text{target}}\bar{T}$, where $t_{k+s}^{(0)}$ is given by Equation (10).

After the application of the perturbation pulse, the LFPs of both areas were recorded and stored. An analysis of the inter-areal phase-locking pattern after stimulation was then performed offline and compared to the phase-locking assessed before stimulation. In case of failed switching, either the same linear model was used to extrapolate directly the time t_{ON} of a further stimulation pulse, or a new testing stage was initiated, verifying that oscillations were still ongoing or waiting for the next oscillatory epoch to begin.

The decision between a prediction scheme based on the AR(1) model and a simpler linear extrapolation scheme depends ultimately on the correlation statistics of the series of period lengths. It can be shown that the prediction error of the estimated phase is reduced by the AR(1) prediction scheme compared to linear extrapolation by a maximal amount of $100\%/\sqrt{1-a^2}$ (and by exactly this amount for Gaussian distributed samples). If the AR(1) parameter a estimated from the recordings during the monitoring window is small (as a rule of thumb, $a < 0.3$), then the performance improvement is negligible and advantage can be taken from the faster computation of the simpler linear extrapolation. Unfortunately, this criterion requires the evaluation of a. Nevertheless, the analysis of **Figure 7E** indirectly suggests that the AR(1) coefficient depends non-monotonically on the synchrony level, and that it increases going from low to intermediate synchrony indices χ, but drops again going toward higher χ. The choice of a high power threshold during the testing stage guarantees a high level of synchrony and, therefore, small values of a during the monitoring stage. This allows one to adopt the computationally faster step (5) instead of (4). However, a tradeoff should be made between the need of a fast prediction and the probability to detect a number of oscillatory epochs sufficient for meeting the testing stage criteria.

RESULTS

DATA-CONSTRAINED MODEL OF ChR2-PHOTOCURRENT

In order to assess from *in silico* experiments the efficacy of optogenetic stimulation in inducing changes of local phase or of inter-areal phase relations, we first derived a realistic and fully data-constrained model of the evoked ChR2 conductance. To do so, we first performed an experimental characterization of photocurrents evoked in living cells *in vitro* by light stimulation over a broad range of light intensities spanning two decades of power (see section Materials and Methods). Then, based on this systematic set of measurements, we fitted to the whole dataset a unique conductance-based model that describes the evoked time-dependent photocurrent, and hence the conductance, as the product of activation and inactivation factors.

The light-activated ChR2 ion channel mediates a current that is carried mostly by Na^+, K^+, and H^+ with contributions of Ca^{2+}. Its reversal potential is typically around 0 mV and therefore it is depolarizing at neuronal resting potential. We found that upon illumination onset, a current built up with a nearly exponential time course with a time constant τ_{act} ranging from 10 ms, for very weak light intensities that barely evoked any current response, to below 1 ms for high intensities. For a large range of intensities the current displayed a transient behavior and its amplitude, after reaching a peak, decayed over tens of milliseconds to reach a plateau. This inactivation behavior was biphasic and its time constants were not dependent on light intensity, unlike the activation time constant. Finally, when the light was switched off, the current decayed back to baseline with a time course that was well described by a single exponential with a 10 ms time constant.

Figure 1A depicts inward currents induced by a light pulse of moderate intensity (approximately 3 mW/mm^2 for 10 ms) in a cultured hippocampal neuron transduced with ChR2. Even such a weak light pulse was able to elicit an action current, as the axon escaped the voltage-clamp (**Figure 1A**, black line). The ChR2 photocurrent could be isolated, by blocking Na-channels with tetrodotoxin (**Figure 1A**, red line).

To achieve an improved characterization of the photocurrent time-course, we systematically analyzed recordings over (non-spiking) transfected kidney cells (**Figure 1B**) using a very large range of light power densities for the characterization of ChR2 activation and inactivation kinetics. We found that the peak and steady state photocurrent do not increase monotonically with light power density. A maximal peak current is achieved around 10–20% of the maximum power density (see section Discussion). For applications, where such power densities can be attained, for instance with a laser or a strongly focused LED, a careful tuning of the applied light intensity could thus potentially reduce the minimum transduction rate needed to efficiently drive the local oscillations in a target area.

As detailed in section Materials and Methods, it was possible to capture the time-course of the evoked ChR2 current with a single conductance-based model with light-dependent parameters. The simulated photocurrents generated by the model in response to a single square pulse of light lasting 3 ms are shown in **Figure 1C** for various light intensities (corresponding to the typical short pulse length used in the simulations of next sections). As evident from **Figure 1C**, our data-constrained model was able to capture the non-monotonic dependence of peak photocurrent on the light intensity, leading to the largest peak photocurrent for a light intensity of approximately 18% the largest deliverable intensity W_{max}.

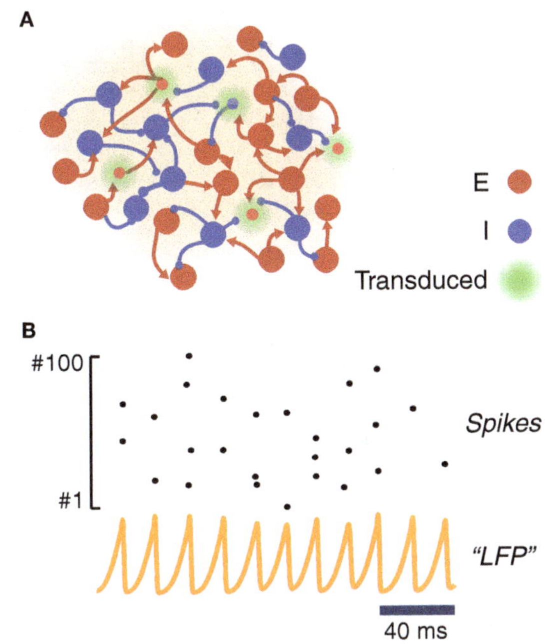

FIGURE 2 | Model of a ChR2-transduced population. (A) Graphic cartoon of a randomly-connected network of inhibitory and excitatory spiking neurons. In order to model the effects of local ChR2 transduction a variable fraction of the neurons is endowed with a ChR2 photoconductance. **(B)** Sample activity from the local circuit model of panel **(A)**. Due to strong and delayed recurrent mutual inhibition, the network undergoes a collective oscillatory activity with a frequency in the gamma range. Even when oscillations at the population level are very regular (see an example "LFP"—i.e., average membrane potential—time series), individual neurons spike very irregularly with a much lower firing rate (see raster plot of the activity of 100 excitatory neurons).

SPIKING NETWORK MODELS OF TRANSDUCED OSCILLATING AREAS

To study the response to light stimulation of systems involving transfected neuronal areas, we simulated the activity of simple canonic circuits composed of just one local area or of two local areas mutually coupled with equal strength. Each area was modeled as a large network of randomly interconnected excitatory and inhibitory neurons. As shown in **Figure 2A**, a fraction of these excitatory and inhibitory model neurons were equipped with ChR2 photoconductances, inducing depolarization in response to simulated light stimulation.

For most of the analyses reported in this study, we adopted within each local area strong and delayed inhibition and a sufficiently strong background drive (see **Table 2**). With such a choice of parameters, local circuits underwent—through an "ING"-type (i.e., "interneuron-generated") mechanism (Whittington et al., 2000; Brunel and Wang, 2003; Brunel and Hansel, 2006; Tiesinga and Sejnowski, 2009) a marked and persistent oscillatory activity, well visible in the traces of a LFP-like signal. The collective frequency of oscillation was in the gamma range. Since driving was provided by background Poisson noise, the spiking activity of individual neurons was very irregular and characterized by a weaker firing rate (cf. **Figure 2B**). Weak pairwise correlations between spike trains coexisted thus with stronger pairwise correlations between membrane potential fluctuations (Yu and Ferster, 2010; Battaglia and Hansel, 2011). While inhibitory connections were confined within each local area, excitatory neurons could additionally establish long-range connections between distant local areas (**Figure 5A**). In this case, the gamma oscillations generated by each local circuit were set into one of many possible multistable phase-locked states (**Figure 5B**).

The dynamical features of the simulated neural activity, including in particular its degree of oscillatory synchrony, depended sensibly on the noisy drive to the network and on the strength of local inhibition. For increased drive intensity and/or stronger inhibitory interactions, a smooth transition occurred toward a dynamic regime characterized by elevated collective synchronization (**Figure 3A**). In this synchronous regime, the frequencies of the network oscillation were in the gamma range, varying between 40 and 70 Hz (**Figure 3B**), while the average firing rate of individual excitatory neurons varied between 1 and 3 Hz (**Figure 3C**) and of inhibitory neurons between 2 and 7 Hz (**Figure 3D**).

Starting from a very wide range of parameters including the probability of inhibitory connections and the strength of the external driving force (**Figure 3**), oscillatory synchrony can be robustly boosted by enhancing the external drive to the network. Qualitatively reproducing existing experimental findings (Adesnik and Scanziani, 2010; Akam et al., 2012), our simulations showed that slowly ramping or constant low-intensity optogenetic stimulation can be used to "switch on" a markedly oscillatory behavior. As shown by **Figure 3E** a network with poorly synchronous activity can be optogenetically driven toward higher oscillatory synchrony, as evident not only from LFP spectrograms but also visually from LFP traces.

In the following, we will mainly consider model networks tuned to generate strong LFP gamma oscillations. However, such

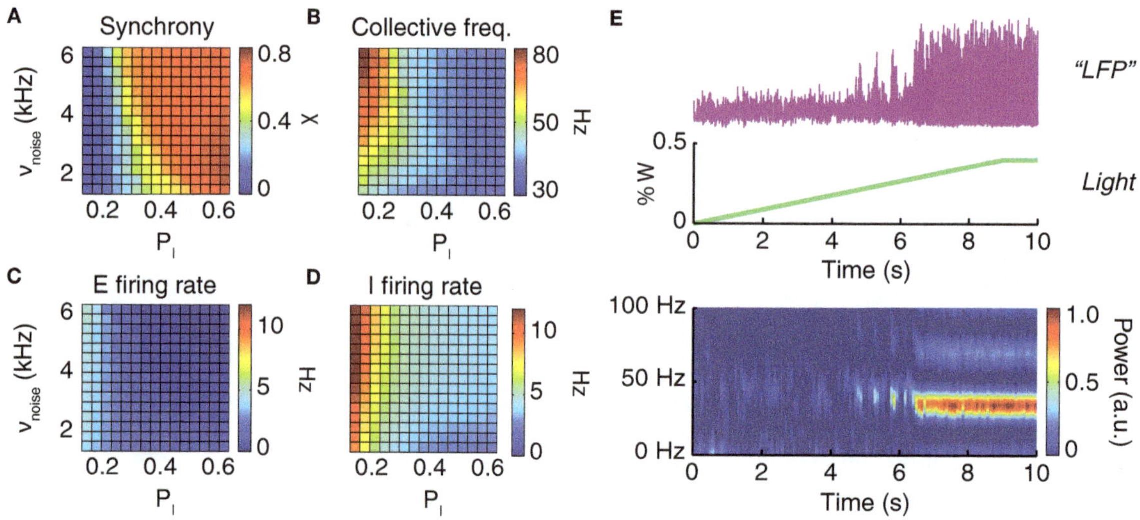

FIGURE 3 | Driving the network toward coherent oscillations. The dynamical regime of a neuronal population depends on the strength of local inhibition (parameterized by the probability p_I of inhibitory connections) and on the strength of an external driving force (parameterized by the rate ν_{noise} of background inputs). Shown are the synchronization index **(A)** which has values in the unit interval (0 corresponds to asynchronous and 1 to perfectly synchronous dynamics); the oscillation frequency of collective activity **(B)**; and the average firing rates of excitatory **(C)** and inhibitory **(D)** neurons. All four quantities are presented in their dependence on the probability of inhibitory connections, P_I, and the rate of background noise input, ν_{noise}. **(E)** Constant or slowly ramping optogenetic stimulation increases the external drive to a neuronal population. This results in intensified collective oscillations and enhanced synchronization at the population level. From top to bottom: LFP time-series (purple) observed during a slowly ramping photostimulation (green); the associated spectrogram (graph at the bottom) indicates the development of highly coherent gamma oscillations as an effect of continuous photostimulation.

a choice is not an arbitrary restriction. Indeed, high synchrony regimes—either spontaneously emergent or induced artificially by continuous photostimulation—are particularly suited for analyses of phase shifting and locking.

SHIFTING THE PHASE OF AN ONGOING LOCAL OSCILLATION

It is well known that the effect of a perturbation to an oscillating system depends on the phase at which the perturbation is applied (Pikovsky et al., 2001). To explore the phase dependency of light stimulation, we applied simulated stimulation pulses with different durations T_{light} to local populations with different transduction rates P_{ChR2} (**Figure 4**). Light intensity was always set to the optimum value of $W_{light} = 18\%\ W_{max}$, which led to maximum evoked peak photocurrents.

For all the explored conditions, we always found strongest effects on the phase of an ongoing oscillation when the perturbation was applied at a phase half-way between the trough and the peak of the collective population oscillation (**Figure 4B**). In this case the phase of the perturbed oscillation was advanced with respect to the unperturbed case (**Figures 4C,D**). Short pulses lasting 1 or 3 ms led only to phase advance effects. As shown in **Figure 4C**, phase advances of the order of one quarter of a cycle could be achieved using such short pulses, over a very wide range of transduction rates, going from very high (100%) down to moderate (25%). Noticeable phase advance effects (although reduced to just one tenth of a cycle) could even be detected for transduction rates as low as 5%.

As displayed by **Figure 4D**, longer stimulation durations also led to phase lagging effects. These effects occurred in different ranges of perturbation application phases than for phase advancing effects. However, phase lagging effects were always weaker than phase advancing effects. For instance, for a transduction rate of 25%, pulses lasting 10 ms could induce phase advances of over a quarter of cycle, but only phase laggings of less than one tenth of cycle.

The positive peaks of the *phase response curves* (PRCs) plotted in **Figures 4C,D** were aligned across all conditions. The strongest phase shifting effects were always observed when the perturbation was applied in proximity of the phase $\phi = 0.17$. We also mention that for the short stimulation duration used, the evoked photocurrent was dominated by the fast activation time-course. Inactivation played no role in determining the response. As a matter of fact, the effect of the fast initial rise of the photocurrent was to evoke a spike in the transduced neurons, as in panel 1A, and additional synchronous spikes evoked in a subpopulation of cells were the dynamic cause of the induced phase shift, as in Battaglia et al. (2012).

PERTURBING PHASE RELATIONS BETWEEN DIFFERENT OSCILLATING POPULATIONS

After the controlled shifting of the phase of a local oscillation, we explored whether precisely phased stimulation could be used to manipulate phase relations between different local oscillating circuits. To do so, we considered a canonic circuit of two coupled oscillating areas, interconnected by long-range random excitatory projections (**Figure 5A**). In general, when driven into a synchronous regime, motifs of a few local areas mutually connected with equal strength can give rise to different phase-locked states.

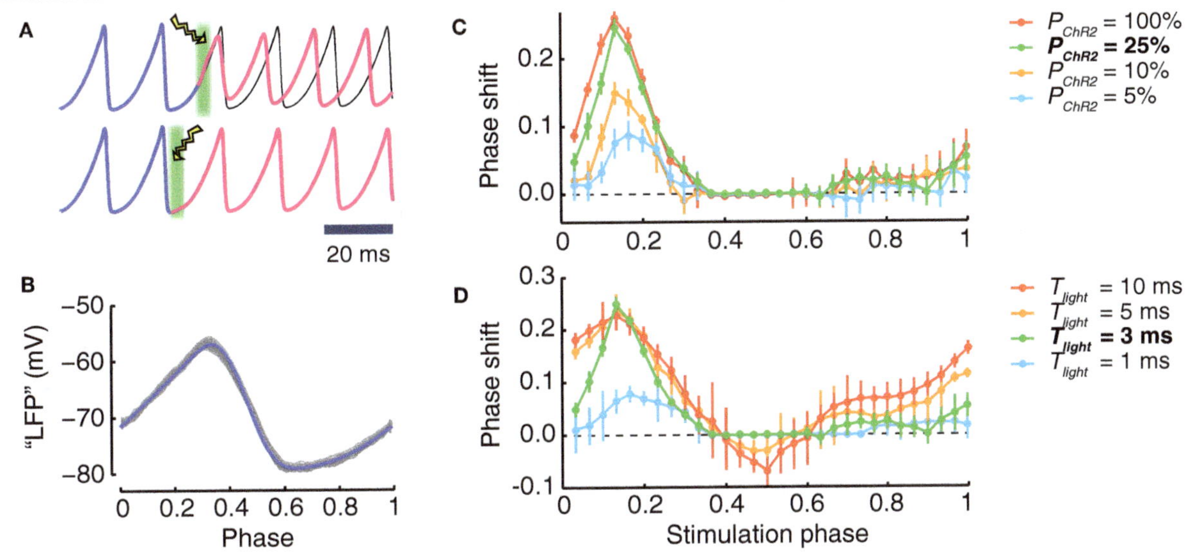

FIGURE 4 | Phase shifts induced by photostimulation. (A) Examples of phase shifts induced by a single light pulse. Top: the phase (blue curve) of the oscillation of the transduced population is shifted by light perturbation (illustrated as a lightning symbol with green background) and, afterwards (magenta curve), remains advanced with respect to the unperturbed oscillation (gray curve). Bottom: such a phase shift cannot be seen when the timing of the light perturbation corresponds to other differently chosen oscillation phases. **(B)** Waveform of the oscillating LFP in dependence on the Hilbert phase. Shown are 500 oscillation cycles (gray) of a LFP and their average waveform (blue). By our conventions, the phase ranges in the unit interval. The maximum of the LFP is obtained for (Hilbert) phase values close to 0.3 while the minimum occurs for phase values close to 0.6. **(C,D)** phase shifts caused by light pulses applied at different (Hilbert) phases of the ongoing LFP oscillation. An optimal light intensity of 18% W_{max} is used. **(C)** Dependence of the phase shift on the transduction rate P_{ChR2} of the population (for a stimulus duration $T_{light} = 3$ ms). **(D)** Dependence of the phase shift on the stimulus duration T_{light} (for a fixed transduction rate of $P_{ChR2} = 25\%$). Bold characters in the legend denote the "reference" phase shift, i.e., $P_{ChR2} = 25\%$ and $T_{light} = 3$ ms of stimulus duration (green curves). In panels **(C)** and **(D)**, error bars are standard deviation of the phase shifts obtained for different perturbations applied in a same time-bin.

These states are associated to different patterns of inter-areal phase relations, which are maintained in a relatively stable manner over long time intervals (Battaglia et al., 2007, 2012).

The specific bi-areal network of **Figure 5A** generated two multi-stable phase-locked states. In the unperturbed system, background noise caused spontaneous switching between these two states (i.e., from one configuration of inter-areal phase relations to another). The result of these stochastic fluctuations was a clearly bimodal distribution of the instantaneous phase difference between the two areas (**Figure 5B**). The actual phase relations in the phase-locked modes depend ultimately on the PRC of the coupled populations. As discussed in Battaglia et al. (2007, 2012), the PRCs associated to our network model are such that they lead to *out-of-phase* locking for sufficiently strong inhibition (unless long-range synaptic delays are tuned *ad-hoc* within narrow intervals associated to in- or anti-phase configurations). Out-of-phase locking is found also in more general systems of pulse-coupled neurons (or neuronal masses) under certain conditions on synaptic delays (Woodman and Canavier, 2011; Wang et al., 2012).

In out-of-phase locked modes, it is always possible to identify one area (leader) whose oscillations lead in phase over the oscillations of the other area (laggard). This leads to anisotropic directed functional influences between local circuits (Battaglia et al., 2012), in agreement with the communication-through-coherence hypothesis (Fries, 2005), despite the fact that inter-areal connections are reciprocal and of equal strength in both directions. Switching between alternative phase-locking configurations would thus correspond to changes in the dominant direction of inter-areal functional influences. Spontaneous switching was a relatively rare event in the high synchrony regime explored here (the average waiting time for spontaneous switching was over 60 periods). Nevertheless, optogenetic stimulation could be used to actively trigger switching events (**Figure 5C**).

Inter-areal phase relations after the application of a single perturbation pulse were compared to the average locked phase difference before the pulse itself. We studied how both transient short-term and persistent long-term effects depend on the phase of perturbation onset. **Figure 5D** shows the probability that the average inter-areal phase difference for the five cycles directly following the perturbation has increased or reduced by at least 10% relative to the average phase difference prior to the perturbation. For a wide range of phases of stimulation onset, such probability was larger than 50% and remarkably larger than the level accounted for by spontaneous fluctuations of the inter-areal phase difference.

The dependency on the perturbation phase was more pronounced for long-term effects. **Figure 5E** shows the probability of a switch in phase locking, i.e., that the average inter-areal phase difference over a long time window beginning ten cycles after the perturbation has changed its sign (note, indeed, that the two phase-locked configurations of the simulated bi-areal motif are characterized by average phase-differences of $\Delta\phi = \pm\Delta\phi_{locked}$,

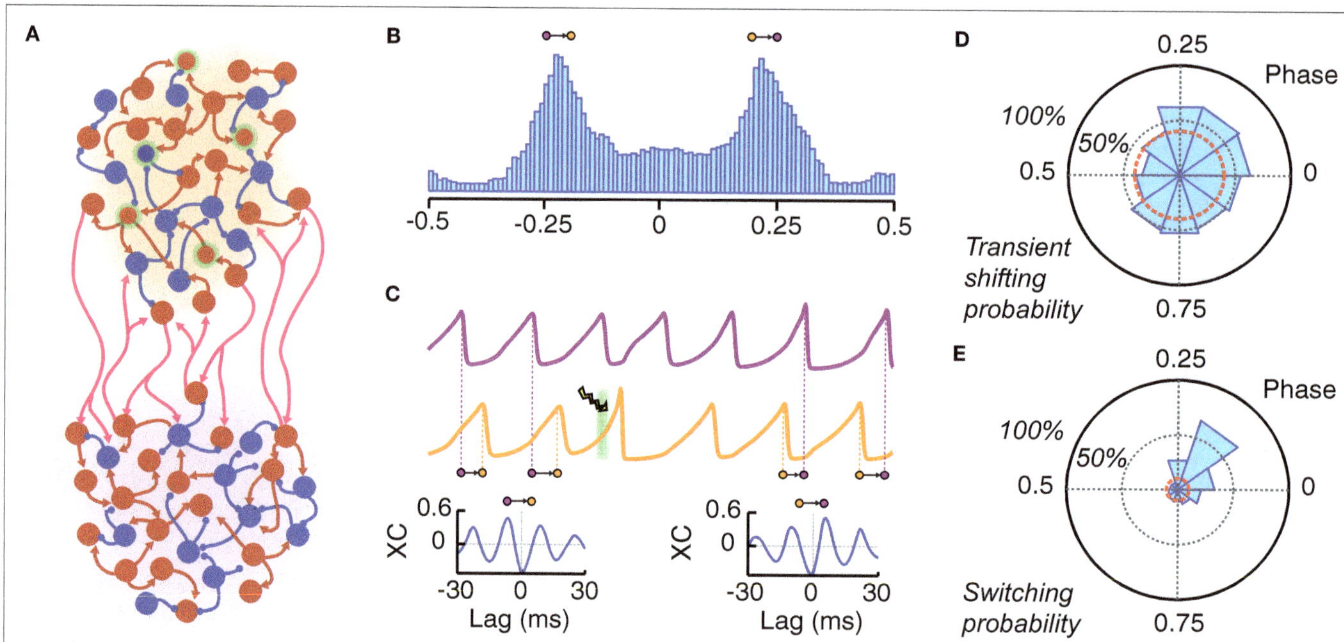

FIGURE 5 | Local photostimulation can reorganize long-range phase-locking patterns. (A) Cartoon of two local populations (each of them with an individual background color: orange and violet) coupled by long-range excitatory connections. **(B)** Both populations oscillate in a non-regular way but with the same main frequency. A histogram of the instantaneous phase difference is shown for a pair of very long LFP time series (over 50,000 oscillation cycles). This distribution is clearly bimodal, indicating the existence of two favorite modes of approximate out-of-phase locking (with the orange population leading in phase over the violet, or the other way around). **(C)** LFP traces of two phase-locked populations. The application of a light pulse stimulation (denoted by a green background and a lightning symbol) can induce switching to another phase-locked mode. This is shown by the qualitative changes between the crosscorrelogram (XC, computed over 500 ms) of the two LFPs before (left) and after (right) light stimulation. Note the changed sign of the lag of the highest XC peak, which corresponds to an inversion of the direction of functional connectivity. **(D)** Probability of changing the average inter-population phase difference of more than 10% during five oscillation cycles after light stimulation ($P_{ChR2} = 25\%$, $T_{light} = 3$ ms). This probability is presented by a polar histogram in dependence on the phase of the onset of the light stimulation (with respect to the leader population). The red circle indicates the probability of similarly large spontaneous phase shifts (i.e., without photostimulation). **(E)** Phase difference averaged over 50 cycles starting 10 cycles after the light pulse. A switching is considered as successful if the sign of this average phase difference has changed (see panel **B**). The probability of successful phase switching is given by a polar histogram, as in panel **(D)**. The red circle indicates the probability of spontaneous switching in the case of non-stimulated activity. Ignoring transient effects, switching can be induced with high probability only if the perturbation is applied within a specific narrow phase range.

cf. **Figure 5B**). In contrast to short-term shifting, the probability of actual switching was concentrated in a narrow phase interval centered on the peak of the single-area PRC, as expected from theory (Battaglia et al., 2012). The switching probability for other phase bins dropped quickly to the level of spontaneous switching.

Our simulations show that the peak probability of optogenetically-induced switching could rise above 60% even for small transduction rates of 25%. However, this happened only if the phase of the perturbation onset was precisely selected. Indeed, the comparison of **Figures 5D,E** shows that many of the short-term shifting effects observed for randomly phased perturbations did not develop into lasting changes in phase-locking. To conclude, we would like to mention that a similar pulse-induced reorganization of inter-areal phase relations could be achieved even when the perturbation was applied to the laggard rather than to the leader area [not shown, but see (Battaglia et al., 2012)].

CLOSING THE LOOP

As discussed in the last section, the controlled switching of inter-areal phase-locking—and, hence, of functional connectivity—required perturbations optimally phased with respect to ongoing oscillations. To increase the probability to induce switching, the timing of perturbation must thus be determined based on phase information extracted from recordings of the recent population activity. We suggest here a possible closed-loop protocol for the online prediction of the timing of stimulation achieving an optimal switching rate. The workflow of the proposed idealized experiment is outlined by a schematic time bar (**Figure 6A**) and a corresponding flow chart (**Figure 6B**). The potential performance of such protocol was studied by simulating the induction of switching in the bi-areal network of **Figure 5A**.

In contrast to this well behaved *in silico* model, oscillatory coherence *in vivo* or *in vitro* recordings is usually transient and confined to specific epochs. There is nevertheless experimental evidence that epochs of phase synchronization at fast gamma frequencies can persist over several hundreds of ms *in vivo* (Varela et al., 2001; Pesaran et al., 2002; Gregoriou et al., 2009; Bosman et al., 2012; Grothe et al., 2012). Detecting the onset of one of such oscillatory epochs was precisely the aim of the *testing stage*, in which LFPs in both areas of the bi-areal motif were recorded and their spectral characteristics extracted in real-time to verify that LFP power and inter-areal coherence with respect to a common

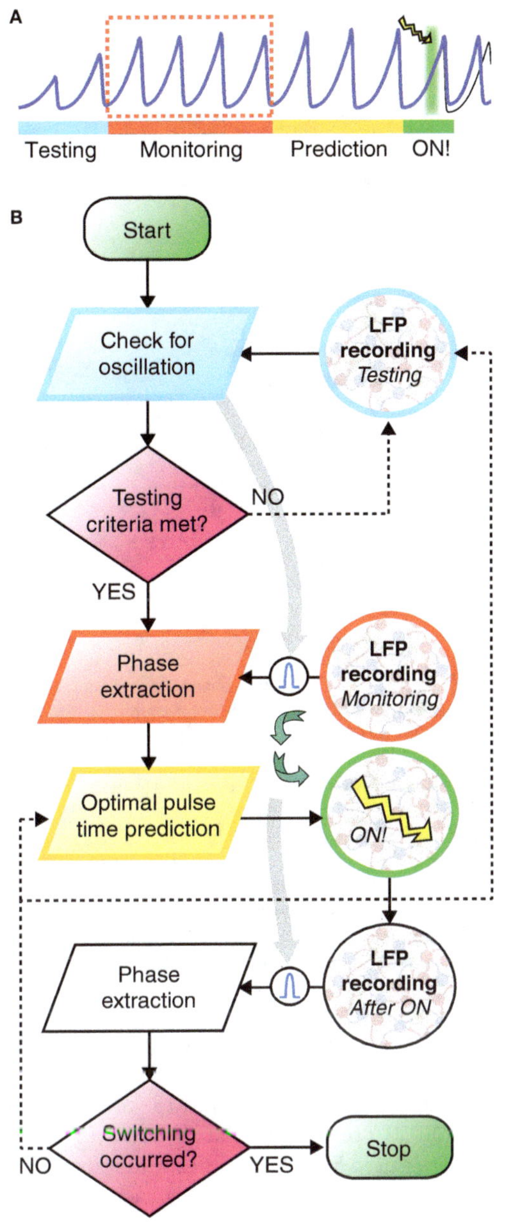

FIGURE 6 | Closed loop strategy for precisely phased photostimulation. (A) Schematic illustration of the proposed experimental protocol. During the *testing stage* (light blue) the LFP is recorded and tested for sufficiently strong power in the gamma-range. If the gamma band power is high enough, then a bandpass-filter is tailored to its peak frequency (light gray arrow). In the *monitoring* stage (red), phases are extracted from the band-passed LFP. Based on these observations, during the *prediction stage* (yellow), lasting only a very few oscillation periods, a linear model of phase evolution is extrapolated to predict the time at which the target phase of the oscillation will occur next. A light pulse is then delivered at this predicted time (green background with lightning symbol). **(B)** The workflow of the closed loop experiment is presented as a flow chart, with the left swim lane presenting computation and decision steps and the right swim lane showing recording and stimulation of the transfected neuronal population. Curved green arrows highlight the closed-loop nature of the workflow, i.e., the light pulse stimulation delivered at a time depending on the phase evolution of LFP oscillations during the monitoring window.

frequency (band) rose above a minimum threshold (see section Materials and Methods).

The *monitoring stage* was entered immediately after the detection of an epoch of reliable inter-areal coherence. During this monitoring stage, LFP signals were recorded, filtered in real time through a low-order band-pass filter with a pass frequency optimized during the testing window and, finally, stored.

A fast online analysis of the phase dynamics of the stored LFP of only the target area was then performed during the following *prediction stage.* Its aim was to predict the timing of one of the next occurrences of the target phase, solely from the phase information acquired during the monitoring stage. To keep the prediction window as short as possible, we propose to use computationally cheap and consequently linear techniques for phase extrapolation. Indeed, the "real" phase values (given by Hilbert Transform of the LFP signal, see section Materials and Methods) and a simple linear descriptor of the phase are strongly correlated (**Figure 7B**) and non-linear effects can be neglected in a first-order approximation.

The phase-locking between LFPs recorded after the stimulation application was finally compared with the locking existing before the stimulation to verify the successful induction of state switching.

Figure 7 analyzes the simulated performance of the proposed protocol, when applied to *in silico* recordings from the bi-areal network motif of **Figure 5**. **Figure 7C** shows how the predicted onset phases of light stimulation concentrate around the actual target phase given by the peak PRC value of $\phi_{\text{target}} = 0.18$. The scattering of predicted phases is computed by hypothesizing prediction stages with different possible (short) durations. This estimate was done with two prediction schemes which both have fast implementations: a simple linear extrapolation based on the average period length and a first-order autoregressive model [AR(1)] (see section Materials and Methods), accounting for correlations between the durations of successive oscillation cycles, at least approximately. For increasing lengths of the prediction window, the median and the average value of the predicted Hilbert phase remained very close to the target (**Figure 7C**). However, the distribution of extrapolated phase values broadened, as indicated by their increasing dispersion. Nevertheless, for a prediction window lasting three oscillation cycles—a sufficiently long time to perform the fast computation required for linear extrapolation (see section Discussion)—the interquartile range of predicted phase values was still contained in the width of the reference PRC. Consequently, we still expect an enhanced effectiveness of light stimulation pulses applied at the inferred time t_{ON}, compared to randomly timed pulses.

The error made in predicting a target phase depends necessarily on the quality of the recorded oscillation. The dynamical regime of the simulations in **Figures 5** and **7C** was strongly synchronous. As previously discussed, the degree of synchrony of the collective response depends on the external driving force to the network and on the strength of local inhibition (**Figure 3A**). We performed phase prediction based on recordings of simulated dynamics with different degrees of synchrony. As shown in **Figure 7D**, stronger synchrony was associated to smaller prediction errors. Interestingly, prediction errors remained moderate

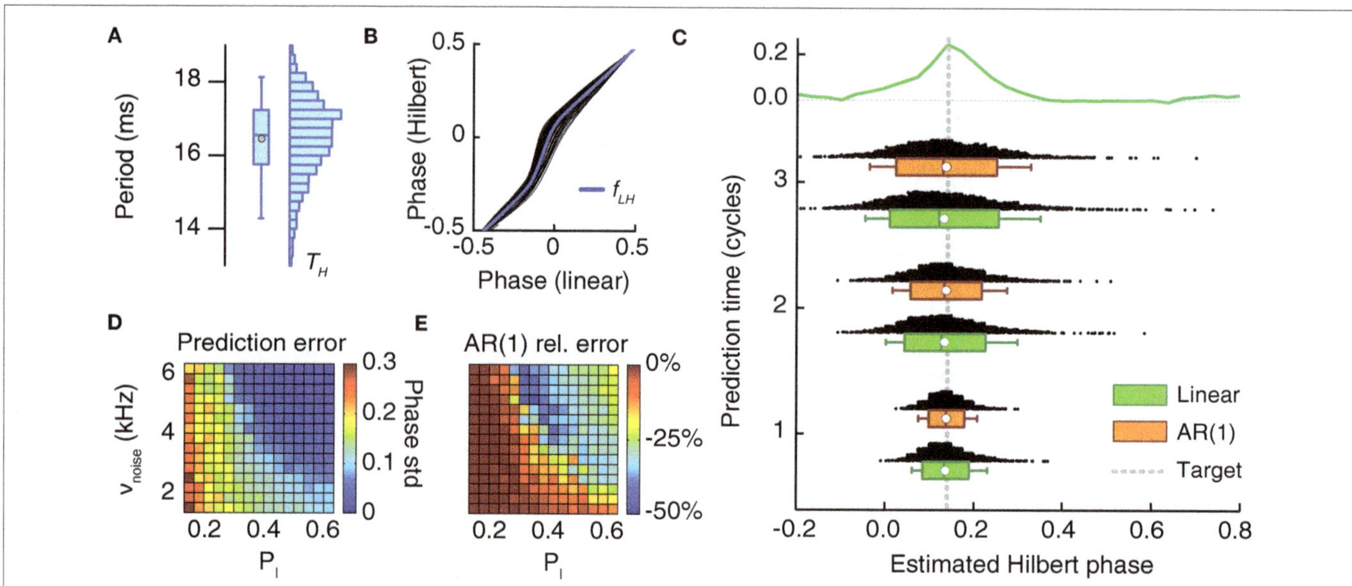

FIGURE 7 | Online prediction of the phase of stimulation onset. (A) The period length of LFP oscillations fluctuates from cycle to cycle and has a broad-range uni-modal distribution (here shown for period lengths as estimated from the Hilbert phases). **(B)** Hilbert phase versus linear phase for a sample LFP time series. To speed-up the computation of t_{ON} in the prediction stage, the Hilbert phase can be approximated by a linear phase, since, as here shown, they are strongly correlated and the mild static non-linearity f_{LH} linking them can be neglected. **(C)** Distribution of the phase of t_{ON} predicted by two different methods and for different lengths of the prediction window (measured in oscillation cycles). Shown are histograms and box plots (box giving median and interquartile range, white circle the mean value and whiskers the 5-th and 95-th percentiles) of the predicted phase of light stimulation $\phi(t_{ON})$ for two prediction methods—pure linear extrapolation based on the average period length (green) and first order autoregressive [AR(1)] models (orange)—applied to period lengths recorded during the monitoring stage. Both the median and the mean of predicted Hilbert phase are in good agreement with the exact target phase (leading with highest probability to a phase shift) with a dispersion not larger than the width of the positive part of the reference phase-shift response curve (reproduced from **Figures 4C,D** on the top of the panel). **(D)** The prediction error (i.e., the standard deviation of the inferred phase $\phi(t_{ON})$ of photostimulation onset) depends on the synchronization level of the neuronal population activity (cf. **Figure 3A**). The prediction error based on linear extrapolation (measured in units of average oscillation period lengths) is shown for different probabilities of local inhibitory connection p_I and background noise rates ν_{noise}. Larger synchronization leads to better prediction. **(E)** The ratio of the prediction error based on the AR(1) model and the prediction error based on linear extrapolation in dependence on the same parameters. For intermediate synchrony levels, the prediction error can be consistently reduced by the use of an AR(1) model.

even when considering regimes "at the edge of synchrony." Furthermore adopting a more elaborate AR(1) approach yielded the strongest performance improvement with respect to simpler linear extrapolation precisely for these intermediate synchrony values (**Figure 7E**).

In contrast, prediction errors associated to weak synchronous dynamics were larger and even the AR(1) approach failed to improve over linear extrapolation in these cases. However, in these regimes, the dynamics rarely displayed long-lasting oscillatory epochs and the probability of spontaneous switching was comparable to the one of induced switching, thus invalidating our analysis protocol. In these cases, therefore, continuous photostimulation should be used to enhance the degree of coherence of the coupled populations activity (analogously to **Figure 3E**).

DISCUSSION

FROM POWER BOOSTING TO RELIABLE PHASE CONTROL

Optogenetic stimulation has been successfully applied to boost the power of fast neural oscillations *in vivo* and *in vitro*. In Cardin et al. (2006), pulsed optogenetic stimulation *in vivo* was used to highlight the existence of a resonance at gamma range frequencies of local inhibitory cortical microcircuits. Adesnik and Scanziani (Adesnik and Scanziani, 2010) and Akam et al. (2012) experimented with ramped light stimulation to induce long-lasting oscillatory episodes in slices.

Beyond controlling oscillation power, the experiments by Akam et al. (2012) are closely related to the first part of our model study. They used 5 ms-long light stimulation pulses to shift local oscillation phases and quantify the phase response curves (PRCs) of oscillations in hippocampal slices, analogously to the simulated experiment of **Figure 4**. The hippocampal PRC measured by Akam et al. (2012) was distinctly biphasic, leading to phase advancement or phase delaying, depending on the phase of application of the stimulation. Such biphasic PRC shape is in qualitative and approximately in quantitative agreement with the PRCs extracted from our local population model for stimulation pulses of comparable lengths (cf. **Figure 4D**, orange curve for 5 ms-long pulses and red curve for 10 ms-long pulses).

Interestingly, however, the PRCs extracted from our model for shorter stimulation durations lacked phase-delaying regions and displayed only a narrow phase range leading to consistent phase advancement. Furthermore, they were characterized by a relatively broad range of application phases for which light stimulation was completely ineffective. These features of the PRC shapes are robustly obtained if the circuit mechanism for the generation of oscillations dominantly relies on delayed mutual interactions within interneuronal networks (Battaglia et al., 2007, 2012). One can actually use very different neuronal models to obtain oscillatory and phase-locking behaviors that qualitatively match those observed. For instance, spatially structured networks of integrate-and-fire neurons (Battaglia and Hansel, 2011) have dynamical regimes that tightly correspond to those of homogeneous networks of the conductance-based neurons (Battaglia et al., 2007) that we adopt here. We predict therefore that similarly looking PRCs could be obtained in the case of Kainate-induced *in vitro* oscillations in slices, in which excitatory neurons are entrained by a coherently oscillating interneuronal population but are not actively involved in the generation of the local rhythm (Fisahn et al., 2004; Bartos et al., 2007; Andersson et al., 2012).

Narrow phase ranges associated to large PRC values reduce the probability of inducing stable phase shifting by applying stimulation at arbitrary times. However such narrow intervals become a desirable resource when optogenetic stimulation is precisely phased conditional to ongoing oscillations, as executable in perspective with a closed-loop setup. Indeed, PRC shapes like the reference PRC discussed in **Figure 3** (green curve for $P_{ChR2} = 25\%$, and $T_{\text{light}} = 3$ ms light-pulses) could allow an "all-or-none" control of phase shifting, in which strong effects are obtained only if the stimulation is applied within a specific target range of phases, but in which undesired switching triggered by noise or by a misapplied input is largely suppressed.

A SIMPLE ChR2 MODEL CAPTURES NON MONOTONIC PHOTORESPONSE

The light-activated cation channel ChR2 activates more rapidly and supports larger peak current amplitudes for increasing light intensities. Therefore, we speculated that brief, high intensity light pulses would provide the optimal stimulation for our purposes. To our knowledge there were no studies that systematically documented ChR2 current responses for stimuli with light intensities above 20 mW/mm^2 (Ishizuka et al., 2006; Ernst et al., 2008; Lin et al., 2009). At this intensity the activation rate is still light sensitive and we aimed to increase it even more using light intensities as high as approximately 130 mW/mm^2. While the activation rate did indeed decrease further, the fact that the peak current amplitude *decreased* for intensities above approximately 20 mW/mm^2 came to us as a surprise (**Figures 1B,C**). This behavior has not been reported before, to the best of our knowledge, though the measurements published in Lin et al. (2009) hint at a decreasing peak amplitude for the highest intensity applied there, which was approximately 19.8 mW/mm^2.

Such phenomenon might be reminiscent of the photoreactive P480b intermediate state, which can be converted by blue light to the early P500 intermediate state. This transition was proposed as a shortcut of the photocycle from a spectroscopic study of ChR2 channels (Ritter et al., 2008). Since previously published models of ChR2 currents (Nikolic et al., 2006, 2009) could not account for this non-monotonic light response, it was necessary to deploy a novel model. Our simple conductance-based model correctly captures the existence of an optimal light intensity for photostimulation, without need to incorporate elaborate details about the ChR2 molecular structure and dynamics. Note that the application of our model is not limited to brief light pulses, but can also predict light-induced conductance in response to ramps of light (cf. **Figure 3E**).

Our model is also accurately data-constrained. To calibrate model parameters, light induced changes of ChR2 conductance were measured in voltage clamp. If the voltage can be clamped throughout a cell, any changes in the whole-cell current can be attributed to ChR2 conductances. In differentiated neurons, however, this perfect voltage control cannot be attained. This is obvious from the recording in **Figure 1A** (black trace), where the activation of ChR2 depolarized the axon sufficiently to activate voltage-dependent sodium channels, which created an unclamped spike. Even when sodium channels are blocked, the conditions are not optimal for a precise biophysical characterization. Using essentially passive and electrotonically compact cells, such as HEK-293 cells (Nikolic et al., 2009), provided optimal recording conditions (**Figure 1B**). The smaller amplitude of the photocurrents in these cells reflected differences in cell surface and expression levels, while the biophysical properties of ChR2 were most likely identical to those expressed in neurons.

TECHNICAL FEASIBILITY

As discussed above, the extraction of PRCs describing the collective response of a transduced neuronal population to light stimulation was already achieved *in vitro* (Akam et al., 2012). Our modeling study suggests that a similar approach could be successfully applied *in vivo*, since phase-shifting effects can be robustly obtained with high and low transduction rates, covering the wide range achievable with different experimental techniques (Adamantidis et al., 2007; Petreanu et al., 2007; Wang et al., 2007; Takahashi et al., 2012). The success rate will depend on a suitably tuned light intensity and on the ability to select the phase of the stimulation onset conditional on ongoing oscillation dynamics. Another factor that might enhance the controllability of phases is the use of faster variants of Chr2, such as ChETA (Gunaydin et al., 2010) and the E123T/T159C (Berndt et al., 2011) mutants.

A closed-loop approach is required for determining the optimal timing of pulse stimulations. **Figure 7C** shows that if the time required for the prediction stage is of the order of a few oscillation cycles, then the discrepancy between the target and the actual perturbation phase is comparable to the width of the peak of the PRC. Consequently the resulting phase shifting should remain close to the optimum. The prediction strategy that we propose (**Figure 6**) is based uniquely on a small number of linear computations, which are particularly suited for ultrafast (millisecond scale) implementation on reconfigurable hardware chips (Zhuo and Prasanna, 2008; Sadrozinski and Wu, 2011) or on GPU architectures (Owens et al., 2008; Volkov and Demmel, 2008) on which FFT algorithms can be efficiently implemented (Bhattacharyya et al., 2010). As a matter of fact, hardware implementations of period extraction (Waskito et al., 2010) and autoregressive modeling of biologic signals (Marinkovic et al., 2005; Kim and Rosen, 2010) have already proven to be order(s) of magnitude faster than on conventional CPUs. Taking into account these high levels of performance and the approximations we propose to implement, a length of the prediction window of ~50 ms that corresponds to approximately three cycles of a 40–70 Hz rhythm appears completely realistic.

Our simulated oscillations constitute an idealized model for neuronal rhythms measured *in vivo* or *in vitro*. In our model, especially when the synchronization index is very high, cycle-to-cycle period length fluctuations are positively correlated with weak to intermediate correlation strength. In real neuronal oscillations, however, adaptation or other phenomena might introduce more complex correlation patterns between the lengths of different periods. Nevertheless, such correlations might still be captured by AR(1) modeling, as hinted to by the better performance of AR(1) in dynamic regimes at the "edge of synchrony" (**Figure 7E**), in which period length fluctuations are more strongly correlated.

Under specific experimental conditions, long-lasting oscillatory epochs might be a rare event. It would then become difficult to meet the conditions for the applicability of our protocol (i.e., the testing stage of **Figure 6** might never be passed). In this case, continuous optogenetic stimulation could be used to stabilize and boost oscillations, as simulated in **Figure 3E**. Then, similarly to the approach of Akam et al. (2012), precisely timed "kicks," superposed on this continuous light stimulation, could be used to perturb the instantaneous phase. In this sense, optogenetic stimulation is more promising than electric micro-stimulation. First, it allows combining continuous and pulsed stimulation within a single setup. Second, it can control with high selectivity the degree of synchronization, not only by providing an unspecific drive to the entire network, but also enhancing the drive to specific neuronal subpopulations, like for instance FS-PV cells which provide the phasic inhibition crucial for rhythm generation (Cardin et al., 2006; Sohal et al., 2009).

Finally, we are optimistic that the network models of transduced neural populations that were pioneered by Talathi et al. (2011) and further developed in this study are powerful tools, which will be increasingly adopted to conduct, optimize and accelerate the design and the calibration of closed-loop optogenetic experimental protocols.

PROBING PHASE-CODING AND COMMUNICATION-THROUGH-COHERENCE

Reliable optogenetic manipulation of the phase dynamics of oscillating neuronal populations would open the way to an interventional exploration of phase coding schemes. In the phase coding framework, it is argued that the phase of spikes relative to a "reference clock"—paced either by a stimulus-locked (De Charms and Merzenich, 1996; Arabzadeh et al., 2006) or an internally-generated oscillation (O'Keefe and Recce, 1993; Siegel et al., 2009)—carry information, which is independent from and multiplexed with the one conveyed by rate fluctuations (Montemurro et al., 2008). Anticipating or delaying the ticks of such a "reference clock," as the one putatively framed by slow cortical oscillations (Kayser et al., 2012), should perturb the decoding of phase-based representations.

Beyond the control of the phase of a local oscillation, inter-areal phase correlations could be disrupted transiently by unspecific optogenetic stimulation (**Figure 5D**). Furthermore, precisely-phased perturbations determined within a closed-loop system could induce persistent switching between alternative phase-locked dynamic patterns (Tiesinga and Sejnowski, 2010; Battaglia et al., 2012). In this sense, the realization of an experiment inspired by the idealized analysis of **Figure 4**, would provide a direct testing of the communication-through-coherence hypothesis (Fries, 2005). More specifically, it would allow experimental testing of whether different sets of inter-areal phase relations lead to different inter-areal functional interactions and to an altered balance between bottom-up and top-down information flows, as predicted by theory (Battaglia et al., 2012).

A reorganization of phase relations between distant neuronal populations might have perceptual or behavioral consequences. Selective alteration of inter-population phase relations, for instance between areas FEF and V4 (Gregoriou et al., 2009) or areas V1 and V4 (Grothe et al., 2012), might be used to suppress or boost attentional effects or even to emulate reorienting of attention. Furthermore, our theoretical investigations suggest that stimulation applied locally to a single area might induce distributed reorganization of phase relations between other more distant areas (Battaglia et al., 2012). Closed-loop optogenetic stimulation might then in perspective be used to trigger system-level switching between global brain states (Deco et al., 2009; Freyer et al., 2011).

AUTHOR CONTRIBUTIONS

Agostina Palmigiano and Demian Battaglia performed the simulations. Annette Witt, Agostina Palmigiano, and Demian Battaglia analyzed the simulations. Andreas Neef and Ahmed El Hady performed and analyzed the experiments. Annette Witt, Andreas Neef, Fred Wolf, and Demian Battaglia designed the models and the study. Annette Witt, Agostina Palmigiano, Andreas Neef, Ahmed El Hady, Fred Wolf, and Demian Battaglia wrote the manuscript.

ACKNOWLEDGMENTS

The authors thank Pascal Fries, Alexander Gail, Theo Geisel, Andreas Kreiter, Shy Shoham, and Walter Stühmer for inspiring discussions. Annette Witt was supported by the Stifterverband für die deutsche Wissenschaft and by the Claussen-Simon-Stiftung. We all acknowledge financial support by the German Federal Ministry of Education and Research (BMBF) via the Bernstein Center for Computational Neuroscience—Göttingen (01GQ1005B, 01GQ0430, 01GQ07113), the Bernstein Focus Neurotechnology—Göttingen (01GQ0811) and the Bernstein Focus Visual Learning (01GQ0921, 01GQ0922), the German Israel Research Foundation and the VolkswagenStiftung (ZN2632) and the Deutsche Forschungsgemeinschaft through CRC-889 (906-17.1/2006).

REFERENCES

Adamantidis, A. R., Zhang, F., Aravanis, A. M., Deisseroth, K., and de Lecea, L. (2007). Neural substrates of awakening probed with optogenetic control of hypocretin neurons. *Nature* 450, 420–424.

Adesnik, H., and Scanziani, M. (2010). Lateral competition for cortical space by layer-specific horizontal circuits. *Nature* 464, 1155–1160.

Akam, T., Oren, I., Mantoan, L., Ferenczi, E., and Kullmann, D. M. (2012). Oscillatory dynamics in the hippocampus support dentate gyrus-CA3 coupling. *Nat. Neurosci.* 15, 763–768.

Andersson, R., Johnston, A., and Fisahn, A. (2012). Dopamine D4 receptor activation increases hippocampal gamma oscillations by enhancing synchronization of fast-spiking interneurons. *PLoS ONE* 7:e40906. doi: 10.1371/journal.pone.0040906

Arabzadeh, E., Panzeri, S., and Diamond, M. E. (2006). Deciphering the spike train of a sensory neuron: counts and temporal patterns in the rat whisker pathway. *J. Neurosci.* 26, 9216–9226.

Aravanis, A. M., Wang, L. P., Zhang, F., Meltzer, L. A., Mogri, M. Z., Schneider, M. B., et al. (2007). An optical neural interface: *in vivo* control of rodent motor cortex with integrated fibreoptic and optogenetic technology. *J. Neural Eng.* 4, S143–S156.

Bakkum, D. J., Gamblen, P. M., Ben-Ary, G., Chao, Z. C., and Potter, S. M. (2007). MEART: the semi-living artist. *Front. Neurorobot.* 1:5. doi: 10.3389/neuro.12.005.2007

Bandyopadhyay, P. R. (2005). Trends in biorobotic autonomous undersea vehicles. *IEEE J. Oceanic Eng.* 30, 109–139.

Bartos, M., Vida, I., and Jonas, P. (2007). Synaptic mechanisms of synchronized gamma oscillations in inhibitory interneuron networks. *Nat. Rev. Neurosci.* 8, 45–56.

Battaglia, D., Brunel, N., and Hansel, D. (2007). Temporal decorrelation of collective oscillations in neural networks with local inhibition and long-range excitation. *Phys. Rev. Lett.* 99:238106. doi: 10.1103/PhysRevLett.99.238106

Battaglia, D., and Hansel, D. (2011). Synchronous chaos and broad band gamma rhythm in a minimal multi-layer model of primary visual cortex. *PLoS Comp. Biol.* 7:e1002176. doi: 10.1371/journal.pcbi.1002176

Battaglia, D., Witt, A., Wolf, F., and Geisel, T. (2012). Dynamic effective connectivity of inter-areal brain circuits. *PLoS Comp. Biol.* 8:e1002438. doi: 10.1371/journal.pcbi.1002438

Berndt, A., Schoenenberger, P., Mattis, J., Tye, K. M., Deisseroth, K., Hegemann, P., et al. (2011). High-efficiency channelrhodopsins for fast neuronal stimulation at low light levels. *Proc. Natl. Acad. Sci. U.S.A.* 108, 7595–7600.

Bhattacharyya, K., Hazra, A., Hatai, I., and Banerjee, S. (2010). Architectural design of a radix-4 CORDIC-based Radix-4 IFFT algorithm and its FGGA implementation. *Int. J. Sig. Imaging Syst. Eng.* 2, 201–215.

Bosman, C. A., Schoffelen, J.-M., Brunet, N., Oostenveld, R., Bastos, A. M., Womelsdorf, T., et al. (2012). Attentional stimulus selection through selective synchronization between monkey visual areas. *Neuron* 75, 875–888.

Brockwell, P. J., and Davis, R. A. (1996). *Introduction to Time Series and Forecasting.* New York, NY: Springer.

Brovelli, A., Ding, M., Ledberg, A., Chen, Y., Nakamura, R., and Bressler, S. L. (2004). Beta oscillations in a large-scale sensorimotor cortical network: directional influences revealed by Granger causality. *Proc. Natl. Acad. Sci. U.S.A.* 101, 9849–9854.

Brunel, N., and Hakim, V. (1999). Fast global oscillations in networks of integrate-and-fire neurons with low firing rates. *Neural Comput.* 11, 1621–1671.

Brunel, N., and Hansel, D. (2006). How noise affects the synchronization properties of recurrent networks of inhibitory neurons. *Neural Comput.* 18, 1066–1110.

Brunel, N., and Wang, X.-J. (2003). What determines the frequency of fast network oscillations with irregular neural discharges? I. Synaptic dynamics and excitation-inhibition balance. *J. Neurophysiol.* 90, 415–430.

Buffalo, E. A., Fries, P., Landman, R., Buschman, T. J., and Desimone, R. (2011). Laminar differences in gamma and alpha coherence in the ventral stream. *Proc. Natl. Acad. Sci. U.S.A.* 108, 11262–11267.

Cardin, J. A., Carlén, M., Meletis, K., Knoblich, U., Zhang, F., Deisseroth, K., et al. (2006). Driving fast-spiking cells induces gamma rhythm and controls sensory responses. *Nature* 459, 663–667.

De Charms, R. C., and Merzenich, M. M. (1996). Primary cortical representations of sounds by the coordination of action-potential timing. *Nature* 381, 610–613.

Deco, G., Jirsa, V., McIntosh, A. R., Sporns, O., and Kötter, R. (2009). Key role of coupling, delay, and noise in resting brain fluctuations. *Proc. Natl. Acad. Sci. U.S.A.* 106, 10302–10307.

Eckhorn, R., Bauer, R., Jordan, W., Brosch, M., Kruse, W., Munk, M., et al. (1988). Coherent oscillations: a mechanism of feature linking in the visual cortex? Multiple electrode and correlation analyses in the cat. *Biol. Cybern.* 60, 121–130.

Ernst, O. P., Sánchez Murcia, P. A., Daldrop, P., Tsunoda, S. P., Kateriya, S., and Hegemann, P. (2008). Photoactivation of channelrhodopsin. *J. Biol. Chem.* 283, 1637–1643.

Fisahn, A., Contractor, A., Traub, R. D., Buhl, E. H., Heinemann, S. F., and McBain, C. J. (2004). Distinct roles for the kainate receptor subunits GluR5 and GluR6 in kainate-induced hippocampal gamma oscillations. *J. Neurosci.* 24, 9658–9668.

Freyer, F., Roberts, J. A., Becker, R., Robinson, P. A., Ritter, P., and Breakspear, M. (2011). Biophysical mechanisms of multistability in resting-state cortical rhythms. *J. Neurosci.* 31, 6353–6361.

Fries, P. (2005). A mechanism for cognitive dynamics: neuronal communication through neuronal coherence. *Trends Cogn. Sci.* 9, 474–480.

Fries, P., Reynolds, J. H., Rorie, A. E., and Desimone, R. (2001). Modulation of oscillatory neuronal synchronization by selective visual attention. *Science* 291, 1560–1563.

Gabor, V. D. (1946). Theory of communication. *J. IEE* 93, 429–457.

Golomb, D., and Hansel, D. (2000). The number of synaptic inputs and the synchrony of large, sparse neuronal networks. *Neural Comp.* 12, 1095–1139.

Gray, C. M., König, P., Engel, A. K., and Singer, W. (1989). Oscillatory responses in cat visual cortex exhibit inter-columnar synchronization which reflects global stimulus properties. *Nature* 338, 334–337.

Gregoriou, G. G., Gotts, S. J., and Desimone, R. (2012). Cell-type-specific synchronization of neural activity in FEF with V4 during attention. *Neuron* 73, 581–594.

Gregoriou, G. G., Gotts, S. J., Zhou, H., and Desimone, R. (2009). High-frequency, long-range coupling between prefrontal and visual cortex during attention. *Science* 324, 1207–1210.

Grothe, I., Neitzel, S. D., Mandon, S., and Kreiter, A. K. (2012). Switching neuronal inputs by differential modulations of gamma-band phase-coherence. *J. Neurosci.* 32, 16172–16180.

Gunaydin, L. A., Yizhar, O., Berndt, A., Sohal, V. S., Deisseroth, K., and Hegemann, P. (2010). Ultrafast optogenetic control. *Nat. Neurosci.* 13, 387–392.

Ishizuka, T., Kakuda, M., Araki, R., and Yawo, H. (2006). Kinetic evaluation of photosensitivity in genetically engineered neurons expressing green algae light-gated channels. *Neurosci. Res.* 54, 85–94.

Kayser, C., Ince, R. A. A., and Panzeri, S. (2012). Analysis of slow (theta) oscillations as a potential temporal reference frame for information coding in sensory cortices. *PLoS Comp. Biol.* 8:e1002717. doi: 10.1371/journal.pcbi.1002717

Kim, H., and Rosen, J. (2010). Epileptic seizure detection – an AR model based algorithm for implantable device. *Conf. Proc. IEEE Eng. Med. Biol. Soc.* 2010, 5541–5544.

Koepsell, K., Wang, X., Hirsch, J. A., and Sommer, F. T. (2010). Exploring the function of neural oscillations in early sensory systems. *Front. Neurosci.* 4:53. doi: 10.3389/neuro.01.010.2010

Kreiter, A. K., and Singer, W. (1996). Stimulus-dependent synchronization of neuronal responses in the visual cortex of the awake macaque monkey. *J. Neurosci.* 16, 2381–2396.

Lin, J. Y., Lin, M. Z., Steinbach, P., and Tsien, R. Y. (2009). Characterization of engineered channelrhodopsin variants with improved properties and kinetics. *Biophys. J.* 96, 1803–1814.

Lisman, J. (2005). The theta/gamma discrete phase code occuring during the hippocampal phase precession may be a more general brain coding scheme. *Hippocampus* 15, 913–922.

Marinkovic, B., Gillette, M., and Ning, T. (2005). "FPGA implementation of respiration signal classification using a soft-core processor," in *Proceedings of the 31st Annual Northeast Bioengineering IEEE Conference* (New York, NY), 54–55.

Marom, S., and Shahaf, G. (2002). Development, learning and memory in large random networks of cortical neurons: lessons beyond anatomy. *Rev. Biophys.* 35, 63–87.

Melloni, L., Molina, C., Pena, M., Torres, D., Singer, W., and Rodriguez, E. (2007). Synchronization of neural activity across cortical areas correlates with conscious perception. *J. Neurosci.* 27, 2858–2865.

Miranda-Dominguez, O., Gonia, J., and Netoff, T. I. (2010). Firing rate control of a neuron using a linear proportional-integral controller. *J. Neural Eng.* 7:066004. doi: 10.1088/1741-2560/7/6/066004

Montemurro, M. A., Rasch, M. J., Murayama, Y., Logothetis, N. K., and Panzeri, S. (2008). Phase-of-firing coding of natural visual stimuli in primary visual cortex. *Curr. Biol.* 18, 375–380.

Nadasdy, Z. (2010). Binding by asynchrony: the neuronal phase code. *Front. Neurosci.* 4:51. doi: 10.3389/fnins.2010.00051

Nikolic, K., Degenaar, P., and Toumazou, C. (2006). Modeling and engineering aspects of channelrhodopsin-2 system for neural photostimulation. *Conf. Proc. IEEE Eng. Med. Biol. Soc.* 1, 1626–1629.

Nikolic, K., Grossman, N., Grubb, M. S., Burrone, J., Toumazou, C., and Degenaar, P. (2009). Photocycles of channelrhodopsin-2. *Photochem. Photobiol.* 85, 400–411.

Novellino, A., D'Angelo, P., Cozzi, L., Chiappalone, M., Sanguineti, V., and Martinoia, S. (2007). Connecting neurons to a mobile robot: an *in vitro* bidirectional neural interface. *Comput. Intell. Neurosci.* 2007, 1–14.

O'Keefe, J., and Recce, M. L. (1993). Phase relationship between hippocampal place units and the EEG theta rhythm. *Hippocampus* 3, 317–330.

Owens, J. D., Houston, M., Luebke, D., Green, S., Stone, J. E., and Phillips, J. C. (2008). GPU computing. *IEEE Proc.* 96, 879–899.

Percival, D. B., and Walden, A. T. (1993). *Spectral Analysis for Physical Applications.* Cambridge: Cambridge University Press.

Pesaran, B., Pezaris, J. S., Sahani, M., Mitra, P. P., and Andersen, R. A. (2002). Temporal structure in neuronal activity during working memory in macaque parietal cortex. *Nat. Neurosci.* 5, 805–811.

Petreanu, L., Huber, D., Sobczyk, A., and Svoboda, K. (2007). Channelrhodopsin-2-assisted circuit mapping of long range callosal projections. *Nat. Neurosci.* 10, 663–668.

Pikovsky, A. S., Rosenblum, M., and Kurths, J. (2001). *Synchronization – A Universal Concept in Nonlinear Sciences.* Cambridge: Cambridge University Press.

Ritter, E., Stehfest, K., Berndt, A., Hegemann, P., and Bartl, F. J. (2008). Monitoring light-induced structural changes of Channelrhodopsin-2 by UV-visible and Fourier transform infrared spectroscopy. *J. Biol. Chem.* 283, 35033–35041.

Roelfsema, P. R., Engel, A. K., König, P., and Singer, W. (1997). Visuomotor integration is associated with zero time-lag synchronization among cortical areas. *Nature* 385, 157–161.

Rotermund, D., Taylor, K., Ernst, U. A., Kreiter, A. K., and Pawelzik, K. R. (2009). Attention improves object representation in visual cortical field potentials. *J. Neurosci.* 29, 10120–10130.

Sadrozinski, H. F. W., and Wu, J. (2011). *Applications of Field-Programmable Gate Arrays in Scientific Research.* Boca Raton, FL: Taylor and Francis.

Samonds, J. M., and Bonds, A. B. (2004). Gamma oscillation maintains stimulus structure-dependent synchronization in cat visual cortex. *J. Neurophysiol.* 93, 223–236.

Schoenenberger, P., Grunditz, A., Rose, T., and Oertner, T. (2008). Optimizing the spatial resolution of channelrhodopsin-2 activation. *Brain Cell Biol.* 36, 119–127.

Siegel, M., Warden, M. R., and Miller, E. K. (2009). Phase-dependent neuronal coding of objects in short-term memory. *Proc. Natl. Acad. Sci. U.S.A.* 106, 21341–21346.

Sohal, V. S., Zhang, F., Yizhar, O., and Deisseroth, K. (2009). Parvalbumin neurons and gamma rhythms enhance cortical circuit performance. *Nature* 459, 698–702.

Takahashi, H., Sakurai, T., Sakai, H., Bakkum, D. J., Suzurikawa, J., and Kanzaki, R. (2012). Light-addressed single-neuron stimulation in dissociated neuronal cultures with sparse expression of ChR2. *Biosystems* 107, 106–112.

Talathi, S. S., Carney, P. R., and Khargonekar, P. P. (2011). Control of neural synchrony using channelrhodopsin-2: a computational study. *J. Comput. Neurosci.* 31, 87–103.

Tallon-Baudry, C., Bertrand, O., Delpuech, C., and Pernier, J. (1996). Stimulus specificity of phase-locked and non-phase-locked 40 Hz visual responses in human. *J. Neurosci.* 16, 4240–4249.

Tiesinga, P., and Sejnowski, T. J. (2009). Cortical enlightenment: are attentional gamma oscillations driven by ING or PING? *Neuron* 63, 727–732.

Tiesinga, P. H., and Sejnowski, T. J. (2010). Mechanisms for phase shifting in cortical networks and their role in communication through coherence. *Front. Hum. Neurosci.* 4:196. doi: 10.3389/fnhum.2010.00196

Varela, F., Lachaux, J. P., Rodriguez, E., and Martinerie, J. (2001). The brainweb: phase synchronization and large-scale integration. *Nat. Rev. Neurosci.* 2, 229–239.

Volkov, V., and Demmel, J. W. (2008). "Benchmarking GPUs to tune dense linear algebra," in *The International Conference for High Performance Computing, Networking, Storage, and Analysis (SC 2008)* (Piscataway, NJ), 1–11.

Wagenaar, D. A., Madhavan, R., Pine, J., and Potter, S. M. (2005). Controlling bursting in cortical cultures with closed-loop multi-electrode stimulation. *J. Neurosci.* 25, 680–688.

Wallach, A., Eytan, D., Gal, A., Zrenner, C., and Marom, S. (2011). Neuronal response clamp. *Front. Neuroeng.* 4:3. doi: 10.3389/fneng.2011.00003

Wang, H., Peca, J., Matsuzaki, M., Matsuzaki, K., Noguchi, J., Qiu, L., et al. (2007). High-speed mapping of synaptic connectivity using photostimulation in channelrhodopsin-2 transgenic mice. *Proc. Natl. Acad. Sci. U.S.A.* 104, 8143–8148.

Wang, S., Chandrasekaran, L., Fernandez, F. R., White, J. A., and Canavier, C. C. (2012). Short conduction delays cause inhibition rather than excitation to favor synchrony in hybrid neuronal networks of the entorhinal cortex. *PLoS Comp. Biol.* 8:e1002306. doi: 10.1371/journal.pcbi.1002306

Wang, X. J. (2010). Neurophysiological and computational principles of cortical rhythms in cognition. *Physiol. Rev.* 90, 1195–1268.

Wang, X. J., and Buzsáki, G. (1996). Gamma oscillation by synaptic inhibition in a hippocampal interneuronal network model. *J. Neurosci.* 16, 6402–6413.

Waskito, P., Miwa, S., Mitsukura, Y., and Nakajo, H. (2010). "Parallelizing Hilbert-Huang Transform on a GPU," in *Proceedings of the 2010 First International Conference on Networking and Computing (ICNC 2010)* (Washington, DC), 184–190.

Whittington, M. A., Traub, R. D., and Jefferys, J. G. (1995). Synchronized oscillations in interneuron networks driven by metabotropic glutamate receptor activation. *Nature* 373, 612–615.

Whittington, M. A., Traub, R. D., Kopell, N., Ermentrout, G. B., and Buhl, E. H. (2000). Inhibition-based rhythms: experimental and mathematical observation on network dynamics. *Int. J. Psychophysiol.* 38, 315–336.

Womelsdorf, T., Schoffelen, J.-M., Oostenveld, R., Singer, W., Desimone, R., Engel, A. K., et al. (2007). Modulation of neuronal interactions through neuronal synchronization. *Science* 316, 1609–1612.

Woodman, M. M., and Canavier, C. C. (2011). Effects of conduction delays on the existence and stability of one to one phase locking between two pulse-coupled oscillators. *J. Comput. Neurosci.* 31, 401–418.

Yu, J., and Ferster, D. (2010). Membrane potential synchrony in primary visual cortex during sensory stimulation. *Neuron* 68, 1187–1201.

Zhuo, L., and Prasanna, V. K. (2008). High-performance designs for linear algebra operations on reconfigurable hardware. *IEEE Trans. Comput.* 57, 1057–1071.

18

Adaptive stimulus optimization for sensory systems neuroscience

Christopher DiMattina[1]* and Kechen Zhang[2]

[1] Program in Psychology, Florida Gulf Coast University, Fort Myers, FL, USA
[2] Department of Biomedical Engineering, The Johns Hopkins University School of Medicine, Baltimore, MD, USA

Edited by:
Ahmed El Hady, Max Planck Institute for Dynamics and Self Organization, Germany

Reviewed by:
Demian Battaglia, Max Planck Institute for Dynamics and Self-Organization, Germany
Tim Gollisch, University Medical Center Göttingen, Germany

***Correspondence:**
Christopher DiMattina, Program in Psychology, Florida Gulf Coast University, 10501 FGCU Boulevard South, Fort Myers, FL 33965-6565, USA
e-mail: chris_dimattina@yahoo.com

In this paper, we review several lines of recent work aimed at developing practical methods for adaptive on-line stimulus generation for sensory neurophysiology. We consider various experimental paradigms where on-line stimulus optimization is utilized, including the classical *optimal stimulus* paradigm where the goal of experiments is to identify a stimulus which maximizes neural responses, the *iso-response* paradigm which finds sets of stimuli giving rise to constant responses, and the *system identification* paradigm where the experimental goal is to estimate and possibly compare sensory processing models. We discuss various theoretical and practical aspects of adaptive firing rate optimization, including optimization with stimulus space constraints, firing rate adaptation, and possible network constraints on the optimal stimulus. We consider the problem of system identification, and show how accurate estimation of non-linear models can be highly dependent on the stimulus set used to probe the network. We suggest that optimizing stimuli for accurate model estimation may make it possible to successfully identify non-linear models which are otherwise intractable, and summarize several recent studies of this type. Finally, we present a two-stage stimulus design procedure which combines the dual goals of model estimation and model comparison and may be especially useful for system identification experiments where the appropriate model is unknown beforehand. We propose that fast, on-line stimulus optimization enabled by increasing computer power can make it practical to move sensory neuroscience away from a descriptive paradigm and toward a new paradigm of real-time model estimation and comparison.

Keywords: sensory coding, optimal stimulus, adaptive data collection, neural network, parameter estimation

INTRODUCTION

One classical approach in sensory neurophysiology has been to describe sensory neurons in terms of the stimuli that are most effective to drive these neurons. The stimulus that elicits the highest response is often referred to as the *optimal stimulus* (Albrecht et al., 1980; Stork et al., 1982; DiMattina and Zhang, 2008). Although the optimal stimulus provides a simple and intuitive means of characterizing a sensory neuron, positively identifying the optimal stimulus may be technically difficult for high-dimensional stimuli, and simply knowing the optimal stimulus without adequately exploring responses to other stimuli may provide limited information about sensory function (Olshausen and Field, 2005). Due to these practical and conceptual limitations of characterizing neurons by the optimal stimulus, many researchers have recently taken engineering-inspired approaches to studying neural coding, for example, by characterizing neurons in terms of the mutual information between sensory stimuli and a neuron's responses (Machens, 2002; Sharpee et al., 2004; Machens et al., 2005; Chase and Young, 2008), by characterizing iso-response surfaces in stimulus parameter spaces (Bölinger and Gollisch, 2012; Horwitz and Hass, 2012), or by fitting predictive mathematical models of neural responses to neurophysiology data (Wu et al., 2006). However, just like the classical optimal stimulus paradigm, these engineering-inspired methods also give rise to non-trivial high-dimensional stimulus optimization problems.

With recent advances in desktop computing power, it has become practical to perform stimulus optimization adaptively in real-time during the course of an experiment (Benda et al., 2007; Newman et al., 2013). In this review, we consider several recent lines of work on adaptive on-line stimulus optimization, focusing on single-unit recording *in vivo* for systems-level sensory neuroscience. Other kinds of closed-loop neuroscience experiments like dynamic patch clamping or closed-loop seizure interventions are considered elsewhere (Prinz et al., 2004; Newman et al., 2013). We first discuss the concept of the optimal stimulus and consider how its properties may be constrained by the underlying functional model describing a neuron's stimulus–response relation. We then discuss how adaptive stimulus optimization has been utilized experimentally to find complex high-dimensional stimuli which optimize a neuron's firing rate, including promising recent studies using evolutionary algorithms. We also discuss a different kind of study where stimuli are "optimized" to elicit a desired constant firing rate so that iso-response contours of the stimulus–response function may be obtained, as well as studies seeking maximally informative stimulus ensembles. Finally, we discuss how adaptive stimulus optimization can be utilized for effective estimation of the parameters of sensory processing models, as well as for effective model comparison. In conclusion, we suggest that adaptive stimulus optimization cannot only make the classical optimal stimulus paradigm more tractable, but can potentially move sensory neuroscience toward a fundamentally new experimental paradigm of real-time model estimation and comparison.

THE OPTIMAL STIMULUS

DEFINING THE OPTIMAL STIMULUS

In order for a sensory neuron to be useful to an organism, there must be a consistent functional relationship between the parameters of sensory stimuli and neural responses. Although this relationship may be highly complex and non-linear, for any set of stimuli defined by parameters $\mathbf{x} = (x_1, \ldots, x_n)^T$ we may think abstractly of the expected neural responses being described by some function $r = f(\mathbf{x})$. For simplicity and definiteness, in this section we will focus our discussion of the optimal stimulus on the most common case where r is a scalar quantity which represents the firing rate of a single neuron, and will assume that the expected firing rate is entirely a function of the stimulus parameters, ignoring variables such as spiking history and stimulus-specific adaptation by assuming that they are kept constant (Ulanovsky et al., 2003; Bartlett and Wang, 2005; Asari and Zador, 2009).

Given this formulation, the problem of finding the optimal stimulus $\mathbf{x}_0$ is simply the problem of maximizing the function $f(\mathbf{x})$. Perhaps the simplest and most intuitive notion of the optimal stimulus is that of a firing rate peak in stimulus parameter space centered at $\mathbf{x}_0$, as illustrated in **Figure 1A**. Here f is maximized at $\mathbf{x}_0$, and for any stimulus perturbation $\Delta\mathbf{x}$ we have $f(\mathbf{x}_0 + \Delta\mathbf{x}) < f(\mathbf{x}_0)$. However, for high-dimensional stimulus spaces like image pixel space (Simoncelli et al., 2004) or auditory frequency space (Yu and Young, 2000; Barbour and Wang, 2003a) this intuitive notion of the optimal stimulus as a response peak is hardly the only possibility. In the example shown in **Figure 1B**, the neuron is tuned along one direction in the stimulus space, but is untuned along an orthogonal direction. In this case, there is not a single optimal stimulus $\mathbf{x}_0$ as in **Figure 1A**, but rather a continuum of optimal stimuli lying along a ridge containing $\mathbf{x}_0$ (**Figure 1B**, thick green line). Another theoretical possibility is the saddle-shaped response surface in **Figure 1C**, where depending on the dimension chosen for exploration, the same stimulus $\mathbf{x}_0$ can be either a firing rate peak or a valley.

For high-dimensional stimulus spaces, a full factorial exploration is impossible since the number of stimuli needed grows exponentially with the dimension, a problem referred to colloquially as the *curse of dimensionality* (Bellman, 1961). In many experiments, stimulus spaces are explored in a restricted subset of dimensions. The behaviors of neuron in the unexplored stimulus dimensions may have various possibilities including the ones considered above. One cannot assume that the stimulus–response relationship must always be a single peak as in **Figure 1A**. Indeed, one of the challenges of sensory neurophysiology is that without prior knowledge about the neuron under study, there are no constraints whatsoever on the possibilities for the optimal stimulus, which must be found in a process of trial-and-error with no way to conclusively prove global optimality (Olshausen and Field, 2005). We now briefly discuss a recent theoretical study describing possible constraints on the optimal stimulus which arise from general anatomical properties of underlying functional circuitry.

CONSTRAINTS FROM UNDERLYING FUNCTIONAL CIRCUITRY

Ultimately, the stimulus–response relationship function $f(\mathbf{x})$ is generated by the underlying neural circuitry connecting the sensory periphery to the neuron under study, but in general this circuitry is highly complex (Felleman and Van Essen, 1991; Shepherd, 2003) and not generally known to the experimenter. Nevertheless, recent theoretical work suggests that very basic anatomical properties of the neural circuitry may be able to provide experimentally useful constraints on the possibilities for the optimal stimulus (DiMattina and Zhang, 2008).

Consider the simple hypothetical sensory network shown in **Figure 2A** (left panel) which receives synaptic inputs from two

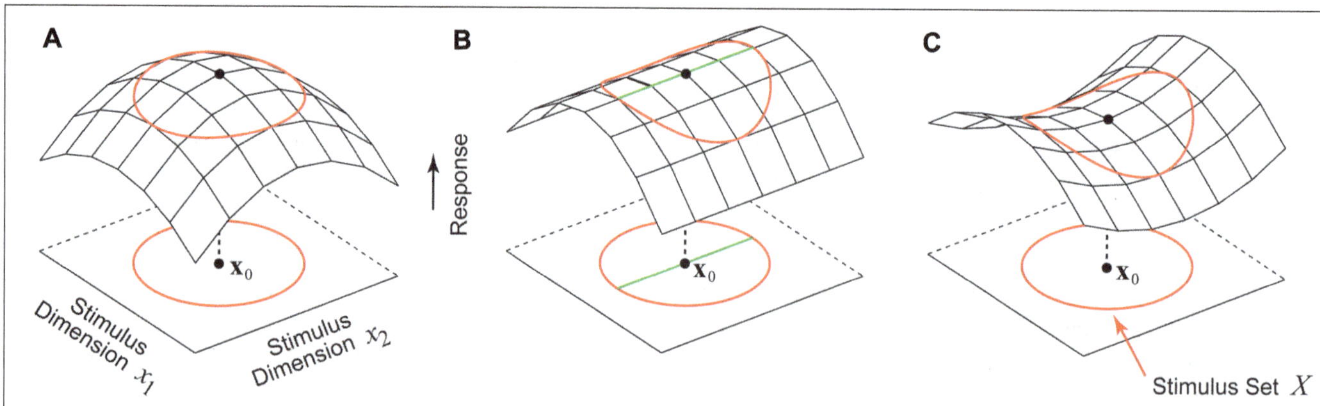

FIGURE 1 | Hypothetical stimulus–response relationships for a sensory neuron. The red circle represents the boundary of the set of permissible stimuli. **(A)** Stimulus $\mathbf{x}_0$ is a firing rate peak which corresponds to the intuitive notion of the optimal stimulus where any perturbation away from $\mathbf{x}_0$ results in a decrease in the firing rate. **(B)** This neuron is tuned to one stimulus dimension but is insensitive to the second dimension. Instead of a single optimal stimulus $\mathbf{x}_0$ there is a continuum of optimal stimuli (green line). **(C)** A neuron whose stimulus–response function around the point $\mathbf{x}_0$ is saddle-shaped. Along one stimulus dimension $\mathbf{x}_0$ is a firing rate maximum, and along the other stimulus dimension $\mathbf{x}_0$ is a minimum.

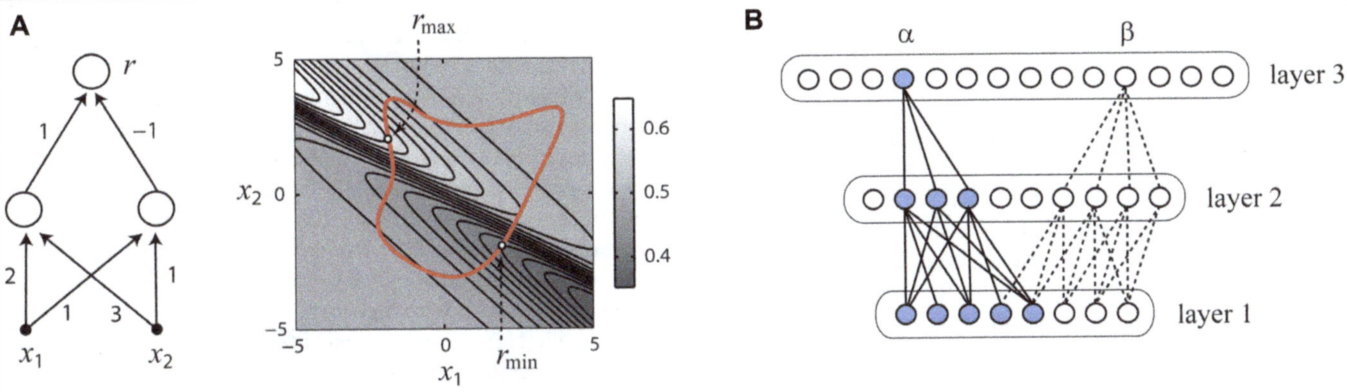

FIGURE 2 | How the optimal stimulus properties of sensory neurons may be constrained by network architecture. Panels **(A,B)** adapted with permission from DiMattina and Zhang (2008). **(A)** A simple neural network (left) and its responses to inputs x_1, x_2 (right). The optimal stimulus for this network must lie on the boundary of any closed set of stimuli (right panel, thick red line). **(B)** The functional network connecting a single neuron (α or β) to the sensory periphery may have fewer units in successive processing layers (convergent), even if the overall number of neurons in successive processing layers is increasing (divergent).

peripheral sensory receptors (filled black circles) which linearly transduce stimulus the variables x_1, x_2 and pass their outputs to a pair of interneurons, which in turn converge onto the output neuron from which responses r are measured. Since there are physical limits on the intensities of stimuli which can be generated by laboratory equipment, we may reasonably assume that the collection X of permissible stimuli is some closed subset of the real plane consisting of an interior and boundary (rightmost panel, thick red line). We may also reasonably assume that each neuron's input–output property is a described by an increasing gain function $g(u)$. With these reasonable assumptions, it is simple to show that that the gradient of the function $f(\mathbf{x})$ implemented by this circuit cannot vanish, and thus an optimal stimulus which is a firing rate peak as in **Figure 1A** is impossible. Therefore, it follows that optimal stimulus must lie on the boundary of X (**Figure 2A**, right panel), with the exact location depending on the synaptic weights and other parameters of the network.

In general, it can be shown that for hierarchical neural networks which can be arranged into layers that if the gain functions are increasing, the number of neurons in successive layers is decreasing or constant, and weight matrices connecting successive layers are non-degenerate, then it is impossible for the optimal stimulus for any neuron in this network to be a firing rate peak like that illustrated in **Figure 1A** (DiMattina and Zhang, 2008). It is important to note that this result requires that the stimuli be defined in the space of activities of the input units to the neural network, such as image pixel luminances which are the inputs to the network. One interesting corollary of this result is that if the space X of permissible stimuli is bounded by a maximum power constraint $\sum_{i=1}^{n} x_i^2 \leq E$, the optimum firing rate will be obtained for a stimulus $\mathbf{x} \in X$ having the greatest power or contrast, since this stimulus will lie on the boundary. Indeed, for many sensory neurons in the visual, auditory, and somatosensory modalities, increasing the stimulus contrast monotonically increases the firing rate response (Albrecht and Hamilton, 1982; Cheng et al., 1994; Oram et al., 2002; Barbour and Wang, 2003b; Ray et al., 2008), which is interesting considering that convergent networks satisfying the conditions of the theorem can model the functional properties of many sensory neurons (Riesenhuber and Poggio, 1999, 2000; Lau et al., 2002; Prenger et al., 2004; Cadieu et al., 2007).

At first, this result may seem to be of limited applicability since it is well known that the numbers of neurons in successive processing stages can be widely divergent (Felleman and Van Essen, 1991). However, the theorem applies only to the *functional network* which connects a given neuron to the sensory periphery. For instance, in the example shown in **Figure 2B**, the functional network connecting neuron a to the input layer is a convergent network with the number of units decreasing from layer to layer (blue), whereas the full network is divergent with the number of units increasing from layer to layer. Similarly, it is important to note that the neural network to which we apply the theorem may not be a literal description of the actual neural circuit, but simply a mathematical description of the functional relationship between the stimulus parameters and the neural response. For instance, a standard functional model of the ventral visual stream postulates a feedforward architecture similar to the models of complex cells postulated by Hubel and Wiesel (Riesenhuber and Poggio, 1999, 2000), and the theorem can be applied to neurons in these models. Similarly, divisive normalization models postulated for visual and auditory neurons (Heeger, 1992b; Koelling and Nykamp, 2012) can be re-written in a form to which the theorem applies and shown to have a non-vanishing gradient (Koelling and Nykamp, 2012).

ADAPTIVE OPTIMIZATION OF FIRING RATE

Despite the conceptual difficulties with the notion of an optimal stimulus, it provides sensory neuroscience with an intuitive first-pass description of neural function when an appropriate quantitative model is unknown. In this section, we discuss adaptive stimulus optimization methods which have been utilized experimentally for optimizing the firing rate of sensory neurons in high-dimensional stimulus spaces where a full factorial exploration would be intractable. Mathematically, the optimization problem may be specified as that of finding

$$\mathbf{x}^* = \arg\max_{\mathbf{x}\in X} f(\mathbf{x}), \quad (1)$$

where $\mathbf{x}^*$ is the optimal stimulus, f is the (unknown) stimulus–response function, and X is the set of allowable stimuli. Methods to optimize firing rate fall into two general categories: those that ascend the local gradient of the stimulus–response function, and those which utilize genetic or evolutionary approaches. We discuss each of these approaches and their relative merits, along with issues of adaptation and constrained stimulus spaces.

LOCAL HILL-CLIMBING

Due to the inherent variability in neural responses (Tolhurst et al., 1983; Rieke et al., 1997), optimizing the firing rate of sensory neurons is a difficult stochastic optimization problem (Spall, 2003). Early work on adaptive stimulus optimization was performed by Harth and Tzanakou (1974), who applied a method of stochastic gradient ascent known as ALOPEX, or "Algorithm of Pattern Extraction" to neurons in the frog visual tectum (Tzanakou et al., 1979). This method works by computing correlations between random perturbations of the current stimulus and changes in firing rate and using these correlations to iteratively update the current stimulus to increase the expected firing rate, eventually converging to the optimal stimulus. More recently, related methods have been employed to optimize the responses of neurons in the primary visual (Foldiak, 2001) and auditory (O'Connor et al., 2005) cortices, providing independent verification of previously described receptive field properties like orientation selectivity (Hubel and Wiesel, 1962) or inhibitory sidebands (Shamma et al., 1993). Variations of ALOPEX have also been utilized to quickly find the best frequency for auditory nerve fibers, an essential first step in many auditory neurophysiology experiments (Anderson and Micheli-Tzanakou, 2002).

In addition to these correlation-based approaches, numerous other computational methods have been utilized for firing rate optimization. One approach is to iteratively make local linear or quadratic approximations to the neural responses around a reference stimulus (Bandyopadhyay et al., 2007a; Koelling and Nykamp, 2008, 2012), which can then be used to determine a good search directions in the stimulus space. This approach has been utilized by Young and colleagues in order to determine that the optimal stimulus for neurons in the dorsal cochlear nucleus is a spectral edge centered at the neuron's best frequency (Bandyopadhyay et al., 2007b), consistent with suggestions from previous studies (Reiss and Young, 2005). An alternative optimization method which does not require estimating the local response function gradient is the Nelder–Mead simplex search (Nelder and Mead, 1965), which has been used to optimize the responses of neurons in cat auditory cortex to four-tone complexes (Nelken et al., 1994).

GENETIC ALGORITHMS

One limitation of the stimulus optimization methods above is that they are local searches which iteratively update the location of a single point (or simplex of points). Therefore, it is certainly possible for optimization runs to end up stuck at local firing rate maxima. Furthermore points of vanishing gradient do not necessarily indicate maxima (Koelling and Nykamp, 2012), as we can see from the examples in **Figure 1**. Furthermore, local search methods only identify a single optimal stimulus, and do not sample the stimulus space richly enough to fully describe neural coding. One possible alternative adaptive optimization method used in previous neurophysiological studies which can potentially surmount both of these problems is a *genetic algorithm* (Goldberg, 1989). A genetic algorithm works by populating the stimulus space widely with many stimuli (analogous to "organisms"), which survive to the next generation with a probability proportional to the firing rate they elicit (analogous to their "fitness"). The parameters of the surviving stimuli are combined at random in a factorial manner ("crossing-over") and mutated in order to produce a new generation of different stimuli based on the properties of the current generation. Over several iterations of this algorithm, a lineage of stimuli will evolve which maximizes the firing rate of the neuron under study, and since the sampling of the stimulus space is non-local, genetic algorithms are more likely to avoid the problem of local maxima than hill-climbing methods.

Genetic algorithms were applied to neurophysiology studies by Winter and colleagues, who optimized the parameters of amplitude-modulated tones defined in a four-dimensional space in order to study neural coding in the inferior colliculus (Bleeck et al., 2003). The optimal stimuli found by this method were in agreement with tuning functions found by traditional methods, thereby validating the procedure. More recently, a very powerful demonstration of genetic algorithms as a tool for adaptive optimization was given by Connor and colleagues studying the representation of two-dimensional shape in V4 (Carlson et al., 2011) and three-dimensional shape in the inferotemporal cortex (Yamane et al., 2008; Hung et al., 2012). The parameter space needed to define three-dimensional shapes is immense and impossible to explore factorially, with most of the stimuli in this space being ineffective. Nevertheless, a genetic algorithm was successful at finding shape stimuli having features which were effective at driving neurons, with the optimization results being consistent over multiple runs. Furthermore, because the genetic algorithm cross-over step generates stimuli which factorially combine different stimulus dimensions, it did a sufficiently thorough job of sampling the stimulus space to permit the investigators to fit predictive models which accurately described the tuning of the neurons to arbitrary shape stimuli (Yamane et al., 2008).

As reviewed above, the different methods developed for automatically optimizing firing rate responses of sensory neurons differ greatly, both in their general search strategy (i.e., gradient ascent versus genetic algorithms) as well as their exact methods for implementing that strategy (Nelken et al., 1994; Foldiak, 2001; Koelling and Nykamp, 2012). Furthermore, it is important to note that while genetic algorithms are a commonly chosen alternative to gradient ascent in the existing literature (Bleeck et al., 2003; Yamane et al., 2008; Chambers et al., 2012; Hung et al., 2012), a wide variety of alternative optimization methods could in principle be applied as well, such as simulated annealing (Kirkpatrick et al., 1983), and particle swarm optimization (Kennedy and Eberhart, 1995). However, without direct comparisons of algorithms on benchmark problems using numerical simulation, it is hard to directly and fairly compare these various methods. As automated stimulus optimization becomes more widely used in physiological experiments, systematic comparison of optimization methods on benchmark problems is certainly an interesting avenue for future research in computational neuroscience.

STIMULUS SPACE CONSTRAINTS

Quite often, one may wish to optimize neuronal responses in a constrained stimulus space for constraints which are more complex than simple upper and lower bounds on stimulus dimensions. For many neurons one can always increase the firing rate simply by increasing the stimulus energy or contrast (Albrecht and Hamilton, 1982; Cheng et al., 1994; Oram et al., 2002), so it is of interest to optimize the stimulus with the constraint of fixed stimulus energy. In Eq. 1, the optimal stimulus is defined over the set of all allowable stimuli, X, which depends on the constraints in the stimulus space. When each component of the stimulus $\mathbf{x} = (x_1, \ldots, x_n)^T$ is constrained between an upper bound and a lower bound (e.g., the luminance of image pixels has a limited range of possible values), the set X is a hypercube:

$$X = \left\{\mathbf{x} : a_i \leq x_i \leq b_i,\ i = 1, \ldots, n\right\}. \quad (2)$$

With a quadratic energy constraint, the allowable stimulus set X should become a hyper-sphere:

$$X = \left\{\mathbf{x} : \sum_{i=1}^{n} x_i^2 = E\right\}. \quad (3)$$

For example, Lewi et al. (2009) derived a fast procedure for optimization for effective model estimation under stimulus power constraints. Optimizing the stimulus in Eq. 1 subject to an energy constraint is an optimization problem for which there are many numerical methods for solutions (Douglas et al., 2000; Nocedal and Wright, 2006).

In special cases where there is prior information about the functional form of $f(\mathbf{x})$, the constrained optimization problem may permit numerically elegant solutions for finding optimal stimuli subject to non-linear constraints, as well as finding invariant transformations of a stimulus which leave responses unchanged. A recent study (Berkes and Wiskott, 2006, 2007) considered the problem of optimizing the responses of any neuron whose functional properties are given by an inhomogeneous quadratic form $f(\mathbf{x}) = \mathbf{x}^T\mathbf{A}\mathbf{x} + \mathbf{b}^T\mathbf{x} + c$, subject to an energy constraint $\mathbf{x}^T\mathbf{x} = E$. This study presented a very efficient algorithm for computing the optimal stimulus $\mathbf{x}^*$ which requires only a bounded one-dimensional search for a Lagrange multiplier, followed by analytical calculation of the optimal stimulus. In addition, they demonstrated a procedure for finding approximate invariant transformations in the constrained stimulus space, which for complex cells amount to shifts in the phase of a Gabor patch. As quadratic models have become popular tools for characterizing non-linear sensory neurons (Heeger, 1992a; Yu and Young, 2000; Simoncelli et al., 2004; Berkes and Wiskott, 2005; Bandyopadhyay et al., 2007a), their algorithm offers a useful tool for sensory neuroscience.

NEURAL RESPONSE ADAPTATION

It is well known that when the same stimulus is presented repeatedly to sensory neurons, they exhibit firing rate adaptation, becoming less sensitive to that stimulus over time (Ulanovsky et al., 2003; Asari and Zador, 2009). Similarly, responses to sensory stimuli can often non-stationary and are affected by context provided by preceding stimuli (Bartlett and Wang, 2005). Adaptation potentially presents a difficulty for stimulus optimization methods, since toward the end of the optimization run as the algorithm converges on a (locally) optimal stimulus, a series of very similar stimuli may be presented repeatedly, thereby leading to firing rate adaptation. This phenomena has been observed in studies in the published literature (Yamane et al., 2008) and presents a potential obstacle to studies of adaptive stimulus optimization (Koelling and Nykamp, 2012). Given the suppression of neural responses to stimuli which occur with high probability (Ulanovsky et al., 2003), one way of dealing with adaptation may be to intersperse random stimuli with those generated by the optimization run, so as to reduce adaptation effects. However, this may be an inefficient method for dealing with adaptation, since it increases the number of stimuli needed in an experiment (Koelling and Nykamp, 2012).

Apart from these technical considerations, the problem of firing rate adaptation illustrates a fundamental conceptual limitation of phenomenological sensory neurophysiology. In particular, it demonstrates that the act of probing a sensory neuron with stimuli can potentially changes the response properties of the neuron itself, possibly including its optimal stimulus. Therefore, it may not be conceptually correct to characterize the stimulus optimization problem as it is written in Eq. 1, but rather to characterize it as a far more complicated optimization problem where the function $f(\mathbf{x}, \mathbf{h}(t))$ to be optimized is constantly changing, dependent on both the stimulus $\mathbf{x}$ and response history $\mathbf{h}(t)$. In this case, the optimal stimulus for a given neuron may only be well-defined with respect to a given history of stimuli and responses.

One solution to this problem would be to have a mathematical model of the neuron's stimulus–response function which takes adaptation into account. Indeed, recent work has demonstrated that bilinear models of sensory neurons incorporating adaptation parameters can greatly improve predictions when compared standard linear receptive field models (Ahrens et al., 2008a). Other work has shown that the failure of spectrotemporal receptive field (STRF) models to account fully for neural responses to natural stimuli may be accounted for by rapid synaptic depression (David et al., 2009), further underscoring the importance of including adaptation parameters in neural models. We discuss the issues of neuronal adaptation and stimulus-response history further when we discuss the estimation of neural models using active data collection.

On the whole however, the problem of adaptation does not seem to pose a fatal limitation to adapting firing rate optimization, as it has been applied successfully in many recent studies (Foldiak, 2001; O'Connor et al., 2005). Furthermore, there are many neurons in the brain for which adaptation effects are small and thus do not pose a concern (Ingham and McAlpine, 2004). These methods are potentially of great importance for investigating neural coding of complex stimuli defined in high-dimensional spaces (Yamane et al., 2008), and it is of great interest to better understand how adaptation affects stimulus optimization and receptive field characterization.

ISO-RESPONSE SURFACES AND MODEL COMPARISON

In high-dimensional stimulus spaces, the same response from a sensory neuron can be elicited by a continuum of equally effective optimal stimuli rather than a single optimal stimulus (**Figure 1**). Therefore, in some experiments it may be of interest to find sets of equivalent stimuli known as *iso-response surfaces* which yield the same response. One possible way of formalizing an optimization problem for this class of experiments is to formulate it as finding stimuli

$$\mathbf{x}^* = \arg\min_{\mathbf{x} \in X} d(f(\mathbf{x}), c), \quad (4)$$

which $d(\cdot, \cdot)$ is some metric measure (e.g., squared error) quantifying the discrepancy between the desired response c and the neuronal response $f(\mathbf{x})$. Multiple optimization runs from different starting locations and for different values of the desired constant response c permit the experimenter to determine families of iso-rate surfaces for the neuron under study. The geometrical shapes of the iso-rate surfaces can help to determine how stimulus variables $x_1, \ldots, x_n$ are integrated, and thus provide a useful tool for comparison of hypothetical models. For instance, linear integration of stimulus energy would yield iso-response surfaces which are hyperplanes of the form $\sum_{i=1}^{n} x_i = c$, whereas non-linear integration would yield non-planar iso-response surfaces. **Figure 3** illustrates iso-response surfaces for two different hypothetical sensory processing models.

The iso-response surface method was used by Gollisch et al. (2002) to test several competing hypotheses about how spectral energy is integrated in locust auditory receptors. The iso-response contours to combinations of two or three pure tone stimuli with fixed frequencies and variable amplitudes were of elliptical shape, consistent with an energy-integrator model of spectral integration. Further work extended the iso-response method to incorporate temporal integration, yielding a complete cascade model of auditory transduction (Gollisch and Herz, 2005).

A more recent study applied this technique to study the integration of visual contrast over space in salamander retinal ganglion cells, revealing a threshold-quadratic non-linearity in the receptive field center as well as a subset of ganglion cells most sensitive to spatially homogeneous stimuli (Bölinger and Gollisch, 2012). The iso-response surface method has also been applied fruitfully in mammalian sensory systems as well. A recent study by Horwitz and Hass (2012) utilized this procedure to study integration of color signals from the three retinal cone types in single neurons in the primary visual cortex. It was found that half of the neurons had planar iso-response surfaces, consistent with linear integration of cone signals. However, the other half showed a variety of non-linear iso-response surfaces, including cup-shaped surfaces indicating sensitivity to only narrow regions of color space.

Although the iso-response surface method has been applied successfully in stimulus spaces of low dimensionality (two or three dimensions), tracing out level hyper-surfaces in higher-dimensional spaces may pose a formidable computational challenge (Han et al., 2003; Willett and Nowak, 2007). In future research, dimensionality reduction procedures might be useful for extending the iso-response surface method to high-dimensional stimulus spaces like pixel space or auditory frequency space (Yu and Young, 2000), as well as for high-dimensional spaces defining complex naturalistic stimuli like 3D shapes or species-specific communication sounds (DiMattina and Wang, 2006; Yamane et al., 2008).

MAXIMALLY INFORMATIVE STIMULUS ENSEMBLES

It has been proposed that one of the major goals of sensory coding is to efficiently represent the natural environment (Barlow, 1961; Simoncelli, 2003). In this spirit, another class of closed-loop stimulus optimization methods has been developed to find the optimal *ensemble* of sensory stimuli for maximizing the mutual information between stimuli and neural responses (Machens, 2002). This method differs from efforts to find the optimal stimulus or efforts to find iso-response surfaces because the goal is not to find an individual stimulus $\mathbf{x}^*$ which optimizes the desired criterion (i.e., Eq. 1), but rather to find the optimal distribution $p^*(\mathbf{x})$ which optimizes the mutual information $I(y; \mathbf{x})$, where y denotes the observed neural response (typically the firing rate of a single neuron). Mathematically, we write

$$p^*(\mathbf{x}) = \arg\max_{p(\mathbf{x}) \in P} I(y; \mathbf{x}) = \int_X \int_Y p(y \mid \mathbf{x}) p(\mathbf{x}) \ln \frac{p(y \mid \mathbf{x})}{p(y)} d\mathbf{x} dy, \quad (5)$$

where P is the space of probability densities on the stimulus space X, and $p(y \mid \mathbf{x})$ and $p(y)$ are determined experimentally by observing neural responses to stimuli. In practice, one starts with an assumption of a uniform distribution with finite support and then applies the Blahut–Arimoto algorithm (Blahut, 1972; Arimoto, 1972) to iteratively update the sampling weights (Machens, 2002). This method has been applied experimentally to characterize grasshopper auditory receptor neurons, demonstrating optimality for processing behaviorally relevant species-specific communication sounds (Machens et al., 2005; Benda et al., 2007).

ADAPTIVE OPTIMIZATION FOR SENSORY MODEL ESTIMATION

An ideal gold standard for sensory neuroscience is to obtain a complete and accurate functional stimulus–response model of the neuron under study. In theory, once such a model is attained, one can then numerically or analytically calculate from this model the neuron's optimal stimulus, its iso-response surfaces, and its maximally informative stimulus ensembles. That is, if one identifies the system, one gets "for free" other information one may be interested in. However, despite its conceptual appeal, the problem of system identification is of great practical difficulty. This is because one needs to specify an accurate yet experimentally tractable model whose parameters can be estimated from data obtained during the available observation time. Unfortunately, research in computational neuroscience has shown that tractable (e.g., linear and quadratic) models are not accurate, whereas more biologically accurate models (deep, multiple layer neural networks incorporating dynamics, recurrence, etc.) often pose intractable parameter estimation problems.

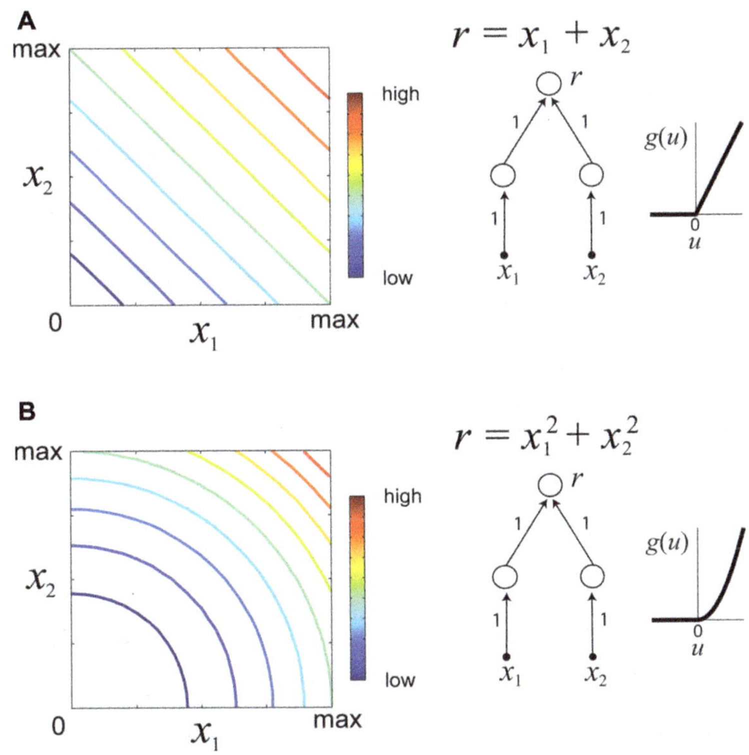

FIGURE 3 | Examples of iso-responses surfaces for two hypothetical sensory processing models. (A) Iso-response contours (left) of a sensory neuron which linearly integrates stimulus variables $x_1, x_2 \geq 0$. The response r of this neuron is a summation of the outputs of two neurons in the lower layer with a threshold-linear gain function (right). Colors in the contour plot represent neural firing rates from low to high. **(B)** Iso-responses contours (right) of a sensory neuron which non-linearly integrates stimulus variables $x_1, x_2 \geq 0$ with a threshold-quadratic gain function (right).

It is well known from the fields of statistics and machine learning that one can more quickly and accurately estimate the parameters of a function using adaptive data collection, where new observations are generated in an iterative, adaptive manner which optimize the expected utility of the responses given the goal of estimating the model parameters (Lindley, 1956; Bernardo, 1979; MacKay, 1992). Mathematically, the optimization problem is to find at each iteration

$$\mathbf{x}_{n+1}^{*} = \arg\max_{\mathbf{x} \in X} U_n^{(E)}(\mathbf{x}), \qquad (6)$$

where $U_n^{(E)}(\mathbf{x})$ is the estimation utility function based on the data of the first n stimulus–response pairs. There are many choices for this function, including expected squared error (Müller and Parmigiani, 1995), expected prediction error (Sugiyama, 2006), and mutual information between stimuli and model parameters (Paninski, 2005). The generic name for this strategy is *optimal experimental design* or OED (Federov, 1972; Atkinson and Donev, 1992; Cohn et al., 1996), and it is often studied in a Bayesian framework (MacKay, 1992; Chaloner and Verdinelli, 1995). Recent theoretical and experimental work has shown that such methods can potentially be fruitfully applied in neuroscientific experiments (Paninski, 2005; Paninski et al., 2007; Lewi et al., 2009, 2011; DiMattina and Zhang, 2011). Not only can optimal experimental design make the estimation of high-dimensional models practical (Lewi et al., 2009), but can also make it tractable to estimate highly non-linear models which cannot be readily identified from random "white noise" data of the kind typically used in system identification experiments (DiMattina and Zhang, 2010, 2011). We first discuss the application of such methods in psychology and cognitive science, and then discuss recent theoretical and experimental work on applications of OED methods to sensory neurophysiology experiments

ADAPTIVE STIMULUS OPTIMIZATION IN PSYCHOLOGY AND COGNITIVE SCIENCE

Psychophysics has long utilized adaptive data collection, with the classic example being the staircase method for threshold estimation (Cornsweet, 1962). More recently, an adaptive Bayesian approach to threshold estimation (QUEST) which chooses new stimuli for each trial at the current Bayesian estimate of the threshold was developed (Watson and Pelli, 1983), and subsequent work extended this approach to permit simultaneous estimation of both the threshold and slope of the psychometric function (Snoeren and Puts, 1997). Another line of work applied an information-theoretic approach to estimating the slope and threshold parameters, where stimuli were chosen at each trial to maximize the expected information gained about the slope and threshold parameters (Kontsevich and Tyler, 1999). More sophisticated methods of this kind have been utilized for psychometric functions defined on two-dimensional stimuli (Kujala and Lukka, 2006), with these procedures being applied for estimating contrast sensitivity functions (Lesmes et al., 2010) and color sensitivity of human observers (Kujala and Lukka, 2006). In addition to finding widespread application in sensory psychophysics, adaptive methods have also been used more broadly in the cognitive sciences (Wixted and Ebbesen, 1991; Rubin and Wenzel, 1996; Nosofsky and Zaki, 2002; Opfer and Siegler, 2007; Kujala et al., 2010; McCullough et al., 2010).

GENERALIZED LINEAR MODELS AND BIOPHYSICAL MODELS

More recently, investigators in computational neuroscience have demonstrated that adaptive information-theoretic sampling where stimuli are chosen to maximize the expected information gain between a stimulus and the model parameters can be a highly effective means of estimating the parameters of sensory processing models (Paninski, 2005; Paninski et al., 2007). A fast information-theoretic algorithm has been developed for the generalized linear model which applies a static non-linearity to the output (Lewi et al., 2009). The generalized linear model has been utilized in numerous studies (Simoncelli et al., 2004) and enjoys a likelihood function with no local maxima (Paninski, 2004). Their algorithm relied on a Gaussian approximation to the posterior density, permitting fast recursive updates, with the calculations for finding the optimal stimulus growing only as the square of the stimulus space dimensionality. Numerical simulations demonstrated that their procedure was asymptotically efficient, with the empirically computed variance of the posterior density converging to the minimum theoretically possible variance.

One issue which potentially affects studies of stimulus optimization is neuronal adaptation due to the stimulus history (Ulanovsky et al., 2003; Asari and Zador, 2009). In sensory neurons, this may be manifested as the system actually changing its underlying parameters which we seek to estimate as the experiment progresses. However, the procedure developed by Lewi et al. (2009) was demonstrated to be robust to parameter drift in numerical simulations, suggesting the ability to compensate for changes to the system brought about by adaptation effects. Furthermore, their model also permits the estimation of a spike-history filter, allowing neuronal response history to influence predictions to new stimuli.

A further study by this group applied this algorithm to fitting generalized linear models to avian auditory neurons probed with conspecific song samples, and it was found that accurate estimation could be obtained using vastly fewer samples when they were chosen adaptively using the algorithm then when they were chosen non-adaptively (Lewi et al., 2011). Although this procedure has yet to be applied in real on-line experiments, it provides experimenters working on a variety of systems with a powerful tool for quickly characterizing neurons whose responses are well described by generalized linear models (Chichilnisky, 2001) or related models (Pillow et al., 2008).

More recently, this group has also applied optimal experimental design to the cellular neuroscience problem of accurately estimating voltages from dendritic trees using measurements suffering from low signal-to-noise ratio (Huggins and Paninski, 2012). Using simulated compartmental models, these authors demonstrated that by adaptively choosing observation locations which minimize the expected squared error of the voltage measurement, a substantial improvement in accuracy was obtained compared to random sampling. This procedure is potentially of great experimental usefulness because techniques like two-photon imaging permit spatially complete observations of dendrites, but with low signal-to-noise ratios (Djurisic et al., 2008; Canepari et al., 2010).

MULTIPLE LAYER NEURAL NETWORKS

Since many sensory neurons are non-linear (Young et al., 2005; Wu et al., 2006), it is of interest to characterize neurons using various non-linear models, including quadratic and bilinear models (Yu and Young, 2000; Berkes and Wiskott, 2006; Ahrens et al., 2008a,b), neural networks (Lau et al., 2002; Prenger et al., 2004; Cadieu et al., 2007) and basis function networks (Poggio and Girosi, 1990). A generalized linear model is also a non-linear model because it employs a static non-linearity at the output stage. Although a generalized linear model allows limited non-linearities, it enjoys tractable and consistent estimation procedures without problems of local minima (Paninski, 2004). Identifying more complex non-linear models like hierarchical neural networks from physiological data tends to be harder due to problems like local minima and plateaus in the error surface (Amari et al., 2006; Cousseau et al., 2008; Wei and Amari, 2008; Wei et al., 2008).

For studies aimed at estimating generalized linear models, the use of a fixed white-noise stimulus set is often quite effective and is theoretically well-justified (Chichilnisky, 2001; Paninski, 2004; Wu et al., 2006). However, recent theoretical work suggests that using fixed stimulus sets like white noise may be deeply problematic for efforts to identify non-linear hierarchical network models due to *continuous parameter confounding* (DiMattina and Zhang, 2010). This problem is illustrated for a very simple non-linear neural network model shown in **Figure 4A**. In this example, the goal is to recover the parameters (w,v) of the network by performing maximum likelihood (ML) estimation given noisy stimulus–response observations. When the input stimuli x only drive the hidden unit over a region of its gain function which can be well approximated by a power function (**Figure 4B**, top), the estimates obtained by ML for different datasets lie scattered along the continuum $vw^{\alpha} = C$, as one would expect for a power law gain function $g(u) = Au^{\alpha}$ (**Figure 4C**, top). (Here the constant $C = v_T w_T^{\alpha}$, where w_T and v_T are the true values of the input and output weights.) In contrast, when the input stimuli x drive the hidden unit over a full range of its gain so that the power law approximation is poor (**Figure 4B**, bottom), the true parameters are accurately recovered for different datasets (**Figure 4C**, bottom).

A hypothetical experiment which suffers from this problem is illustrated in **Figure 5**. We see that when the network in **Figure 5A** is probed with random stimuli (**Figure 5B**, right), the hidden unit is driven over a limited range of its gain function which may be well approximated by an exponential, so that the sigmoidal gain (**Figure 5C**, black curve) may *de facto* be replaced by a new exponential gain function $g(u) = Ae^{\alpha u}$ (**Figure 5C**, red curve). With this new gain, it follows that a continuum of different values of the output weight v and bias w_0 lying on the curve $ve^{\alpha w_0} = C$ will yield models whose responses to the training data are

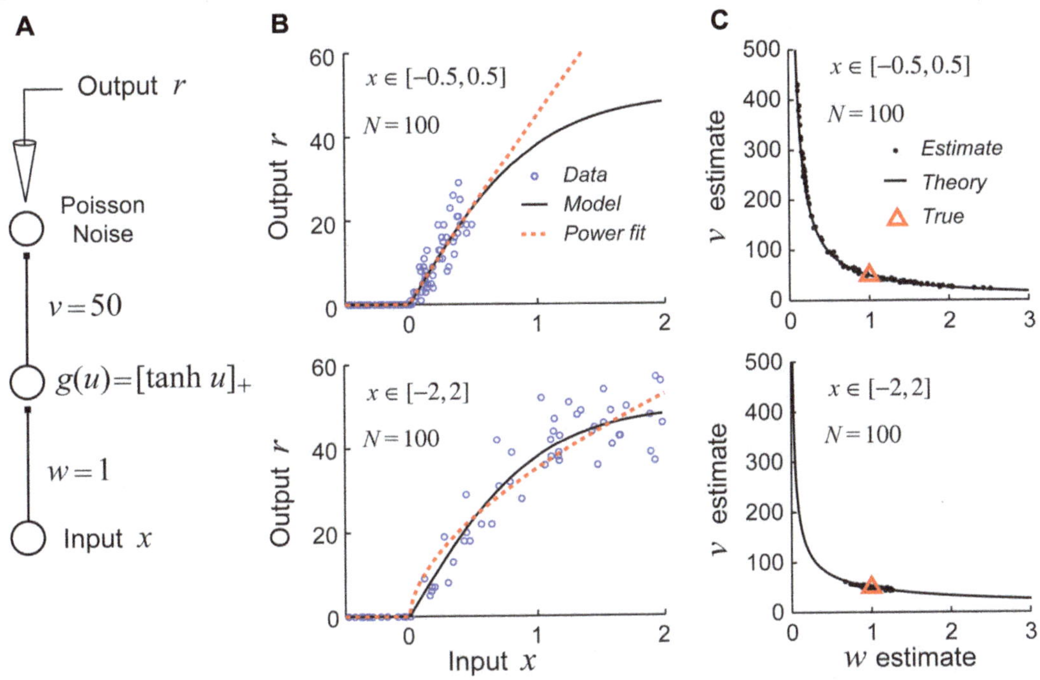

FIGURE 4 | Example of continuous parameter confounding in a simple non-linear neural network model. Adapted with permission from DiMattina and Zhang (2010). **(A)** A simple three layer neural network whose input and output weight parameters (w, v) we wish to estimate from noisy stimulus–response data. Noise is drawn from a Poisson distribution. **(B)** *Top*: The input stimuli $x \in [-0.5, 0.5]$ only drive the hidden unit over a limited region of its gain function (black curve) which may be well approximated by a power law function (red dashed line). *Bottom*: The input stimuli $x \in [-2, 2]$ drive the hidden unit over a larger region of its gain function which is poorly approximated by a power law function. **(C)** *Top*: When trained with sets of stimuli like that in the top of **Figure 4B**, the estimates (black dots) lie scattered along the curve predicted by the power law confounding theory. *Bottom*: When trained with sets of stimuli like those in the bottom panel of **Figure 4B**, the true parameter values (red triangle) are more reliably recovered.

indistinguishable and therefore multiple estimates of these parameters from different random training sets will lie scattered along this curve (**Figure 5D**). (Here the constant $C = v_T e^{\alpha w_{0T}}$ where V_T and w_{0T} are the true values of the output weight and hidden unit bias.)

Adaptive stimulus optimization methods like information-theoretic sampling (Paninski, 2005) can in principle overcome this problem of continuous parameter confounding, as we see in **Figure 5D** where the correct network parameters are reliably recovered when optimally designed stimuli (**Figure 5B**, left) are used. This simple example suggests that adaptive stimulus optimization may make it tractable to reliably recover the parameters of complex hierarchical networks needed to model non-linear neurons, whereas it is much harder to recover these networks using standard stimulus sets like white noise.

Many previous studies in the statistics and machine learning literature have demonstrated that faster convergence and smaller generalization error may be obtained when neural networks are trained adaptively using optimally designed stimuli (Lindley, 1956; MacKay, 1992; Cohn et al., 1994). Recently, we have developed a practical method for implementing the information-theoretic stimulus optimization approach derived for generalized linear models (Lewi et al., 2009) for arbitrary non-linear models like hierarchical neural networks. Although this method employs numerous approximations, it has been shown in simulated experiments to be effective at recovering non-linear neural networks having multiple hidden units, and is fast enough to utilize in real experiments (Tam et al., 2011; Dekel, 2012; Tam, 2012).

ADAPTIVE OPTIMIZATION FOR SENSORY MODEL COMPARISON

Quite often the appropriate model for describing a sensory neuron or perceptual quantity is unknown. Therefore, an important experimental goal may be to discriminate between two or more competing models. Mathematically, the optimization problem is to iteratively find stimuli

$$\mathbf{x}_{n+1}^{*} = \arg\max_{\mathbf{x}} U_n^{(C)}(\mathbf{x}), \tag{7}$$

which optimize a model comparison utility function $U_n^{(C)}(\mathbf{x})$, one choice of which may be the expected reduction in model space entropy (Cavagnaro et al., 2010; DiMattina and Zhang, 2011). This equation may be regarded as the optimal comparison counterpart of the equation for optimal estimation (Eq. 6). We now briefly discuss recent studies making use of adaptive stimulus optimization for model selection.

PSYCHOPHYSICAL MODEL COMPARISON

Although standard model comparison methods like the Bayesian Information Criterion (BIC; Schwarz, 1978) or predictive

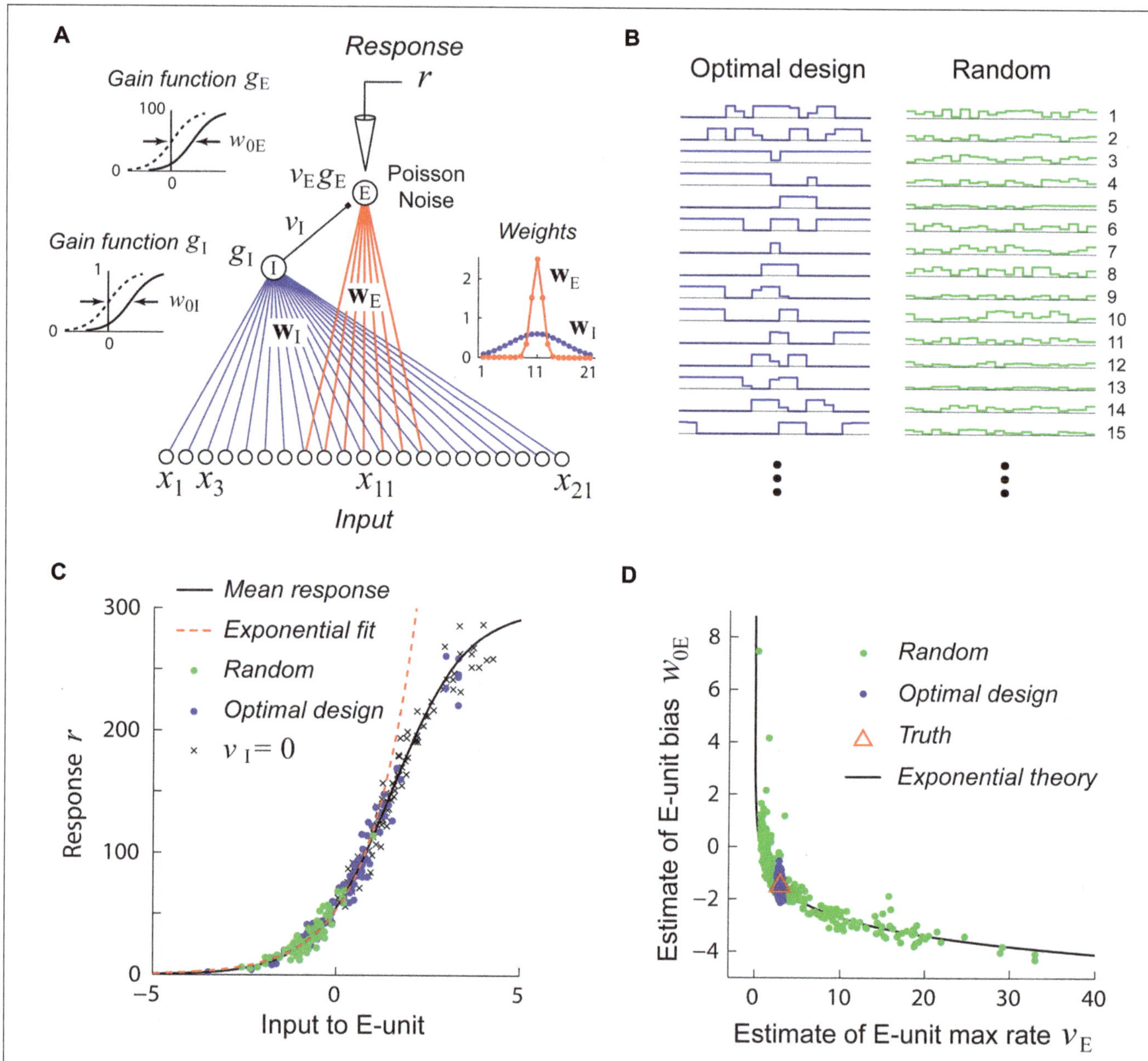

FIGURE 5 | Stimuli which are adaptively optimized for accurate parameter estimation can be more effective than random stimuli for recovering non-linear models. Adapted with permission from DiMattina and Zhang (2011). **(A)** A simple center-surround neural network consisting of a narrowly integrating excitatory output unit (E-unit) which receives inhibitory input from a broadly integrating interneuron (I-unit). **(B)** Examples of optimally designed (left) and random (right) stimuli. Note that the optimally designed stimuli exhibit complex correlated structure. **(C)** Random stimuli (green dots) only drive the E-unit over a limited range of its gain function (black curve) which may be well approximated by an exponential function (red dashed line). This is due to inhibition from the I-unit, as can be seen by setting $v_I = 0$ (crosses). By contrast, optimally designed stimuli (blue dots) drive the gain function over its full range. **(D)** Estimates attained from training with random stimuli (green dots) exhibit continuous parameter confounding between the output weight and bias, as predicted by the exponential theory (black curve). In contrast, estimates attained from optimally designed stimuli accurately recover the true parameters (red triangle).

cross-validation may be applied *post hoc* (Vladusich et al., 2006; Wu et al., 2006), numerous studies suggest that performing experiments using stimuli optimized for model comparison may be far more effective (Atkinson and Fedorov, 1975a,b). One method for model comparison developed recently for psychophysical experiments is known as MAximum Differentiation (MAD) competition (Wang and Simoncelli, 2008). Given two perceptual models which relate stimulus parameters to a perceptual quantity, this method generates a pair of stimuli which maximizes/minimizes the response of one model while holding the other model's response fixed. Next, this procedure is repeated with the role of the two models reversed. Testing human subjects on the two pairs of synthesized stimuli can determine which model is "better" in the sense of telling us which model's max/min pairs are simpler to discriminate. This procedure has been fruitfully applied to comparing image quality assessment models which aim to predict human perception of image quality (Wang and Bovik, 2006)

An information-theoretic method for model comparison was recently derived by Cavagnaro et al. (2010). Given a set of models with the i-th model having prior probability $P_0(i)$, stimuli are chosen to maximize the mutual information between the stimulus and the model index i by minimizing the expected model space entropy in a manner directly analogous to information-theoretic model estimation (Paninski, 2005), except that in this case the unknown variable is a discrete model index i rather than a continuous parameter value $\boldsymbol{\theta}$. This method was applied to competing models of memory retention from the cognitive science literature (Rubin et al., 1999) and was shown to permit much more accurate discrimination than standard non-adaptive methods.

NEURAL MODEL COMPARISON

In general, the correct parameters of competing sensory processing models are not known beforehand. Therefore, it is of interest to consider how to conduct experiments which estimate and discriminate competing models. Typically, investigators in neurophysiology and neuroimaging have applied model-comparison techniques *post hoc* (David and Gallant, 2005; Vladusich et al., 2006; Penny, 2012), particularly in the system identification literature (Prenger et al., 2004; David and Gallant, 2005; Wu et al., 2006; Sharpee et al., 2008; Rabinowitz et al., 2012; Schinkel-Bielefeld et al., 2012). However, a fundamental limitation with *post hoc* analysis is that it is not possible to generate and test critical stimuli which are optimized for model comparison, as this is only possible while the system is under observation. This limitation can only be overcome by fitting multiple models to a sensory neuron during the course of an experiment and then using the fitted models to generate and present critical stimuli which are optimized to best discriminate the models. Although previous work has presented stimuli on-line to test or verify a single model (deCharms et al., 1998; Touryan et al., 2002), very little work in single-unit *in vivo* sensory neurophysiology has presented stimuli optimized for model comparison in real-time (Tam et al., 2011).

A recent study considered a two-stage approach for combining the goals of model estimation and comparison in neurophysiology experiments, illustrated schematically in **Figure 6A** (DiMattina and Zhang, 2011). In the first stage, stimuli are adaptively optimized for parameter estimation, with the optimal stimulus for each model being presented in turn. In the second stage, stimuli are generated adaptively in order to optimally discriminate competing models making use of an information-theoretic criterion (Cavagnaro et al., 2010) or a likelihood-based criterion. In the special case of two models $f_1(\mathbf{x}, \boldsymbol{\theta}_1)$, $f_2(\mathbf{x}, \boldsymbol{\theta}_2)$ and Gaussian response noise, it can be shown that under a likelihood criterion the best stimulus for model discrimination is the stimulus which maximizes the quantity $\left[f_1(\mathbf{x}, \boldsymbol{\theta}_1) - f_2(\mathbf{x}, \boldsymbol{\theta}_2)\right]^2$, and furthermore this stimulus will maximally increase the BIC in favor of the best model (DiMattina and Zhang, 2011).

Figure 6 illustrates a numerical experiment making use of this two-stage procedure for the problem of discriminating an additive and multiplicative model of neural responses (**Figure 6B**), where the additive model is assumed to be the true model. After the estimation phase, the BIC does not have a strong preference for either model, only being correct about half the time (**Figure 6C**). However, after presenting 500 stimuli optimized for discriminating the additive and multiplicative model and applying the BIC to all available data, the correct (additive) model is preferred for 24 of 25 Monte Carlo trials (red curve). As a control, presenting additional stimuli optimized for model estimation only improves final model selection moderately (blue curve), while presenting random stimuli does not at all improve model selection performance (green curve). This procedure has now been applied in neurophysiology experiments to generate critical stimuli to distinguish between two competing models of spectral processing by single neurons in the primate inferior colliculus (Tam et al., 2011; Tam, 2012).

DISCUSSION

With increasing computer power, it is becoming practical for neuroscience experiments to utilize adaptive stimulus optimization where stimuli are generated in real-time during the course of the experiment (Benda et al., 2007; Newman et al., 2013). Various experiments have utilized adaptive stimulus optimization in order to break the "curse of dimensionality" and find the optimal stimulus for a sensory neuron in spaces which are too large for factorial exploration (O'Connor et al., 2005; Yamane et al., 2008). However, simply characterizing the optimal stimulus for a sensory neuron provides at best only a partial description of neural coding (Olshausen and Field, 2005). Therefore, in addition to helping to find the optimal stimulus, adaptive stimulus optimization makes it possible to pursue engineering-inspired approaches to sensory neurophysiology which may yield greater functional insights, for instance finding stimulus ensembles maximizing information between stimuli (Machens, 2002; Machens et al., 2005) and neural responses or fitting and comparing multiple non-linear models to neural responses (Lewi et al., 2009; DiMattina and Zhang, 2011). **Table 1** summarizes the various closed-loop stimulus optimization paradigms discussed in this review, and **Figure 7** schematically illustrates the closed-loop experimental approach.

The vast majority of the work to date has applied closed-loop methods to studying scalar firing rate responses measured from single neurons. However, as closed-loop approaches are continuing to develop, and as new techniques like optical imaging (Ohki et al., 2005; Bock et al., 2011) are making it increasingly feasible to observe large numbers of neurons simultaneously, it is of great interest for future investigations to apply these methods to neural populations and to measurements beyond scalar firing rate. Here we briefly discuss some possible directions for future research.

While the notion of the optimal stimulus is well-defined for single neurons, it is not well-defined for neural populations. However, an alternative approach to stimulus optimization for a population of neurons is to find the stimulus at which the population is best at discriminating nearby stimuli, as opposed to the stimulus yielding the highest firing rate response. Indeed, it has been suggested by a number of investigators that high-slope regions of tuning curves, where nearby stimuli are best

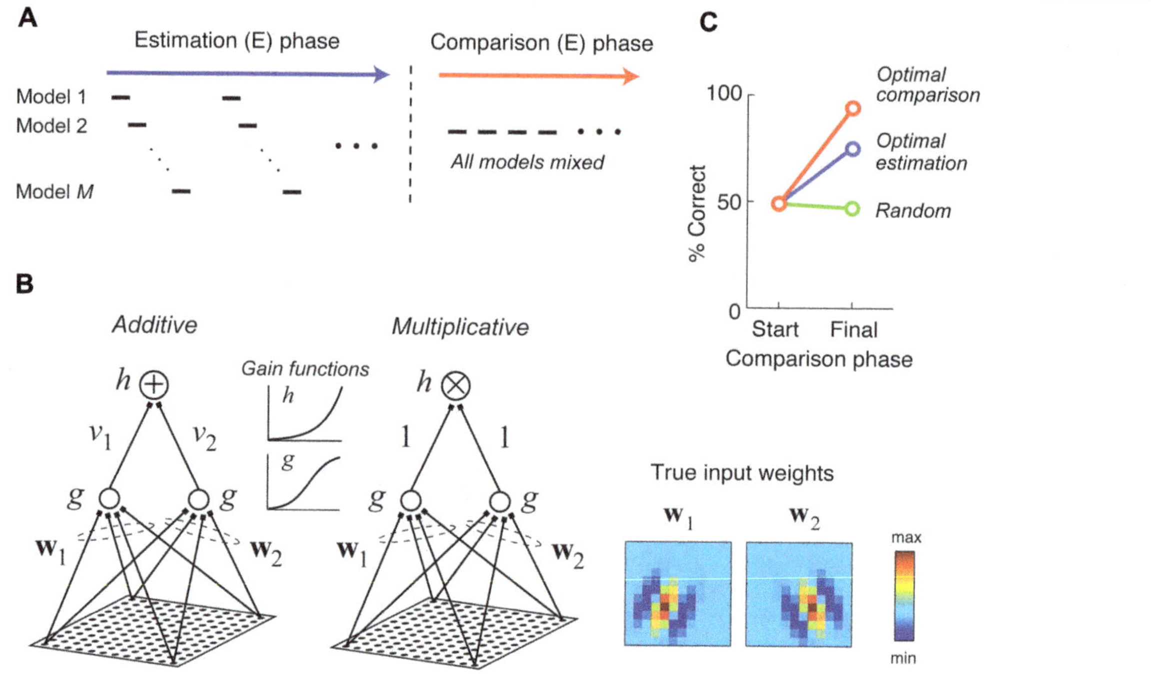

FIGURE 6 | Stimuli which are adaptively optimized for model comparison can lead to more accurate model selection. Adapted with permission from DiMattina and Zhang (2011). **(A)** A hypothetical two phase procedure for estimating and comparing multiple competing models. During the estimation (E) phase, stimuli are optimized in turn for estimating each model. During the comparison (C) phase, stimuli are optimized for comparing all of the models. **(B)** Two candidate models were fit to data generated by a true additive model whose input weights (w_1 and w_2) were 12 × 12 Gabor patches shown at the right. The two competing models differ only in their method of integrating subunit activities (additive versus multiplicative). **(C)** At the end of the estimation phase ("Start"), the BIC does not consistently prefer either model. Presenting additional stimuli optimized for model discrimination yields almost perfect model selection (red curve), while presenting additional random stimuli (green curve), or stimuli optimized for model estimation (blue curve) either does not improve or only somewhat improves model selection.

discriminated, are much more important in sensory coding than tuning curve peaks (Seung and Sompolinsky, 1993; Harper and McAlpine, 2004; Butts and Goldman, 2006; Bonnasse-Gahot and Nadal, 2008). Under reasonable assumptions of independent Poisson responses, the one-dimensional stimulus x at which a neural population can best discriminate nearby stimuli $x + \delta x$ is the stimulus which maximizes the Fisher information $I_F(x) = \sum_{i=1}^{N} [f_i'(x)]^2 / f_i(x)$, where $f_i(x)$ is the tuning curve of the i-th neuron (Dayan et al., 2001). It is relatively straightforward to extend this Fisher information formalism to higher dimensional stimulus spaces (Zhang and Sejnowski, 1999; Johnson et al., 2001; Bethge et al., 2002). Local approximation of the Fisher information matrix has been used in previous work aimed at stimulus optimization in a single neuron (Bandyopadhyay et al., 2007b), and this technique could readily generalize to find the stimulus which is best discriminated from nearby stimuli by a population code.

Extension of the definition of iso-response surfaces (Gollisch et al., 2002) to multiple neurons is relatively straightforward. In particular, if we can view each neuron as implementing a function $f(\mathbf{x})$ on the stimulus space, then the region of stimulus space which simultaneously satisfies multiple constraints $f_1(\mathbf{x}) = c_1, \cdots, f_N(\mathbf{x}) = c_N$ should simply be the (possibly empty) intersection of the regions of stimulus space satisfying each individual constraint. It would be interesting to extend the maximally informative ensemble approach (Machens, 2002) to multiple neurons as well. One potential difficulty is that the number of possible responses which one needs to measure to compute

Table 1 | Summary of various closed-loop stimulus optimization approaches utilized in sensory systems neuroscience.

Optimization goal	Equation	Example references
Firing rate optimization	1	Nelken et al. (1994); O'Connor et al. (2005), Yamane et al. (2008); Koelling and Nykamp (2012)
Iso-response surfaces	4	Gollisch et al. (2002); Bölinger and Gollisch (2012), Horwitz and Hass (2012)
Maximally informative stimulus ensembles	5	Machens (2002); Machens et al. (2005)
On-line model estimation	6	Lewi et al. (2009, 2011), DiMattina and Zhang (2011)
On-line model comparison	7	Cavagnaro et al. (2010); DiMattina and Zhang (2011)

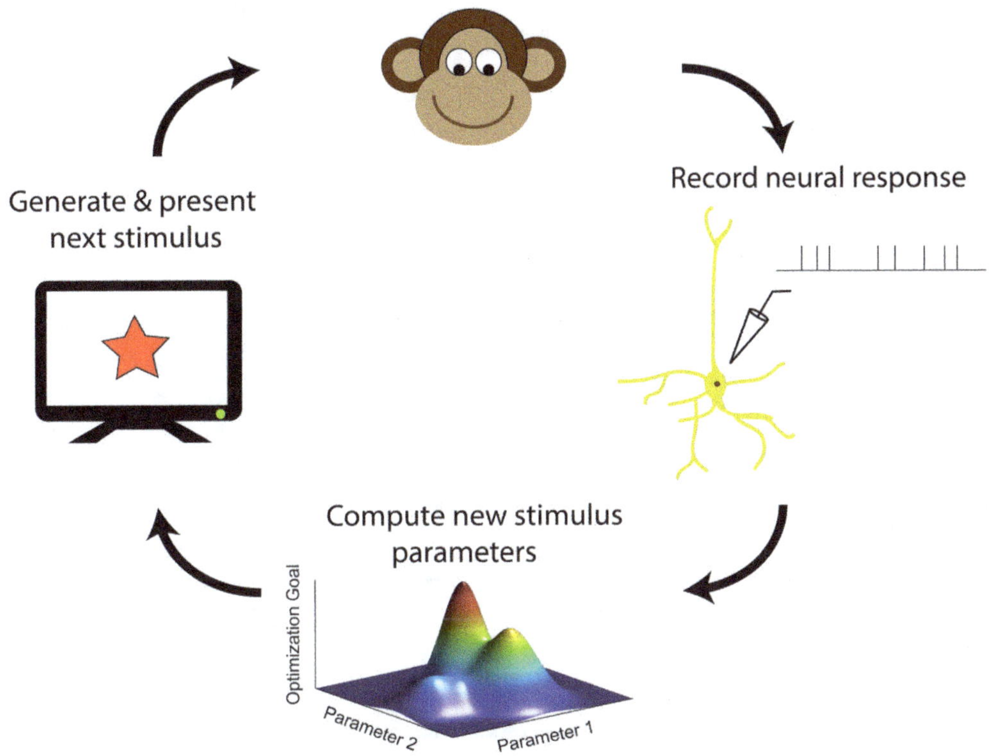

FIGURE 7 | A schematic summary of closed-loop approaches in sensory neurophysiology. Neural responses to previous stimuli are used in order to choose new stimuli, by maximizing an objective function for accomplishing a desired experimental goal (see also **Table 1**).

the probability distribution $p(y|\mathbf{x})$ increases exponentially with the number of neurons in the population. Indeed, this exponential increase in the number of symbols with the dimensionality of the response space is a well-known problem with applications of information-theoretic methods in neuroscience (Rieke et al., 1997). It would be desirable to develop more efficient computational techniques for studying neuronal populations in the future (Yarrow et al., 2012).

In addition to considering neural populations, another direction for extending the closed-loop paradigm is to consider neural responses more sophisticated than firing rates, for instance the temporal patterns of neural responses (Optican and Richmond, 1987; Victor and Purpura, 1996), first spike latency (VanRullen et al., 2005; Gollisch and Meister, 2008), or synchronous responses in neural populations (Brette, 2012). Since a temporal pattern is a vector but not a scalar, one needs to extract a scalar quantity from a temporal pattern in order to define the optimal stimulus. For example, synchrony can be defined as a scalar quantity (Steinmetz et al., 2000) and can in principle be optimized over a stimulus space in the same manner as firing rate. The iso-response paradigm (Gollisch et al., 2002) would generalize quite well to both spike pattern and synchrony measures. In this case of spike pattern, the goal would be to find the equivalence class of all stimuli which could elicit a desired pattern of spiking, and theoretical efforts have demonstrated that it is possible to design stimuli to produce a desired spike pattern (Ahmadian et al., 2011). Similarly, for iso-synchrony curves one could find equivalence classes of stimuli yielding the same degree of synchrony in the population by utilizing algorithms similar to those developed for firing rate.

One of the most powerful applications of the closed-loop paradigm is the ability to move sensory neurophysiology toward a model-based paradigm, where experiments are performed with the goal of identifying and comparing multiple competing nonlinear models (Paninski, 2005; Lewi et al., 2009; DiMattina and Zhang, 2011; Tam et al., 2011). One advantage of model identification is that successful identification gives the experimenter a variety of biologically important information about the neuron or neuronal population "for free." That is, once one has determined an accurate model for a sensory neuron, the optimal stimulus for maximizing firing rate, the iso-response surfaces, or the stimulus ensemble maximizing information transmission can be predicted from this model, and these predictions can be tested experimentally. However, the model-based approach is not without its difficulties, as many sensory neurons are poorly described by tractable linear and quadratic models and may be better described by more complex models like basis functions and neural networks. Recent work has demonstrated that in principle, adaptive stimulus optimization methods long utilized in machine learning and psychophysics can be applied in sensory neurophysiology for purposes of model estimation and comparison (Paninski, 2005; Lewi et al., 2009; DiMattina and Zhang, 2011). In particular, our recent study has presented a practical two-stage experimental method for generating stimuli which are optimal for estimating the parameters of multiple non-linear models and then generating stimuli on-line in order to critically compare the predictions of different models (DiMattina and Zhang, 2011). This method is presently being applied in ongoing auditory neurophysiology studies (Tam et al., 2011; Dekel, 2012; Tam, 2012), and may be applicable to a broad variety of sensory systems.

ACKNOWLEDGMENTS

Supported by grant NSF IIS-0827695. Thanks to Sarah Osmer DiMattina for her assistance with graphic design.

REFERENCES

Ahmadian, Y., Packer, A. M., Yuste, R., and Paninski, L. (2011). Designing optimal stimuli to control neuronal spike timing. *J. Neurophysiol.* 106, 1038–1053.

Ahrens, M. B., Linden, J. F., and Sahani, M. (2008a). Nonlinearities and contextual influences in auditory cortical responses modeled with multilinear spectrotemporal methods. *J. Neurosci.* 28, 1929–1942.

Ahrens, M. B., Paninski, L., and Sahani, M. (2008b). Inferring input nonlinearities in neural encoding models. *Network* 19, 35–67.

Albrecht, D. G., DeValois, R. L., and Thorell, L. G. (1980). Visual cortical neurons: are bars or gratings the optimal stimuli? *Science* 207, 88–90.

Albrecht, D. G., and Hamilton, D. B. (1982). Striate cortex of monkey and cat: contrast response function. *J Neurophysiol.* 48, 217–237.

Amari, S.-I., Park, H., and Ozeki, T. (2006). Singularities affect dynamics of learning in neuromanifolds. *Neural Comput.* 18, 1007–1065.

Anderson, M. J., and Micheli-Tzanakou, E. (2002). Auditory stimulus optimization with feedback from fuzzy clustering of neuronal responses. *IEEE Trans. Inf. Technol. Biomed.* 6, 159–170.

Arimoto, S. (1972). An algorithm for computing the capacity of arbitrary discrete memoryless channels. *IEEE Trans. Inf. Theory* 18, 14–20.

Asari, H., and Zador, A. M. (2009). Long-lasting context dependence constrains neural encoding models in rodent auditory cortex. *J. Neurophysiol.* 102, 2638–2656.

Atkinson, A., and Fedorov, V. (1975a). The design of experiments for discriminating between two rival models. *Biometrika* 62, 57–70.

Atkinson, A., and Fedorov, V. (1975b). Optimal design: experiments for discriminating between several models. *Biometrika* 62, 289–303.

Atkinson, A. C., and Donev, A. N. (1992). *Optimum Experimental Designs.* Oxford: Clarendon Press.

Bandyopadhyay, S., Reiss, L. A. J., and Young, E. D. (2007a). Receptive field for dorsal cochlear nucleus neurons at multiple sound levels. *J. Neurophysiol.* 98, 3505–3515.

Bandyopadhyay, S., Young, E. D., and Reiss, L. A. J. (2007b). "Spectral edges as optimal stimuli for the dorsal cochlear nucleus," in *Hearing – From Basic Research to Applications,* eds B. Kollmeier, G. Klump, V. Hohmann, U. Langemann, M. Mauermann, S. Upperkamp, et al. (New York: Springer-Verlag), 39–45.

Barbour, D. L., and Wang, X. (2003a). Auditory cortical responses elicited in awake primates by random spectrum stimuli. *J. Neurosci.* 23, 7194–7206.

Barbour, D. L., and Wang, X. (2003b). Contrast tuning in auditory cortex. *Science* 299, 1073–1075.

Barlow, H. B. (1961). "Possible principles underlying the transformation of sensory messages," in *Sensory Communication,* ed. W. A. Rosenblith (Cambridge, MA: MIT Press), 217–234.

Bartlett, E. L., and Wang, X. (2005). Long-lasting modulation by stimulus context in primate auditory cortex. *J. Neurophysiol.* 94, 83–104.

Bellman, R. (1961). *Adaptive Control Processes: A Guided Tour.* Princeton, NJ: Princeton University Press.

Benda, J., Gollisch, T., Machens, C. K., and Herz, A. V. (2007). From response to stimulus: adaptive sampling in sensory physiology. *Curr. Opin. Neurobiol.* 17, 430–436.

Berkes, P., and Wiskott, L. (2005). Slow feature analysis yields a rich repertoire of complex cell properties. *J. Vis.* 5, 579–602.

Berkes, P., and Wiskott, L. (2006). On the analysis and interpretation of inhomogeneous quadratic forms as receptive fields. *Neural Comput.* 18, 1868–1895.

Berkes, P., and Wiskott, L. (2007). Analysis and interpretation of quadratic models of receptive fields. *Nat. Protoc.* 2, 400–407.

Bernardo, J. (1979). Expected information as expected utility. *Ann. Stat.* 7, 686–690.

Bethge, M., Rotermund, D., and Pawelzik, K. (2002). Optimal short-term population coding: when fisher information fails. *Neural Comput.* 14, 2317–2751.

Blahut, R. (1972). Computation of channel capacity and rate-distortion functions. *IEEE Trans. Inf. Theory* 18, 460–473.

Bleeck, S., Patterson, R. D., and Winter, I. M. (2003). Using genetic algorithms to find the most effective stimulus for sensory neurons. *J. Neurosci. Methods* 125, 73–82.

Bock, D. D., Lee, W.-C. A., Kerlin, A. M., Andermann, M. L., Hood, G., Wetzel, A. W., et al. (2011). Network anatomy and in vivo physiology of visual cortical neurons. *Nature,* 471, 177–182.

Bölinger, D., and Gollisch, T. (2012). Closed-loop measurements of iso-response stimuli reveal dynamic nonlinear stimulus integration in the retina. *Neuron* 73, 333–346.

Bonnasse-Gahot, L., and Nadal, J. P. (2008). Neural coding of categories: information efficiency and optimal population codes. *J. Comput. Neurosci.* 25, 169–187.

Brette, R. (2012). Computing with neural synchrony. *PLoS Comput. Biol.* 8:e1002561. doi: 10.1371/journal.pcbi.1002561

Butts, D. A., and Goldman, M. S. (2006). Tuning curves, neuronal variability, and sensory coding. *PLoS Biol.* 4:e92. doi: 10.1371/journal.pbio.0040092

Cadieu, C., Kouh, M., Pasupathy, A., Connor, C. E., Riesenhuber, M., and Poggio, T. (2007). A model of v4 shape selectivity and invariance. *J. Neurophysiol.* 98, 1733–1750.

Canepari, M., Willadt, S., Zecevic, D., and Vogt, K. (2010). Imaging inhibitory synaptic potentials using voltage sensitive dyes. *Biophys. J.* 98, 2032–2040.

Carlson, E. T., Tasquinha, R. J., Zhang, K., and Connor, C. E. (2011). A sparse object coding scheme in area v4. *Curr. Biol.* 21, 288–293.

Cavagnaro, D. R., Myung, J. I., Pitt, M. A., and Kujala, J. V. (2010). Adaptive design optimization: a mutual information-based approach to model discrimination in cognitive science. *Neural Comput.* 22, 887–905.

Chaloner, K., and Verdinelli, I. (1995). Bayesian experimental design: a review. *Stat. Sci.* 10, 273–304.

Chambers, A., Hancock, K. E., and Polley, D. B. (2012). An adaptive stimulus search method for rapid characterization of multidimensional receptive fields in auditory cortex of awake animals. *Soc. Neurosci. Abstr.* 460, 15.

Chase, S. M., and Young, E. D. (2008). Cues for sound localization are encoded in multiple aspects of spike trains in the inferior colliculus. *J. Neurophysiol.* 99, 1672–1682.

Cheng, K., Hasegawa, T., Saleem, K. S., and Tanaka, K. (1994). Comparison of neuronal selectivity for stimulus speed, length, and contrast in the prestriate visual cortical areas v4 and mt of the macaque monkey. *J. Neurophysiol.* 71, 2269–2280.

Chichilnisky, E. J. (2001). A simple white noise analysis of neuronal light responses. *Network* 12, 199–213.

Cohn, D., Atlas, L., and Ladner, R. (1994). Improving generalization with active learning. *Mach. Learn.* 15, 201–221.

Cohn, D. A., Ghahramani, Z., and Jordan, M. I. (1996). Active learning with statistical models. *J. Artif. Intell. Res.* 4, 129–145.

Cornsweet, T. N. (1962). The staircase method in psychophysics. *Am. J. Psychol.* 75, 485–491.

Cousseau, F., Ozeki, T., and Amari, S.-I. (2008). Dynamics of learning in multilayer perceptrons near singularities. *IEEE Trans. Neural Netw.* 19, 1313–1328.

David, S., and Gallant, J. (2005). Predicting neuronal responses during natural vision. *Network* 16, 239–260.

David, S., Mesgarani, N., Fritz, J., and Shamma, S. (2009). Rapid synaptic depression explains nonlinear modulation of spectro-temporal tuning in primary auditory cortex by natural stimuli. *J. Neurosci.* 29, 3374–3386.

Dayan, P., Abbott, L. F., and Abbott, L. (2001). *Theoretical Neuroscience: Computational and Mathematical Modeling of Neural Systems.* Cambridge, MA: MIT Press.

deCharms, R. C., Blake, D., and Merzenich, M. (1998). Optimizing sound features for cortical neurons. *Science* 280, 1439–1444.

Dekel, E. (2012). *Adaptive On-line Modeling in the Auditory System: In Vivo Implementation of the Optimal Experimental Design Paradigm.* Master's thesis, Department of Biomedical Engineering, Johns Hopkins University, Baltimore, MD.

DiMattina, C., and Wang, X. (2006). Virtual vocalization stimuli for investigating neural representations of species-specific vocalizations. *J. Neurophysiol.* 95, 1244–1262.

DiMattina, C., and Zhang, K. (2008). How optimal stimuli for sensory neurons are constrained by network architecture. *Neural Comput.* 20, 668–708.

DiMattina, C., and Zhang, K. (2010). How to modify a neural network gradually without changing its input–output functionality. *Neural Comput.* 22, 1–47.

DiMattina, C., and Zhang, K. (2011). Active data collection for efficient estimation and comparison of nonlinear neural models. *Neural Comput.* 23, 2242–2288.

Djurisic, M., Popovic, M., Carnevale, N., and Zecevic, D. (2008). Functional structure of the mitral cell dendritic tuft in the rat olfactory bulb. *J. Neurosci.* 28, 4057–4068.

Douglas, S. C., Amari, S., and Kung, S. Y. (2000). On gradient adaptation with unit norm constraints. *IEEE Trans. Signal Proc.* 48, 1843–1847.

Federov, V. V. (1972). *Theory of Optimal Experiments.* New York: Academic Press.

Felleman, D. J., and Van Essen, D. C. (1991). Distributed hierarchical processing in the primate cerebral cortex. *Cereb. Cortex* 1, 1–47.

Foldiak, P. (2001). Stimulus optimisation in primary visual cortex. *Neurocomputing* 38–40, 1217–1222.

Goldberg, D. (1989). *Genetic Algorithms in Search, Optimization, and Machine Learning.* Upper Saddle River, NJ: Addison-Wesley Professional.

Gollisch, T., and Herz, A. (2005). Disentangling sub-millisecond processes within an auditory transduction chain. *PLoS Biol.* 3:e8. doi: 10.1371/journal.pbio.0030008

Gollisch, T., and Meister, M. (2008). Rapid neural coding in the retina with relative spike latencies. *Science* 319, 1108–1111.

Gollisch, T., Schütze, H., Benda, J., and Herz, A. V. M. (2002). Energy integration describes sound-intensity coding in an insect auditory system. *J. Neurosci.* 22, 10434–10448.

Han, X., Xu, C., and Prince, J. (2003). A topology preserving level set method for geometric deformable models. *IEEE Trans. Pattern Anal. Mach. Intell.* 25, 755–768.

Harper, N. S., and McAlpine, D. (2004). Optimal neural population coding of an auditory spatial cue. *Nature* 430, 682–686.

Harth, E., and Tzanakou, E. (1974). Alopex: a stochastic method for determining visual receptive fields. *Vis. Res.* 14, 1475–1482.

Heeger, D. J. (1992a). Half-squaring in responses of cat striate cells. *Vis. Neurosci.* 9, 427–443.

Heeger, D. J. (1992b). Normalization of cell responses in cat striate cortex. *Vis. Neurosci.* 9, 181–197.

Horwitz, G. D., and Hass, C. A. (2012). Nonlinear analysis of macaque v1 color tuning reveals cardinal directions for cortical color processing. *Nat. Neurosci.* 15, 913–919.

Hubel, D. H., and Wiesel, T. N. (1962). Receptive fields, binocular interaction and functional architecture in the cat's visual cortex. *J. Physiol.* 160, 106–154.

Huggins, J., and Paninski, L. (2012). Optimal experimental design for sampling voltage on dendritic trees in the low-SNR regime. *J. Comput. Neurosci.* 32, 347–366.

Hung, C. C., Carlson, E. T., and Connor, C. E. (2012). Medial axis shape coding in macaque inferotemporal cortex. *Neuron* 74, 1099–1113.

Ingham, N., and McAlpine, D. (2004). Spike-frequency adaptation in the inferior colliculus. *J. Neurophysiol.* 91, 632–645.

Johnson, D. H., Gruner, C. M., Baggerly, K., and Seshagiri, C. (2001). Information-theoretic analysis of neural coding. *J. Comput. Neurosci.* 10, 47–69.

Kennedy, J., and Eberhart, R. (1995). "Particle swarm optimization," in *Proceedings of the IEEE International Conference on Neural Networks,* Vol. 4 (Washington, DC: IEEE), 1942–1948.

Kirkpatrick, S., Gelatt, C. D. Jr., and Vecchi, M. P. (1983). Optimization by simulated annealing. *Science* 220, 671–680.

Koelling, M. E., and Nykamp, D. Q. (2008). Computing linear approximations to nonlinear neuronal response. *Network* 19, 286–313.

Koelling, M. E., and Nykamp, D. Q. (2012). Searching for optimal stimuli: ascending a neuron's response function. *J. Comput. Neurosci.* 33, 449–473.

Kontsevich, L. L., and Tyler, C. W. (1999). Bayesian adaptive estimation of psychometric slope and threshold. *Vis. Res.* 39, 2729–2737.

Kujala, J., and Lukka, T. (2006). Bayesian adaptive estimation: the next dimension. *J. Math. Psychol.* 50, 369–389.

Kujala, J., Richardson, U., and Lyytinen, H. (2010). A Bayesian-optimal principle for learner-friendly adaptation in learning games. *J. Math. Psychol.* 54, 247–255.

Lau, B., Stanley, G. B., and Dan, Y. (2002). Computational subunits of visual cortical neurons revealed by artificial neural networks. *Proc. Natl. Acad. Sci. U.S.A.* 99, 8974–8979.

Lesmes, L. A., Lu, Z.-L., Baek, J., and Albright, T. D. (2010). Bayesian adaptive estimation of the contrast sensitivity function: the quick CSF method. *J. Vis.* 10, 17.1–17.21.

Lewi, J., Butera, R., and Paninski, L. (2009). Sequential optimal design of neurophysiology experiments. *Neural Comput.* 21, 619–687.

Lewi, J., Schneider, D. M., Woolley, S. M. N., and Paninski, L. (2011). Automating the design of informative sequences of sensory stimuli. *J. Comput. Neurosci.* 30, 181–200.

Lindley, D. (1956). On a measure of the information provided by an experiment. *Ann. Math. Stat.* 27, 986–1005.

Machens, C. K. (2002). Adaptive sampling by information maximization. *Phys. Rev. Lett.* 88, 228104.

Machens, C. K., Gollisch, T., Kolesnikova, O., and Herz, A. V. M. (2005). Testing the efficiency of sensory coding with optimal stimulus ensembles. *Neuron* 47, 447–456.

MacKay, D. (1992). Information-based objective functions for active data selection. *Neural Comput.* 4, 590–604.

McCullough, M. E., Luna, L. R., Berry, J. W., Tabak, B. A., and Bono, G. (2010). On the form and function of forgiving: modeling the time-forgiveness relationship and testing the valuable relationships hypothesis. *Emotion* 10, 358–376.

Müller, P., and Parmigiani, G. (1995). Optimal design *via* curve fitting of Monte Carlo experiments. *J. Am. Stat. Assoc.* 90, 1322–1330.

Nelder, J., and Mead, R. (1965). A simplex method for function minimization. *Comput. J.* 7, 308–313.

Nelken, I., Prut, Y., Vaadia, E., and Abeles, M. (1994). In search of the best stimulus: an optimization procedure for finding efficient stimuli in the cat auditory cortex. *Hear. Res.* 72, 237–253.

Newman, J., Zeller-Townson, R., Fong, M., Desai, S., Gross, R., and Potter, S. (2013). Closed-loop, multichannel experimentation using the open-source neurorighter electrophysiology platform. *Front. Neural Circuits* 6:98. doi: 10.3389/fncir.2012.00098

Nocedal, J., and Wright, S. (2006). *Numerical Optimization. Springer Series in Operations Research and Financial Engineering,* 2 Edn. New York: Springer.

Nosofsky, R., and Zaki, S. (2002). Exemplar and prototype models revisited: response strategies, selective attention, and stimulus generalization. *J. Exp. Psychol. Learn. Mem. Cogn.* 28, 924–940.

O'Connor, K. N., Petkov, C. I., and Sutter, M. L. (2005). Adaptive stimulus optimization for auditory cortical neurons. *J. Neurophysiol.* 94, 4051–4067.

Ohki, K., Chung, S., Ch'ng, Y. H., Kara, P., and Reid, R. C. (2005). Functional imaging with cellular resolution reveals precise microarchitecture in visual cortex. *Nature* 433, 597–603.

Olshausen, B. A., and Field, D. J. (2005). How close are we to understanding v1? *Neural Comput.* 17, 1665–1699.

Opfer, J., and Siegler, R. (2007). Representational change and children's numerical estimation. *Cogn. Psychol.* 55, 169–195.

Optican, L. M., and Richmond, B. J. (1987). Temporal encoding of two-dimensional patterns by single units in primate inferior temporal cortex. III. Information theoretic analysis. *J. Neurophysiol.* 57, 147–161.

Oram, M. W., Xiao, D., Dritschel, B., and Payne, K. R. (2002). The temporal resolution of neural codes: does response latency have a unique role? *Philos. Trans. R. Soc. Lond. B Biol. Sci.* 357, 987–1001.

Paninski, L. (2004). Maximum likelihood estimation of cascade point-process neural encoding models. *Network* 15, 243–262.

Paninski, L. (2005). Asymptotic theory of information-theoretic experimental design. *Neural Comput.* 17, 1480–1507.

Paninski, L., Pillow, J., and Lewi, J. (2007). Statistical models for neural encoding, decoding, and optimal stimulus design. *Prog. Brain Res.* 165, 493–507.

Penny, W. (2012). Comparing dynamic causal models using AIC, BIC and free energy. *Neuroimage* 59, 319–330.

Pillow, J. W., Shlens, J., Paninski, L., Sher, A., Litke, A. M., Chichilnisky, E. J., et al. (2008). Spatio-temporal correlations and visual signalling in a complete neuronal population. *Nature* 454, 995–999.

Poggio, T., and Girosi, F. (1990). Networks for approximation and learning. *Proc. IEEE* 78, 1481–1497.

Prenger, R., Wu, M. C.-K., David, S. V., and Gallant, J. L. (2004). Nonlinear v1 responses to natural scenes revealed by neural network analysis. *Neural Netw.* 17, 663–679.

Prinz, A., Abbott, L., and Marder, E. (2004). The dynamic clamp comes of age. *Trends Neurosci.* 27, 218–224.

Rabinowitz, N., Willmore, B., Schnupp, J., and King, A. (2012). Spectrotemporal contrast kernels for neurons in primary auditory cortex. *J. Neurosci.* 32, 11271–11284.

Ray, S., Hsiao, S. S., Crone, N. E., Franaszczuk, P. J., and Niebur, E. (2008). Effect of stimulus intensity on the spike-local field potential relationship in the secondary somatosensory cortex. *J. Neurosci.* 28, 7334–7343.

Reiss, L. A. J., and Young, E. D. (2005). Spectral edge sensitivity in neural circuits of the dorsal cochlear nucleus. *J. Neurosci.* 25, 3680–3691.

Rieke, F., Warland, D., de Ruyter van Steveninck, R., and Bialek, W. (1997). *Spikes: Exploring the Neural Code.* Cambridge: MIT Press.

Riesenhuber, M., and Poggio, T. (1999). Hierarchical models of object recognition in cortex. *Nat. Neurosci.* 2, 1019–1025.

Riesenhuber, M., and Poggio, T. (2000). Models of object recognition. *Nat. Neurosci.* 3(Suppl.), 1199–1204.

Rubin, D., Hinton, S., and Wenzel, A. (1999). The precise time course of retention. *J. Exp. Psychol.* 25, 1161–1176.

Rubin, D., and Wenzel, A. (1996). One hundred years of forgetting: a quantitative description of retention. *Psychol. Rev.* 103, 734–760.

Schinkel-Bielefeld, N., David, S., Shamma, S., and Butts, D. (2012). Inferring the role of inhibition in auditory processing of complex natural stimuli. *J. Neurophysiol.* 107, 3296–3307.

Schwarz, G. (1978). Estimating the dimension of a model. *Ann. Stat.* 6, 461–464.

Seung, H., and Sompolinsky, H. (1993). Simple models for reading neuronal population codes. *Proc. Natl. Acad. Sci. U.S.A.* 90, 10749–10753.

Shamma, S. A., Fleshman, J. W., Wiser, P. R., and Versnel, H. (1993). Organization of response areas in ferret primary auditory cortex. *J. Neurophysiol.* 69, 367–383.

Sharpee, T., Miller, K., and Stryker, M. (2008). On the importance of static nonlinearity in estimating spatiotemporal neural filters with natural stimuli. *J. Neurophysiol.* 99, 2496–2509.

Sharpee, T., Rust, N., and Bialek, W. (2004). Analyzing neural responses to natural signals: maximally informative dimensions. *Neural Comput.* 16, 223–250.

Shepherd, G. (2003). *The Synaptic Organization of the Brain,* 5 Edn. New York: Oxford University Press.

Simoncelli, E. (2003). Vision and the statistics of the visual environment. *Curr. Opin. Neurobiol.* 13, 144–149.

Simoncelli, E. P., Pillow, J. W., Paninski, L., and Schwartz, O. (2004). "Characterization of neural responses with stochastic stimuli," in *The Cognitive Neurosciences III,* ed. M. Gazzaniga (Cambridge, MA: MIT Press), 327–338.

Snoeren, P. R., and Puts, M. J. H. (1997). Multiple parameter estimation in an adaptive psychometric method: MUEST, an extension of the quest method. *J. Math. Psychol.* 41, 431–439.

Spall, J. (2003). *Introduction to Stochastic Search and Optimization.* Hoboken, NJ: Wiley-Interscience.

Steinmetz, P. N., Roy, A., Fitzgerald, P., Hsiao, S., Johnson, K., and Niebur, E. (2000). Attention modulates synchronized neuronal firing in primate somatosensory cortex. *Nature* 404, 187–190.

Stork, D. G., Levinson, J. Z., Albrecht, D. F., DeValois, R. L., and Thorell, L. G. (1982). Receptive fields and the optimal stimulus. *Science* 216, 204–205.

Sugiyama, M. (2006). Active learning in approximately linear regression based on conditional expectation of generalization error. *J. Mach. Learn. Res.* 7, 141–166.

Tam, W. (2012). *Adaptive Modeling of Marmoset Inferior Colliculus Neurons In Vivo.* PhD thesis, Department of Biomedical Engineering, Johns Hopkins University, Baltimore, MD.

Tam, W., Dekel, E., DiMattina, C., Young, E. D., and Zhang, K. (2011). Using optimal experimental design for capturing parameters of neural networks in the inferior colliculus of the common marmoset. *Soc. Neurosci. Abstr.* 480.10.

Tolhurst, D. J., Movshon, J. A., and Dean, A. F. (1983). The statistical reliability of signals in single neurons in cat and monkey visual cortex. *Vis. Res.* 23, 775–85.

Touryan, J., Lau, B., and Dan, Y. (2002). Isolation of relevant visual features from random stimuli for cortical complex cells. *J. Neurosci.* 22, 10811–10818.

Tzanakou, E., Michalak, R., and Harth, E. (1979). The alopex process: visual receptive fields by response feedback. *Biol. Cybern.* 35, 161–174.

Ulanovsky, N., Las, L., and Nelken, I. (2003). Processing of low-probability sounds by cortical neurons. *Nat. Neurosci.* 6, 391–398.

VanRullen, R., Guyonneau, R., and Thorpe, S. J. (2005). Spike times make sense. *Trends Neurosci.* 28, 1–4.

Victor, J. D., and Purpura, K. P. (1996). Nature and precision of temporal coding in visual cortex: a metric-space analysis. *J. Neurophysiol.* 76, 1310–1326.

Vladusich, T., Lucassen, M. P., and Cornelissen, F. W. (2006). Do cortical neurons process luminance or contrast to encode surface properties? *J. Neurophysiol.* 95, 2638–2649.

Wang, Z., and Bovik, A. (2006). *Modern Image Quality Assessment.* New York: Morgan & Claypool Publishers.

Wang, Z., and Simoncelli, E. P. (2008). Maximum differentiation (MAD) competition: a methodology for comparing computational models of perceptual quantities. *J. Vis.* 8, 8.1–8.13.

Watson, A. B., and Pelli, D. G. (1983). Quest: a Bayesian adaptive psychometric method. *Percept. Psychophys.* 33, 113–20.

Wei, H., and Amari, S.-I. (2008). Dynamics of learning near singularities in radial basis function networks. *Neural Netw.* 21, 989–1005.

Wei, H., Zhang, J., Cousseau, F., Ozeki, T., and Amari, S.-I. (2008). Dynamics of learning near singularities in layered networks. *Neural Comput.* 20, 813–843.

Willett, R., and Nowak, R. (2007). Minimax optimal level-set estimation. *IEEE Trans. Image Proc.* 16, 2965.

Wixted, J., and Ebbesen, E. (1991). On the form of forgetting. *Psychol. Sci.* 2, 409.

Wu, M. C.-K., David, S. V., and Gallant, J. L. (2006). Complete functional characterization of sensory neurons by system identification. *Annu. Rev. Neurosci.* 29, 477–505.

Yamane, Y., Carlson, E. T., Bowman, K. C., Wang, Z., and Connor, C. E. (2008). A neural code for three-dimensional object shape in macaque inferotemporal cortex. *Nat. Neurosci.* 11, 1352–60.

Yarrow, S., Challis, E., and Series, P. (2012). Fisher and Shannon information in finite neural populations. *Neural Comput.* 24, 1740–1780.

Young, E. D., Yu, J. J., and Reiss, L. A. J. (2005). Non-linearities and the representation of auditory spectra. *Int. Rev. Neurobiol.* 70, 135–68.

Yu, J. J., and Young, E. D. (2000). Linear and nonlinear pathways of spectral information transmission in the cochlear nucleus. *Proc. Natl. Acad. Sci. U.S.A.* 97, 11780–11786.

Zhang, K., and Sejnowski, T. J. (1999). Neuronal tuning: to sharpen or broaden? *Neural Comput.* 11, 75–84.

19

High-density microelectrode array recordings and real-time spike sorting for closed-loop experiments: an emerging technology to study neural plasticity

Felix Franke*, David Jäckel, Jelena Dragas, Jan Müller, Milos Radivojevic, Douglas Bakkum* and *Andreas Hierlemann

Department of Biosystems Science and Engineering, ETH Zürich, Basle, Switzerland

Edited by:
Steve M. Potter, Georgia Institute of Technology, USA

Reviewed by:
Suguru N. Kudoh, Kwansei Gakuin University, Japan
Michela Chiappalone, Italian Institute of Technology, Italy

****Correspondence:***
Felix Franke, Department of Biosystems Science and Engineering, ETH Zürich, 4058 Basle, Switzerland.
e-mail: felfranke@gmail.com

Understanding plasticity of neural networks is a key to comprehending their development and function. A powerful technique to study neural plasticity includes recording and control of pre- and post-synaptic neural activity, e.g., by using simultaneous intracellular recording and stimulation of several neurons. Intracellular recording is, however, a demanding technique and has its limitations in that only a small number of neurons can be stimulated and recorded from at the same time. Extracellular techniques offer the possibility to simultaneously record from larger numbers of neurons with relative ease, at the expenses of increased efforts to sort out single neuronal activities from the recorded mixture, which is a time consuming and error prone step, referred to as spike sorting. In this mini-review, we describe recent technological developments in two separate fields, namely CMOS-based high-density microelectrode arrays, which also allow for extracellular stimulation of neurons, and real-time spike sorting. We argue that these techniques, when combined, will provide a powerful tool to study plasticity in neural networks consisting of several thousand neurons *in vitro*.

Keywords: closed-loop, real-time, spike sorting, multielectrode arrays, neural cultures

INTRODUCTION

The understanding of neural circuits and their activities is to a major extent based on measurements with extracellular electrodes. This is due to the fact that extracellular recordings are relatively easy to perform and very well established. In contrast to single cell measurements with intracellular recording techniques, extracellular electrodes pick up the action potentials (spikes) of all neurons in their vicinity. This is a blessing as well as a curse. An advantage is that in principle several neurons can be measured simultaneously using a single extracellular electrode, but the price to pay is the need to assign single spikes to their putative neuronal sources. This problem is referred to as spike sorting and it is known to be difficult and error-prone (Lewicki, 1998), and spike sorting often involves a highly time consuming, manual component.

Depending on the experiment, time consuming spike sorting can be regarded as a mere inconvenience, and many studies have focused on the development of spike sorting algorithms for the offline analysis of the recordings after performing the experiment (see e.g., Letelier and Weber, 2000; Shoham and Fellows, 2003; Delescluse and Pouzat, 2006). For real-time closed-loop experiments and brain machine interfaces (BMI), however, it is absolutely necessary to obtain spike trains already during the recording so that time consuming spike sorting is not only a problem but essentially prohibits performing such experiments. Therefore, spike sorting is usually avoided in those experiments by detecting just the presence of action potentials, e.g., by applying a voltage threshold, which can be relatively easy and efficiently implemented also in hardware (Guillory and Normann, 1999). Real-time spike detection allows for studying closed-loop feedback of neural activity, for example, through the implementation of visual feedback to an awake monkey (Fetz, 1969), or by applying electrical stimulation to neurons in an awake animal (Jackson et al., 2006). Electrical stimulation of neurons that depends on the activity of other neurons (see also **Figure 1**) was also successfully used in neural cultures on top of multi-electrode arrays (MEAs): electrical feedback stimuli have been used to control the bursting activity of cultured neurons in Wagenaar et al. (2005) and the connection strengths between neurons in Müller et al. (in review). The closed-loop approach can also be used to connect a neural network to a robot (Bontorin et al., 2007; Potter, 2010). For a review of real-time closed-loop electrophysiology see, e.g., Arsiero et al. (2007). These studies, however, were all realized without using spike sorting, either by limiting the number of single neurons that were recorded from (by trying to detect only one specific neuron per electrode), or by using multi-unit activities.

Recent developments in measurement techniques and in spike sorting algorithms make it now possible to overcome some of the limitations of extracellular recordings. A possible setup using spike sorting for closed-loop stimulation of specific neurons is shown in **Figure 1**. To use the closed loop, e.g., to investigate spike-timing-dependent plasticity, the real-time spike-sorting-induced latency may not exceed a few milliseconds. In the following, we will review the advances in MEA recording technology with a special focus on high-density MEAs and show

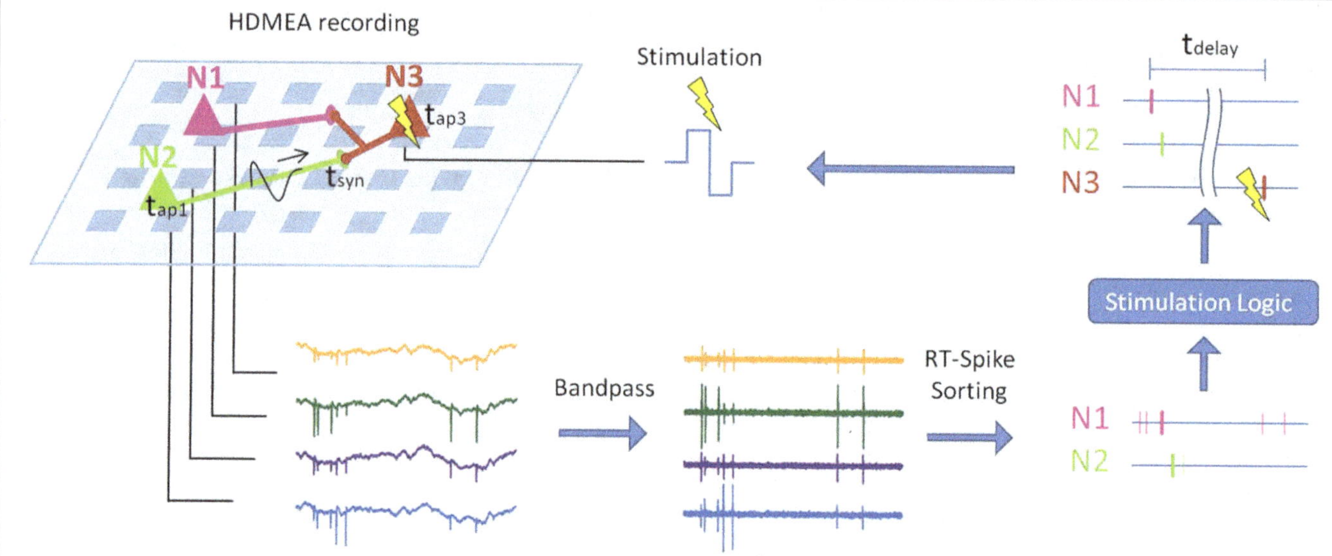

FIGURE 1 | Principle of real-time closed-loop experiments with spike sorting. Sketch of a potential real-time closed-loop stimulation on an HDMEA, combined with spike sorting. The electrical activity of three neurons (colored triangles) is measured by a high-density array of electrodes (light blue squares). First, the recorded signal is bandpass-filtered. In a second step, spike sorting is applied to compute the spike times of the single neurons. Depending on the sorted spike trains and the stimulation logic, the postsynaptic neuron (N3) is stimulated (Müller et al., in review). If the stimulation latency (t_{delay}) is short enough, the stimulation can be timed with respect to the arrival of the action potentials of N1 and N2 at their synapses to N3 (t_{syn}). This can be used to change the synapse characteristics via spike-timing-dependent plasticity (Feldman, 2012). Parts of this graph were adopted from Einevoll et al. (2011).

that the high-density of the electrodes provides unprecedented signal quality that holds the promise to enable clear and reliable assignment of single spikes to putative neurons (Litke et al., 2004; Prentice et al., 2011; Jäckel et al., 2012).

MEA RECORDING TECHNOLOGY

Planar MEAs are two-dimensional arrangements of recording electrodes for *in vitro* extracellular measurements of cultured neuronal cells or slice preparations. They allow for recording of electrical activity simultaneously on many electrodes at high temporal resolution. Thus, they represent an important tool to study the dynamics in neuronal networks (e.g., Potter et al., 2006; Bontorin et al., 2007; Chao et al., 2007; Rolston et al., 2010; Müller et al., in review).

An important parameter of MEAs is the inter-electrode distance (IED). For multi-electrode arrangements on shafts of needles, such as tetrode configurations (Eckhorn and Thomas, 1993; O'Keefe and Recce, 1993), this distance is small enough (less than 20 μm) that a single action potential can be simultaneously detected on several electrodes. The maximal distance between a neuron and an electrode, at which the action potentials of the neuron can be still measured, is assumed to be smaller than 50–70 μm although this greatly depends on the recording setup and the respective preparation (Buzsáki, 2004; Frey et al., 2009b). For traditional, commercially available MEAs, however, the IED was usually much larger [100–200 μm IED and 60–200 metal electrodes on a glass substrate (Stett et al., 2003)] so that MEA recordings constituted, in principle, multiple simultaneous single-electrode recordings. In other words, the distance between the electrodes was too large to detect activity of the same single neuron on multiple electrodes.

From the signal processing point of view, this is an unfavorable recording situation, as recording the same action potential with more than one electrode was shown to strongly increase spike sorting performance (Gray et al., 1995). Furthermore, many neurons will lie in between electrodes and not be measured at all. To ensure that neurons lie close to the electrodes, additional measures can be taken during the preparation of the cultures, such as patterning the cells at electrode locations (Shein et al., 2009), but this adds complexity to the experimental procedure.

Recent advances in microtechnology, especially the realization of MEAs in complementary metal–oxide–semiconductor (CMOS) technology (Berdondini et al., 2009; Lambacher et al., 2010; Hierlemann et al., 2011), made it possible to greatly increase the number of electrodes per MEA, for example to 4096 in Berdondini et al. (2009), 11,011 in Frey et al. (2010) or 16,384 in Lambacher et al. (2010), while decreasing the IED to less than 20 μm, a distance comparable to that of the previously mentioned electrode ensembles on needles (e.g., tetrodes). Additionally, this technology provides increased signal quality through on-chip amplification and digitization circuits. Using on-chip multiplexing schemes, high-density MEAs (HDMEA) systems have been realized, which enable to read out large numbers of electrodes, arranged at high spatial density (Eversmann et al., 2003; Berdondini et al., 2005; Hutzler et al., 2006; Frey et al., 2009a).

The closely spaced microelectrodes of HDMEAs enable that virtually every neuron on the array is detected by multiple electrodes. Along with the additional information where the signal originated from, the high electrode density greatly improves spike sorting (Gray et al., 1995; Harris et al., 2000; Einevoll et al., 2011; Prentice et al., 2011). **Figure 2** shows an example of such a recording.

However, HDMEAs do not only improve recording but also stimulation capabilities. Localized, reliable stimulation of single cells (Hottowy et al., 2012) is a powerful tool for plasticity experiments (Müller et al., in review). Indeed, subcellular sized electrodes have been shown to provide reliable stimulation of individual neurons *in vitro*. This has been demonstrated using MEAs with particularly high electrode densities that feature only stimulation capabilities, such as (Braeken et al., 2010; Lei et al., 2011). Procedures how to optimally stimulate a given neuron by using multiple electrodes and complex stimulation patterns are currently under investigation.

HDMEAs featuring recording and stimulation circuitry (Frey et al., 2010; Eversmann et al., 2011) combine the advantages of reliable spike sorting and localized single neuron stimulation,

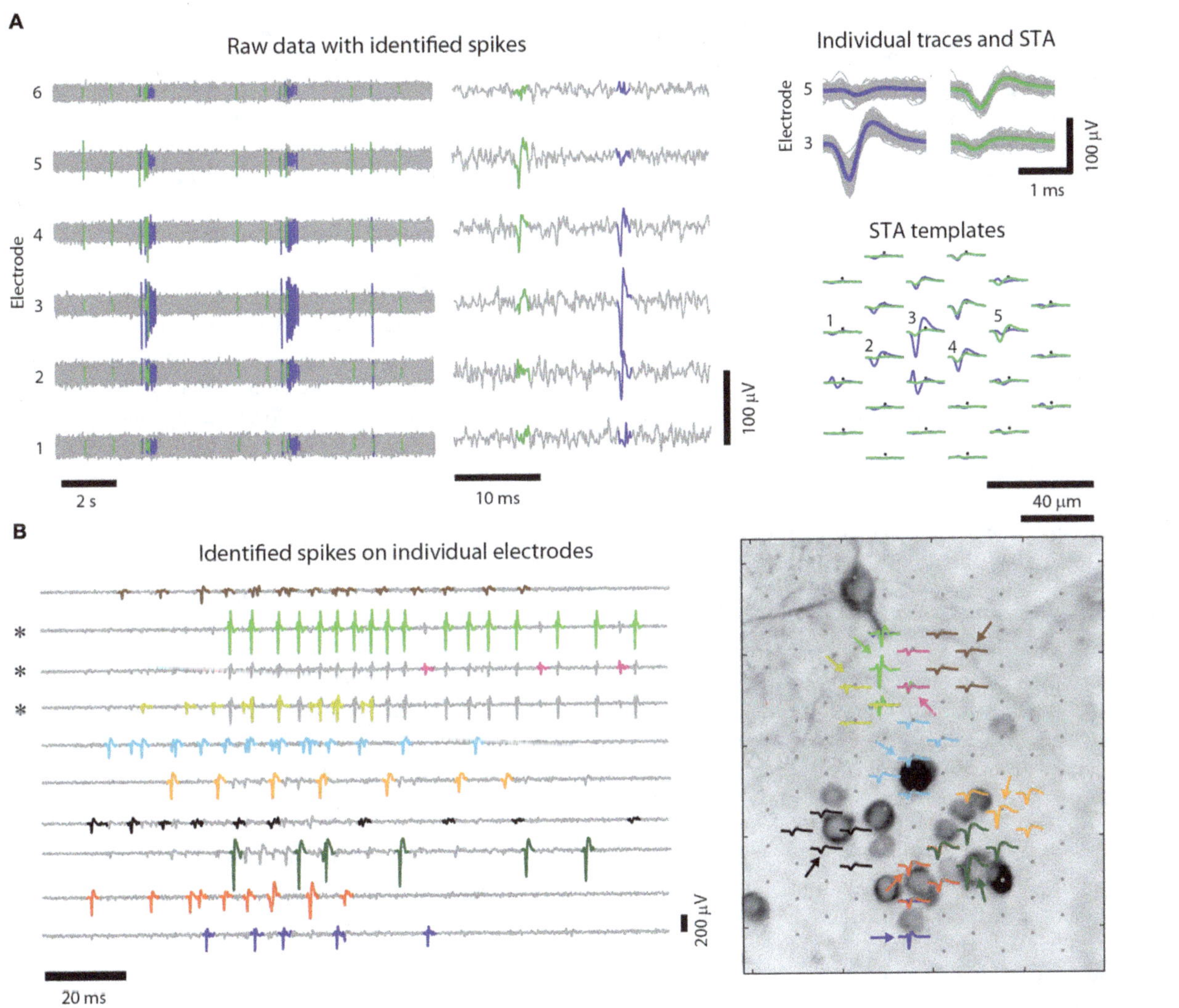

FIGURE 2 | Spike sorting for high-density multi-electrode recordings of cultured neurons. (A) Example recording of 6 out of 102 electrodes of a HDMEA (left), where mainly two neurons were recorded from, and a close up on two spikes (middle) (similar figure as in Frey et al. (2009a), however, with cultured cortical neurons). Spikes of individual neurons are recorded by multiple electrodes. Colored traces are identified spikes from two neurons. Note that on the trace of electrode 4, the two spikes are hardly distinguishable and that only combining the information of different channels enables unambiguous spike assignment, see also (Fiscella et al., 2012). (Right top) Several superimposed spike traces of the two neurons. The colored traces are the spike-triggered averages (STAs) of the two neurons on the respective electrodes. The templates of the two neurons (green and violet) spatially overlap (right bottom) indicating that the same set of electrodes recorded from both neurons. **(B)** Spikes (left) and templates (right) for 10 identified neurons (colored traces). For each neuron, the electrode was chosen, where its template had the largest peak-to-peak amplitude (indicated by the colored arrows in the right panel). Note that some of the spikes are visible on more than one electrode (three channels marked by asterisks) and that high-amplitude spikes on one electrode can overlap with spikes on another electrode. Right: for illustration purposes the identified templates are superimposed onto a MAP2 staining of the culture they were recorded from Bakkum et al. (in review). Note that the electrodes have a similar IED than the distance between neurons.

which paves the way to truly bidirectional experiments on single-cell level within the network context.

REAL-TIME SPIKE SORTING ALGORITHMS

The overall spike sorting process consists of a number of non-trivial processing steps (for a schematic of the spike sorting process see, e.g., Einevoll et al., 2011). First, spikes need to be detected in the noisy signals. For multi-electrode-shaft and HDMEA recordings, a single action potential can be detected on multiple electrodes. Then, a short piece of data is usually cut out around the detected events (potentially on multiple electrodes) and structured into a vector in a high dimensional space. Spike features are then extracted from this piece using, e.g., principle component analysis (Lewicki, 1998). This step aims at reducing the dimension of the vector space in order to keep dimensions that carry most information about the origin of the spikes and to remove dimensions that only carry noise. The goal of the feature space representation and dimensionality reduction is that spikes from the same neuron, i.e., appear to be similar to each other, are located closely together while being distant from spikes of other neurons. The most demanding step, achieved by using a clustering routine, is to determine how many neurons were recorded from, and which spike was produced by which neuron. Since most standard spike sorting procedures (e.g., Harris et al., 2000; Shoham and Fellows, 2003; Quiroga et al., 2004) need to store all individual spikes before the clustering step, they are not applicable for online spike sorting with the notable exceptions of Öhberg et al. (1996), where a neural network is used for real-time spike sorting, and (Rutishauser and Schuman, 2006), where the clusters are formed in an online procedure. The output of the spike sorting consists of the number of neurons, the individual neuronal spike trains, and the prototypic spike waveforms (called templates) for every neuron.

Since some data from a certain preparation can already be recorded and stored prior to a specific experiment, templates can be pre-computed using an offline spike sorter. This way, fast and efficient classifiers can be designed based on stored templates that are able to sort spikes in real-time. It does not come as a surprise that almost all research efforts in the direction of real-time spike sorting follow this approach (Friedman, 1968; Mishelevich, 1970; Roberts and Hartline, 1975; Stein et al., 1979; Salganicoff et al., 1988; Yang and Shamma, 1988; Gozani and Miller, 1994; Santhanam et al., 2004; Asai et al., 2005; Takahashi and Sakurai, 2005; Vollgraf et al., 2005; Biffi et al., 2010; Franke, 2011), although not all of these approaches explicitly make use of templates to derive spike classifiers.

So far, real-time spike sorting was mainly achieved by deriving simple hardware-implementable decision rules, based on the spike templates. One such rule is to check, if the spike voltage sample at a given time lies between a lower and an upper threshold relative to the peak of the spike waveform (a so called hoop), as described in Santhanam et al. (2004). Such decision rules are also used in commercially available recording systems and were individually applied to single electrodes (Nicolelis et al., 1997; Wessberg et al., 2000; Taylor et al., 2002; Guenther et al., 2009).

However, there have been only few applications of these approaches to multielectrode arrays in real-time scenarios, such as Takahashi and Sakurai (2005), where independent-component analysis was used to separate individual neuronal activities. The information of several recording channels must be efficiently combined for multi-electrode recordings. Extending a spike sorting method that works for single electrodes to multi-electrodes is not a trivial task and might not be possible for all methods.

As already discussed, HDMEAs impose even higher demands on the methods due to the large overall number of simultaneously recorded neurons and the large number of electrodes that are available per single neuron. There are a number of approaches to spike sorting of HDMEA data (Meister et al., 1994; Litke et al., 2004; Jäckel et al., 2011, 2012; Prentice et al., 2011; Fiscella et al., 2012) but none of those has been evaluated with respect to low latency real-time spike sorting so far. There is also no commercial system with real-time spike sorting available, and it is currently unclear how effective the application of the "hoop"-approach (Santhanam et al., 2004) is. Another ICA-based real-time approach has been described in Takahashi and Sakurai (2005), but the performance of ICA to separate all neurons of HDMEA data sets was found to be limited (Jäckel et al., 2012).

LINEAR FILTERS FOR SPIKE SORTING

Linear-filter-based spike sorting approaches rely on linear filters that preferentially respond to one template that is considered to represent spikes from a single neuron (Roberts and Hartline, 1975; Stein et al., 1979; Gozani and Miller, 1994; Vollgraf and Obermayer, 2006; Franke et al., 2010; Franke, 2011). Spikes can then be detected by thresholding the filter outputs. An alternative method was suggested in Vollgraf et al. (2005), where a preprocessing filter was designed to be tuned to the average spike waveform of all spikes. However, detected spikes have subsequently to be clustered in the filter output space, which introduces a complex problem after the filtering. Filter-based methods hold the promise to be suitable even for low-latency real-time spike sorting of MEA: linear filters can be efficiently implemented in hardware and they scale well with the number of recording electrodes. Firstly, all electrodes can be processed in parallel, and, secondly, if spikes of one neuron cannot be detected on a given electrode, this electrode can be ignored for the corresponding filter (Jäckel et al., 2011).

It was argued that linear-filter-based spike sorting provides only moderate performance in terms of sorting quality (Wheeler and Heetderks, 1982; Lewicki, 1994; Guido et al., 2006), but it was shown more recently that this could be due to the fact that the candidate filters have been derived in the frequency domain, which was shown to be non-optimal (Vollgraf and Obermayer, 2006).

REAL-TIME IMPLEMENTATION

Numeric computations behind linear filters are based on multiply-accumulate (MAC) operations. For every recording electrode, a set of filter coefficients has to be multiplied with the most recent samples of the recordings, and all multiplications over all electrodes are then summed up. Since multiplications are independent of each other, they can be done in parallel on a digital signal processor (DSP) as a single processing step. DSPs are well suited for implementing MAC-based algorithms, but filter-based spike sorting algorithms can consist of more complex operations [like buffering the filter outputs, thresholding, and estimation of the filter with the maximal output (Franke, 2011)], which requires more flexibility than provided by DSPs. Such more complex operations can, however, be implemented by using field-programmable gate arrays (FPGAs). The digital interface of a MEA can be controlled by these fast and reprogrammable microcontrollers. By integrating data analysis modules, as well as stimulation logics directly on the FPGA, the complete closed-loop experiment can be realized in "programmable hardware" (Hafizovic et al., 2007). This obviates the necessity to route the signal path through a PC, which would increase latency and jitter. Another advantage of FPGAs is the relatively large available memory to store filter coefficients.

OVERLAPPING SPIKES

When two spikes occur nearly at the same time, they can cause problems for the spike sorting: The overlapping signals could be detected as a single spike instead of being recognized as two spikes, and the distorted overall waveform can lead to misclassifications. With multi-electrode recordings, there can be two different types of spike overlaps: (1) temporal overlaps include spikes that occur nearly at the same time but on different electrodes, while (2) spatio-temporal overlaps occur nearly at the same time and also on the same electrodes. Purely temporal overlaps do not cause any problems for filter-based methods, as the filters corresponding to one neuron can be made "blind" to the electrodes of another neuron and can be treated separately. Spatio-temporal overlaps (see **Figure 2**), however, will distort the filter outputs of both filters. A way to solve this problem is to remove the corresponding waveform from the data, once a spike was detected, and to then recompute the filter outputs (Gozani and Miller, 1994; Franke, 2011). This approach is not well suited for a challenging real-time implementation, since it will generate a larger delay for overlapping spikes than for non-overlapping ones. The realization of an efficient overlap resolution technique for high-electrode-density data of real-time applications is still an open issue.

DISCUSSION/OUTLOOK

A number of issues in implementing real-time spike sorting still remain unsolved. It would be desirable to make the linear filters as short as possible to achieve the smallest possible delay (the delay of a causal filter is directly related to its length) (Vollgraf and Obermayer, 2006). However, it was not investigated yet, how short the filters for HDMEA recordings can be, while still ensuring a high spike sorting quality. Furthermore, the filters described in Roberts and Hartline (1975) are, in principle, more powerful than a simple matched filter (Vollgraf et al., 2005; Franke, 2011), since they try to suppress spikes from other neurons. This may be useful to resolve overlapping spikes but comes at a price: the filters might be less robust to noise, since they are under stronger constraints. Additionally, spike waveforms of two different neurons may not necessarily be linearly independent, which poses a problem for this kind of linear filters.

Given the high spatial resolution of HDMEAs, it will be interesting to investigate, how the quality of the results obtained by using simple spike sorting algorithms compares to that of more complex ones. Promising algorithms for use with high electrode density include the aforementioned "hoop"-approach (Santhanam et al., 2004), or a sorting that is solely based on the identities of the electrodes, on which a spike was detected.

An important issue for spike sorting is the occurrence of bursts. Here, a neuron produces potentially many spikes with successively decreasing amplitudes and, possibly, varying waveforms (Fee et al., 1996). For most algorithms, it is not known, how the spike sorting error rate is affected by bursts. HDMEAs seem to offer the potential to correctly sort spikes according to their relative amplitude distribution over many electrodes, which may be a robust feature also preserved during bursts (Rinberg et al., 1999).

HDMEAs are a valuable tool to study neural networks, and in combination with real-time spike sorting, hold great promise for new closed-loop experiments to study, e.g., neural plasticity. We have discussed the potential applicability of spike-sorting algorithms for this purpose and come to the conclusion that the combination of hardware-optimized algorithms with HDMEA recordings may possibly enable high performance spike sorting of more than hundred neurons with latencies in the range that is required to stimulate and control synaptic plasticity (Feldman, 2012). This may allow for experiments similar to those reported in Fetz (1969); Jackson et al. (2006); Bontorin et al. (2007); Rebesco et al. (2010), however, with the possibility to use sophisticated feedback stimuli upon occurrence of defined signature signals of single neurons within a local population.

ACKNOWLEDGMENTS

This work was financially supported by the European Community through the ERC Advanced Grant 267351, "NeuroCMOS" and the Swiss National Science Foundation through the Ambizione Grant PZ00P3_132245. Felix Franke acknowledges individual support through an EU-funded Marie Curie Training Network of FP6: CT 2006-035854, CELLCHECK.

REFERENCES

Arsiero, M., Lüscher, H.-R., and Giugliano, M. (2007). Real-time closed-loop electrophysiology: towards new frontiers in *in vitro* investigations in the neurosciences. *Arch. Ital. Biol.* 145, 193–209.

Asai, Y., Aksenova, T. I., and Villa, A. E. P. (2005). On-line real-time oriented application for neuronal spike sorting with unsupervised learning. *Lect. Notes Comput. Sci.* 3696, 109–114.

Berdondini, L., Imfeld, K., Maccione, A., Tedesco, M., Neukom, S., Koudelka-Hep, M., et al. (2009). Active pixel sensor array for high spatio-temporal resolution electrophysiological recordings from single cell to large scale neuronal networks. *Lab Chip* 9, 2644–2651.

Berdondini, L., van der Wal, P. D., Guenat, O., de Rooij, N. F., Koudelka-Hep, M., Seitz, P., et al. (2005). High-density electrode array for imaging *in vitro* electrophysiological activity. *Biosens. Bioelectron.* 21, 167–174.

Biffi, E., Ghezzi, D., Pedrocchi, A., and Ferrigno, G. (2010). Development and validation of a spike detection and classification algorithm aimed at implementation on hardware devices. *Comput. Intell. Neurosci.* 2010:659050. doi: 10.1155/2010/659050

Bontorin, G., Renaud, S., Garenne, A., Alvado, L., Le Masson, G., and

Tomas, J. (2007). A real-time closed-loop setup for hybrid neural networks. *Conf. Proc. IEEE Eng. Med. Biol. Soc.* 2007, 3004–3007.

Braeken, D., Huys, R., Loo, J., Bartic, C., Borghs, G., Callewaert, G., et al. (2010). Localized electrical stimulation of *in vitro* neurons using an array of sub-cellular sized electrodes. *Biosens. Bioelectron.* 26, 1474–1477.

Buzsáki, G. (2004). Large-scale recording of neuronal ensembles. *Nat. Neurosci.* 7, 446–451.

Chao, Z. C., Bakkum, D. J., and Potter, S. M. (2007). Region-specific network plasticity in simulated and living cortical networks: comparison of the center of activity trajectory (CAT) with other statistics. *J. Neural Eng.* 4, 294–308.

Delescluse, M., and Pouzat, C. (2006). Efficient spike-sorting of multi-state neurons using inter-spike intervals information. *J. Neurosci. Methods* 150, 16–29.

Eckhorn, R., and Thomas, U. (1993). A new method for the insertion of multiple microprobes into neural and muscular tissue, including fiber electrodes, fine wires, needles and microsensors. *J. Neurosci. Methods* 49, 175–179.

Einevoll, G. T., Franke, F., Hagen, E., Pouzat, C., and Harris, K. D. (2011). Towards reliable spike-train recordings from thousands of neurons with multielectrodes. *Curr. Opin. Neurobiol.* 27, 1–7.

Eversmann, B., Jenkner, M., Hofmann, F., Paulus, C., Brederlow, R., Holzapfl, B., et al. (2003). A 128 x 128 cmos biosensor array for extracellular recording of neural activity. *IEEE J. Solid-State Circ.* 38, 2306–2317.

Eversmann, B., Lambacher, A., Gerling, T., Kunze, A., Fromherz, P., and Thewes, R. (2011). "A neural tissue interfacing chip for *in-vitro* applications with 32k recording/stimulation channels on an active area of 2.6 mm^2," in *Proceedings ESSCIRC* (Helsinki), 211–214. Available online at: http://ieeexplore.ieee.org/xpls/absall.jsp?arnumber=6044902&tag=1

Fee, M. S., Mitra, P. P., and Kleinfeld, D. (1996). Variability of extracellular spike waveforms of cortical neurons. *J. Neurophysiol.* 76, 3823–3833.

Feldman, D. E. (2012). The spike-timing dependence of plasticity. *Neuron* 75, 556–571.

Fetz, E. E. (1969). Operant conditioning of cortical unit activity. *Science* 163, 955–958.

Fiscella, M., Farrow, K., Jones, I. L., Jäckel, D., Müller, J., Frey, U., et al. (2012). Recording from defined populations of retinal ganglion cells using a high-density CMOS-integrated microelectrode array with real-time switchable electrode selection. *J. Neurosci. Methods* 211, 103–113.

Franke, F. (2011). *Real-Time Analysis of Extracellular Multielectrode Recordings*. PhD Thesis, Technische Universität Berlin, Berlin.

Franke, F., Natora, M., Boucsein, C., Munk, M. H. J., and Obermayer, K. (2010). An online spike detection and spike classification algorithm capable of instantaneous resolution of overlapping spikes. *J. Comput. Neurosci.* 29, 127–148.

Frey, U., Egert, U., Heer, F., Hafizovic, S., and Hierlemann, A. (2009a). Microelectronic system for high-resolution mapping of extracellular electric fields applied to brain slices. *Biosens. Bioelectron.* 24, 2191–2198.

Frey, U., Egert, U., Jackel, D., Sedivy, J., Ballini, M., Livi, P., et al. (2009b). "Depth recording capabilities of planar high-density microelectrode arrays," in *2009 4th International IEEE/EMBS Conference on Neural Engineering* (Antalya: IEEE), 207–210.

Frey, U., Sedivy, J., Heer, F., Pedron, R., Ballini, M., Mueller, J., et al. (2010). Switch-matrix-based high-density microelectrode array in CMOS technology. *IEEE J. Solid-State Circ.* 45, 467–482.

Friedman, D. H. (1968). *Detection of Signals by Template Matching.* Baltimore, MD: Johns Hopkins Press.

Gozani, S. N., and Miller, J. P. (1994). Optimal discrimination and classification of neuronal action potential waveforms from multiunit, multichannel recordings using software-based linear filters. *IEEE Trans. Biomed. Eng.* 41, 358–372.

Gray, C. M., Maldonado, P. E., Wilson, M., and McNaughton, B. (1995). Tetrodes markedly improve the reliability and yield of multiple single-unit isolation from multi-unit recordings in cat striate cortex. *J. Neurosci. Methods* 63, 43–54.

Guenther, F. H., Brumberg, J. S., Wright, E. J., Nieto-Castanon, A., Tourville, J. A., Panko, M., et al. (2009). A wireless brain-machine interface for real-time speech synthesis. *PloS ONE* 4:e8218. doi: 10.1371/journal.pone.0008218

Guido, R. C., Slaets, J. F. W., Köberle, R., Almeida, L. O. B., and Pereira, J. C. (2006). A new technique to construct a wavelet transform matching a specified signal with applications to digital, real time, spike, and overlap pattern recognition. *Digit. Signal Process.* 16, 24–44.

Guillory, K. S., and Normann, R. A. (1999). A 100-channel system for real time detection and storage of extracellular spike waveforms. *J. Neurosci. Methods* 91, 21–29.

Hafizovic, S., Heer, F., Ugniwenko, T., Frey, U., Blau, A., Ziegler, C., et al. (2007). A CMOS-based microelectrode array for interaction with neuronal cultures. *J. Neurosci. Methods* 164, 93–106.

Harris, K. D., Henze, D. A., Csicsvari, J., Hirase, H., and Buzsáki, G. (2000). Accuracy of tetrode spike separation as determined by simultaneous intracellular and extracellular measurements. *J. Neurophysiol.* 84, 401–414.

Hierlemann, A., Frey, U., Hafizovic, S., and Heer, F. (2011). Growing cells atop microelectronic chips: interfacing electrogenic cells *in vitro* with CMOS-based microelectrode arrays. *Proc. IEEE* 99, 252–284.

Hottowy, P., Skoczeń, A., Gunning, D. E., Kachiguine, S., Mathieson, K., Sher, A., et al. (2012). Properties and application of a multichannel integrated circuit for low-artifact, patterned electrical stimulation of neural tissue. *J. Neural Eng.* 9:066005. doi: 10.1088/1741-2560/9/6/066005

Hutzler, M., Lambacher, A., Eversmann, B., Jenkner, M., Thewes, R., and Fromherz, P. (2006). High-resolution multitransistor array recording of electrical field potentials in cultured brain slices. *J. Neurophysiol.* 96, 1638–1645.

Jäckel, D., Muller, J., Khalid, M. U., Frey, U., Bakkum, D., and Hierlemann, A. (2011). High-density microelectrode array system and optimal filtering for closed-loop experiments. in *2011 16th International Solid-State Sensors, Actuators and Microsystems Conference (IEEE)*, (Beijing, China), 1200–1203.

Jackson, A., Mavoori, J., and Fetz, E. E. (2006). Long-term motor cortex plasticity induced by an electronic neural implant. *Nature* 444, 56–60.

Jäckel, D., Frey, U., Fiscella, M., Franke, F., and Hierlemann, A. (2012). Applicability of independent component analysis on high-density microelectrode array recordings. *J. Neurophysiol.* 108, 334–348.

Lambacher, A., Vitzthum, V., Zeitler, R., Eickenscheidt, M., Eversmann, B., Thewes, R., et al. (2010). Identifying firing mammalian neurons in networks with high-resolution multi-transistor array (MTA). *Appl. Phys. A* 102, 1–11.

Lei, N., Ramakrishnan, S., Shi, P., Orcutt, J. S., Yuste, R., Kam, L. C., et al. (2011). High-resolution extracellular stimulation of dispersed hippocampal culture with high-density CMOS multielectrode array based on non-Faradaic electrodes. *J. Neural Eng.* 8, 044003.

Letelier, J. C., and Weber, P. P. (2000). Spike sorting based on discrete wavelet transform coefficients. *J. Neurosci. Methods* 101, 93–106.

Lewicki, M. S. (1998). A review of methods for spike sorting: the detection and classification of neural action potentials. *Network* 9, R53–R78.

Lewicki, M. S. (1994). Bayesian modeling and classification of neural signals. *Neural Comput.* 6, 1005–1030.

Litke, A. M., Bezayiff, N., Chichilnisky, E. J., Cunningham, W., Dabrowski, W., Grillo, A. A., et al. (2004). What does the eye tell the brain?: development of a system for the large-scale recording of retinal output activity. *IEEE Trans. Nucl. Sci.* 51, 1434–1440.

Meister, M., Pine, J., and Baylor, D. A. (1994). Multi-neuronal signals from the retina: acquisition and analysis. *J. Neurosci. Methods* 51, 95–106.

Mishelevich, D. J. (1970). On-line real-time digital computer separation of extracellular neuroelectric signals. *IEEE. Trans. Biomed. Eng.* 17, 147–150.

Nicolelis, M. A., Ghazanfar, A. A., Faggin, B. M., Votaw, S., and Oliveira, L. M. (1997). Reconstructing the engram: simultaneous, multisite, many single neuron recordings. *Neuron* 18, 529–537.

Öhberg, F., Johansson, H., Bergenheim, M., Pedersen, J., and Djupsjöbacka, M. (1996). A neural network approach to real-time spike discrimination during simultaneous recording from several multi-unit nerve filaments. *J. Neurosci. Methods* 64, 181–187.

O'Keefe, J., and Recce, M. L. (1993). Phase relationship between hippocampal place units and the EEG theta rhythm. *Hippocampus* 3, 317–330.

Potter, S. M. (2010). Closing the loop between neurons and neurotechnology. *Front. Neurosci.* 4:15. doi: 10.3389/fnins.2010.00015

Potter, S. M., Wagenaar, D. A., and DeMarse, T. B. (2006). "Closing the loop: stimulation feedback systems for embodied MEA cultures," in *Advances in Network Electrophysiology* (New York, NY: Springer), 215–242.

Prentice, J. S., Homann, J., Simmons, K. D., Tkačik, G., Balasubramanian, V., and Nelson, P. C. (2011). Fast, scalable, Bayesian spike identification for multi-electrode arrays. *PloS ONE* 6:e19884. doi: 10.1371/journal.pone.0019884

Quiroga, R. Q., Nadasdy, Z., and Ben-Shaul, Y. (2004). Unsupervised spike detection and sorting with wavelets and superparamagnetic clustering. *Neural Comput.* 16, 1661–1687.

Rebesco, J. M., Stevenson, I. H., Körding, K. P., Solla, S. A., and Miller, L. E. (2010). Rewiring neural interactions by micro-stimulation. *Front. Syst. Neurosci.* 4:39. doi: 10.3389/fnsys.2010.00039

Rinberg, D., Davidowitz, H., and Tishby, N. (1999). "Multi-electrode spike sorting by clustering transfer functions," in *Advances in Neural Information Processing Systems 11: Proceedings of the 1998 Conference* (Cambridge, MA: MIT Press), 146–152.

Roberts, W. M., and Hartline, D. K. (1975). Separation of multi-unit nerve impulse trains by a multi-channel linear filter algorithm. *Brain Res.* 94, 141–149.

Rolston, J. D., Gross, R. E., and Potter, S. M. (2010). Closed-loop, open-source electrophysiology. *Front. Neurosci.* 4:31. doi: 10.3389/fnins.2010.00031

Rutishauser, U., and Schuman, E. (2006). Online detection and sorting of extracellularly recorded action potentials in human medial temporal lobe recordings, *in vivo*. *J. Neurosci.* 154, 204–224.

Salganicoff, M., Sarna, M., Sax, L., and Gerstein, G. L. (1988). Unsupervised waveform classification for multi-neuron recordings: a real-time, software-based system. I. Algorithms and implementation. *J. Neurosci. Methods* 25, 181–187.

Santhanam, G., Sahani, M., Ryu, S. I., and Shenoy, K. V. (2004). "An extensible infrastructure for fully automated spike sorting during online experiments," in *Engineering in Medicine and Biology Society, 2004. IEMBS'04. 26th Annual International Conference of the IEEE (IEEE)*, (San Francisco, CA), 4380–4384.

Shein, M., Greenbaum, A., Gabay, T., Sorkin, R., David-Pur, M., Ben-Jacob, E., et al. (2009). Engineered neuronal circuits shaped and interfaced with carbon nanotube microelectrode arrays. *Biomed. Microdevices* 11, 495–501.

Shoham, S., and Fellows, M. (2003). Robust, automatic spike sorting using mixtures of multivariate t-distributions. *J. Neurosci. Methods* 172, 112–121.

Stein, R. B., Andreassen, S., and Oguztöreli, M. N. (1979). Mathematical analysis of optimal multichannel filtering for nerve signals. *Biol. Cybern.* 32, 19–24.

Stett, A., Egert, U., Guenther, E., Hofmann, F., Meyer, T., Nisch, W., et al. (2003). Biological application of microelectrode arrays in drug discovery and basic research. *Anal. Bioanal. Chem.* 377, 486–495.

Takahashi, S., and Sakurai, Y. (2005). Real-time and automatic sorting of multi-neuronal activity for sub-millisecond interactions *in vivo*. *Neuroscience* 134, 301–315.

Taylor, D. M., Tillery, S. I. H., and Schwartz, A. B. (2002). Direct cortical control of 3D neuroprosthetic devices. *Science* 296, 1829–1832.

Vollgraf, R., Munk, M. H. J., and Obermayer, K. (2005). Optimal filtering for spike sorting of multi-site electrode recordings. *Network* 16, 85–113.

Vollgraf, R., and Obermayer, K. (2006). Improved optimal linear filters for the discrimination of multichannel waveform templates for spike-sorting applications. *IEEE Signal Process. Lett.* 13, 121–124.

Wagenaar, D. A., Madhavan, R., Pine, J., and Potter, S. M. (2005). Controlling bursting in cortical cultures with closed-loop multi-electrode stimulation. *J. Neurosci.* 25, 680–688.

Wessberg, J., Stambaugh, C. R., Kralik, J. D., Beck, P. D., Laubach, M., Chapin, J. K., et al. (2000). Real-time prediction of hand trajectory by ensembles of cortical neurons in primates. *Nature* 408, 361–365.

Wheeler, B. C., and Heetderks, W. J. (1982). A comparison of techniques for classification of multiple neural signals. *IEEE Trans. Biomed. Eng.* 29, 752–759.

Yang, X. W., and Shamma, S. A. (1988). A totally automated system for the detection and classification of neural spikes. *IEEE Trans. Biomed. Eng.* 35, 806–816.

Permissions

All chapters in this book were first published in CLANS, by Frontiers; hereby published with permission under the Creative Commons Attribution License or equivalent. Every chapter published in this book has been scrutinized by our experts. Their significance has been extensively debated. The topics covered herein carry significant findings which will fuel the growth of the discipline. They may even be implemented as practical applications or may be referred to as a beginning point for another development.

The contributors of this book come from diverse backgrounds, making this book a truly international effort. This book will bring forth new frontiers with its revolutionizing research information and detailed analysis of the nascent developments around the world.

We would like to thank all the contributing authors for lending their expertise to make the book truly unique. They have played a crucial role in the development of this book. Without their invaluable contributions this book wouldn't have been possible. They have made vital efforts to compile up to date information on the varied aspects of this subject to make this book a valuable addition to the collection of many professionals and students.

This book was conceptualized with the vision of imparting up-to-date information and advanced data in this field. To ensure the same, a matchless editorial board was set up. Every individual on the board went through rigorous rounds of assessment to prove their worth. After which they invested a large part of their time researching and compiling the most relevant data for our readers.

The editorial board has been involved in producing this book since its inception. They have spent rigorous hours researching and exploring the diverse topics which have resulted in the successful publishing of this book. They have passed on their knowledge of decades through this book. To expedite this challenging task, the publisher supported the team at every step. A small team of assistant editors was also appointed to further simplify the editing procedure and attain best results for the readers.

Apart from the editorial board, the designing team has also invested a significant amount of their time in understanding the subject and creating the most relevant covers. They scrutinized every image to scout for the most suitable representation of the subject and create an appropriate cover for the book.

The publishing team has been an ardent support to the editorial, designing and production team. Their endless efforts to recruit the best for this project, has resulted in the accomplishment of this book. They are a veteran in the field of academics and their pool of knowledge is as vast as their experience in printing. Their expertise and guidance has proved useful at every step. Their uncompromising quality standards have made this book an exceptional effort. Their encouragement from time to time has been an inspiration for everyone.

The publisher and the editorial board hope that this book will prove to be a valuable piece of knowledge for researchers, students, practitioners and scholars across the globe.

List of Contributors

Jacob T. Robinson
Departments of Electrical and Computer Engineering and Bioengineering, Rice University, Houston, TX, USA

Marsela Jorgolli
Department of Physics, Harvard University, Cambridge, MA, USA

Hongkun Park
Department of Physics, Harvard University, Cambridge, MA, USA
Department of Chemistry and Chemical Biology, Harvard University, Cambridge, MA, USA

Avner Wallach
Department of Neurobiology, Weizmann Institute of Science, Rehovot, Israel

Alexey Pimashkin
Department of Neurodynamics and Neurobiology, Lobachevsky State University of Nizhny Novgorod, Nizhny Novgorod, Russia

Arseniy Gladkov and Irina Mukhina
Department of Neurodynamics and Neurobiology, Lobachevsky State University of Nizhny Novgorod, Nizhny Novgorod, Russia
Normal Physiology Department, Nizhny Novgorod State Medical Academy, Nizhny Novgorod, Russia

Victor Kazantsev
Department of Neurodynamics and Neurobiology, Lobachevsky State University of Nizhny Novgorod, Nizhny Novgorod, Russia
Laboratory of Nonlinear Processes in Living Systems, Institute of Applied Physics of the Russian Academy of Science, Nizhny Novgorod, Russia

A. Hanuschkin and R. H. R. Hahnloser
Institute of Neuroinformatics, University of Zurich and ETH Zurich, Zurich, Switzerland
Neuroscience Center Zurich (ZNZ), Zurich, Switzerland

S. Ganguli
Department of Applied Physics, Stanford University, Stanford, USA

Ted Brookings and Eve Marder
Volen Center and Biology Department, Brandeis University,Waltham, MA, USA

Rachel Grashow
Environmental Health Department, Harvard School of Public Health, Boston, MA, USA

Mike Skocik
Department of Physics, Pennsylvania State University, University Park, PA, USA

Alexay Kozhevnikov
Department of Physics, Pennsylvania State University, University Park, PA, USA
Department of Psychology, Pennsylvania State University, University Park, PA, USA

Rishi R. Dhingra
Division of Pulmonary, Critical Care and Sleep Medicine, Department of Medicine, Case Western Reserve University, Cleveland, OH, USA
Department of Neurosciences, CaseWestern Reserve University, Cleveland, OH, USA

Yenan Zhu and Roberto F. Galán
Department of Neurosciences, CaseWestern Reserve University, Cleveland, OH, USA
Systems Biology and Bioinformatics Program, CaseWestern Reserve University, Cleveland, OH, USA

Frank J. Jacono
Division of Pulmonary, Critical Care and Sleep Medicine, Department of Medicine, CaseWestern Reserve University, Cleveland, OH, USA
Louis Stokes Veterans Affairs Medical Center, CaseWestern Reserve University, Cleveland, OH, USA

David M. Katz
Department of Neurosciences, CaseWestern Reserve University, Cleveland, OH, USA

Thomas E. Dick
Division of Pulmonary, Critical Care and Sleep Medicine, Department of Medicine, CaseWestern Reserve University, Cleveland, OH, USA

Armin Walter and Wolfgang Rosenstiel
Department of Computer Engineering, Wilhelm-Schickard-Institute, Eberhard Karls Universität Tübingen, Tübingen, Germany

Ander R. Murguialday
Institute of Medical Psychology and Behavioural Neurobiology, University Hospital Tübingen, Tübingen, Germany
Health Technologies Department, TECNALIA, San Sebastian, Spain

Christopher DiMattina
Program in Psychology, Florida Gulf Coast University, Fort Myers, FL, USA

Niels Birbaumer
Institute of Medical Psychology and Behavioural Neurobiology, University Hospital Tübingen, Tübingen, Germany
Ospedale San Camillo, IRCCS, Venice, Italy

Martin Bogdan
Department of Computer Engineering, Wilhelm-Schickard-Institute, Eberhard Karls Universität Tübingen, Tübingen, Germany
Department of Computer Engineering, University of Leipzig, Leipzig, Germany

Gregory J. Brewer
Department of Medical Microbiology, Immunology and Cell Biology, Southern Illinois University School of Medicine, Springfield, IL, USA
Department of Neurology, Southern Illinois University School of Medicine, Springfield, IL, USA

Michael D. Boehler
Department of Medical Microbiology, Immunology and Cell Biology, Southern Illinois University School of Medicine, Springfield, IL, USA

Stathis Leondopulos
Department of Medical Microbiology, Immunology and Cell Biology, Southern Illinois University School of Medicine, Springfield, IL, USA
Pruitt Family Department of Biomedical Engineering, University of Florida, Gainesville, FL, USA

Liangbin Pan, Sankaraleengam Alagapan, Thomas B. DeMarse and Bruce C. Wheeler
Pruitt Family Department of Biomedical Engineering, University of Florida, Gainesville, FL, USA

Paolo Bonifazi and Miri Goldin
School of Physics and Astronomy, Tel Aviv University, Tel Aviv, Israel

Francesco Difato, Gian L. Breschi, Valentina Pasquale, Marta Bisio, Jacopo Tessadori, Stefano Taverna and Michela Chiappalone
Department of Neuroscience and Brain Technologies, Istituto Italiano di Tecnologia, Genova, Italy

Paolo Massobrio and Mariateresa Tedesco
Department of Informatics, Bioengineering, Robotics and System Engineering, University of Genova, Genova, Italy

Timothée Levi and Yannick Bornat
IMS laboratory, UMR CNRS 5218, University of Bordeaux, Talence, France

Sivan Kanner and Ronit Galron
Department of Neurobiology, George S. Wise Faculty of Life Sciences, Sagol School of Neuroscience, Tel Aviv University, Tel-Aviv, Israel

Steve I. Perlmutter and Eberhard E. Fetz
Department of Physiology & Biophysics, University of Washington, Seattle, WA, USA
Washington National Primate Research Center, University ofWashington, Seattle,WA, USA

Ioan Opris, Joshua L. Fuqua, Robert E. Hampson and Sam A. Deadwyler
Department of Physiology and Pharmacology, Wake Forest University School of Medicine, Winston-Salem, NC, USA

Peter F. Huettl and Greg A. Gerhardt
Department of Anatomy and Neurobiology, University of Kentucky, Lexington, KY, USA

Theodore W. Berger
Department of Biomedical Engineering, University of Southern California, Los Angeles, CA, USA

Naveed Ejaz
Institute of Cognitive Neuroscience, University College London, London, UK
Department of Bioengineering, Imperial College London, London, UK

Holger G. Krapp and Reiko J. Tanaka
Department of Bioengineering, Imperial College London, London, UK

Daniel Y. Little
Department of Molecular and Cell Biology, Redwood Center for Theoretical Neuroscience, University of California, Berkeley, CA, USA

Friedrich T. Sommer
Redwood Center for Theoretical Neuroscience, Helen Wills Neuroscience Institute, University of California, Berkeley, CA, USA

Min-Chi Hsiao
Department of Biomedical Engineering, University of Southern California, Los Angeles, CA, USA

Dong Song
Department of Biomedical Engineering, Center for Neural Engineering, University of Southern California, Los Angeles, CA, USA

Lilach Bareket-Keren and Yael Hanein
School of Electrical Engineering, Tel-Aviv University, Tel-Aviv, Israel
Tel-Aviv University Center for Nanoscience and Nanotechnology, Tel-Aviv University, Tel-Aviv, Israel

Annette Witt
Cognitive Neuroscience Department, German Primate Center, Bernstein Center for Computational Neuroscience, Max Planck Institute for Dynamics and Self-Organization, Göttingen, Germany

Agostina Palmigiano and Demian Battaglia
Bernstein Center for Computational Neuroscience, Max Planck Institute for Dynamics and Self-Organization, Göttingen, Germany

Andreas Neef, Ahmed El Hady and Fred Wolf
Max Planck Institute for Dynamics and Self-Organization, Bernstein Center for Computational Neuroscience and Bernstein Focus Neurotechnology, CRC-889, Germany
Cellular Basis of Sensory Processing, Göttingen, Germany

Kechen Zhang
Department of Biomedical Engineering, The Johns Hopkins University School of Medicine, Baltimore, MD, USA

Felix Franke, David Jäckel, Jelena Dragas, Jan Müller, Milos Radivojevic, Douglas Bakkum and Andreas Hierlemann
Department of Biosystems Science and Engineering, ETH Zürich, Basle, Switzerland

Yukio Nishimura
Department of Physiology & Biophysics, University of Washington, Seattle, WA, USA
Washington National Primate Research Center, University of Washington, Seattle, WA, USA
Precursory Research for Embryonic Science and Technology, Japan Science and Technology Agency, Tokyo, Japan

Theodore W. Berger
Department of Biomedical Engineering, Program in Neuroscience, and Center for Neural Engineering, University of Southern California, Los Angeles, CA, USA

Index

www.ingramcontent.com/pod-product-compliance
Lightning Source LLC
LaVergne TN
LVHW061514220926
848485LV00018B/1029